Advances in Animal Alternatives for Safety and Efficacy Testing

Advances in Animal Alternatives for Safety and Efficacy Testing

Edited by

Harry Salem
U.S. Army Edgewood Research Development and Engineering Center
Aberdeen Proving Ground, Maryland

Sidney A. Katz
Rutgers University
Camden, New Jersey

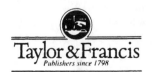

Taylor&Francis
Publishers since 1798

USA	Publishing Office:	Taylor & Francis
		1101 Vermont Avenue, N.W., Suite 200
		Washington, DC 20005-2531
		Tel: (202) 289-2174
		Fax: (202) 289-3665
	Distribution Center:	Taylor & Francis
		1900 Frost Road, Suite 101
		Bristol, PA 19007-1598
		Tel: (215) 785-5800
		Fax: (215) 785-5515
UK		Taylor & Francis Ltd
		1 Gunpowder Square
		London EC4A 3DE
		Tel: 171 583 0490
		Fax: 171 583 0581

The authors and editors have made every effort to ensure the accuracy of the information herein, particularly with regard to drug selection and dose. However, appropriate information sources should be consulted, especially for new or unfamiliar procedures. It is the responsibility of every practitioner to evaluate the appropriateness of a particular opinion in the context of actual clinical situations and with due considerations of new developments. The authors, editors, and the publishers cannot be held responsible for errors or for any consequences arising from the use of the information contained herein. The opinions in this book are personal to the authors and do not represent those of the U.S. Army or Department of Defense.

ADVANCES IN ANIMAL ALTERNATIVES FOR SAFETY AND EFFICACY TESTING

1 2 3 4 5 6 7 8 9 0 BRBR 9 0 9 8 7

This book was set in Times Roman The production editors were Christine Williams and Laura Haefner. The copy editor was Beth Dugger. Cover design by Ed Atkeson, Berg Design.

A CIP catalog record for this book is available from the British Library.
⊗ The paper in this publication meets the requirements of the ANSI Standard Z39.48-1984 (Permanence of Paper)

Library of Congress Cataloging-in-Publication Data
Advances in animal alternatives for safety and efficacy testing /
    editors, Harry Salem, Sidney A. Katz.
        p. cm.
    Expanced ed. of: Animal test alternatives. New York: M. Dekker,
c 1995.
    1. Toxicity testing—In vitro. I. Salem, Harry.
II. Katz, Sidney A.   III. Animal test alternatives.
RA1199.4.I5A38   1997
615.9'07—dc21   97-5402
                                                                    CIP

ISBN 1-56032-623-9 (case)

Our expressions of gratitude go to our colleagues for their contributions to *Advances in Animal Alternatives for Safety and Efficacy Testing,* and to Carolyn Ormes for guiding its development. We dedicate this book to our loved ones: Flo, Jerry, Amy, Joel, and Marshall; Sheila, Craig, Ji, and Kevin; and Jeff and Wendy, who continue to encourage and inspire us to follow our dreams, and to those who respect all forms of life.

TABLE OF CONTENTS

PART I
DERMAL TOXICITY

CONTRIBUTORS

Michael Aschner, Ph.D.
Department of Physiology and
Pharmacology, Bowman Gray School of
Medicine, Winston-Salem, NC 27157-1083

Steven I. Baskin, Pharm.D., Ph.D.
U.S. Army Medical Research Institute of
Chemical Defense, Aberdeen Proving
Ground, Maryland

Dale J. Beck, Ph.D.
Department of Surgery, School of Medicine,
Washington University, St. Louis, MO
63110

L. I. Bernstam, M.D.
Department of Environmental and Industrial
Health (Toxicology Program), The
University of Michigan, Ann Arbor, MI
48109-2029

I. A. Bernstein, Ph.D.
Department of Biological Chemistry and
Department of Environmental and
Industrial Health (Toxicology Program), The
University of Michigan, Ann Arbor, MI
48109-2029

Benjamin W. Blake
Health Designs, Inc., Rochester, NY 14604

J. A. Blank, Ph.D., D.A.B.T.
Battelle Memorial Institute, 505 King
Avenue, Columbus, OH 43201-2693

J. L. Borowitz, Ph.D.
Department of Medicinal Chemistry and
Molecular Pharmacology, Purdue University,
West Lafayette, IN 47906

Nicole Bournias-Vardiabasis, Ph.D.
Department of Biology, California State
University at San Bernardino, 5500
University Parkway, San Bernardino, CA
92407-2397

J. von Bredow, Ph.D.
Division of Experimental Therapeutics,
WRAIR, Washington, DC

T. Brewer, M.D.
Division of Experimental Therapeutics,
WRAIR, Washington, DC

B. V. Bronk, Ph.D.
U.S.A.F. Armstrong Laboratory, U.S. Army
ERDEC, Aberdeen, MD 21010-5423

Clarence A. Broomfield, Ph.D.
Pharmacology Division, U.S. Army Medical
Research Institute of Chemical Defense,
Aberdeen Proving Ground, MD 21010-5425

L. D. Brown, D.V.M.
Division of Experimental Therapeutics,
WRAIR, Washington, DC

Robert D. Bruce, M.S.
The Procter & Gamble Company, Miami
Valley Laboratories, Cincinnati, OH 45239

Piet Bruijnzeel, M.D., Ph.D.
Department of Pharmacology, TNO Prins
Maurits Laboratory, Lance Kleiweg 137,
P.O. Box 45, 2280 AA Rijswijk,
THE NETHERLANDS

C. L. Cannon
MatTek Corporation, 200 Homer Avenue,
Ashland, MA 01721

Florence A. Caputo, Ph.D.
Sierra Biomedical, Inc., 587 Dunn Circle,
Sparks, NV 89431

James R. Carter
Health Designs, Inc., Rochester, NY 14604

D. Cerven
MB Research Laboratories, Inc., P.O. Box
178, Spinnerstown, PA 18968

Byong Han (Paul) Chin, Ph.D.
Office of Pesticide Programs (7509C), U.S.
Environmental Protection Agency,
Washington, DC 20460

Ih Chu, Ph.D.
Environmental Health Centre, Tunneys
Pasture, Ottawa K1A OL2, CANADA

Tae-Wook Chun
Johns Hopkins University, School of
Medicine, Baltimore, MD 21205

Offie E. Clark, B.S.
Pharmacology Division, U.S. Army Medical
Research Institute of Chemical Defense,
Aberdeen Proving Ground, MD 21010-5425

David K. Cohoon
43 Skyline Drive, Glen Mills, PA 19342

P. Contard
Department of Dermatology, Mount Sinai
School of Medicine, New York, NY 10029

Joseph A. Cotruvo, Ph.D.
NSF International/WHO Collaborating
Center for Water Safety and Technology,
Washington, DC 20005

Fred M. Cowan, B.S.
Pharmacology Division, U.S. Army Medical
Research Institute of Chemical Defense,
Aberdeen Proving Ground, MD 21010-5425

Raymond J. Cronise
NASA Marshall Space Flight Center, ES-76,
Huntsville, AL 35812

R. D. Curren
Microbiological Associates, Inc.,
Rockville, MD

J. Czégé, Ph.D.
Biomedical Instrumentation Center,
Uniformed Services University of the
Health Sciences, Bethesda, MD 20814-4799

Tracy A. Donnelly
Advanced Tissue Sciences, Inc., 10933 N.
Torrey Pines Road, La Jolla, CA 92037

Joanna M. Doyle, M.S.
Clairol, Inc., Bristol-Myers Squibb Division,
2 Blatchley Road, Stamford, CT 06922

William E. Dressler, Ph.D.
Clairol, Inc., Bristol-Myers Squibb Division,
2 Blatchley Road, Stamford, CT 06922

Susan M. Edwards
Advanced Tissue Sciences, Inc., 10933 N.
Torrey Pines Road, La Jolla, CA 92037

Marion Ehrich, Ph.D., D.A.B.T.
Virginia-Maryland Regional College of
Veterinary Medicine, Blacksburg, VA
24061-0442

Graham Elliott, Ph.D.
Department of Pharmacology, TNO Prins
Maurits Laboratory, Lance Kleiweg 137, P.O.
Box 45, 2280 AA Rijswijk, THE
NETHERLANDS

Craig A. Elmets
Department of Dermatology and Oncology,
Case Western Reserve University,
University Hospitals of Cleveland, 11100
Euclid Avenue, Cleveland, OH 44106-
5028

Kurt Enslein
Health Designs, Inc., Rochester, NY 14604

Leonardo D. Epstein, Ph.D.
Center for Alternatives to Animal Testing,
School of Hygiene and Public Health,
Johns Hopkins University, 111 Market Place,
Suite 840, Baltimore, MD 21202-6709

R. Fleischmajer
Department of Dermatology, Mount Sinai
School of Medicine, New York, NY, 10029

Gordon L. Flynn, Ph.D.
College of Pharmacy, The University of
Michigan, Ann Arbor, MI 48109-1065

Shayne C. Gad, Ph.D., D.A.B.T.
GAD Consulting Services, 1818 White Oak
Road, Raleigh, NC 27608

E. Gasiciel, M.S.
Department of Environmental and Industrial
Health (Toxicology Program), The
University of Michigan, Ann Arbor, MI
48109-2029

Anthony A. Gaspari, M.D.
Department of Dermatology, School of
Medicine and Dentistry, University of
Rochester, Box 697, Rochester, NY 14642

Michael J. Goddard, Ph.D.
Environmental Health Centre, Tunneys
Pasture, Ottawa K1A OL2, CANADA

Alan M. Goldberg, Ph.D.
Center for Alternatives to Animal Testing,
School of Hygiene and Public Health,
Johns Hopkins University, 111 Market Place,
Suite 840, Baltimore, MD 21202-6709

Vijay K. Gombar, Ph.D.
Health Designs, Inc., Rochester, NY 14604

C. M. Gonzalez
University of Maryland School of Medicine,
Aquatic Pathology Center, Baltimore,
MD 21201

Virgina C. Gordon, Ph.D.
Saftey Associates, 1385C Warner Ave.,
Tustin, CA 92780

Sidney Green, Ph.D.
Covance Laboratories Inc., 9200 Leesburg
Pike, Vienna, VA 22182-1699

Stanley B. Gross, Ph.D., D.A.B.T., C.I.H.
U.S. Environmental Protection Agency
(7905C), Washington, DC 20460

Clark L. Gross, M.S.
Pharmacology Division, U.S. Army Medical
Research Institute of Chemical Defense,
Aberdeen Proving Ground, MD 21010-5425

J. W. Harbell, Ph.D.
Microbiological Associates, Inc.,
Rockville, MD

K. Harris
Dermatology Department, Box 0989, School
of Medicine University of California, San
Francisco, CA 94143-0989

Richard N. Hill, M.D., Ph.D.
U. S. Environmental Protection Agency,
Office of Prevention, Pesticides and Toxic
Substances (7401), Washington, DC 20460

D. W. Hobson, Ph.D., D.A.B.T.
Healthpoint Medical, 307 E. Josephine, San
Antonio, TX 78015

Keri Hopkins
Biology Department, California State
University at San Bernardino, 5500
University Parkway, San Bernardino, CA
92407-2397

Kuyng-Won Huh
Biology Department, California State
University at San Bernardino, 5500
University Parkway, San Bernardino, CA
92407-2397

Gary E. Isom, Ph.D.
Department of Medicinal Chemistry and
Molecular Pharmacology, Purdue University,
West Lafayette, IN 47907

Jacqueline U. Johnson, M.D., M.S.
Department of Food Science and Animal
Industries, Alabama A & M University,
Normal, AL 35762

Donald L. Kaminski
Surgical Research Institute, St. Louis
University Health Sciences Center, 3635
Vista at Grand Avenue, St. Louis, MO 63110

A. Kaminskis, Ph.D.
Division of Drug Assessment, Institute of
Chemical Defense, Aberdeen Proving Ground,
Aberdeen, MD 21010-5425

A. G. Kanthasamy, Ph.D.
Department of Neurology, University of
California at Irvine, Irvine, CA 92717-
4279

Robert J. Kavlock
Reproductive Toxicology Division, MD-71,
U.S. Environmental Protection Agency,
Research Triangle Park, NC 27711

Ian Kimber, Ph.D.
Zeneca Central Toxicology Laboratory,
Alderley Park, Macclesfield, Cheshire,
SK10 4TJ, UNITED KINGDOM

S. D. Kirby, B.S.
Pharmacology Division, U.S. Army Medical
Research Institute of Chemical Defense,
3100 Ricketts Point Road, Aberdeen Proving
Ground, MD 21010-5425

M. Klausner
MatTek Corporation, 200 Homer Avenue,
Ashland, MA 01721

Norman W. Klein, Ph.D.
Center for Environmental Health, Box U-39,
Department of Animal Science, 3636
Horsebarn Road, University of Connecticut,
Storrs, CT 06268

Albert M. Kligman, M.D., Ph.D.
Department of Dermatology, School of
Medicine, University of Pennsylvania,
Philadelphia, PA 19104

D. W. Korte, Jr., Ph.D., D.A.B.T.
Concordia University, 12800 North Lake
Shore Drive, Mequon, WI 53097

A. Kotlyar, B.S.
Department of Environmental and Industrial Health (Toxicology Program), The University of Michigan, Ann Arbor, MI 48109-2029

J. Kubilus
MatTek Corporation, 200 Homer Avenue, Ashland, MA 01721

K. Lamintausta, M.D.
Department of Dermatology, University of California Hospital, San Francisco, CA 94143

Jan de Lange
Department of Pharmacology, TNO Prins Maurits Laboratory, Lance Kleiweg 137, P.O. Box 45, 2280 AA Rijswijk, THE NETHERLANDS

Albert P. Li, Ph.D.
In Vitro Technologies, Inc., 1450 S. Rolling Rd., Baltimore, MD 21227

Zhao Z. Li, M.D.
Uniformed Services University of the Health Sciences, Bethesda, MD 20814-4799

P. P. Lin, Ph.D.
Department of Environmental and Industrial Health (Toxicology Program), The University of Michigan, Ann Arbor, MI 48109-2029

Robert L. Lipnick, Ph.D.
U. S. Environmental Protection Agency, Office of Prevention, Pesticides and Toxic Substances (7403), Washington, DC 20460

Loren L. Looger
Stanford University, Stanford, CA

Linda J. Loretz, Ph.D.
Grand Metropolitan/Pillsbury, 330 University Avenue SE, Minneapolis, MN 55414

E. D. MacDonald
Department of Dermatology, Mount Sinai School of Medicine, New York, NY 10029

J. S. Madren-Whalley
Pharmacology Division, U.S. Army Medical Research Institute of Chemical Defense, 3100 Ricketts Point Road, Aberdeen Proving Ground, MD 21010-5425

Edward U. Maduh, Ph.D.
Allsig Health and Toxicology, Inc., 1825 I St. NW, Suite 400, Washington, DC 20006

Howard I. Maibach, M.D.
Department of Dermatology, University of California Hospital, San Francisco, CA 94143

M. T. Marino, M.D.
Division of Experimental Therapeutics, WRAIR, Washington, DC

Margaret E. Martens, Ph.D.
Pharmacology Division, U.S. Army Medical Research Institute of Chemical Defense, Aberdeen Proving Ground, MD 21010-5425

Helen C. Matsos
NASA Marshall Space Flight Center, ES-76, Huntsville, AL 35812

D. R. Mattie, Ph.D.
Toxicology Division, Armstrong Laboratory, OL AL HSC/OETB Building 79, 2856 G Street, Wright-Patterson AFB, OH 45433-7400

James N. McDougal, Ph.D.
Geo-Centers Inc., OL AL HSC/OETB Building 79, 2856 G Street, Wright-Patterson AFB, OH 45433-7400

Ronald G. Menton, Ph.D.
Battelle Memorial Institute, 505 King Avenue, Columbus, OH 43201-2693

Jill C. Merrill, Ph.D., D.A.B.T.
Gillette Capital Corporation, 401 Professional Drive, Gaithersburg, MD 20879

Soheila Mirhashemi
In Vitro International, 16632 Millikan Avenue, Irvine, CA 92714

M. A. E. Mol, Ph.D.
Department of Pharmacology, TNO Nutrition, P.O. Box 5815, 2280 HV Rijswijk, THE NETHERLANDS

O. Moreno
MB Research Laboratories, Inc., P.O. Box 178, Spinnerstown, PA 18968

Roy C. Myers, B.S., D.A.B.T.
Brown & Root Environmental, Foster Plaza VII, 661 Andersen Drive, Pittsburgh, PA 15220-2745

P. J. Neal
MatTek Corporation, 200 Homer Avenue, Ashland, MA 01721

David A. Noever
NASA Marshall Space Flight Center, ES-76, Huntsville, AL 35812

C. T. Olson, D.V.M., Ph.D.
Battelle Memorial Institute, 505 King Avenue, Columbus, OH 43201-2693

Sunita Patil, Ph.D.
Department of Dermatology, University of California Hospital, San Francisco, CA 94143

J. S. Perlish
Department of Dermatology, Mount Sinai School of Medicine, New York, NY 10029

Y. P. Pu, M.D., Ph.D.
Department of Environmental and Industrial Health (Toxicology Program), The University of Michigan, Ann Arbor, MI 48109-2029

S. R. Rachui, M.S.
Thomas J. Stephens & Associates, Inc., 3310 Keller Springs Road, Carrollton, TX 75006-5057

Asenath Rasmussen, M.S.
Monsanto Company, St. Louis, MO 63167

R. Reimschuessel
University of Maryland School of Medicine, Aquatic Pathology Center, Baltimore, MD 21201

Rachna A. Relwani
NASA Marshall Space Flight Center, ES-76, Huntsville, AL 35812

Lawrence A. Rheins
Advanced Tissue Sciences, Inc., 10933 N. Torrey Pines Road, La Jolla, CA 92037

Saura C. Sahu
U.S. Food and Drug Administration, Beltsville, MD 20708

Harry Salem, Ph.D.
U. S. Army Edgewood Research, Development, and Engineering Center, Aberdeen Proving Ground, MD 21010-5425

Andrew C. Scallet, Ph.D.
Division of Neurotoxicology, National Center for Toxicological Research/FDA, 3900 NCTR Drive, Jefferson, AR 72079

Govert van der Schans, Ph.D.
Department of Pharmacology, TNO Prins Maurits Laboratory, Lance Kleiweg 137, P.O. Box 45, 2280 AA Rijswijk, THE NETHERLANDS

Larry M. Segal, Ph.D.
Environmental Health Centre, Tunneys Pasture, Ottawa K1A 0L2, CANADA

William J. Smith, Ph.D.
Pharmacology Division, U.S. Army Medical Research Institute of Chemical Defense, Aberdeen Proving Ground, MD 21010-5425

T. H. Snider, B.S., D.A.B.T.
Battelle Memorial Institute, 505 King Avenue, Columbus, OH 43201-2693

Janet A. Springer, Ph.D.
U. S. Food and Drug Administration, Center for Food Safety and Nutrition, Washington, DC 20204

H. M. Stahr, Ph.D.
Analytical Toxicology, Veterinary Diagnostic Lab, College of Veterinary Medicine, Iowa State University, Ames, IA 50011-1250

Katherine A. Stitzel, Ph.D.
The Procter & Gamble Company, Miami Valley Laboratories, P.O. Box 538707, Cincinnati, OH 45253-8707

T. S. C. Sun, Ph.D.
Chemistry, Veterinary Diagnostic Lab, College of Veterinary Medicine, Iowa State University, Ames, IA 50011-1250

R. James Swanson, Ph.D.
Department of Biology, Old Dominion University, 1014 Jamestown Crescent, Norfolk, VA 23508-1233

W. P. Van De Merwe, Ph.D.
Uniformed Services University of the Health Sciences, Bethesda, MD 20814-4799

F. L. Vaughan, Ph.D.
Department of Environmental and Industrial Health (Toxicology Program), The University of Michigan, Ann Arbor, MI 48109-2029

Bellina Veronesi, Ph.D.
U.S. EPA, National Health Effects and Environmental Research Laboratories, Neurotoxicology Division, MD74B, Research Triangle Park, NC 27711

J. A. Vick
Research and Testing, Center for Drug
Evaluation, FDA, 8301 Muirkirk Road,
Laurel, MD 20708

Arthur P. Walker, Ph.D.
Apojay Consultancy, Tyne and Wear,
NE26 3DU, UNITED KINGDOM

W.-D. Wang, Ph.D.
Frontier Herbs, P.O. Box 299,
Norway, IA 52318

Rosalind Wei
In Vitro International, 16632 Millikan
Avenue, Irvine, CA 92714

Robert J. Werrlein, Ph.D.
Pharmacology Division, U.S. Army Medical
Research Institute of Chemical Defense,
3100 Ricketts Point Road, Aberdeen Proving
Ground, MD 21010-5425

Patricia P. Wilcox
School of Public Health, The Ohio State
University, Columbus, OH 43210

Lilly Xu, Ph.D.
Surgical Research Institute, St. Louis
University Health Sciences Center, 3635
Vista at Grand Avenue, St. Louis, MO 63110

Y. Yang, M.D.
Department of Environmental and Industrial
Health (Toxicology Program), The
University of Michigan, Ann Arbor, MI
48109-2029

Ronald J. Young, Ph.D.
Toxicology, SCBRD-RTL, Bldg E3220,
Room 113, APG, MD 21010

Joanne Zurlo, Ph.D.
Center for Alternatives to Animal Testing,
School of Hygiene and Public Health,
Johns Hopkins University, 111 Market Place,
Suite 840, Baltimore, MD 21202-6709

PREFACE

Advances in Animal Alternatives for Safety and Efficacy Testing is a timely and relevant expansion of *Animal Test Alternatives* (Marcel Dekker, 1995) in which more recent developments with greater depth and broader scope are presented. The contents of *Advances in Animal Alternatives for Safety and Efficacy Testing* address some of the important ramifications from the National Institutes of Health (NIH) Revitalization Act of 1993 (Public Law No. 103-43, Section 1301), in which the U.S. Congress instructed the NIH to research into replacement, reduction, and refinement alternatives, and to establish criteria for the validation and regulatory acceptance of alternatives, and to recommend a process through which scientifically validated alternative methods can be accepted for regulatory use. Subsequently, an ad hoc Interagency Coordinating Committee on the Validation of Alternative Methods was established in 1994 to develop a report recommending criteria and processes for validation and regulatory acceptance. Fifteen federal regulatory and research agencies and organizations participated in this effort. In addition, *Advances in Animal Alternatives for Safety and Efficacy Testing* addresses some of the ramifications from the European Union's Cosmetic Directive, which bans marketing of animal-tested cosmetics in Europe after 1997 if validated alternatives are available. Clearly, the legislative bodies in North America and in Western Europe have recognized the value of and the need for developing and validating replacement, reduction, and refinement alternatives to animal testing. *Advances in Animal Alternatives for Safety and Efficacy Testing* contains descriptions of the results from validation studies on recently developed, commercially available in vitro methodologies as well as the applications of computer and computational models for the assessment of toxicity. Nearly 50 individual contributions from over 150 international experts are grouped into five categories: Dermal; Developmental/Reproductive; Immunotoxicity; Neurotoxicity; and Oral/Dermal/Ocular Validation.

Advances in Animal Alternatives for Safety and Efficacy Testing has added a fourth R for *responsibility* to the traditional three R's of reduction, refinement, and replacement. The Edgewood Research, Development, and Engineering Center (ERDEC) has demonstrated responsibility through its commitment to pursue the application of alternatives to animal testing for reasons of humaneness, time, and economics. ERDEC has an additional responsibility of promoting technology transfer for the three R's of alternatives to animal testing.

The three R's of alternatives to animal testing are *reduction* in the number of animals used; *refinement* in emphasizing relief of pain, maximizing information obtained from each animal, and utilizing animals lower on the phylogenetic tree; and *replacement* of animals with in vitro cultures, chemical reactions (such as those used to determine pregnancy), and computer models. The third R, replacement, will continue slowly as alternatives are developed and validated to assure that safety and efficacy can be predicted without compromising public and environmental health and welfare. Until such time as development and validataion are completed, alternatives must be utilized to complement and/or supplement whole-animal testing.

Toxicity assessment using animal testing must be conducted at facilities that are accredited by the American Association for the Accreditation of Laboratory Animal Care (AAALAC), consistent with the National Institutes of Health Guide for the Care and Use of Laboratory Animals, subject to review by a laboratory animal use committee, and in compliance with the Animal Welfare Act, the Code of Ethics of the Society of Toxicology, and Good Laboratory Practices.

Scientists from the academic, governmental, and industrial sectors contributed to *Advances in Animal Alternatives for Safety and Efficacy Testing*. Their contributions made possible the achievement of objectives to present state-of-the-art concepts and approaches to the theory and practice of alternatives to animal testing and to promote transfer of the technology.

We are grateful to our Department of Defense sponsors, the participants, the steering committee, the coordinating scientific societies, members of ERDEC: Dean Bona, Dianne Bratton, Kenneth Cameron, Dale Heitkamp, James Manthei, Dianne Merkel, and Dr. Eugene Olajos. In addition, we express our thanks to the CBIAC staff: Charles P. Baumgart, Valentia McVey, and Kimberly G. Oyler. The success of *Advances in Animal Alternatives for Safety and Efficacy Testing* is the result of diligence, perseverance, and hard work by these competent and committed colleagues.

Harry Salem
Sidney A. Katz

PART I

DERMAL TOXICITY

Chapter One

PSEUDO-EPIDERMIS: AN IN VITRO SURROGATE FOR THE STUDY OF CUTANEOUS SULFUR MUSTARD TOXICITY

I. A. Bernstein, L. I. Bernstam, E. Gasiciel, A. Kotlyar, P. P. Lin, Y. P. Pu, F. L. Vaughan, and Y. Yang

Pseudo-epidermis, generated from a purified population of human or rodent germinative cutaneous keratinocytes and similar to the intact epidermis in morphology and biochemistry, can be a convenient and versatile surrogate for the tissue in studies of the molecular mechanisms by which environmental chemicals produce toxic cutaneous responses in animals and humans. This stratified, cornified culture, in association with submerged mono- and multilayer cultures of keratinocytes, has proven useful in investigating the mechanisms responsible for the destruction of the epidermal basal layer in human skin exposed to bis(β-chloroethyl) sulfide (BCES) in vivo. It has been demonstrated that topical application of BCES to human pseudo-epidermis results in the dose- and time-responsive inhibition of DNA synthesis and destruction of the basal layer as occurs in exposed epidermis. Exposure of monolayer cultures of rodent keratinocytes to relatively low levels of BCES has been shown to cause proliferative cells to become committed to differentiation leading to programmed cell death. It has been proposed that differentiation, as well as necrosis, accounts for the loss of proliferative capacity among the basal cells of the exposed epidermis. The formation of adducts in DNA and cellular attempts to repair the damage form the central entities in a proposed mechanism to explain the destruction of the germinative population.

INTRODUCTION

Scavarelli-Karantsavelos et al.[1] have proposed that pseudo-epidermis be used as a model system for the study of the molecular mechanisms by which environmental chemicals produce toxic responses in the epidermis of animals and humans. In addition, they have suggested that this

This project was supported by the U. S. Army Medical Research Institute of Chemical Defense under contract DAMD17-90-C-0031. The views, opinions, or findings contained in this chapter, however, are those of the authors and should not necessarily be construed to represent the position, policy, or decision of the agency supporting the work. The authors are sincerely grateful to Dr. H. P. Benschop of the TNO Prins Maurits Laboratory in the Netherlands for his gift of authentic samples of the N^7-monoadduct and the diguanyl adduct of guanine, and to Dr. D. R. Ludlum of the University of Massachusetts Medical School for his gift of an authentic sample of the monoadduct of guanine. The authors acknowledge with thanks the assistance of Dr. Don Gordon Davis, Kathleen Ellwood, and Karen Domiansky of the Michigan Capital Medical Center in Lansing, who obtained and provided the human skin from which some of the human pseudo-epidermis was derived. Human skin was also provided by the Cooperative Human Tissue Network, supported by the National Cancer Institute of the National Institutes of Health. The technical assistance of Amir Cohen is gratefully acknowledged.

stratified, cornified culture system[2,3] can be used to quantify parameters of toxicity resulting from topical chemical exposures. Since it is grown and maintained at the air–liquid interface, the pseudo-epidermis can be exposed to chemicals under conditions similar to those that occur in vivo.

The pseudo-epidermis and submerged monolayer and multilayer cultures of keratinocytes have been used to probe the molecular and cellular mechanisms associated with vesication in skin exposed to bis(β-chloroethyl) sulfide (BCES, sulfur mustard, HD). Pseudo-epidermis, grown from primary rat[2] or human[3] keratinocytes, provides a convenient and versatile system for studying and quantifying interactions between BCES and the initial target tissue, without the complications resulting from secondary systemic responses. Furthermore, the pseudo-epidermis, which is similar to intact epidermis in morphology and biochemistry,[3,4] can be used to ascertain the pathogenic relevance of data obtained, using submerged cultures, or to define or test the efficacy of proposed preventive or therapeutic strategies.

Destruction of the basal layer in the epidermis is a major component of the vesication resulting when human skin is exposed to BCES.[5] The blister is formed as a result of the accumulation of systemic fluid in the position formerly occupied by the basal cells, and is capped by the residual differentiated layers.

A mechanism (Figure 1) for the BCES-mediated destruction of the epidermal proliferative compartment has been formulated.[6] The hypothesis assumes that alkylation of epidermal DNA by BCES and subsequent cellular efforts to repair these molecular lesions are the primary dose- and time-dependent steps in the pathogenic process culminating in cutaneous vesication. It is proposed that as the dose increases, the ability of the cell to repair its DNA with high fidelity is compromised, leading to the production of heterotypic DNA, that is, DNA containing base sequences abnormal for the cell. This results in a change in the informational content of the cell and loss of proliferative capacity with consequent commitment to keratinization and programmed cell death. As the dose is further increased, the damage is too extensive to permit repair (e.g., as a result of the presence of cross-links) and cell necrosis occurs. Therefore, loss of proliferative competence in the epidermis occurs as a result of both commitment to differentiation and necrosis in the germinative population, depending on the level of BCES to which the cells are exposed.

Figure 1 attempts to formalize these ideas into three stages of toxicity labeled I, II, and III. In Stage I, at the lowest level of exposure, damaged DNA is completely repaired. In Stage II, at an intermediate level of exposure, damaged DNA is repaired, but inappropriate bases are inserted. In Stage III, at the highest dose, repair cannot cope with the extensive damage and repair is minimal or absent.

This presentation marshals available information in support of the proposed mechanism for destruction of the epidermal basal layer in skin exposed to BCES. Dose- and time-dependent data derived from exposed pseudo-epidermis and submerged cultures of keratinocytes are included. Since it is difficult to compare the levels of exposure when BCES is applied topically to pseudo-epidermis and when the mustard is added to the medium of submerged cultures, parameters of toxicity identified as occurring after a particular dose of BCES in submerged cultures need to be studied in pseudo-epidermis to establish that they do occur in this organized tissue and to determine the level of exposure to the mustard at which they occur.

METHODS

Growth of Submerged Cultures and Pseudo-Epidermis

Primary submerged monolayer cultures of keratinocytes derived from rat skin were prepared as previously described.[7] A similar technique was used for human keratinocytes, except that culture dishes were first coated with calf skin collagen. Pseudo-epidermis was prepared from human keratinocytes, as described by Bernstam et al.[3]

Exposure of Cultures to BCES

Monolayer cultures, after being washed with phosphate-buffered saline (PBS), were exposed to BCES by the addition of the mustard diluted to the desired concentration in PBS. Pseudo-

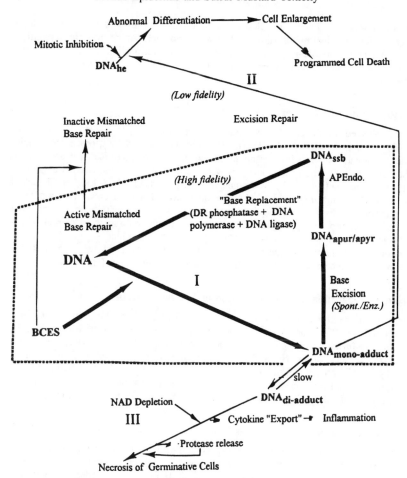

Figure 1. Hypothetical scheme for cellular toxicity in basal cells of human pseudo-epidermis. DNAhe, heterotypic DNA, that is, DNA with an abnormal base sequence or containing an adduct(s); DNAssb, DNA with a single-strand break(s); DNAapur/apyr, DNA having an apurinic or apyrimidinic site(s); DNAmono-adduct, DNA having an alkylated base(s); DNAdi-adduct, DNA having an inter- or intrastrand cross-link(s); Spont/enz, spontaneous or enzymatically catalyzed depurination(s) or depyrimidination(s); APendo, apurinic (or apyrimidinic) endonuclease; DR phosphatase, deoxyribose phosphatase; NAD, nicotinamide adenine dinucleotide; I, II, III, stages of toxicity (see text for definition).

epidermis was exposed to BCES by the topical application of the mustard in PBS. Exposures were carried out for 30 min at 35°C. BCES was provided by the U.S. Army Medical Research Institute of Chemical Defense.

Isolation and Separation of Keratin Proteins from Cultures of Keratinocytes

In the case of monolayer cultures, keratinocytes were detached from the plastic dish by scraping. In the case of pseudo-epidermis and whole epidermis, the entire preparation was usually pulverized in liquid nitrogen. When it was desired to obtain differentiated and basal cells separately, trypsinization was used as previously described.[4] In all cases, preparations were extracted with

Tris buffer containing 2% sodium dodecyl sulfate (SDS). The extract was submitted to SDS polyacrylamide gel electrophoresis (PAGE) on 7% polyacrylamide gels for separation of the proteins. After electrophoresis, proteins were transferred to nitrocellulose membranes for staining with 7B4 monoclonal antibody. A second antibody, with attached peroxidase, was used to monitor the presence of 7B4.

Isolation and Hydrolysis of DNA

DNA was isolated from exposed cells grown in the presence of [³H]- or [¹⁴C]guanosine ([³H]- or [¹⁴C]GR) to label the nucleic acid. The nucleic acid was isolated by a procedure utilizing SDS, sodium perchlorate, and a "silica" technique (Nucleon II by Scotlab, Kirkshaws Rd., Coatbridge, Strathclyde, Scotland). Briefly, keratinocytes were washed with PBS and lysed with 6 ml of 0.4 M Tris, pH 8, containing 0.06 M ethylenediamine tetraacetic acid (EDTA), 0.15 M NaCl, and 1% SDS. The lysate was then mixed with 1.5 ml of 5 M sodium perchlorate and incubated at room temperature for 15 min followed by 70°C for 25 min. The mixture was extracted with 5.5 ml of cold chloroform (stored at −20°C prior to use) for 10 min at room temperature on a rotary shaker, after which 800 µl of Nucleon Silica suspension was added. After centrifugation to separate the aqueous and nonaqueous layers, the upper aqueous layer, which contained the DNA, was removed. The DNA was recovered by precipitation with 2 volumes of cold absolute ethanol and centrifugation.

Isolation, Separation, and Identification of Adducts in DNA

After isolation, the alkylated DNA was submitted to hydrolysis at pH 3.5 and 70°C for 30 min[8] or in 1N HCl at 100°C for 15 min and gel permeated on a column of BioRad P2. Fractions thought to contain adducts were combined and submitted to HPLC on a C_{18} RP-ODS 2 Spherisorb column (Phase Separations, Norwalk, CT) with elution programmed as follows: an isocratic elution by 50 mM phosphate, pH 4.4, for 4 min, followed by addition of methanol in a linear gradient from 0 to 15% over 4 min, continued elution at 15% methanol/50 mM phosphate for 10 min, linear reduction of methanol to 0% over 5 min, and 50 mM phosphate for 5 min.

Determination of Interstrand Cross-Links in DNA from Cells Exposed to BCES

DNA interstrand cross-links were determined using the ethidium bromide fluorescence technique described by Brent.[9] Two milliliters of a solution of ethidium bromide (1 µg/ml) in 0.02 M potassium phosphate, pH 12, and containing 0.002 M EDTA was added to about 100 µl of solution containing 10 µg DNA. Fluorescence was measured at 600 nm with excitation at 525 nm prior to and following denaturation. DNA was denatured by heating for 8 min at 100°C followed by rapid cooling to room temperature (i.e., within 10 min). In control samples of DNA, fluorescence was nearly completely lost as a result of denaturation. After exposure to BCES, the presence of cross-links allowed the DNA to renature even though the sample was cooled rapidly and fluorescence was retained. The percentage of cross-linking in the DNA was calculated according to Garcia et al.[10]

Determination of IL-1α in Cells Exposed to BCES

Each well in 96-well plates was coated with monoclonal anti-human interleukin-1α (IL-1α) antibody by addition of 100 µl of 0.05 M carbonate–bicarbonate buffer, pH 9.6, containing 1.5 µg antibody/ml, and incubation at 4°C overnight. Then the plates were coated with bovine serum albumin to minimize nonspecific binding of protein. After being extensively washed with PBS containing 0.05% Tween 20, 100 µl of a cell suspension was added to the well, and the plate was incubated at 37°C for 1 h. Then the plates were again extensively washed and 100 µl of polyclonal rabbit anti-human IL-1α antibody was added. After incubation at 37°C for 1 h, the plates were washed, and 100 µl of peroxidase-conjugated goat anti-rabbit immunoglobulin G (IgG) was added. Finally, after incubation at 37°C for 30 min and washing, 100 µl peroxidase substrate was added to each well. After 10 min, the reaction was stopped with 50 µl of 2.5 M sulfuric acid, and the absorbance at 450 nm was determined using a Titertek Multiscanner.

Assay of Cell Viability

Cell viability was determined by exclusion of trypan blue.

RESULTS

Parameters Originally Defined in Monolayer Cultures That Have Been Confirmed in Pseudo-Epidermis: Dose- and Time-Responsive Inhibition of DNA and Protein Synthesis

A prolonged depression of the incorporation of [³H]thymidine ([³H]TdR) into cellular DNA occurs when monolayer cultures of keratinocytes derived from the epidermis of the newborn rat are exposed to increasing levels of BCES. In the data shown in Figure 2, inhibition was evident immediately after exposure to 0.625 μM BCES, but recovery had begun by 72 h postexposure. A similar picture was seen after exposure to 1.25 μM and, possibly, to 2.5 μM BCES. On the basis that the cell tries to restore integrity of its damaged DNA before replicating the nucleic acid,[11] it seems reasonable to assume that complete repair had occurred prior to 72 h postexposure to as much as 2.5 μM BCES. After an exposure to 5 μM BCES, DNA synthesis had not resumed by 72 h after exposure.

A similar picture was seen when human pseudo-epidermis was topically exposed to BCES (Table 1). The incorporation of [³H]TdR was slightly reduced immediately after applying 0.19 nmol/cm², but DNA synthesis appeared to be normal by 24 h after exposure. A dose of 0.56 nmol/cm² unquestionably reduced the incorporation of this tracer at zero time, but normality appeared to have been achieved by 48 h postexposure. After applying 1.1 nmol/cm², resumption of the incorporation of [³H]TdR had not returned to the normal level even by 48 h postexposure.

Although the incorporation of [¹⁴C]leucine was affected in pseudo-epidermis exposed to BCES, higher doses were necessary and recovery was quicker than was the case with [³H]TdR (Table 1).

Dose- and Time-Dependent Destruction of the Germinative (Basal) Cells

As noted earlier, the destruction of the basal layer of germinatively competent cells in the epidermis is a major endpoint of blister formation in human skin exposed to BCES. Figure 3

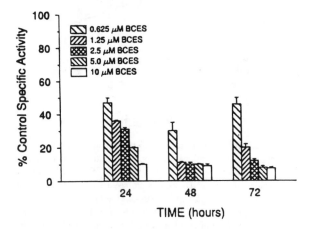

Figure 2. Prolonged depression of the incorporation of [³H]TdR in exposed monolayer cultures of keratinocytes from the skin of the newborn rat. For culture protocol see the text. Cultures were exposed 24 h after seeding. Cultures were pulse-labeled for 1 h with [³H]TdR at the indicated times, harvested, and the acid-insoluble ³H determined. From Ribeiro et al.[13] with permission.

Table 1. Effect of Topical Exposure to BCES on the Incorporation of [³H]TdR into DNA and [¹⁴C]Leucine ([¹⁴C]leu) into Protein in Pseudo-Epidermis Topically Exposed to BCES

	Control value (+SD)					
	[³H]TdR			[¹⁴C]leu		
BCES (nmol/cm²)	0 h	24 h	48 h	0 h	24 h	48 h
0.19	86 + 8	94 + 21	103 + 26			
0.56	54 + 10	61 + 12	96 + 33			
1.1	23 + 6	12 + 6	55 + 17	97 + 16	97 + 4	111 + 16
1.9				89 + 10	89 + 22	109 + 13
2.6				62 + 17	68 + 15	103 + 14

Note. For growth protocol and exposure procedure see the text.

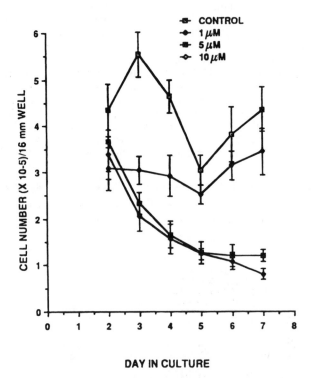

DAY IN CULTURE

Figure 3. Effect of exposure to BCES on the kinetics of cell production in a proliferating submerged monolayer culture of keratinocytes from the skin of the newborn rat. Cultures of isolated, purified populations of germinative cells were seeded in plastic dishes at 4–5 × 10⁵ cells/cm², grown in 0.08–0.11 mM Ca²⁺ and exposed for 30 min to 1, 5, and 10 µM BCES after 1 d in culture. At each time point, cultures were harvested and the number of cells determined using a hemocytometer (n = 4). From Ku and Bernstein[7] with permission.

shows the effect of exposure to BCES on the number of cells in a proliferating submerged monolayer culture of keratinocytes from the newborn rat. Normally in such a culture, as shown in this figure, the number of cells increases until d 3 in culture, after which there is a major sloughing of cells until d 5, when a progressive increase in cell number begins again. After exposure to 1 μM BCES, the increase in cell number occurring normally between 2 and 3 d was eliminated. However, the increase seen in control cultures after 5 d of cultivation did occur. On the other hand, after exposure to 5 or 10 μM BCES, the total number of cells in exposed cultures continually decreased between 1 and 6 d postexposure as the formation of new cells apparently did not compensate for the loss of cells. These data suggest that at an exposure between 1 μM and 5μM BCES, the nature of the damage from BCES and the cellular response changed from what it was at a lower exposure. It appears reasonable to assume that at this higher level of exposure, toxicity had reached Stage II or III.

The photomicrographs in Figure 4 clearly demonstrate a dose- and time-dependent destruction of the basal layer in human pseudo-epidermis topically exposed to 50 or 100 nmol BCES/cm^2. The destructive effect was observed at 24 h posttreatment in cultures exposed to the higher dose (Figure 4d), but foci of necrosis were clearly evident at 24 h postexposure to 50 nmol/cm^2 (Figure 4b). Stage III toxicity had probably been reached in pseudo-epidermis after a topical exposure to 50 nmol BCES/cm^2.

Parameters That Have Been Defined in Monolayer Cultures and Are Now Being Studied in Pseudo-Epidermis: Abnormal Differentiation of Cells in the Germinative Population

The hypothesis for BCES-mediated toxicity in epidermis shown in Figure 1 proposes that at Stage II, cells in the proliferative population become committed to differentiation. A test of this

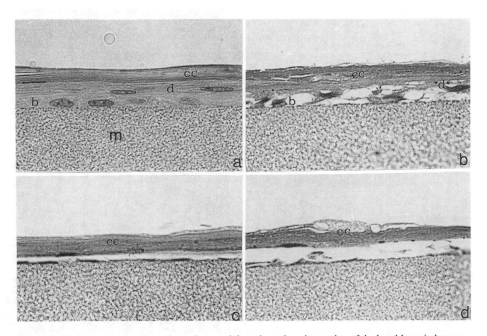

Figure 4. Photomicrographs illustrating a time- and dose-dependent destruction of the basal layer in human pseudo-epidermis topically exposed to BCES. (a) Control; (b) 24 h after exposure to 50 nmol BCES/cm^2; (c) 48 h after exposure to 50 nmol BCES/cm^2; (d) 24 h after exposure to 100 nmol BCES/cm^2. cc, Cornified layer; d, differentiated layers; b, basal layer; m, membrane. Growth protocol described by Bernstam et al.[3] Cultures exposed by topical application of BCES in PBS for 30 min. Sections stained with H&E, $\times$ 590.

proposal would be evidence of differentiation in a proliferating monolayer culture of keratinocytes after exposure to BCES.

Monoclonal antibody, 7B4, was generated in mice against keratin derived from the epidermis of the newborn rat. The photomicrographs in Figure 5 show the localization of that antibody in cross sections of skin (Figure 5b) and in pseudo-epidermis (Figure 5d) grown from cutaneous keratinocytes from the newborn rat. Fluorescence from goat anti-mouse antibody conjugated with fluorescein isothiocyanate (FITC) marked the sites where 7B4 was present. Fluorescence was restricted to the cornified layer in both epidermis and pseudo-epidermis. Figures 5a and 5c are photomicrographs of similar sections stained with hematoxylin and eosin.

As expected from the finding that the 7B4 antigen was localized in the stratum corneum, 7B4 did not decorate cells in a normal submerged monolayer culture of rat keratinocytes (Figure 6a). However, as Figure 6e shows, when a culture exposed to 5 μM BCES was assayed for 7B4 binding at 48 h postexposure, nearly every cell was stained. This was not the case at 24 h postexposure (Figure 6b). However, nearly every cell was stained 24 h after exposure to 20 μM BCES (Figure 6f). Unless exposure to BCES altered a previously synthesized keratin so that the antibody reacted with 7B4, this observation suggested that BCES caused a population of proliferating cells to precociously differentiate.

In an effort to resolve this uncertainty, 7B4-reactive protein was isolated from control and exposed monolayer cultures. As shown in Figure 7, submission of such extracts to SDS-PAGE followed by Western blotting resulted in the finding that even the extracts from control cells had a band of 7B4-reactive material with a size of about 58 kD. The fact that cells in control monolayer cultures were not decorated with 7B4 suggests that the 7B4-reactive epitope on the 58-kD protein is structurally "blocked" in situ so that it cannot react with the antibody. An additional band at about 55 kD was present in the extracts from cultures exposed to 10 μM

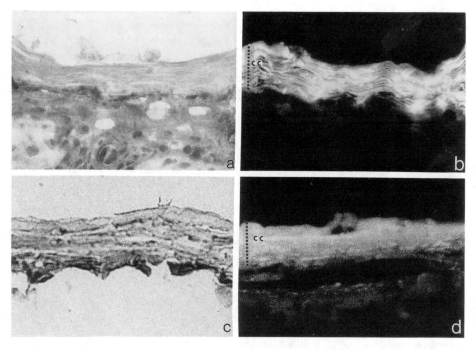

Figure 5. Staining of epidermis and pseudo-epidermis derived from rat skin by 7B4 monoclonal antibody. For growth protocol of pseudo-epidermis, see legend in Figure 4. Cryostat cross sections of newborn rat skin (a & b) and pseudo-epidermis (c & d) stained with H&E (a & c) or 7B4 antibody followed by a second antibody conjugated with fluorescein isothiocyanate (FITC) (b & d). cc, Cornified cells, × 640.

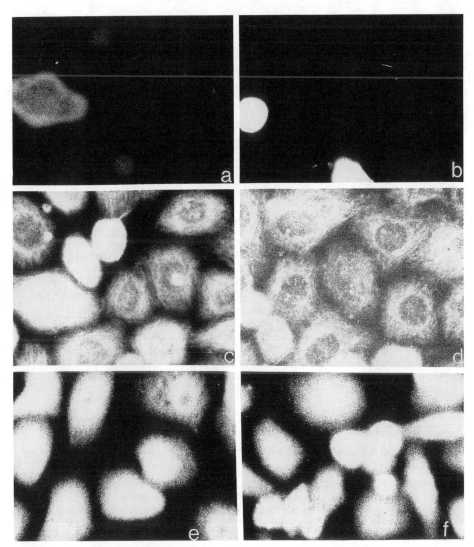

Figure 6. Appearance of fluorescence from 7B4-FITC on submerged monolayer cultures resulting from exposure to BCES. For growth protocol, see legend to Figure 4. For staining procedure, see legend to Figure 4. (a,b,e,f) Cells visualized by indirect fluorescence; (a) fluorescent cell, probably a contaminating differentiated cell; (c,d) same fields as in (a) and (b) without the fluorescence filter; (a,c) control culture; (b,d) 24 h postexposure to 5 μM BCES; (e) 48 h postexposure to 5 μM BCES; (f) 24 h postexposure to 20 μM BCES, $\times$ 816.

BCES. Figure 7 also shows Western blots of 7B4-reactive proteins isolated from various fractions of control pseudo-epidermis. Extraction of basal cells did not yield any 7B4-reactive protein. However, extraction of either the differentiated layers alone or the entire pseudo-epidermis yielded both 55- and 58-kD 7B4-reactive proteins. Interestingly, as also shown in Figure 7, no 58-kD 7B4-reactive protein was observed in extracts of basal cells from the entire epidermis and no 55-kD 7B4-reactive protein was observed in any epidermal fraction. Clearly, the 7B4 antibody can be a useful marker in the study of BCES-mediated differentiation, but the metabolic sequence of events involving the 7B4-reactive protein is not obvious.

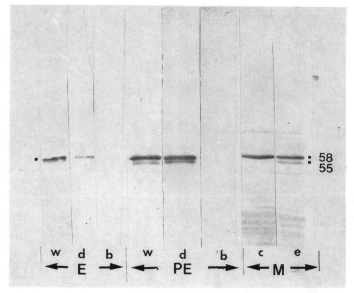

Figure 7. Western blots of proteins isolated from unexposed epidermis and pseudo-epidermis and from unexposed and exposed monolayer cultures derived from newborn rat skin. Numbers indicate μM_r in kD. For culture protocol, see legend for Figure 3. E, from epidermis; PE, from pseudo-epidermis, M, from monolayer; b, from basal cells; d, from differentiated cells; w, from whole tissue or culture; c, control; e, exposed.

Parameters That Are Still Being Studied in Submerged Mono- or Multilayer Cultures and Have Not Been Investigated in Pseudo-Epidermis

Formation of Adducts in the DNA of Cells in Multilayer Submerged Cultures Exposed to BCES

As indicated in Figure 1, monoadducts and diadducts in DNA are postulated to represent critical elements in the epidermal toxicity of BCES. The latter species would be expected to lead to necrosis of cells, while the former could be repaired with "high fidelity" by base replacement if only a few adducts exist or with less fidelity by repair of sequences of damaged bases leading to "heterotypic" DNA if the number of adducts is more extensive. Heterotypic DNA would result from the insertion of noncomplementary bases that are inadequately removed by a mismatched-base repair system that is inefficient in cells exposed to BCES.[12] Support for this hypothesis comes from the observation that in monolayer cultures of proliferating keratinocytes exposed to 1 μM BCES, single-strand breaks in the DNA are completely repaired by 24 h postexposure,[13] but the cells in the culture do not resume replication of DNA until 72 h postexposure and show an abnormally high percentage of differentiated cells, many of which are unusually large.[7] Although replication of DNA does resume, the number of cells participating in the process is small compared with control cultures.[7]

To gain further insight into the role of adducts in the process of toxicity from exposure to BCES, DNA was isolated from cultures of human keratinocytes that had been grown in the presence of [8-³H]GR and exposed for 30 min to 1 μM BCES. Tomasz[14] had reported that alkylation at the N7-position of guanine labilized the proton at the C8-position of this purine and that the appearance of ^3H_2O could be used as an indicator of this alkylation. Therefore, the isolated tritiated DNA was treated for 30 min at 70°C and pH 3.5 to maximize the tritiated proton exchange with the aqueous medium and the mixture was then passed through a column of BioRad P2 to collect the ^3H_2O that would be retarded on the column of BioRad P2 [i.e., would appear at the imbibed volume (V_i)] while the high-molecular-weight residual DNA would be excluded from the column (i.e., would appear at the V_0). In fact, as shown in Figure 8, a peak of tritium was seen at fraction 29, the position of water (as confirmed by the appearance of ^3H at 4 min when fractions 26–31 were submitted to HPLC, cf., Figure 9) suggesting that an exposure of a culture of human keratinocytes to even 1 μM BCES, under the conditions used, results in an alkylation of a significant fraction of the guanine residues.

Figure 10 shows that when such tritiated DNA was isolated, then exposed to different concentrations of BCES from 50 to 5000 μM, and analyzed on a column of BioRad P2, a dose-responsive increase of tritium in fractions 26–30 was observed indicating a dose-responsive increase in proton exchange and, therefore, in the formation of N7-alkylated guanine residues in the DNA. When the DNA was labeled in the cell with [^{14}C]GR, isolated, then exposed to 300 μM BCES, submitted to hydrolysis in 1N HCl at 100° for 15 min to depurinate the nucleic acid, and analyzed on a column of BioRad P2 (Figure 11), labeled monoadduct was observed. Analysis of the combined fractions 37–38 by HPLC (Figure 12) confirmed the identity of the adduct as the N7-monoadduct of guanine.

More recently, an experiment with cultured human keratinocytes in which the cells were grown in the presence of [8-^{14}C]guanosine and exposed to 600 μM BCES for only 15 min followed by application of the same analytical procedures indicated that about 2% of the guanine residues had been converted to [^{14}C]N7-monoadducts of this base. Further work needs to be done to evaluate the role of this adduct in the toxicity of BCES.

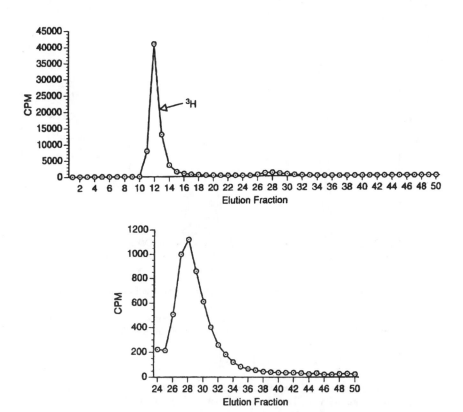

Figure 8. Gel permeation profile of a sample of [^3H]DNA hydrolysate, derived from multilayer cultures of human keratinocytes that were exposed to 1 μM BCES for 30 min. Column matrix: BioRad P2. Insert is an enlargement of the profile for fractions 24–50 of the upper diagram. Fractions 12–14 represent the DNA. Fractions 26–34 include the ^3H_2O resulting from exposure to BCES.

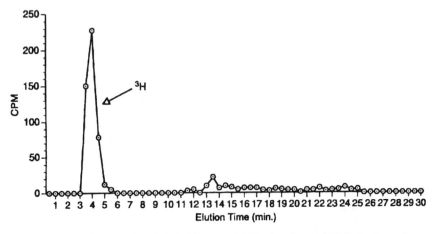

Figure 9. HPLC elution profile of pooled fractions 26–31 taken from the BioRad column shown in Figure 8. For methodology, see the text.

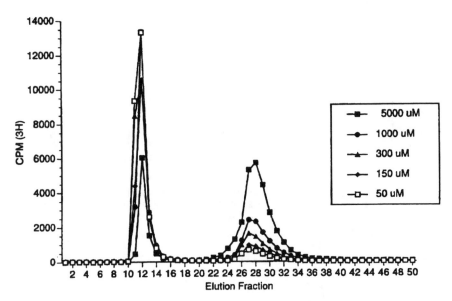

Figure 10. Gel permeation profile of a hydrolyzed sample of human [³H]DNA, derived from cultures of human keratinocytes grown in the presence of [³H]GR and exposed to different doses of BCES after isolation from the culture. Column matrix: BioRad P2. Fractions 10–14 represent residual DNA. The major fraction of ³H eluted between fractions 24 and 34 at all doses utilized. For methodological details, see the text.

Relationship of Interstrand Cross-Links in DNA, Production of Interleukin-1α (IL-1α), and Cytotoxicity in Human Keratinocytes Exposed to BCES

Although there is evidence for the repair of cross-links in DNA,[10] the presence of a high level of diguanyl derivatives in cellular DNA exposed to BCES suggests the possibility that this adduct might be strongly associated with cell death. To test this point, experiments with monolayer cultures of human keratinocytes were carried out in which the levels of cross-linkage in DNA

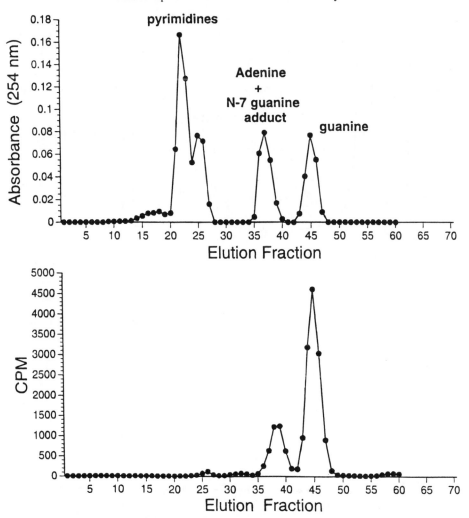

Figure 11. The gel permeation profile of a hydrolyzed sample of [^{14}C]DNA, derived from submerged multilayer cultures of rat keratinocytes grown in the presence of [^{14}C]GR and exposed to 300 μM BCES after isolation from the culture. Column matrix: BioRad P2. For methodological details, see the text.

(as indicated by the intercalation of ethidium bromide), the levels of IL-1α (as measured by an enzyme-linked immunosorbent assay technique with monoclonal antibody to human IL-1α), and cell viability (as measured by exclusion of trypan blue) were compared. Cultures grown submerged as monolayers for 4 d were exposed to different concentrations of BCES at 37°C for 30 min. Cross-linked DNA was determined immediately. IL-1α and viability were determined at 72 h postexposure.

Interstrand cross-linking showed a linear increase between 1 and 13% of the DNA as the concentration of BCES was increased from 10 to 100 μM. Since 1% was the control value, interstrand cross-linking became significant only at a concentration above 10 μM BCES. Significant loss of viable cells became apparent at 24 h postexposure to 10 μM BCES and showed a progressive increase thereafter up to 72 h. At higher exposures, loss of viability among cells in exposed cultures became apparent earlier. The level of IL-1α also showed a linear increase with

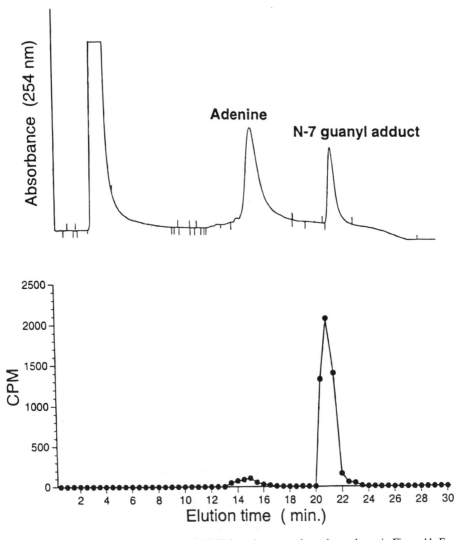

Figure 12. HPLC elution profile of fractions 37–38 from the permeation column shown in Figure 11. For procedural details, see the text.

exposures between 10 and 100 μM BCES. Below an exposure to 10 μM, the level of IL-1α was not significantly different from control. Figure 13 shows the positive correlation ($r = .96$) between the increase in the amount of IL-1α in the cells and the degree of cross-linking in the cellular DNA, while Figure 14 shows the inverse correlation ($r = .96$) between the amount of IL-1α in the cells and cell viability. Thus, it is possible to predict the degree of cytotoxicity that a culture exposed to BCES will exhibit at 72 h postexposure by determining the degree of interstrand cross-linking immediately after exposure.

DISCUSSION

The loss of proliferative capability that accompanies destruction of the basal layer in the epidermis is a major concomitant of the vesication occurring after a delay when human skin is exposed

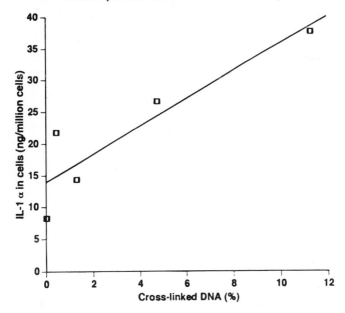

Figure 13. Correlation curve of the IL-1α found in cells exposed to BCES and the degree of cross-linking in the DNA of such cells. For details of procedure, see the text; $r = .96$. From Pu et al.[17] with permission.

to BCES in vivo.[5] An understanding of the mechanism(s) involved in this phenomenon should provide insight into the nature of the initial interactions between sulfur mustard and the skin. Pseudo-epidermis, a stratified, cornified culture of cutaneous keratinocytes grown at the air–liquid interface, exhibits a response after topical exposure to BCES similar to that seen in the epidermis, and thus should be useful for the study of these primary interactions. As shown in Figure 4, the loss of the germinative layer in an exposed human pseudo-epidermis is both dose and time dependent. The time dependency of the response suggests that generalized necrosis cannot be entirely responsible for the destruction of the basal cells in an epidermal system exposed topically to BCES. Figure 1 proposes enhanced differentiation as an additional mechanism for loss of proliferative capacity in an exposed epidermal system, particularly at lower levels of exposure. Differentiation, which represents a form of programmed cell death and occurs over a period of time, can be a factor in the delay that is observed between the application of BCES and the appearance of the blister.

The division of the hypothetical scheme, shown in Figure 1, into Stages I, II, and III is not meant to propose that there are sharp delineations between the various facets of the scheme as the level of exposure to BCES is increased. Rather, it is meant to suggest that at the lowest doses, repair is complete (Stage I) but as the dose of BCES increases, the sequences of events in Stages II and III come increasingly into play.

Stage II is postulated to be a phase of toxicity involving commitment to differentiation by previously proliferative cells that cannot divide, because of the presence of heterotypic DNA in their genome. Although these cells become committed to differentiation, the course of their differentiation is abnormal. For example, they undergo abnormal enlargement before they are lost from the culture.[7] Using a monoclonal antibody, 7B4, which was generated against a preparation of keratins isolated from the epidermis of the newborn rat, this hypothesis was tested. 7B4 was shown to decorate predominantly the cornified layer in unexposed rat skin or pseudo-epidermis derived from the epidermis of the newborn rat (Figure 5). Monolayer cultures of keratinocytes derived from rat skin, which showed no reactivity with 7B4 followed by goat anti-mouse IgG coupled with fluorescein isothiocyanate (FITC), showed fluorescence with this

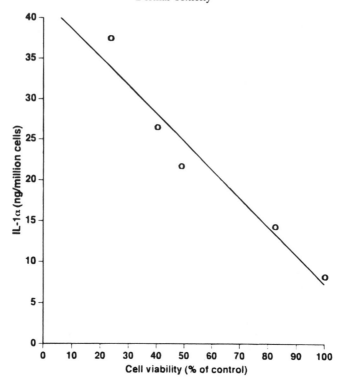

Figure 14. Correlation curve of the amount of IL-1α found in cells exposed to BCES and the viability of such cells. For details of procedure, see the text; $r = .96$. From Pu et al.[17] with permission.

combination of antibodies after the cultures were exposed to BCES (Figure 6). This effect was time and dose dependent. Clearly, these observations can be interpreted to support the view that exposure to BCES can lead to enhanced differentiation among basal cells, which would have the effect of decreasing the number of germinatively-competent cells in the culture. In fact, at 2 d postexposure to 5 μM BCES, nearly all cells bound 7B4 and, by this criterion, had differentiated. Ku and Bernstein[7] have previously shown that at 6 d postexposure to 5 μM BCES, replication of DNA, an absolute prerequisite for mitosis, is essentially absent in monolayer cultures. Unfortunately, the effort to isolate the keratin protein responsible for 7B4 binding resulted in ambiguous data. Extracts of both exposed and unexposed monolayer cultures revealed a 58-kD protein that bound 7B4. However, extracts of exposed cells also had a smaller 7B4-reactive protein whose size was 55 kD. To rationalize these latter data with the results from the fluorescence study of unexposed and exposed cells, one has to assume that, in the cell, the 58-kD protein is "blocked," so that it cannot react with the antibody, and that the extraction technique "frees" the epitope to react with 7B4. Further complicating the picture is the observation that the 55-kD protein was detected in extracts of differentiated cells in pseudo-epidermis, but not in extracts of whole epidermis. Perhaps the technique of isolation is responsible for the ambiguities. Obviously, further work will be necessary to clarify the situation. Nevertheless, it appears reasonable to consider that exposure to BCES causes cells capable of division to become committed to differentiation, thus decreasing the germinative pool of keratinocytes.

According to Figure 1, formation of diadducts in DNA—especially cross-linking diadducts—should be correlated with cellular destruction. Presumably, diadducts in DNA should prevent either transcription or translation of the nucleic acid. As shown by the data in Figures 13 and 14, the insertion of interstrand cross-links leads to loss of viability in submerged monolayer cultures exposed to BCES. An increase in the degree of interstrand cross-linking observed immediately after exposure correlated with an increase in the percentage of nonviable cells at 3 d postexposure. If repair of interstrand cross-links does occur, it does not appear to enhance the survival of cells significantly. In this context, it is interesting to note that the presumed diguanyl adduct was not detected in the DNA of human keratinocytes exposed to 1 μM or to any level of BCES. However, the analytical techniques utilized in these studies may have been inadequately sensitive to detect the presence of a small amount of diadduct, especially the amount of diadduct likely to have resulted from exposure to 1 μM BCES.

Although no diguanyl residues have been detected as yet in these studies, significant formation of monoguanyl adduct has been shown even after a very low exposure of human keratinocytes to BCES. As shown by the technique of proton exchange (cf., Figures 8 and 9), monoguanyl residues in the DNA are alkylated when human keratinocytes are exposed to 1 μM BCES for 30 min. Data in the literature (see Ref. 15) suggest that the ratio of the percentage of diadduct relative to the percentage of monoadduct of guanine should be of the order of 0.2. It is unlikely that the techniques used in this study would be sensitive enough to measure diadduct at this level. Higher specific activity radioactive precursor might be successfully utilized for this purpose.

The finding that the production of IL-1α in exposed cells correlated with loss of cell viability provides a useful parameter for monitoring cell death. Presumably, the appearance of the cytokine in the cell, which is paralleled by an increase of IL-1α in the medium (data not shown), would signal the initiation of the inflammatory response[16] if it occurred in the intact skin. If a similar response is seen in pseudo-epidermis exposed to BCES, the system can be used to elucidate the role played by the cytokine in the response of keratinocytes to injury.

From the data in hand, it is possible to begin to estimate the limits of exposure relating to the proposed three stages of toxicity from BCES for human pseudo-epidermis. The upper limit of exposure for Stage I seems to be about 1 nmol BCES/cm^2. Stage III is certainly reached by an exposure to 50 nmol/cm^2. These conclusions are based upon the morphological data shown in Figure 4. Presumably, Stage II starts at a level of 1 nmol/cm^2, but its upper limit cannot be estimated. Additional dose-response studies of parameters of BCES-mediated toxicity should provide data for further delineating the exposure levels within which each stage occurs in human pseudo-epidermis. This culture appears to be a promising model system for investigating the pathogenesis of human cutaneous vesication.

REFERENCES

1. Scavarelli-Karantsavelos, R. M., Saroya, S. Z., Vaughan, F. L., and Bernstein, I. A. 1990. Pseudoepidermis, constructed in vitro, for use in toxicological and pharmacological studies. *Skin Pharmacol.* 3:115–125.
2. Vaughan, F. L., Gray, R. H., and Bernstein, I. A. 1986. Growth and differentiation of primary rat keratinocytes on synthetic membranes, *In Vitro Cell. Dev. Biol.* 22:141–149.
3. Bernstam, L. I., Vaughan, F. L., and Bernstein, I. A. 1990. Stratified cornified primary cultures of human keratinocytes grown on microporous membranes at the air-liquid interface. *J. Dermatol. Sci.* 1:173–181.
4. Bernstam, L. I., Vaughan, F. L., and Bernstein, I. A. 1986. Keratinocytes grown at the air-liquid interface. *In Vitro Cell. Dev. Biol.* 22:695–705.
5. Papirmeister, B., Gross, C. L., Meier, H. L., Petrali, J. P., and Johnson, J. B. 1985. Molecular basis for mustard-induced vesication. *Fundam. Appl. Toxicol.* 5:S134–S149.
6. Bernstein, I. A., Bernstam, L. I., Yang, Y. H., Lin, P. P., and Vaughan, F. L. 1993. Pseudo-epidermis: A model system for investigating molecular and cellular pathways of cutaneous epidermal toxicity from sulfur mustard. *Proc. 1993 Medical Defense Bioscience Rev., USAMRDC*, pp. 97–104.
7. Ku, W. W., and Bernstein, I. A. 1988. Bis-(β-chloroethyl)sulfide (BCES)-induced changes in epidermal cell homeostasis *in vitro. Toxicol. Appl. Pharmacol.* 95:397–411.
8. Ludlum, D. B., Austin-Ritchie, P., Hagopian, M., Niu, T. G. Q., and Yu, D. 1994. Detection of sulfur mustard-induced DNA modifications. *Chem. Biol. Interact.* 91:39–49.
9. Brent, T. P. 1984. Suppression of cross-link formation in chloroethylnitrosourea-treated DNA by an activity in extracts of human leukemic lymphoblasts. *Cancer Res.* 44:1887–1892.
10. Garcia, S. T., McQuillan, A., and Panasci, L. 1988. Correlation between the cytotoxicity of melphalan and DNA crosslinks as detected by the ethidium bromide assay in F1 variant of B16 melanoma cells. *Biochem. Pharmacol.* 34:3189–3192.
11. Papirmeister, B., and Davison, C. L. 1964. Elimination of sulfur mustard-induced products from DNA of *Escherichia coli. Biochem. Biophys. Res. Commun.* 17:608–617.

12. Fan, L., and Bernstein, I. A. 1991. Effect of bis(β-chloroethyl)sulfide (BCES) on base mismatch repair of DNA in monkey kidney cells. *Toxicol. Appl. Pharmacol.* 111:233–241.

13. Ribeiro, P. L., Mitra, R. S., and Bernstein, I. A. 1991. Assessment of the role of DNA damage and repair in the survival of primary cultures of rat cutaneous keratinocytes exposed to bis(2-chloroethyl) sulfide. *Toxicol. Appl. Pharmacol.* 111:342–351.

14. Tomasz, M. 1970. Extreme lability of the C-8 proton: A consequence of 7-methylation of guanine residues in model compounds and in DNA and its analytical application. *Biochim. Biophys. Acta* 199:18–28.

15. Papirmeister, B., Feister, A. J., Robinson, S. I., and Ford, R. D. 1991. *Medical defense against mustard gas, toxic mechanisms and pharmacological implications.* Boca Raton, FL: CRC Press.

16. Nickoloff, B. J. 1992. Cytokine networks in skin disease. In *Cytokines in health and disease,* eds. S. L. Kunkel and D. G. Remick, chap. 23. Basel: Marcel Dekker.

17. Pu, Y., Lin, P., Vaughan, F. L., and Bernstein, I. A. 1995. Appearance of interleukin 1*ga relates DNA interstrand cross-links and cytotoxicity in cultured human kertainocytes exposed to bis-(2-chloroethyl)sulfide.

Chapter Two

REFINEMENT OF AN ENDPOINT FOR MEASURING SKIN DECONTAMINANT EFFICACY

J. A. Blank, Ronald G. Menton, C. T. Olson, D. W. Hobson, T. H. Snider, and D. W. Korte, Jr.

Battelle's Medical Research and Evaluation Facility (MREF) has developed, validated, and implemented the measurement of red blood cell acetylcholinesterase activity levels to evaluate candidate skin decontaminants against percutaneous organophosphonate exposure. The procedure was validated by comparing results with previously collected experimental lethality data for a standard decontaminant. This refined endpoint allows animals to be anesthetized during studies while obtaining quantitative data. Animal use is reduced further through the use of statistical analytical procedures such as group sequential stopping rules and stagewise dose allocation.

INTRODUCTION

In the past, skin decontaminants for the treatment of organophosphonate (OP) exposure were experimentally evaluated using lethality as an endpoint. As acetylcholinesterase (AChE) inhibition is an effect of acute OP intoxication, monitoring erythrocyte AChE activity following OP exposure may be an alternative endpoint to lethality for evaluating the effectiveness of candidate decontaminants. This quantitative measurement can be made on serial blood samples from the same animal. The purpose of this work was to examine the feasibility of using erythrocyte AChE measurements as a means for experimentally assessing skin decontaminant effectiveness against percutaneous OP exposures.

METHODS

Male New Zealand white rabbits weighing 2–4 kg were obtained from Hazleton Research Animals (Denver, PA). Soman in a methylacrylate thickener (TGD), VX, and XE-555 skin decontaminating resin were obtained from the U.S. Army Medical Research Institute of Chemical Defense.

AChE Inhibition Studies

AChE inhibition studies were used to determine the extent of erythrocyte AChE inhibition that occurs following absorption of percutaneously applied OP. Blood samples were drawn from rabbits 5 min prior to OP exposure to establish baseline AChE activity values, and at 30, 60, and 120 min following application of an OP. At time zero, animals were dosed with an OP and treated with XE-555 resin 2 min following exposure. Treatment was performed by briskly wiping the exposed area with the resin for 10 s.

A stagewise adaptive dose allocation design[1] was used to select doses for studies to estimate the median inhibitory doses (MID) of OP in the presence or absence of decontaminant treatment. OP doses on all but the first day of experimentation were selected based on estimates of the slope and percentiles of the dose-response relationship between the OP and AChE inhibition. As data were obtained, all information available was used to select the OP doses for the next day or stage of experimentation. This approach permitted OP dose–AChE inhibition response estimation with a minimal number of animals.

The slope and intercept of the dose-response relationship were estimated using special-purpose programs based on the nonlinear regression procedure (PROC NLIN) in the Statistical Analyses System (SAS, Version 6.03). For these calculations, the percent AChE inhibition was assumed to be linearly related to the logarithm of the OP dose [$\log_{10}$(OP dose)] through the cumulative distribution function of the normal distribution.[2] This relationship is expressed as:

$$\rho = \phi \, [\alpha + \beta* \log_{10}(\text{OP dose})]$$

where

α = intercept of the dose-response relationship
β = slope of the dose-response relationship
ρ = percent AChE inhibition exhibited at $\log_{10}$(OP dose)
ϕ = cumulative distribution function for the normal distribution

Estimated parameters from the OP dose–AChE inhibition response relation were used to calculate the TGD and VX MID doses. Confidence intervals for the percentiles of the dose-response relationship were computed using Fieller's method.[2]

Candidate Resin Evaluation

Candidate decontaminant resins were compared to XE-555 resin for effectiveness against TGD exposure. Animals were exposed to a TGD dose that caused 50% AChE inhibition in XE-555 decontaminated animals. Two minutes following a TGD exposure, animals were decontaminated either with XE-555 resin or with candidate resin. These evaluations were performed using a sequential stopping rule.[3] If a significant difference in the two treatments existed after 2 d of evaluation, then testing procedures were stopped. Otherwise, a third evaluation day was performed and the groups were statistically compared.

AChE Activity Analysis

Heparinized blood samples were centrifuged and 10 μl of the red blood cell pellet was solubilized in a Triton X-100 solution. The samples were centrifuged and the supernatant was analyzed for AChE activity. Formation of a hydrolytic product of acetylthiocholine iodide (ATCI), which reacts with dithionitrobenzoic acid (DTNB) to form a yellow product, was monitored spectrophotometrically as described by Ellman and co-workers.[4] This procedure was automated by slightly modifying the procedure for use on a Cobas Fara™ centrifugal analyzer (Roche Diagnostics). Control charting of rabbit erythrocyte baseline AChE activity was performed for assay quality control purposes.

RESULTS

Figures 1 and 2 illustrate AChE data for animals percutaneously exposed to TGD or VX and either not decontaminated or decontaminated with XE-555 resin. Decontamination of exposed animals shifted the dose-response curves to the right for both AChE inhibition and lethality measurements, indicating decontaminant effectiveness.

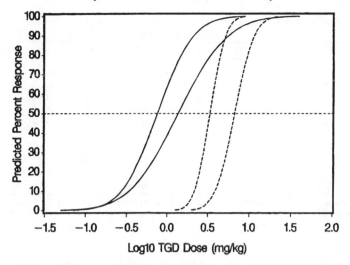

Figure 1. TGD dose-response curves for percent acetylcholinesterase inhibition (——) and lethality (- - - -) in XE-555 decontaminated and control animals. Animals were dosed with TGD and either not decontaminated or decontaminated with XE-555 resin. AChE activity was measured prior to and 60 min following application, and the percent AChE inhibition relative to baseline levels was calculated. Lethality was examined at 24 h postexposure. From Blank et al.[5] with permission.

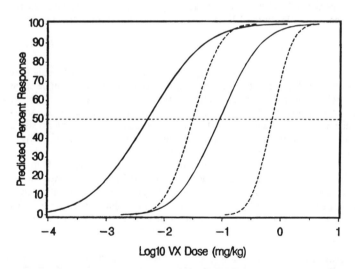

Figure 2. VX dose-response curves for percent acetylcholinesterase inhibition (——) and lethality (- - - -) in XE-555 decontaminated and control animals. Animals were dosed with VX and either not decontaminated or decontaminated with XE-555 resin. AChE activity was measured prior to and 120 min following exposure, and the percent AChE inhibition was calculated. Lethality was evaluated at 24 h postexposure. From Blank et al.[5] with permission.

Table 1. Effect of XE-555 Treatment on VX- and TGD-Induced Acetylcholinesterase Inhibition and Lethality in the Rabbit

Agent	TX	MID/MLD	LL	UL	N	PR	Slope (SE)
			AChE inhibition				
TGD	None	0.76	0.61	0.92	23	—	2.89 (0.57)
TGD	XE-555	1.37	1.13	1.66	32	1.8	2.11 (0.29)
VX	None	0.005	0.003	0.006	38	—	1.28 (0.21)
VX	XE-555	0.089	0.073	0.106	37	17.8	1.78 (0.23)
			24-h lethality				
TGD	None	3.35	3.15	3.59	208	—	6.89 (1.18)
TGD	XE-555	6.67	6.05	7.37	160	2.0	5.41 (1.13)
VX	None	0.031	0.020	0.103	136	—	2.73 (0.79)
VX	XE-555	0.708	0.567	0.814	206	22.8	3.79 (0.64)

Note. From Blank et al.[5] with permission. TX, treatment. MID, median inhibitory dose (mg/kg). LL, lower 95% confidence limit. UL, upper 95% confidence limit. PR, protective ratio (MLD or MID of treated rabbits/MLD or MID of control rabbits). MLD, Median lethal dose (mg/kg).

The MID and medial lethal doses (MLD) along with the 95% confidence limits and the protective ratio (PR; ratio of the MID or MLD of treated rabbits to the respective MID or MLD of TGD/VX-exposed control rabbits) are presented in Table 1. The PR obtained for XE-555 resin against TGD and VX exposure using the AChE activity endpoint is similar to the corresponding values obtained using lethality measurements.

Five experimental decontaminants were evaluated relative to the XE-555 resin for effectiveness against TGD (Table 2). The TGD MID for XE-555 resin-treated animals was used as the fixed challenge. After 2 d of evaluations, interim statistical analyses revealed that no differences between the experimental decontaminants and the XE-555 resin were present. A third evaluation day was then performed and the data were again analyzed. All experimental resins were found to be equivalent ($p > .05$) to the XE-555 resin in protection from TGD exposure.

CONCLUSIONS

In contrast to lethality measurements, AChE activity analyses can provide quantitative measurements for each animal as a function of time. AChE activity values also can be standardized for each animal relative to preexposure baseline activity values. For evaluating the effectiveness of skin decontaminants, AChE activity determinations provide advantages. An experimental evaluation can be performed within a few hours, as opposed to 24-h lethality assessments. During exposures and AChE activity evaluations, animals can be maintained in a fully anesthetized state, making the experimental procedures more humane.

For AChE activity studies, two statistical procedures were applied to help reduce animal utilization. First, stagewise experimental design was used for dose-response studies. Although lethality measurements performed prior to implementation of this statistical procedure required as many as 200 animals per MLD determination, it was possible to obtain a good MID estimate using 40 or fewer animals with the stagewise experimental design. Second, a statistical sequential

Table 2. Effectiveness of Candidate Decontaminants Relative to XE-555 Resin Against TGD Exposure

	Candidate resin			XE-555 resin		
Decontaminant	n	Mean[a]	STD	n	Mean[a]	STD
1513	24	44.4	3.8	24	39.8	5.0
1514	24	44.0	5.8	24	43.5	4.9
1515	24	43.7	4.7	24	51.7	4.1
1516	24	50.9	4.5	24	51.7	4.1
1517	24	52.9	3.1	24	50.8	3.0

[a] Values are percent AChE inhibition.

stopping rule, which implements interim statistical analyses to allow early termination of testing when large differences in treatment group responses are observed, was used. Although this procedure did not result in animal reduction for data presented in this chapter, it is a procedure that can be included in the experimental design of routine testing procedures to help minimize animal use.

REFERENCES

1. Feder, P. I., Hobson, D. W., Olson, C. T., Joiner, R. L., and Matthews, M. C. 1992. Stagewise, group sequential experimental designs for comparisons of quantal response levels obtained with candidate treatment regimens versus those with a concurrent control or a specified standard. In *Biopharmaceutical sequential statistical applications,* ed. K. E. Peace, pp. 87–116. New York: Marcel Dekker.
2. Finney, D. J. 1971. *The comparison of effectiveness. Probit analysis,* 3rd ed., pp. 119–121. New York: Cambridge University Press.
3. Geller, N. L., and Pocock, S. J. 1988. Design and analysis of clinical trials with group sequential stopping rules. In *Biopharmaceutical statistics for drug development,* ed. K. E. Peace, pp. 489–508. New York: Marcel Dekker.
4. Ellman, G. L., Courtney, K. D., Andres, V., Jr., and Featherstone, R. M. 1961. A new and rapid colorimetric determination of acetylcholinesterase activity. *Biochem. Pharmacol.* 7:88–95.
5. Blank, J., Hobson, D., Snider, T., Menton, R., Olson, C., and Korte, D., Jr. 1993. Acetylcholinesterase inhibition measurements for the evaluation of decontaminant efficacy following percutaneous organophosphorous compound exposure. *Toxicol. Methods* 3:252–260.

Chapter Three

AN IN VITRO MODEL FOR SKIN RECONSTRUCTION

R. Fleischmajer, E. D. MacDonald, P. Contard, and J. S. Perlish

This is a report on an in vitro coculture model where fibroblasts grown in a three-dimensional nylon mesh were recombined with human keratinocytes. The cultures were kept for 3 and 5 wk and then processed for electron microscopy and immunochemistry. The epidermis showed a basal layer with hemidesmosomes, a stratified epithelium with tonofilaments and desmosomes, a granular layer with keratinosomes and keratohyaline granules, and a transitional stratum corneum. The epidermis expressed K-10 keratin, trichohyalin, and filaggrin. There was formation of anchoring filaments, lamina densa, anchoring fibrils, bundles of elastin-associated microfibrils (diameter 10 mm), and fine collagen fibrils. The basal lamina contained type IV collagen, laminin, nidogen, and heparan sulfate. Type IV collagen, laminin, and nidogen were also noted in the extracellular matrix. Type VI collagen and fibrillin stained the anchoring zone and also gave a reticulated pattern in the dermis. There was a heavy signal for fibronectin throughout the dermis. The extracellular matrix also revealed type I, III, and V collagens. Decorin was present throughout the dermis but elastin was absent. The present study shows that fibroblasts in a natural environment will support epidermal morphogenesis and differentiation as well as the formation of a basal lamina and anchoring zone.

INTRODUCTION

The role of the microenvironment in morphogenesis and differentiation of tissues has been the subject of numerous investigations.[1] There is considerable evidence that cells transduce signals not only from hormones and growth factors but also from adjacent cells and their surrounding extracellular matrix (ECM). Numerous attempts have been made to create ideal conditions so that cells grown in in vitro conditions may express and retain their phenotype. Cell monolayers cultured on plastic proved to be a useful model to elucidate the flow of information from DNA to a specific protein. However, epithelial cells proliferate but do not fully differentiate when grown on plastic. Fibroblasts proliferate into two-dimensional monolayer cultures; however, this is a nonphysiological environment. These cells in vivo never show a tendency for confluency except during early embryogenesis, wound healing, and following neoplastic transformation. The normal environment for fibroblasts and related mesenchymal cells is the ECM that they help synthesize. The specificity of this ECM varies depending on the function of the tissue, that is, skin, cartilage, bone, etc.

The study of epithelial tissue specificity in in vitro conditions requires a rather complex microenvironment where crucial epithelial–mesenchymal interactions can be preserved. Over the past 20 years, several advances have been made in the development of techniques for growing human keratinocytes in culture.[2] Rheinwald and Green[3] grew human keratinocytes on a feeder layer of lethally irradiated 3T3 fibroblasts and noted proliferation and keratinizing colonies containing tonofilaments, desmosomes, and keratohyalin granules. Freeman et al.[4] cultured human keratinocytes on dead porcine dermis and obtained an epidermal layer that closely resembled the in vivo situation. Similar studies were performed by seeding keratinocytes onto a human dead dermis that retained basal lamina components.[5] These keratinocytes revealed migration, proliferation and expression of a 67-kD keratin, indicative of suprabasal differentiation.[5] Bell et al.[6,7] cultured fibroblasts in a type I collagen gel. Following contraction of the gel, a tissue-like fabric developed that supported proliferation and differentiation of epidermal cells. However, Mauch et al.[8] observed that under such conditions, fibroblasts were metabolically inactive, making only 5% of the normal amount of collagen they were capable of producing. Furthermore, immunoelectron microscopy using antibodies directed against the aminopropeptides of type I and type III procollagens showed no evidence of the release of procollagens or active fibrillogenesis (Fleischmajer and Krieg, unpublished data). Diollan et al.[9] grew epidermal cells in a "sponge" consisting of collagen, glycosaminoglycans, and glycoproteins and obtained partial differentiation. More recently, epidermal cells were grown in a collagen–fibroblast matrix at an air–liquid interface.[10] This model revealed epidermal differentiation by morphogenesis and the induction of a 67-kD keratin. Hirone and Taniguchi[11] grew epidermal cells on collagen gels and plastic and noted development of hemidesmosomes and a less defined basal lamina only in those cultures on collagen gels. David et al.[12] also showed an incomplete basal lamina with mammary epithelial cells grown either on plastic or a type I collagen substrate. Similar results were obtained by Chamson et al.[13] after recombining keratinocytes with collagen gels populated by fibroblasts. Tinois et al.[14] reported keratinocyte differentiation and basal lamina formation when cells were cultured on a substrate consisting of type I and type III collagens coated with type IV collagen.

Naughton et al.[15] described a three-dimensional culture where fibroblasts attached to a mesh, proliferated, and created an ECM similar to that of human dermis.[15-17] Coculture of keratinocytes and this dermal model resulted in epidermal differentiation. In this report, we should review the evidence that this coculture model results in epidermal differentiation, formation of a basal lamina, anchoring zone, and a dermis that closely resembles the "in vivo" situation.

MATERIALS AND METHODS

Keratinocyte/Dermal Model Cocultures

All cultures were grown at Advanced Tissue Sciences and shipped on nutrient agarose to Mount Sinai Medical Center for evaluation. The culture conditions have been previously reported.[15,18,19] Human neonatal foreskin fibroblasts and keratinocytes were isolated by sequential trypsin and collagenase digestion and expanded in monolayer cultures. Fibroblasts were seeded onto nylon mesh (8 × 8 cm) and allowed to grow for 26 d in DMEM containing 10% calf serum and 100 μg/ml ascorbate to form the dermal model. Keratinocytes were seeded onto the dermal model and the coculture was grown submerged for 1 wk, and then at an air–liquid interface in DMEM containing 5% fetal calf serum, 100 μg/ml ascorbate, and 0.5 μg/ml hydrocortisone. After 3–5 wk in culture, the mesh was laser cut into 11 × 11 mm squares, placed on agarose containing growth medium, and shipped at room temperature for overnight delivery. Cultures were removed from the agarose and either fixed for electron microscopy or cryopreserved for immunofluorescence microscopy.

Source of Antibodies

Antibodies used to characterize the epidermal layer, basal lamina-anchoring zone, and the remainder of the extracellular matrix were either purchased or a generous gift. The following antibodies were used: mouse monoclonal anti-human type III collagen antibodies (immunoglobulin M, IgM)[20] and mouse monoclonal antibodies directed against the NC-1 domain of the type VII collagen (IgG)[21-22] (R. E. Burgeson), rabbit polyclonal antibodies to type I collagen (LF-67),[23] decorin (LF-30),[24] and osteonectin[25] (L. W. Fisher and J. D. Termine). Type I antibodies were prepared against a 26-amino-acid residue (unconjugated) of a synthetic C telopeptide of the human L1 (I) chain.[26] Tenascin was a gift of H. Erickson. Decorin antibodies were prepared using synthetic peptides.[27] R. Timpl provided rabbit polyclonal antibodies against the aminopropeptides of type I and type III procollagens,[28] laminin,[29] fibronectin,[30] type VI collagen,[31] heparan sulfate,[32] osteonectin, and nidogen. A rabbit polyclonal antibody against type IV collagen was a gift from H. K. Kleinman.[34] Rabbit polyclonal antibodies against type V collagen were purified from human placenta (D. Hartmann). These antibodies were tested by radioimmunoassay and by immunoblotting. Fibrillin monoclonal antibodies were prepared from crude extracts of human amnion[35] (L. Sakai). Elastin antibodies (mouse monoclonal, IgG) were purchased from Sigma, St. Louis, MO.

The following epidermal antibodies were used: K-10, which is a marker for skin suprabasal cells,[36] trichohyalin,[37] and filaggrin[38] (T. T. Sun). The keratin marker antibodies were all monoclonal, mouse IgG directed against human protein.

Electron Microscopy

The periphery of the mesh was trimmed about 1 mm, leaving only the central portion, and fixed in Karnovsky's solution for 4 h at room temperature,[39] postfixed in ferrocyanide osmium tetroxide for 1 h, then stained en bloc for 1 h each in an aqueous solution of 1% phosphotungstic acid followed by 2% uranyl acetate.[40] After dehydration in graded ethanols, they were embedded in Spurr's resin in a flat embedding mold and rotated at an angle of 45° with the point of each square-shaped opening aligned toward the knife edge; the nylon was then carefully trimmed away from the sides of the chosen opening and ultrathin sections were cut with a diamond knife on a Sorval MT-2b ultramicrotome and examined in a JEOL EM 100 electron microscope.

Immunofluorescence Microscopy

The nylon mesh was cut into small pieces 3–4 mm square, and frozen in Tissue Tech O.C.T. embedding compound (Miles, Inc.). Frozen sections 5–6 μm thick were collected on polylysine-coated slides and fixed for 5 min in cold acetone (−20°C). Following a 5-min wash in 2 changes of phosphate-buffered saline (PBS, Sigma), the sections were challenged with the primary antibody in a moist chamber at 37°C for 30 min. Excess antibody was removed in two changes of PBS. The secondary fluorescein-conjugated antibody was then applied for 30 min at 37°C. After washing twice in PBS, the slides were drained and coverslipped using Aquamount medium (Lerner Laboratories) and examined with a Nikon microscope equipped with epifluorescent illumination.

RESULTS

Electron Microscopy

Three weeks postseeding of keratinocytes cultures revealed a well-developed epidermis and underlying dermal equivalent (Figure 1). Basal cells were cuboidal in shape and contained large nuclei and tonofilaments. The suprabasal layers consisted of flattened cells containing tonofilaments and intercellular desmosomes (Figure 2). A granular layer was observed containing well-developed intracellular keratohyalin and membrane coating granules. Although some of the cornified material was lost in preparation, signs of keratinization were evident in the uppermost layers of the epidermis.[41]

Four-week cultures revealed hemidesmosomes along the cytoplasmic membrane of the basal cells, multiple pinocytotic vesicles, anchoring filaments, a lamina lucida, and a lamina densa (Figure 3). Thin collagen fibers, measuring 24 nm in diameter, were evident in the uppermost dermis. Anchoring fibrils, straight or curved showing typical banding, were seen originating at the lamina densa (Figure 3). Some of these fibers terminated in anchoring plaques.[41]

Collagen fibers in the upper dermis showed typical 67 nm periodicity but appeared to be thin (about 24–48 nm). Microfibrils believed to be those associated with elastic tissue also were seen at the dermal-epidermal junction.

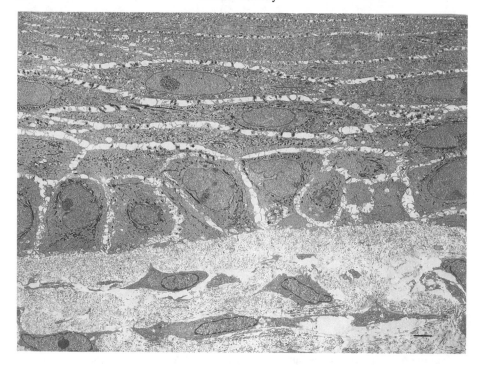

Figure 1. This represents a 3-wk keratinocyte–dermal recombination showing an epidermis consisting of cuboidal basal cells and elongated squamous cells. Note numerous desmosomes between keratinocytes. The dermis shows numerous fibroblasts embedded in a rich extracellular matrix. Bar = 100 nm.

Collagen fibers in the lower dermal equivalent showed typical 67 nm periodicity.[42] However, they were larger in diameter than those in the upper part of the dermal equivalent (about 45–76 nm). Microfibrils, 10 nm in diameter, were dispersed among the collagen fibers and did not form discrete bundles as was observed at the epidermal–dermal junction.

Immunochemistry

Indirect immunofluorescence microscopy was carried out with specimens that contained the nylon mesh and included the epidermal layer, basal lamina, anchoring zone, and extracellular matrix.

K-10 keratin antibodies labeled suprabasal cells up to the granular layer, but did not stain the basal cells. Most suprabasal cells were elongated and showed staining of the cytoplasm except for nuclei. Alpha-trichohyalin stained the upper layers, which consisted of long, narrow, elongated cells. Filaggrin stained similar areas, but the pattern was less continuous, showing various interruptions. Rabbit serum from nonimmunized animals was negative.[43]

The basal lamina stained for type IV collagen, laminin, nidogen, and heparin sulfate.[43] Type IV collagen and laminin stained the basal lamina, and also the entire extracellular matrix, suggesting strong participation by fibroblasts. Heparan sulfate was more restricted to the basal lamina, with a few streaks present in the extracellular matrix. Nidogen stained the basal lamina but there was significant staining of fibroblasts and the ECM. The lower and mid level of the epidermal layer stained homogeneously with osteonectin. Fibroblasts stained with osteonectin, but not the rest of the ECM (Figure 4).

Fibronectin was noted throughout the entire extracellular matrix without predilection for the epidermal–dermal junction (Figure 4). Type VI collagen not only appeared as a distinct band at the anchoring zone, but also showed staining of fibroblasts and a reticulated network throughout

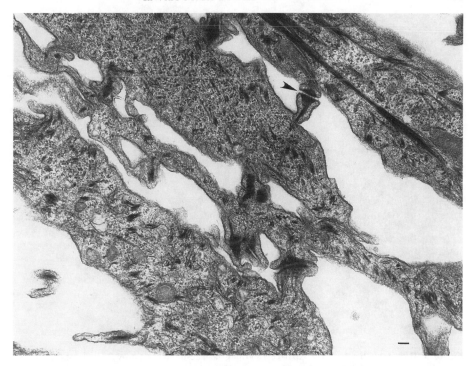

Figure 2. High magnification of keratinocytes showing numerous desmosomes (arrow head) and bundles of tonofilaments (arrows). Bar = 100 nm.

the entire extracellular matrix. Type VII collagen was restricted to the epidermal–dermal junction. Fibrillin was present at the epidermal–dermal junction and throughout the dermis in a reticulated pattern. Elastin was absent.[43]

Interstitial collagen fibers stained for type I, type III, and type V collagens in a similar pattern (Figure 5). Decorin also stained the entire extracellular matrix (Figure 5).

DISCUSSION

In previous studies, it has been shown that fibroblasts grown in a three-dimensional nylon mesh readily attach to the mesh, proliferate, and form a dermal model.[19] The cells arrange themselves in a parallel fashion and create well-demarcated intercellular chambers where a rich ECM is being deposited. The dermis contains collagen fibrils arranged in bundles, large numbers of elastin-associated microfibrils (10 nm), and filamentous and homogeneous electron-dense materials to be identified.[16] There is active fibrillogenesis since collagen fibrils grow from 20 to up to 80 nm in about 50 d in culture.[42] Furthermore, additional evidence of collagen fibril formation is the presence at their surface of the aminopropeptides of type I and type III procollagens.[42]

The present study shows that fibroblasts grown in a nylon mesh produce a rich extracellular matrix, which, when recombined with keratinocytes, will result in epidermal morphogenesis, differentiation, and formation of a basal lamina and an anchoring zone. Furthermore, an epithelial mesenchymal interaction takes place at the epidermal–ECM interface and appears to regulate collagen fibril diameter and to promote aggregation of microfibrils into bundles.

Epidermal differentiation was confirmed by immunocytochemistry of keratins. K-10 keratin was demonstrated in the suprabasal layer. We also demonstrated the presence of trichohyalin and filaggrin in the upper layers.[43]

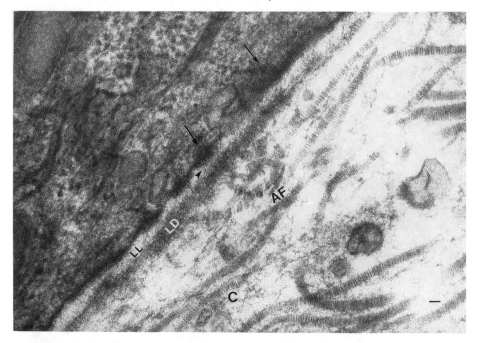

Figure 3. High magnification of a basal cell showing hemidesmosomes (arrows), anchoring filaments (arrowheads), a lamina lucida (LL), a lamina densa (LD), anchoring fibrils (AF), and thin collagen fibrils (C). Bar = 100 nm. From Contard et al.[41] with permission.

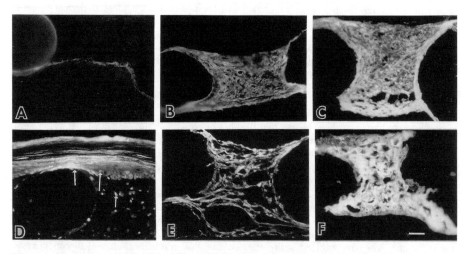

Figure 4. Note staining of type VII collagen at the epidermal-dermal junction (A). Type VI collagen stains the anchoring zone and rest of the dermis (B). Fibronectin stains the entire dermis (C), while osteonectin stains the epidermis (arrow) and fibroblasts (D). Fibrillin stains the epidermal–dermal junction and dermis (E), while elastin was negative. Note strong staining for tenascin throughout the entire dermis (F). Original magnification × 560. Bar = 50 μm. From Fleischmajer et al.[43] with permission.

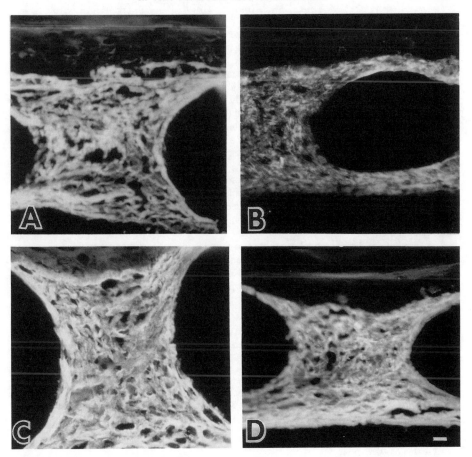

Figure 5. Interstitial collagens stain for type I, III, and V collagens (A, B, C). Note diffuse staining of the ECM with decorin (D). Original magnification × 560. Bar = 25 μm. From Fleischmajer et al.[43] with permission.

The most striking achievement of this model was the development of a basal lamina and an anchoring zone. An incomplete, fragmentary lamina densa was noted using 3-wk cocultures but at 5 wk most areas showed a distinct lamina densa and lamina lucida.

Type IV collagen, laminin, nidogen, and heparan sulfate were present at the interface area. Type IV collagen, laminin, and nidogen showed not only staining of the epidermal–ECM interface but also significant staining in the rest of ECM. Heparin sulfate was restricted mainly to the interface, although it also stained the ECM. It is noteworthy that there is evidence that during embryonic development, type IV collagen and laminin appear to originate from the surrounding mesenchymyme as demonstrated by in situ hybridization studies.[44,45] On the other hand, heparan sulfate appears to originate exclusively from the epithelium.[46] Nidogen was noted at the interface, but a strong signal was also present in the fibroblasts and throughout the dermis.

Type IV collagen was present at the epidermal–dermal junction, in fibroblasts, and also throughout the entire ECM in a reticulated pattern. This distribution is similar to that reported in normal skin.[31] Fibronectin was widely distributed throughout the entire ECM, without any specific predilection for the epidermal–dermal junction. This pattern is similar to that observed in normal skin where fibronectin is found in the papillary layer and within collagen bundles.[47] It is still not clear whether fibronectin interacts with basal lamina in adult tissues, although there is some evidence for such interaction in embryonic tissues.[48]

The anchoring zone in this skin culture model showed anchoring fibrils, bundles of microfibrils, and a network of thin collagen fibers.[49] These last structures appeared to be enlaced within anchoring fibrils. Anchoring fibrils extend from the lamina densa to anchoring placques, and type VII collagen is their major component.

Elastin-associated microfibrils are produced in large quantities when fibroblasts are grown in the absence of other cell types in a three-dimensional nylon mesh.[16] In these cultures, microfibrils are seen as single units or in bundles frequently intermingled with collagen fibrils in a parallel fashion.[16] In the coculture, this pattern persisted throughout the dermal component. The distribution of microfibrils was also studied by immunochemistry with antibodies against fibrillin.[35] Although we did not discern "candelabra" formation at the epidermal–dermal junction, as seen in vivo, there was a band distribution in that area and a reticular network in the rest of the ECM, similar to that seen in normal human skin.

It is noteworthy that the immunochemistry of collagen fibrils revealed type I, III, V, and VII collagens. The fibrils near the epidermal–dermal junction were thin, resembling the in vivo situation where reticulin fibrils are concentrated in the dermal epidermal junction.[50] Decorin appeared to coat all collagen fibrils in our model, as reported previously for embryonic and adult human skin.[24]

The keratinocyte/dermal model coculture corroborates the concept that promotion and maintenance of epidermal morphogenesis and differentiation are greatly dependent upon interactions with the microenvironment. Furthermore, it also suggests that the formation of a basal-lamina anchoring zone is the result of a cooperative process between epidermal cells and their surrounding ECM.

REFERENCES

1. Sanders, E. J. 1988. The roles of epithelial mesenchymal cell interactions in development processes. *Biochem. Cell. Biol.* 66:530–540.
2. Prunieras, M. 1991. To reconstitute skin: Theme and variations. *Matrix* 11:302–305.
3. Rheinwald, J. G., and Green, H. 1975. Serial cultivation of strains of human epidermal keratinocytes: The formation of keratinizing colonies from single cells. *Cell* 6:331–334.
4. Freeman, A. E., Igel, H. J., Herrman, B. J., and Kleinfeld, K. L. 1976. Growth and characterization of human skin epithelial cell cultures. *In Vitro* 12:352–362.
5. Regnier, M., Schweizer, J., Michel, S., Bailly, C., and Prunieras, M. 1986. Expression of high molecular weight (67kD) keratin in human keratinocytes cultured on dead–de-epidermized dermis. *Exp. Cell. Res.* 165:63–72.
6. Bell, E., Ivarsson, B., and Merrill, C. 1979. Production of a tissue-like structure by contraction of collagen lattices by human fibroblasts of different proliferative potential "in vitro." *Proc. Natl. Acad. Sci. USA* 76:1274–1278.
7. Bell, E., Ehrlich, H. P., Buttle, D. J., and Nakatsuji, T. 1981. Living tissue formed "in vitro" and accepted as skin equivalent tissue of full thickness. *Science* 211:1052–1054.
8. Mauch, C., Hatamochi, A., Scharffetter, K., and Krieg, T. 1988. Regulation of collagen synthesis in fibroblasts within a three-dimensional collagen gel. *Exp. Cell Res.* 178:493–503.
9. Doillan, C. J., Wasserman, A. J., Berg, R. A., and Silver, F. H. 1988. Behavior of fibroblasts and epidermal cells cultivated in analogues of extracellular matrix. *Biomaterials* 9:91–96.
10. Asselineau, D., Bernhard, B., Bailly, C., and Darmon, M. 1985. Epidermal morphogenesis and induction of the 67kD keratin polypeptide by culture of human keratinocytes at the liquid–air interface. *Exp. Cell Res.* 159:536–539.
11. Hirone, T., and Taniguchi, S. 1980. Basal lamina formation by epidermal cells in cell culture. *Curr. Probl. Dermatol.* 10:158–169.
12. David, G., Nusgens, B., van der Schueren, B., van Cauwenberge, D., van der Berghe, H., and Lampiere, C. 1987. Collagen metabolism and basement membrane formation in cultures of mouse mammary epithelial cells. *Exp. Cell Res.* 170:402–416.
13. Chamson, A., Germain, N., Claudy, A., Perier, C., and Frey, J. 1989. Study of basement membrane formation in dermal-epidermal recombinants in vitro. *Arch. Dermatol. Res.* 281:267–272.
14. Tinois, E., Tiollier, J., Gaucherand, M., Dumas, H., Turdy, M., and Thivolet, J. 1991. In vitro and post-transplantation differentiation of human keratinocytes grown on human type IV collagen film of a bilayered dermal substitute. *Exp. Cell Res.* 193:310–319.
15. Naughton, G. K., Jacob, L., and Naughton, B. A. 1989. A physiological skin model for in vitro toxicity studies. In *Alternative methods in toxicology*, vol. 7, ed. A. M. Goldberg, pp. 183–189. New York: Mary Ann Liebert.

16. Fleischmajer, R., Contard, P., Schwartz, E., MacDonald, E. D. II, Jacobs, L. II, and Sakai, L. Y. 1991. Elastin-associated microfibrils (10 nm) in a three-dimensional fibroblast culture. *J. Invest. Dermatol.* 97:638–643.

17. Contard, P., Jacobs, L., Perlish, J. S., and Fleischmajer, R. 1991. Fibrillogenesis in a new three dimensional fibroblast culture system (abstr.). *J. Invest. Dermatol.* 96:605.

18. Slivka, S. R., Laudeen, L., Zimber, M. P., and Bartel, R. L. 1991. Biochemical characterization, barrier function and drug metabolism in an in vitro skin model (abstr.). *J. Cell Biol.* 115:236a.

19. Triglia, D., Sherard-Braa, S., Donnelly, T., Kidd, I., and Naughton, G. K. 1991. A three dimensional human dermal model substrate for in vitro toxicological studies. In *Alternative methods in toxicology,* vol. 8, ed. A. M. Goldberg, pp. 351–362. New York: Mary Ann Liebert.

20. Keene, D. R., Sakai, L. Y., Burgeson, R. E., and Bachinger, H. P. 1987. Direct visualization of IgM antibodies bound to tissue antigens using a monoclonal anti-type III collagen IgM as a model system. *J. Histochem. Cytochem.* 35:311–318.

21. Sakai, L. Y., Keene, D. R., Morris, N. P., and Burgeson, R. E. 1986. Type VII collagen is a major structural component of anchoring fibrils. *J. Cell Biol.* 103:1577–1586.

22. Burgeson, R. E., Lunstrum, G. P., Rokosova, B., Rimberg, C. S., Rosenbaum, L. M., and Keene, D. S. 1990. The structure and function of type VII collagen. *Ann. NY Acad. Sci.* 580:32–43.

23. Fleischmajer, R., MacDonald, E. D., Perlish, J. S., Burgeson, R. E., and Fisher, L. W. 1990. Dermal collagen fibrils are hybrids of type I and type III collagen molecules. *J. Struct. Biol.* 105:162–169.

24. Fleischmajer, R., Fisher, L. W., MacDonald, D., Jacobs, L., Jr., Perlish, J. S., and Termine, J. D. 1991. Decorin interacts with fibrillar collagen of embryonic and adult human skin. *J. Struct. Biol.* 106:82–90.

25. Termine, J. D., Kleinman, H. K., Whitson, S. W., Cohn, K. M., McGarvey, M. L., and Martin, G. R. 1981. Osteonectin, a bone-specific protein linking mineral to collagen. *Cell* 26:99–105.

26. Bernard, M. P., Chu, M.-L., Myers, J. C., Ramirez, F., Eikenbery, E. F., and Prockop, D. J. 1983. Nucleotide sequences of complementary deoxyribonucleic acids for the Pro 1 chain of human type I procollagen. Statistical evaluation of structures that are conserved during evolution. *Biochemistry* 22:5213–5223.

27. Krusius, T., and Ruoslahti, E. 1986. Primary structure of an extracellular matrix proteoglycan core protein deduced form cloned cDNA. *Proc. Natl. Acad. Sci. USA* 83:7683–7687.

28. Nowack, H. A., Gay, G., Wick, G., Becker, U., and Timpl, R. 1976. Preparation and use in immunohisto-chemistry of antibodies specific for type I and III collagen and procollagen. *J. Immunol. Methods* 12:117–124.

29. Rohde, H., Wick, G., and Timpl, R. 1979. Immunochemical characterization of the basement membrane glycoprotein laminin. *Eur. J. Biochem.* 102:195–201.

30. Dessau, W., Sasse, R., Timpl, R., Jilek, F., and von der Mark, K. 1978. Synthesis and extracellular deposition of fibronectin in chondrocyte cultures. Response to the removal of extracellular cartilage matrix. *J. Cell Biol.* 79:342–355.

31. von der Mark, H., Aumailley, M., Wick, G., Fleischmajer, R., and Timpl, R. 1984. Immunochemistry, genuine size and tissue localization of collagen VI. *Eur. J. Biochem.* 142:493–502.

32. Dziadek, M., Fujiwara, S., Paulsson, M., and Timpl, R. 1985. Immunological characterization of basement membrane types of heparan sulfate proteoglycan. *EMBO J.* 4:905–912.

33. Fox, J. W., Mayer, U., Nischt, R., Aumailley, M., Reinhardt, D., Wiedemann, H., Mann, K., Timpl, R., Krieg, T., Engel, J., and Chu, M.-L. 1991. Recombinant nidogen consists of three globular domains and mediates binding of laminin to collagen type IV. *EMBO J.* 10:3173–3146.

34. Davis, C. M., Papadopoulos, V., Sommers, C. L., Kleinman, H. K., and Dym, M. 1990. Differential expression of extracellular matrix components in rat Sertoli cells. *Biol. Reprod.* 43:860–869.

35. Sakai, L. Y., Keene, D. R., and Engvall, E. 1986. Fibrillin, a new 350-kD glycoprotein, is a component of extracellular microfibrils. *J. Cell Biol.* 103:2499–2509.

36. Weiss, R. A., Eichner, R., and Sun, T.-T. 1984. Monoclonal antibody analysis of keratin expression in epidermal diseases: A 48- and 56-Kdalton keratin as molecular markers for hyperproliferative keratino-cytes. *J. Cell Biol.* 98:1377–1406.

37. O'Guin, W. M., Manabe, M., and Sun, T.-T. 1989. Association of a basic 25K protein with membrane coating granules of human epidermis. *J. Cell Biol.* 109:2313–2321.

38. Dale, B. A., Holbrook, K. A., Kimball, J. R., Hoff, M., and Sun, T.-T. 1985. Expression of epidermal keratins and filaggrin during human fetal skin development. *J. Cell Biol.* 101:1257–1269.

39. Karnovsky, M. J. 1965. A formaldehyde-glutaraldehyde fixative of high osmolality for use in electron microscopy (abstr.). *J. Cell Biol.* 27:137–138a.

40. Hulmes, D. J. S., Jesior, J.-C., Miller, A., Bethet-Colominas, C., and Wolff, C. 1981. Electron microscopy shows periodic structure in collagen fibril cross sections. *Proc. Natl. Acad Sci. USA* 78:3567–3571.

41. Contard, P., Bartel, R. L., Jacobs, L. II, Perlish, J. S., MacDonald, E. D., Handler, L., Cone, D., and Fleischmajer, R. 1993. Culturing keratinocytes and fibroblasts in a 3-dimensional mesh result in epidermal differentiation and formation of a basal lamina-anchoring zone. *J. Invest. Dermatol.* 100:35–39.

42. Contard, P., Jacobs, L., Perlish, J. S., and Fleischmajer, R. 1993. Collagen fibrillogenesis in a 3-dimensional fibroblast cell culture system. *Cell Tissue Res.* 273:571–575.
43. Fleischmajer, R., MacDonald, E. D., Contard, P., and Perlish, J. S. 1993. Immunochemistry of a keratinocyte-fibroblast co-culture model for reconstruction of human skin. *J. Histochem. Cytochem.* 41:1359–1366.
44. Simon-Assmann, P., Bouziges, F., Freund, J. N., Perrin-Schmitt, F., and Kepinger, M. 1990. Type IV collagen mRNA accumulates in the mesenchymal compartment at early stages of murine developing intestine. *J. Cell Biol.* 110:849–857.
45. Senior, P. V., Critchley, D. R., Beck, F., Walker, R. A., and Varley, J. M. 1988. The localization of laminin mRNA and protein in the post implantation embryo and placenta of the mouse: An "in situ" hybridization and immunocytochemical study. *Development (Camb.)* 104:P431–446.
46. Simon-Assmann, P., Bouziges, F., Vigny, M., and Keginger, M. 1989. Origin and deposition of basement membrane heparan sulfate proteoglycan in the developing intestine. *J. Cell Biol.* 109:1837–1848.
47. Stenman, S., and Vaheri, A. 1978. Distribution of a major connective tissue protein, fibronectin in normal human tissues. *J. Exp. Med.* 147:1054–1064.
48. Fleischmajer, R., and Timpl, R. 1984. Ultrastructural localization of fibronectin to different anatomic structures of human skin. *J. Histochem. Cytochem.* 32:315–321.
49. Fleischmajer, R., Jacobs, L. II, Schwartz, E., and Sakai, L. Y. 1991. Extracellular microfibrils (10 nm in diameter) are increased in localized and systemic scleroderma skin. *Lab. Invest.* 64:791–798.
50. Fleischmajer, R., Jacobs, L. II, Perlish, J. S., Katchen, B., Schwartz, E., and Timpl, R. 1992. Immunochemistry of human kidney reticulin. *Am. J. Pathol.* 140:1225–1235.

Chapter Four

CRITIQUE OF CELL CULTURE METHODS IN SKIN PERMEABILITY ASSESSMENT

Gordon L. Flynn

There are many reasons why we might elect to assess the rates at which chemicals pass through the skin. For instance, the delivery of drugs into and through the skin is critical to the performance of dermatological and transdermal dosage forms, and scientists who design topical dosage forms have skin permeation uppermost in their thoughts. In another quarter, environmentalists are concerned with permeation of the skin by industrial chemicals that find their ways into the water we bathe and swim in. In armed forces laboratories a concern exists that incapacitating or lethal chemicals might be sprayed on the skin in warfare. And in yet another sphere, scientists who design cosmetic products must know which chemical attributes keep substances from being drawn into the skin so that the formulations they prepare can be as safe as possible. In vitro assessments of skin permeability are performed to better understand and deal with all these issues. Animals, particularly hairless varieties, are a common source of skin for such investigations, although human skin in the forms of cadaver skin and waste surgical skin is also used. Human skin is difficult to obtain and the supply is invariably conditional. Therefore, it tends to be stockpiled and stored in desiccated or frozen state. Long storage and extreme storage conditions raise questions concerning its representativeness. By all accounts animal tissue is even less paradigmatic, but at least it is available on demand and therefore can be used in a fresh and metabolically vital state. Thus, when raised, stratified epidermal cultures of human skin came into being, they were warmly received as potential membranes of study by researchers.

To be useful in permeability assessment, raised epidermal cultures must possess a stratum corneum comparable to the natural counterpart. At one level, this means that stratified epidermal cultures and the actual epidermis should appear histologically alike—and they do! The two should be equally consonant at the molecular structural level, for the dimensions, compositions, arrangements, and densities of the constituent phases bestow the barrier properties. Here we can expect problems. Cultured cells grow under what must be considered unnatural, stressed conditions. The exquisitely tuned relationships underlying epidermal differentiation and specialization of actual skin, especially those attending keratinocyte proteogenesis and lipogenesis, seem to be beyond our ability to adequately duplicate in vitro. Thus it comes as no surprise that permeation results to date with cultured epidermal membranes have been largely disappointing. This point and the issues underlying it are to be discussed.

INTRODUCTION

There are many questions in the biological sphere that cannot be answered satisfactorily without recourse to animal experiments, here including clinical studies, and our goal as researchers should be to use animals (including humans) in research only after establishing that there is not an alternative for resolving a particular, justifyingly important problem. This guiding principle should apply as much to dermatological research as it does to any other sphere of medical research.

Assessment of skin permeability is one activity under the banner of dermatological research where large numbers of research animals have tended to be consumed. It is the purpose of this chapter to examine whether this use of animals is prudent and necessary in light of the fact that stratified human epidermal membranes can be prepared via culturing.

Before evaluating the question, it is important to acknowledge that membranes prepared by culturing epidermal cells do lend themselves to answering many basic research questions. Cultured cells are an integrated system of cells capable of metabolizing chemical substances in much the same manner as the native epidermis metabolizes the substances. Thus cells in culture can be used to assess the structural fates of chemicals, endogenous or exogenous, that might find their ways into the epidermis. Cultured cells necessarily communicate with one another to organize and effect their differentiation. Likenesses in the differentiated structures of cultured membranes and the actual epidermis indicate that strong parallels in biomolecular messaging have to exist between them. One can thus presume a priori that a great deal might be learned about the events that control cell differentiation using cultures. But are the fully differentiated cultures—specifically meaning the membranes obtained upon culturing—suitable for permeability assessment? One must consider this question with an eye to the purposes of permeability assessment, and we will. And it is important to keep in mind that an already existing presumption of many in the skin permeation field is that certain animal skins, especially those of hairless and sparsely haired species like the hairless mouse, the pig, the monkey and the fuzzy rat, are good barrier surrogates for human skin. It is within the mission of this essay to also critically examine this premise.

Let's for the moment allow that permeation data obtained using cultured skin membranes might offer an accurate depiction of the permeability of human skin under circumstances where accurate, quantitative permeability information is needed. Let's allow that data obtained using animal skins might provide the same advantage. What would we use the information for? For one reason, pharmaceutical researchers often evaluate permeability coefficients and permeation lag times to decide which drug within a family of drugs is the best to develop for topical or transdermal use. Similarly, toxicologists and environmentalists need accurate data to properly quantify the threat a chemical poses when it is brought in contact with the skin. Only after we deal with these uses of membranes can we put the reasonableness of the premise concerning cultures to test and, side by side, examine the identical premise built around the use of membranes prepared from animal skins. We can accept or reject either of these types of membranes as being suitable for a particular type of skin permeability research based upon the purposes of the research and the available evidence regarding how such membranes fulfill these purposes.

PURPOSES OF PERMEABILITY ASSESSMENT

Let's consider in detail some of the reasons why skin permeability is often at issue and why we might wish to generate permeability coefficients and related information. As with all membranes, the relationship between chemical structure and permeability tells much about the barrier function of the membrane. Consider the rather ordinary situation where molecules in aqueous solution pass through a biological membrane and into a second aqueous phase *downstream*. This scene is played out when a substance crosses the thin membrane of an individual cell, whether from cytoplasm to extracellular fluid or the reverse. It applies equally well to the situation where orally ingested foodstuffs and drugs transit the gastrointestinal lining, from mucosal to serosal sides. The collective literature detailing the barrier function of these membranes and other biological membranes teaches us that biological membranes, as a rule, tend to thermodynamically restrain the passage of polar molecules and favor the passage of nonpolar ones. Consequently, where necessary, special transport mechanisms, including some that consume energy, have evolved to offset such exclusion. Scientists have rightly concluded that most biological membranes function to a good first approximation as lipoidal structures. Semipolar and nonpolar organic molecules are believed to partition into and pass through the lipoidal elements of their complex structures. In support of this view, beginning early in this century, relationships have been drawn between the tendencies of molecules to partition between oil and water (i.e., octanol and water) and to be absorbed. As elementary as all of this may seem, such information is fundamental to our understandings of the workings of the membranes of life, including the skin.

Any membrane to be used as a surrogate of human skin for the purpose of structure-permeability analysis would ideally provide quantitatively correct permeability information (permeability coefficients, lag times, fluxes from solutions of known concentration, etc., that are true reflections of the behavior of intact human skin). However, a surrogate membrane would still be of some use if it reliably rank-ordered the permeabilities of disparate substances. Much published information teaches us that membranes prepared from animal skin cannot be relied upon to give quantitatively correct and faithful estimates of the permeability coefficients (or other comparable transport measures) of human skin, but if the animal lacks hair, the membranes do generate data that are in qualitative and at times even semiquantitative accord with human values. Consequently, hairless and nude mice, fuzzy rats, hairless guinea pigs, pigs, and primates have found favor in skin permeability research. The relative merits of the skins of these species as human surrogates are under ongoing debate. Importantly, whether from human or animal, virtually all displays of permeability coefficients against partition coefficients (octanol/water partition coefficients are popular) or the alkyl chain lengths of homologs etc. teach us that the skin, like the cell membrane and gastrointestinal lining, is a hydrophobic barrier to a good first approximation. It is also a barrier for which permeation is highly sensitive to molecular size. These molecular sensitivities are related directly to the physical chemistry of the skin's principal barrier phase, the stratum corneum. A great deal of literature supports the view that lipophilicity and molecular size together dominate the aggregate permeability picture,[1] dependencies that have been ferreted from data on the relative permeabilities of animal skin as well as data developed using human skin. The broad correspondence of the physical behaviors of human and animal skins clearly lends validity to the use of animals (membranes formed from animal skin) in conceptual skin research. Unfortunately, there are no existing data that would allow us to project with even a modest measure of confidence that cultured epidermal membranes might serve similarly.

As a matter of commercial interest, much research on skin permeability is actually concerned with drug delivery through the skin. The actions of topical dosage forms, which are used to treat skin disorders themselves, and transdermal dosage forms, which take advantage of the skin to access the internal body and its organ systems, depend on the ease by which drugs penetrate either into the skin or through the skin. Either way, topical pharmacological intervention in disease relies on the drug in question being diffusively passed through the surface structure of the skin and into the living tissues beyond. Ease of permeation of the skin is clearly at issue here, and high-quality permeability information is needed to select the best compound for either local or transdermal therapy from the available pool of therapeutic substances. Experience teaches us that molecular sorting like this might reasonably be done with a well-chosen animal membrane. Again, unfortunately, there are no data to suggest that cultured membranes can serve well—can serve at all—in this capacity.

After screening, as just outlined, has identified the choice drug for further development, rigorous work must be undertaken to quantitatively assess the ability of the chosen compound to permeate skin. The goal is to determine the actual feasibility of delivering the drug for its intended purpose. It is no longer enough to just know that the compound is the best penetrant of those considered. Rather, one must come to terms with the adequacy of permeation of the candidate. One also wishes to discover which chemical components might be used to put together a good vehicle for applying the drug. Even further down the development line, issues of bioavailability—delivery of the drug to its site of action—and possibly even bioequivalency— equivalency of delivery relative to an approved and marketed form of the drug—have to be addressed. High-quality information is essential to making prudent business decisions here, irrespective of whether a topical (local effect) or a transdermal delivery (systemic effect) system is in the offing.

What more needs to be said here with respect to drug development is most easily done in the context of development of a transdermal delivery system. All transdermal drugs to date have been old drugs and have had a previous history of use by other routes of administration; their dosages, systemic toxicities, body clearances, etc. have generally been known. Armed with the drug's dosage (scaled to 24 h of therapy and adjusted for lack of oral first-pass loss), its aqueous solubility, and its transcutaneous permeability coefficient measured from an aqueous medium, it is possible to crudely gauge the size (area) of a patch that would be needed to deliver the daily dose (therapeutic requirement) from[2]:

$$A \approx \delta/24PS$$

where A is the patch size (area) estimate, δ is the appropriately adjusted daily dosage (mg), 24 is the hours in a day, P is the permeability coefficient (cm/h), and S is the aqueous solubility (mg/ml). Where weak electrolytes are involved, the pH values of the media used in the solubility and permeability determinations must be the same. If the estimated size is reasonable relative to common transdermal practice or if the pharmacological imperative of providing the drug transdermally is strong enough to allow consideration of a patch of extraordinary size, or both, serious work is begun on the actual system of delivery for the drug. This is an expensive undertaking, as costly resources, manpower, and time are committed when setting a development plan into motion, and the importance of making an early, sound permeability–bioavailability decision prior to actually starting serious transdermal system development cannot be overstressed. A lack of timely attention to this critical aspect of system performance can and usually does lead to the squandering of precious resources. Since membranes prepared from animal skins invariably result in higher than real skin permeability coefficients and/or percutaneous skin fluxes, one is at risk in using them to make such refined judgments. Frankly, the only membrane that can be relied on to give an accurate representation of the permeability of human skin is a membrane formed from human skin itself. This explains why cadaver skin or surgical waste skin is brought into the research at this point to address the feasibility issue. We know from extensive past experience that animal membranes generally perform poorly for the purpose. Importantly and unfortunately, no data exist that support the use of cultured epidermal membranes in such critical decision making.

Another use of permeability information is to foresee the dangers that might be attributable to absorption of toxicants through the skin that might be topically encountered in the environment or, alternatively, that might be inadvertently brought into contact with the skin in the course of their use in research or industrial activities. For this purpose, underestimating the skin's permeability, and therefore potential risks, is generally considered more perilous than overestimating it. Therefore, scientists use conservative premises to judge risks. Consequently, permeability coefficients obtained with animal skins that tend to somewhat exaggerate risks can be put to good use here. This is not to say, however, that reckless overestimation of absorption risk is without its grievous consequences, for if risk is absurdly overblown, the limited resources we have to manage risk, meaning to educate about the problems of risk as well as remedy them, will invariably be inappropriately allocated, misspent, and frittered away. Thus it is again that surrogate membranes used in the estimation of human skin permeability should exhibit a high degree of correspondence in their barrier behavior to human skin. Some animal skins, such as rhesus monkey, pig, and perhaps hairless rodents, exhibit a satisfying degree of correspondence; cultured human cell membranes are, at their best, an unproven human skin surrogate. Those data we do have from cultured membranes are discouraging in their consonance.

It almost goes without saying that the risks associated with chemicals that are to serve as instruments for waging war must be accurately portrayed in laboratory data. Underestimation of risks here can clearly cost lives. Overestimation, on the other hand, can be costly if it results in implementation of gratuitous protections. Thus is seems it would be imprudent to use either animal or cultured membranes to gauge risks in this special sphere.

DESCRIPTION OF THE IN VITRO METHOD OF PERMEABILITY ASSESSMENT[3]

In all of the preceding examples, permeability assessment is presumed to be done on the lab bench with the aid of diffusion cells. There are myriad diffusion cells for the purpose. No one cell of itself is better than another in any fundamental sense, although some cells are clearly superior to others with respect to the study of specific issues. Some may be more convenient to use than others in certain circumstances. In these latter regards, diffusion cells in which a membrane is placed between two well-stirred compartments tend to work best for determining permeability coefficients. These compartments can have discrete volumes from which small, individual samples are periodically taken, or they can be flow-through compartments from which periodic collections are made and assayed. It usually works best from the standpoint of ease of estimation to set up the diffusion experiments to obtain a steady state in flux. Often, however, the actual conditions used for experiments fall somewhat short of this mark, and many if not most researchers gather data obtained in a quasi-steady state. Be this as it may, when skin permeability coefficients are at issue, in the absence of solubility problems, aqueous media are used in both chambers of the diffusion cell simply because water is the least skin-destructive of all possible solvents. Even when low solubility presents a problem, generally other solvents are blended into water only to the extent necessary to resolve the problem while maintaining the media of the diffusion experiment in as aqueous a condition as possible. In some instances, a compound may be applied to the skin as a saturated solution in water or another solvent. This is done, for instance, when determining the flux of a compound for transdermal purposes. The limiting flux of a saturated solution now sets the reference mark, and subsequently, any flux-accelerating influences of organic solvents (or enhancers) known not to be irritating or toxic are welcome. When the permeant is a liquid, its permeation rate as the neat liquid is relevant to risk, as this represents a facsimile of a splashing incident.

Irrespective of the purpose of a study, skin membranes of study are prepared from tissues or cell cultures and positioned in the diffusion cells. Usually, pressure generated by a clamp of some kind is applied to the cell to press its halves tightly together around the membrane periphery, which prevents leakage. The cells may be jacketed and maintained at an even temperature by connecting their outer chambers to a circulating water bath, or they may be placed in a manifold or even immersed in a bath to achieve temperature control. The temperature is generally set somewhere between 32 and 37°C, with 32°C being the ostensible surface temperature of actual skin. A medium containing the test substance is layered over the stratum corneum (horizontal, "Franz-type" cell) or placed in or passed through the chamber of the diffusion cell facing the stratum corneum. Generally the medium is a solution or a slurry, with the latter being used to achieve both the limiting concentration of the permeant in the test medium and, through dissolution replenishment, to keep the concentration of the test substance uniform over the course of an experiment. Blank medium is placed in or, alternatively, continuously passed through the downstream chamber (flow-through design). These chambers are respectively referred to as the donor and receptor chambers of the diffusion cell. Net diffusion takes place from the donor phase to the receptor phase. Ordinarily samples are taken periodically from the receptor compartment (zero-order kinetics), but, under some relatively unique circumstances, periodic sampling of the donor compartment may be done to get data reducible to a permeability coefficient (first-order kinetics). In the case of the skin, depending on the permeant, an experiment may last for as little as 6–8 h or for as long as several days. Sampling is done at programmed times over the experimental course, and in the instance of receptor sampling the cumulative amount penetrated is plotted against time. The slope of the best line that can be passed through the data out beyond where the curve is straightening is used to calculate the permeability coefficient. The equation is:

$$P = (\partial M/\partial t)/A\Delta C$$

where P is the permeability coefficient, $\partial M/\partial t$ is the measured steady- or quasi-steady-state flux, A is the effective area of the diffusion cell, and ΔC is the concentration differential expressed across the skin membrane. The latter more often than not is well approximated by the concentration of the permeant in the donor compartment, as the downstream compartment's concentration is usually kept very low. Rarely if ever is sufficient time actually allowed for attainment of a true steady state in flux, about three lag times, when a section of skin is used as a membrane. To do so would push the time for collecting data out into the period where the skin begins to deteriorate because of its continuous immersion in the donor medium.

The critical reader might be wondering how this description of the diffusion experiment relates to the question of suitability of membranes prepared from animal skin and cultured epidermal membranes for the purposes that have been described. One point is that such membranes must withstand the physical handling associated with putting the diffusion cells together. Experience with animal membranes in this regard is good. There are surely less than adequate data on cultured membranes to make a similar judgement about them. The membranes, moreover, must stand up to long periods of exposure to the moving fluids of the diffusion cell. They must resist alteration by hydration as the result of their immersion. We have a great deal of experience with membranes cut from animal skins, and most hold up quite well with respect to having them in the diffusion apparatus. On the other hand, some become waterlogged in relatively short order and, as a consequence, change in their barrier property. We have found, for instance, that hairless mouse skin membranes often evidence dramatic increases in permeability as a result of hydration, often in less than a full day. These changes are inevitably abrupt rather than gradual, suggesting that hydration induces sudden changes in critical membrane phases. For such reasons we don't consider such membranes to be barrier competent if they have been immersed for a long time. Due to a paucity of data, no conclusions can be made concerning the robustness of cultured membranes.

A THEORETICAL VIEW—HOW THE POROSITY OF MEMBRANES AFFECTS THEIR UTILITY

To be useful in diffusion cell work, skin membranes must be free of holes. As will be seen momentarily, any appreciable porosity at all renders them useless. This is not normally a problem with epidermal membranes prepared from cadaver skin, human surgical waste skin, or animal skins. Nevertheless and often, the permeability of [³H]water or another test substance is assessed prior to or along with the main permeant as a check on the integrity of the membrane. Specific membranes are discarded, along with the data obtained using them, when the permeation rate of the control substance comes in above a defined, acceptable limit. Holes (porosity) are a major concern with cultured membranes. Here cultured cells are seeded onto an appropriate substrate (nylon mesh, collagen, etc.) and grown to confluency. Confluency is checked by eye or with a microscope. Even when magnification is used, confluency is not guaranteed, for it is impossible to tell by eye, even under magnification, if the cells have truly tight junctions. In work we have done using a flow-through technique, it was noted that even a slight pressure head led to bulk flow of aqueous solvent through our cultured membranes, a sure sign they were porous, despite the fact that they appeared molecularly continuous when viewed under a microscope.[4]

The impact of even slight porosity can be devastating, a point easily made by theoretical argument. Consider the simple situation where a membrane consisting of two layers, one hydrophobic (the stratum corneum) and one made up of viable tissue (the living epidermis), has its hydrophobic element interrupted here and there with tiny pores. One thus has two parallel, independent pathways existing through the key stratum of the tissue. The resistance of a layer is equal to the reciprocal of the permeability coefficient of the layer; resistances in series are additive. Therefore the total resistance of this laminate would be[5]:

$$R_T = \frac{1}{P_T} = \left(\sum_{i=1}^{n} \frac{1}{P_i} \right)$$

and it follows directly that:

$$\frac{1}{P_T} = \left(\frac{1}{P_{sc}} + \frac{1}{P_{vt}} \right)$$

where the subscripts sc and vt, respectively, designate the stratum corneum and the underlying viable epidermis. The stratum corneum as depicted has two routes through it. For simplicity, we assume they function independently. Consequently, the total amount of substance permeating this stratum of the barrier is simply the sum of what permeates each of its independent routes. Introducing the notion that each individual permeability coefficient is a product of the diffusity through a route, the relative capacity of the route, and the inverse of thickness of the route (i.e., $P_i = D_i K_i / h_i$) and the thought that, when there is more than one route, each route must be couched in terms of the fraction of the total area it provides for diffusion, leads one to the following descriptive equation:

$$\frac{1}{P_T} = \frac{1}{\left[\dfrac{(1 - f_p)D_m K_m}{h_m} + \dfrac{f_p D_p}{h_p} \right]} + \frac{1}{(D_{vt}/h_{vt})}$$

where the subscript m signifies an attribute of the lipoidal phase of the stratum corneum while p signifies a property of its pores. The symbol f designates a fractional area, D is diffusivity, K is a partition coefficient, and h is thickness. No partition coefficients appear explicitly for the pore route or for the viable tissue, as these are, to a good first approximation, aqueous in character and therefore, when the external media are aqueous, K values for them would be on the order of 1.0. We can now consider what happens to the overall resistance (or its reciprocal, the permeability coefficient) when reasonable values for the parameters are substituted into this equation. Based on the literature it is reasonable to set D_{vt} and D_p at about 3.6×10^{-3} cm^2/h (1×10^{-6} cm^2/s). The thickness of the viable tissue layer between the stratum corneum and the outermost capillary plexus of the vascular system is about 200 μm, so $h_{vt} = 200$ μm. Since the stratum corneum is only 10 μm thick, h_p can be assumed to be about 10 μm. A permeability coefficient for the lipoidal fraction of the membrane that is representative of the values found experimentally can be used in lieu of assigning values to the individual parameters associated with this phase. $D_m K_m / h_m$ can thus be set at 1×10^{-4} cm/h, a value typifying what one might find for a semipolar solute having molecular weight above 200.

The values appearing in Table 1 were generated using the specified parameterization. The first column in the table is the key column in the analysis, for it indicates the fractional porosity of the stratum corneum. It can be seen from the information in the first row of the table that a skin membrane with no stratum corneum porosity takes the permeability coefficient of the stratum corneum (compare the second and fourth columns). A fractional stratum corneum area porosity of as little as 1/1,000,000 leads to about a 3.6% distortion of the permeability coefficient value one would otherwise find. Obviously, we could live with this. Increasing the porosity to 1/100,000 of the total area produces an error of 36% in the estimated permeability coefficient, everything else being equal. Even this could be hidden in the variability associated with determinations of permeability coefficients. However, a further order of magnitude increase in the porosity leads to a error in the permeability coefficient of over 500%, which would be intolerable. One part in 1000 pore area produces a 36-fold error, and 1% pore area raises the permeability coefficient about 300 times above what it would be in the absence of pores. With 10% porosity the permeability of the skin approaches that of the permeability of the viable epidermis (0.12 cm/h v. 0.18 cm/h). The table clearly illustrates that there is little tolerance for pores. From the standpoint of using cultured membranes as surrogates for human skin membranes, this issue dominates our concern and is over and above considerations of similarities in histological appearance of the respective tissues.

Toward the end of 1994, G. Flynn, J. Citteur, S. Wiley, and J. Krueger[4] attempted to use cultured membranes to ascertain if ^{125}I-labeled-epidermal growth factor (EGF) passed through the cell mass by a receptor-mediated transcytosis (unpublished data). The cell cultures were grown using time-tested methods on Millipore membranes. Microscopic examination showed the raised cultures to be confluent, highly differentiated, and stratified. In the initial studies with the membranes, a very low level of the iodinated EGF was applied to their stratum corneum surface (using the culture membrane housing as an actual part of the diffusion cell in order that the membranes might be studied in a physically undisturbed state), and an excitingly high permeability was noted. In a second set of studies, a swamping amount of "cold" EGF was added to the medium of application to competitively inhibit transcytosis (as measured in terms

Table 1. Illustration of the Influence of Porosity Through the Stratum Corneum, the Skin Barrier's Principal Barrier Element, on the Skin's Barrier Function

f_p	P_{sc} (cm/h)	P_{vt} (cm/h)	P_T (cm/h)	$\dfrac{P_T}{P_T^{f_p=0}}$
0	1.0×10^{-4}	0.18	1.0×10^{-4}	1.000
1×10^{-6}	1.0×10^{-4}	0.18	1.0×10^{-4}	1.036
1×10^{-5}	1.4×10^{-4}	0.18	1.4×10^{-4}	1.36
1×10^{-4}	4.6×10^{-4}	0.18	5.6×10^{-4}	5.60
1×10^{-3}	3.7×10^{-3}	0.18	3.6×10^{-3}	36.3
1×10^{-2}	3.6×10^{-2}	0.18	3.0×10^{-2}	301
1×10^{-1}	3.6×10^{-1}	0.18	1.2×10^{-1}	1200

of the radioactive label). The radioactive EGF still came pouring through! In the course of these experiments we noticed that there was bulk flow of watery media through the membranes. This could not have occurred through a molecularly continuous, cellularly tight stratum corneum. Disappointingly, the permeability was orders of magnitude higher than was physically achievable with skin sections. We concluded the cultured membranes we were using were porous.

Given the outcomes of the work done at Utah with ^{125}I-labeled-epidermal growth factor,[4] it is not surprising that other investigators have found cultured membranes to be exceedingly permeable. Consider the experiences of Roy et al.[6] These investigators used commercially available Living Skin Equivalent (LSE, Organogenesis, Cambridge, MA) membranes, and compared the results they obtained with these membranes directly against results they obtained using cadaver skin membranes. More specifically, they measured fluxes and calculated permeability coefficients for three alkyl-p-aminobenzoates, namely, the methyl, ethyl, and butyl esters of p-aminobenzoic acid. Selected results of their efforts are presented in Table 2. The symbol J_{ss} in the table represents flux from saturated solutions; P is the calculated permeability coefficient. It is notable that the permeability coefficients obtained for the three compounds with the LSE membranes are not actually different, despite markedly increased lipophilicity, methyl ester to butyl ester. By way of contrast, the skin permeability coefficients for the methyl and ethyl esters are over threefold smaller than for the considerably more lipophilic butyl ester. Qualitatively, this is the expected outcome for a membrane that acts to a good first approximation as a lipoidal barrier. Both the fluxes and permeability coefficients of the methyl and ethyl esters through LSE membranes are about 10 times those found with cadaver skin. This factor drops to about 2 in the case of the butyl ester, an expected narrowing. This is so because the more lipophilic a compound is, the less is the resistance of the stratum corneum to it. Eventually, at a high enough lipophilicity, the stratum corneum's resistance becomes subordinate to the resistances of its underlying tissues. The bottom line here is that the Roy et al. data also suggest that cultured membranes, here membranes prepared by the most experienced people in the business at the time, were substantially porous. They lacked permeselectivity. The Roy et al. principal conclusion was: "The LSE membrane may not quantitatively represent a good human skin model for evaluating skin permeation of a drug from topical or transdermal formulations."

Other investigators have reached similar conclusions. M. Ponec et al.[7] measured the permeation of nitroglycerine and sucrose across raised human keratinocytes cultured using de-epidermized dermis (DED) as the culturing substrate. The permeation rate of glucose was 100 times lower and nitroglycerine 2 times lower than DED membranes alone. At the same time, the penetration rates of the reconstructed epidermis were 3–10 times higher for each compound than for freshly excised human skin. Later, M. Fartasch and M. Ponec[8] stated, "In spite of histological similarities, the barrier function [of cultured cells] seems to be impaired." C. J. Nolte et al.[9] found that transepidermal water loss through cultured cell membranes was >4 mg/cm^2/h throughout the culture period, about 10 times the normal rate. S. R. Slivka et al.[10] determined the permeabilities of a number of compounds through cultured cell membranes using Franz-type diffusion cells and so-called side-by-side diffusion cells. They found the permeability coefficient for water to be of the same order of magnitude as that determined for neonatal foreskin, a membrane for which an exceedingly high permeability had already been established. M. Regnier et al.[11] also found an abnormally high permeability coefficient for water using "reconstituted epidermis," as did M. B. Cumpstone et al.[12] with the latter group demonstrating that water's permeability varied widely over the area of the cultured membrane. A. M. Ernesti et al.[13] also measured diffusion

Table 2. Direct Comparison of Permeability Coefficients Obtained for Three Homologous Alkyl-p-aminobenzoates on Cultured Skin Membranes and Cadaver Skin Membranes

	Methyl ester		Ethyl ester		Butyl ester	
	LSE membrane	Cadaver skin membrane	LSE membrane	Cadaver skin membrane	LSE membrane	Cadaver skin membrane
J_{ss} (μg/cm^2/h)	345	32.9	161.5	18.0	24.1	10.7
P (cm/h)	24.0	2.3	17.8	2.0	20.1	8.9

rates through Organogenesis LSE membranes, finding values for the compounds of study consistently four- to sixfold higher than reported for human abdominal skin. They determined P values for two steroids, estradiol and hydrocortisone, in their studies, finding these to have permeability coefficients 63 times and 187 times, respectively, higher than published values. They concluded that, compared to human skin, LSE membranes have only partial barrier function. Finally, K. Ohkura et al.[14] claimed the order of permeation of nitrophenols across newborn abdominal epidermis to be the opposite of that for their permeation across a cultured cell layer. Any one of these studies could, of course, be misleading of itself. Taken together, however, they teach us that cultured membranes, at least as they existed a few years back, are unrepresentingly permeable. Taken together, they also teach us that the level of agreement between actual skin permeability coefficients (or other measures of permeability) and permeability coefficients obtained using cultured epidermal membranes depends on the compound chosen for study. One can expect the disagreement between values to be striking for large compounds, polar compounds, and ionized compounds.

A TELEOLOGICAL VIEW AND QUESTION CONCERNING THE USE OF RAISED CULTURED MEMBRANES

Are we in an early phase of a technology here that can be significantly improved in time? Can raised cultured membranes ever work? Should raised cultured membranes ever work? One can mount a strong teleological argument that they won't and that, fundamentally, they can't work well for the outlined purposes. This argument begins with a look at the experiences our lab has had with rates of turnover of epidermal tissue that has suffered mild injury and the influences of such injuries on the barrier integrity of the stratum corneum.

In general, mammalian skin that experiences a mild but nevertheless stressful stimulus (chemical, thermal, mechanical, ultraviolet) warms and displays a visible reddening. Both are the result of increased blood perfusion through the peripheral vasculature. Such erythema is invariably followed by a hyperproliferation of keratinocytes within the affected area as part of the natural repair process. There is a stepped up rate of formation of new epidermis to replace that which has been damaged.

We have found that, on hairless mice, the hastily formed stratum corneum resulting from the mildest of injuries (chemical, thermal, and ultraviolet), meaning the stratum corneum that appears several days post injury, tends to be barrier defective, with the level of its impairment being tied to the intensity of the damage.[15] We found that transepidermal water loss rates through such damaged skin ranged from severalfold higher for a barely perceptible injury to as much as 20 times higher for relatively severe second-degree trauma with the degree of increase also depending on the elapsed time between the measurement and the injury. We also measured epidermal turnover times via a technique involving [^{14}C]glycine labeling[16] and, on stained skin cross sections, saw readily visible microscopic changes in the thickness of epidermal layer. With barely perceptible ultraviolet (UV) damage, the healing process, from the moment of injury to the point of full return of normal skin function, took about a week, with the maximum in water flux and other evidence of damage being seen several days into the injury. Specifically, at this midpoint the epidermis was measurably thicker than the normal epidermis, but not quite twice as thick. The rate of epidermal turnover measured by radiotagging at d 2 into the injury was not quite half ($\approx$2.5 d) of what is normal ($\approx$4.2 d). However, with more extended UV applications still well short of those capable of producing visible necrosis, wound repair as measured in barrier compromise and accelerated turnover extended through a second week and well beyond. In these higher than threshold injuries the epidermal thicknesses more than doubled and the turnover rates were more than halved, tissue expressions that were maintained for the aggregate of the time it took the skin to return to normal. In the mildest UV injury we were unable to demonstrate a trauma-induced increase in hydrocortisone's permeability of sections of skin excised so as to contain the wounded tissues. This remained true irrespective of when the treated sections were excised during the healing process. However, doubling the threshold injury resulted in permeability coefficients that were about 10 times those found for control skin sections 4 d into the injury. Trebling the threshold injury led to hydrocortisone permeability coefficients over 100 times higher than normal 4 d into the injury! Yet these wounds were all mild, effectively ranging from minimally perceptible sunburns to what might be painful sunburns. At the worst, the damage done amounted to deep partial thickness injury. Without exception, the injured surfaces healed without a break in the skin and without any lasting visual or other skin defects.

Our overall view of the healing of the mild thermal, chemical, and ultraviolet injuries that we applied to mice was that the hastily formed stratum corneum appearing on the heels of these injuries functioned as one might expect any hastily thrown together fabric to function—badly! This was the general result even though the stratum corneum at the injured surface was formed under conditions as natural as could possibly be engineered, the conditions established by the animal's own physiology. Nevertheless, the tissue was wanting and more permeable than stratum corneum formed at the normal rate in untreated areas. We read into this that stratum corneum formed under stressful circumstances, even the mildest of stresses, will invariably be functionally lacking. We strongly suggest that culturing creates a highly unnatural environment for cell growth and is therefore quite stressful! Having taken this point of view, we find it interesting that M. Ponec et al.[7] claimed that, based on barrier function and the distribution of differentiation markers, their reconstituted epidermis showed a high similarity to hyperproliferating epidermis.

CONCLUSION

Not a single line of evidence supports the idea that cultured epidermal membranes, at their best, share the permeability properties of normal human skin. At times they have seemed to lack permselectivity. At other times they have proven better than membranes lacking stratum corneum, but still have nowhere near the barrier function of normal skin. I suggest that this may never change no matter what amount of research effort goes into improving the preparations of such membranes. I would like my view here to be proven wrong, because such membranes would be enormously useful if they could ever be made to be true surrogates for human skin. For the time being, however, it appears that the prudent researcher will turn to cadaver skin or to waste surgical skin to prepare membranes for drug development studies and most risk evaluation studies. It should be noted that human membranes as described obviate the need for the sacrifice of animals. Thus the issue here concerning cultured membranes is not fundamentally or at least necessarily a matter of animal welfare.

REFERENCES

1. Flynn, G. L. 1989. Mechanism of percutaneous absorption from physicochemical evidence. In *Percutaneous absorption: Mechanisms—Methodology—Drug delivery,* 2nd ed., eds. R. Bronaugh and H. I. Maibach, pp. 27–51. New York: Marcel Dekker.
2. Flynn, G. L., and Stewart, B. 1988. Percutaneous drug penetration: Choosing candidates for transdermal development. *Drug Dev. Res.* 13:169–185.
3. Poulsen, B. J., and Flynn, G. L. 1985. In vitro methods to study dermal delivery and percutaneous absorption. In *Percutaneous absorption: Mechanisms—Methodology—Drug delivery,* eds. R. Bronaugh and H. I. Maibach, pp. 431–460. New York: Marcel Dekker.
4. Flynn, G., Citteur, J., Wiley, S., and Krueger, J., unpublished data, 1994.
5. Flynn, G. L., Yalkowsky, S. H., and Roseman, T. J. 1974. Mass transport phenomena and models: Theoretical aspects. *J. Pharm. Sci.* 63:479.
6. Roy, S. D., Fujiki, J., and Fleitman, J. S. 1993. Permeabilities of alkyl *p*-aminobenzoates through Living Skin Equivalent and cadaver skin. *J. Pharm. Sci.* 82:1266.
7. Ponec, M., Wauben-Penris, P. J., Burger, A., Kempenaar, J., and Boddé, H. 1990. Nitroglycerine and sucrose permeability as quality markers for reconstructed human epidermis. *Skin Pharmacol.* 3:126.
8. Fartasch, M., and Ponec, M. 1994. Improved barrier structure formation in air-exposed human keratinocyte culture systems. *J. Invest. Dermatol.* 102:366. 1994.
9. Nolte, C. J., Oleson, M. A., Bilbo, P. R., and Parenteau, N. L. 1993. Development of a stratum corneum and barrier function in an organotypic skin culture. *Arch. Dermatol. Res.* 285:466.
10. Slivka, S. R., Landeed, L. K., Zeigler, F., Zimber, M. P., and Bartel, R. L. 1993. Characterization, barrier function, and drug metabolism of an in vitro skin model. *J. Invest. Dermatol.* 100:40.
11. Regnier, M., Caron, D., Reichert, U., and Schaefer, H. 1992. Reconstructed human epidermis: A model to study in vitro the barrier function of the skin. *Skin Pharmacol.* 5:49.
12. Cumpstone, M. B., Kennedy, A. H., Harmon, C. S., and Potts, R. O. 1989. The water permeability of primary mouse keratinocyte cultures grown at the air-liquid interface. *J. Invest. Dermatol.* 92:598.

13. Ernesti, A. M., Swiderek, M., and Gay, R. 1992. Absorption and metabolism of topically applied testosterone in an organotypic skin culture. *Skin Pharmacol.* 5:146.
14. Ohkura, K., Iwamoto, K., and Terada, H. 1990. Transcellular permeation of nitrophenols through newborn rat skin epidermal cells in monolayer culture, *Chem. Pharm. Bull.* 38:2788.
15. Han, S. T., Haberkamp, M., and Flynn, G. L., unpublished data, 1989.
16. Haberkamp, M., Flynn, G. L., Han, S. T. R., and Turner, N. 1991. Influence of age on turnover times of normal, ultraviolet-irradiated and tape-burned hairless mouse skin. *J. Toxicol. Cutan. Ocul. Toxicol.* 10:15.

Chapter Five

THE LOCAL LYMPH NODE ASSAY AND OTHER APPROACHES TO THE EVALUATION OF SKIN SENSITIZING POTENTIAL

Ian Kimber

Allergic contact dermatitis is a form of delayed-type hypersensitivity reaction. The induction phase of skin sensitization is characterized by the activation of lymph nodes draining the site of primary exposure to the chemical allergen and the initiation of specific T-lymphocyte responses. The stimulation by chemical allergens of lymphocyte proliferative responses in draining lymph nodes forms the basis of the murine local lymph node assay, an alternative method for the prospective identification of sensitizing chemicals. This method has been the subject of comparisons with guinea pig predictive tests and of extensive interlaboratory validation exercises. Experience to date indicates that the local lymph node assay provides a viable method for assessing skin sensitizing activity and, compared with other test methods, offers a number of important benefits.

INTRODUCTION

Various guinea pig methods for the prospective identification of skin sensitizing chemicals are available.[1] Recently there has been a growing interest in the mouse as a model for investigation of contact sensitization, and several novel predictive test methods have been described using this species.[2] Among these are tests in which skin sensitizing activity is measured as a function of challenge-induced increases in ear thickness in previously sensitized animals: the mouse ear swelling test (MEST) and related methods.[3–6] An alternative approach in mice is the local lymph node assay.[7–9]

THE LOCAL LYMPH NODE ASSAY

The local lymph node assay is based upon an understanding that the induction of contact sensitization is dependent upon the initiation of T-lymphocyte responses to the causative allergen.[7] Such responses are generated first in lymph nodes draining the site of exposure and are characterized by replicative DNA synthesis. There is good evidence that if T lymphocytes are absent or functionally impaired then contact sensitization fails to develop. Also the vigor of proliferative responses induced by chemical allergens in the draining lymph nodes correlates closely with the effectiveness of sensitization.[10,11] The local lymph node assay seeks to identify skin sensitizing chemicals on the basis of proliferative responses provoked in draining lymph nodes following repeated topical exposure of mice to the test material.[8] In the original description of the assay proliferative responses were measured in vitro following culture of draining lymph node cells (LNC) in the presence or absence of the T lymphocyte growth factor interleukin 2.[12,13] Although in vitro analysis of chemical allergen-induced lymph node activation is still employed by some investigators and for some purposes,[14–17] the current procedure of choice requires the assessment of lymph node hyperplastic responses in situ following intravenous injection of tritiated thymidine (^{3}H-TdR).[8,9,18] This version of the local lymph node assay, which obviates the requirement for tissue culture, has been the subject of national interlaboratory validation exercises[8,19–21] and of extensive comparisons with guinea pig test data and the results of human sensitization studies.[19–26]

Experience to date confirms that the local lymph node assay provides a reliable method for the identification of the majority of skin allergens and, in addition, offers a number of important advantages compared with guinea pig predictive tests. The assay is relatively rapid and cost-effective, is unaffected by the color of the test material, and is largely uninfluenced by irritant properties. Unlike the more sensitive guinea pig tests, the local lymph node assay does not require the use of adjuvant. Activity in guinea pig methods is assessed normally by visual evaluation of challenge-induced erythema and/or edema in previously sensitized animals. In contrast to such subjective assessment, the local lymph node assay provides an objective endpoint. Finally, fewer animals are required and, as there is no requirement to elicit contact hypersensitivity reactions, the animals tested are subject to less trauma.

Initiatives currently in progress include the further evaluation of the assay within the context of a five-laboratory international trial and assessment of whether the method is sufficiently robust to accommodate minor procedural modifications without material changes in test performance. Presently the local lymph node assay is used primarily for hazard identification, for which purpose chemicals able to elicit a threefold or greater increase in lymph node proliferation compared with vehicle controls are considered to possess skin sensitizing activity. It may prove possible to use the local lymph node assay also as a means of investigating the relative sensitizing potential of chemicals.[8,9] The proposal is that by measuring, or calculating, the minimum exposure concentration necessary to provoke a defined level of activity in the draining lymph nodes (at this time a stimulation index of 3), it will be possible to compare directly the potential of test materials to cause contact sensitization. Such an approach has already been used with some success in establishing the relative skin sensitizing activity of biocides.[27]

With a growing appreciation of the cellular and molecular mechanisms that result in the effective induction of contact sensitization there may be readouts, other than cellular proliferation, suitable for use in the local lymph node assay and that reflect allergen-induced activation of draining lymph nodes. There is little doubt that cytokines play a pivotal role in immune responses and influence markedly a number of important immunobiological processes. It is now known that topical exposure of mice to skin sensitizing chemicals causes the production, or increased production, of a number of cytokines by draining LNC. Included among these are interleukins 1, 2, 3, 4, and 6 (IL-1, IL-2, IL-3, IL-4, and IL-6).[16,28–33] The value of IL-6 and other cytokines as molecular correlates of immune activation in the local lymph node assay is being considered currently.[16,17,34] In addition to the possible use of inducible cytokine production as an alternative endpoint, several other procedural changes to the assay have been investigated and new applications proposed.[15,35–39] Potentially one of the most important applications is the use of the local lymph node assay for investigation of the chemical basis for skin sensitization and in the derivation of structure–activity relationships.[40]

In summary, the local lymph node assay provides a valuable alternative approach to the identification and characterization of skin sensitizing chemicals.

The induction of draining lymph node activation and the subsequent development of contact sensitization are dependent upon responses provoked by chemical allergens in the skin. It is from an understanding that the skin serves to transduce the signal provided by chemical sensitizers into immunobiological responses that the most realistic opportunities for the development of purely in vitro methods for predictive testing are likely to arise.

EPIDERMAL RESPONSES

The skin is an immunologically active tissue. Many skin cells are able to elaborate cytokines and resident within the epidermis are Langerhans cells (LC).[41–44] It is believed that under normal circumstances LC play a central role in the induction of cutaneous immune responses to chemical allergens. Following skin sensitization, antigen-bearing LC migrate from the epidermis via afferent lymphatics and accumulate in the lymph nodes draining the site of exposure.[45–47] The cells that arrive in draining nodes are functionally mature, have assumed the characteristics of immunocompetent dendritic cells (DC), and are able effectively to present antigen to responsive T lymphocytes and initiate the immune responses necessary for skin sensitization.[41] By analogy with *in vitro* studies it is likely that the acquisition of immunostimulatory properties by LC while in transit to lymph nodes is effected by epidermal cytokines and, in particular, granulocyte/ macrophage colony-stimulating factor (GM-CSF).[48] Recent evidence indicates that the signal for LC to leave the epidermis and begin their journey toward local lymph nodes is provided by another epidermal cytokine, tumor necrosis factor α (TNF-α).[49,50] If the migration and maturation of LC is regulated by skin cytokines, and if these processes are of central importance in the effective induction of cutaneous immune responses to chemical allergens, then one might predict that only those materials that are able to stimulate or upregulate the production by epidermal cells of cytokines such as TNF-α and GM-CSF will elicit contact sensitization. While this may be the case, it does not necessarily follow that the induction of cytokines known to influence LC behavior serves as a selective marker for chemical allergens. Indeed, cutaneous trauma other than that resulting from topical exposure to sensitizing chemicals will result in the increased production of some epidermal cytokines. It is known, for instance, that the nonsensitizing skin irritant sodium lauryl sulfate and irradiation with ultraviolet B (UVB) light each causes the increased production by keratinocytes of TNF-α.[51,52] While some epidermal products such as TNF-α do not represent selective inducible markers for skin allergens, it may nevertheless be the case that chemicals that fail to result in the increased local availability of cytokines necessary for LC migration and functional maturation will be unable to induce contact sensitization.

In addition to those already discussed, epidermal cells, both keratinocytes and LC themselves, produce constitutively, or can be stimulated to produce, a wide variety of cytokines. Those identified to date include interleukins 1 (α and β), 3, 6, 7, 8, and 10, various colony-stimulating factors [GM-CSF, granulocyte colony-stimulating factor (G-CSF), and macrophage colony-stimulating factor (M-CSF)], transforming growth factors α and β (TGF-α and TGF-β), TNF-α, and macrophage inflammatory proteins 1α and 2 (MIP-1α and MIP-2).[52–55] It has been reported recently that certain of these proteins may be regulated selectively by skin sensitizing chemicals. Enk and Katz,[52] using a reverse transcriptase-polymerase chain reaction technique, found that although both contact allergens and skin irritants induced the increased expression by murine epidermal cells of mRNA for TNF-α and GM-CSF, sensitizing chemicals alone caused the upregulation of IL-1β and MIP-2. Subsequent investigations suggested that keratinocyte-derived IL-10 is similarly regulated selectively by chemical allergens.[53] The influence of topical sensitization on epidermal expression of IL-1β is of particular interest. The available data indicate that within epidermal populations this cytokine is produced exclusively by LC,[52,56–58] and that in mice expression by LC of mRNA for IL-1β is upregulated within 15 min of skin painting.[52,59] Moreover, the induction of skin sensitization may be dependent upon the local availability of this cytokine. Intracutaneous injection of mice with a neutralizing anti-IL-1β antibody has been shown to inhibit completely the development of sensitization following skin painting at the same site with the contact allergen picryl chloride.[60] It is suggested, therefore, that an early event following topical exposure to chemical allergens is the increased synthesis by LC of IL-1β and that the activity of this cytokine is essential for the subsequent induction of contact sensitization. One action of IL-1β appears to be the upregulation of other epidermal cytokines, including a significant increase in the expression of keratinocyte-derived TNF-α.[60] It may be that the association of chemical allergens with LC stimulates their increased production of IL-1β, which in turn acts on adjacent keratinocytes to provoke the synthesis of TNF-α necessary for the initiation of LC migration. Whatever the sequence of events, it is relevant that the stimulation of IL-1β synthesis by LC appears to be an exclusive property of chemical allergens, or at least that chemical allergens upregulate IL-1β production by LC more rapidly or more effectively than do other stimuli. If this is the case then clearly there exist opportunities to evaluate contact sensitizing potential at the level of changes induced by chemicals in the skin. If robust associations between skin sensitization and changes in epidermal cytokine expression are borne out by further experimentation with a wider range of chemicals, then this may represent the basis for a realistic approach to the design of in vitro predictive methods.

CONCLUSION

There are now available several comparatively new methods for the prospective identification of skin allergens that may be used in place of conventional guinea pig tests. Exciting and realistic opportunities for the development of in vitro predictive assays are emerging based upon a more sophisticated appreciation of the early events initiated in the skin by chemical allergens and that are associated with, and necessary for, the induction of contact sensitization.

REFERENCES

1. Andersen, K. E., and Maibach, H. I., eds. 1985. *Contact allergy predictive tests in guinea pigs.* Current Problems in Dermatology, Vol. 14. Basel: Karger.
2. Kimber, I., and Dearman, R. J. 1993. Approaches to the identification and classification of chemical allergens in mice. *J. Pharmacol. Toxicol. Methods* 29:11–16.
3. Gad, S. C., Dunn, B. J., Dobbs, D. W., Reilly, C., and Walsh, R. D. 1986. Development and validation of an alternative dermal sensitization test: The mouse ear swelling test (MEST). *Toxicol. Appl. Pharmacol.* 84:93–114.
4. Descotes, J. 1988. Identification of contact allergens: The mouse ear sensitization assay. *J. Toxicol. Cutaneous Ocul. Toxicol.* 7:263–272.
5. Thorne, P. S., Hawk, C., Kaliszewski, S. D., and Guiney, P. D. 1991. The noninvasive mouse ear swelling assay. 1. Refinements for detecting weak contact sensitizers. *Fundam. Appl. Toxicol.* 17:790–806.
6. Sailstad, D. M., Tepper, J. S., Doerfler, D. L., and Selgrade, M. K. 1993. Evaluation of several variations of the mouse ear swelling test (MEST) for detection of weak and moderate contact sensitizers. *Toxicol. Methods* 3:169–182.
7. Kimber, I. 1989. Aspects of the immune response to contact allergens: Opportunities for the development and modification of predictive test methods. *Food Chem. Toxicol.* 27:755–762.
8. Kimber, I., and Basketter, D. A. 1992. The murine local lymph node assay: A commentary on collaborative studies and new directions. *Food Chem. Toxicol.* 30:165–169.
9. Kimber, I., Dearman, R. J., Scholes, E. W., and Basketter, D. A. 1994. The local lymph node assay: Developments and applications, *Toxicology.* 93:13–31.
10. Kimber, I., and Dearman, R. J. 1991. Investigation of lymph node cell proliferation as a possible immunological correlate of contact sensitizing potential. *Food Chem. Toxicol.* 29:125–129.
11. Kimber, I. 1992. Contact sensitivity. In *Principles and practice of immunotoxicology,* eds. K. Miller, J. Turk, and S. Nicklin, pp. 104–124. Oxford: Blackwell Scientific.
12. Kimber, I., Mitchell, J. A., and Griffin, A. C. 1986. Development of a murine local lymph node assay for the determination of sensitizing potential. *Food Chem. Toxicol.* 24:585–586.
13. Kimber, I., and Weisenberger, C. 1989. A murine local lymph node assay for the identification of contact allergens. Assay development and results of an initial validation study. *Arch. Toxicol.* 63:274–282.
14. Ikarashi, Y., Tsuchiya, T., and Nakamura, A. 1993. Evaluation of contact sensitivity of rubber chemicals using the murine local lymph node assay. *Contact Dermatitis* 28:77–80.
15. Ikarashi, Y., Tsuchiya, T., and Nakamura, A. 1993. A sensitive mouse lymph node assay with two application phases for detection of contact allergens. *Arch. Toxicol.* 67:629–636.
16. Dearman, R. J., Hope, J. C., Hopkins, S. J., Debicki, R. J., and Kimber, I. 1993. Interleukin 6 (IL-6) production by lymph node cells: An alternative endpoint for the murine local lymph node assay. *Toxicol. Methods* 3:268–278.
17. Dearman, R. J., and Kimber, I. 1994. Cytokine production and the local lymph node assay. In *In vitro skin toxicology,* eds. A. Rougier, A. M. Goldberg, and H. I. Maibach, pp. 367–372. New York: Mary Ann Liebert.
18. Kimber, I., Hilton J., and Weisenberger, C. 1989. The murine local lymph node assay for identification of contact allergens: A preliminary evaluation of in situ measurement of lymphocyte proliferation. *Contact Dermatitis* 21:215–220.
19. Kimber, I., Hilton, J., Botham, P. A., Basketter, D. A., Scholes, E. W., Miller, K., Robbins, M. C., Harrison, P. T. C., Gray, T. J. B., and Waite, S. J. 1991. The murine local lymph node assay: Results of an interlaboratory trial. *Toxicol. Lett.* 55:203–213.
20. Basketter, D. A., Scholes, E. W., Kimber, I., Botham, P. A., Hilton, J., Miller, K., Robbins, M. C., Harrison, P. T. C., and Waite, S. J. 1991. Interlaboratory evaluation of the local lymph node assay with 25 chemicals and comparison with guinea pig test data. *Toxicol. Methods* 1:30–43.
21. Scholes, E. W., Basketter, D. A., Sarll, A. E., Kimber, I., Evans, C. D., Miller, K., Robbins, M. C.,

Harrison, P. T. C., and Waite, S. J. 1992. The local lymph node assay: Results of a final interlaboratory validation under field conditions. *J. Appl. Toxicol.* 12:217–222.

22. Kimber, I., Hilton, J., and Botham, P. A. 1990. Identification of contact allergens using the murine local lymph node assay: Comparisons with the Buehler occluded patch test in guinea pigs. *J. Appl. Toxicol.* 10:173–180.

23. Basketter, D. A., Scholes, E. W., Cumberbatch, M., Evans, C. D., and Kimber, I. 1992. Sulphanilic acid: Divergent results in the guinea pig maximization test and the local lymph node assay. *Contact Dermatitis* 27:209–213.

24. Basketter, D. A., and Scholes, E. W. 1992. Comparison of the local lymph node assay with the guinea-pig maximization test for the detection of a range of contact allergens. *Food Chem. Toxicol.* 30:65–69.

25. Basketter, D. A., Selbie, E., Scholes, E. W., Lees, D., Kimber, I., and Botham, P. A. 1993. Results with OECD recommended positive control sensitizers in the maximization, Buehler and local lymph node assays. *Food Chem. Toxicol.* 31:63–67.

26. Basketter, D. A., Scholes, E. W., and Kimber, I. 1994. The performance of the local lymph node assay with chemicals identified as contact allergens in the human maximization test. *Food Chem. Toxicol.* 32:543–547.

27. Botham, P. A., Hilton, J., Evans, C. D., Lees, D., and Hall, T. J. 1991. Assessment of the relative skin sensitizing potency of 3 biocides using the murine local lymph node assay. *Contact Dermatitis* 25:172–177.

28. Hopkins, S. J., Humphreys, M., Kinnaird, A., Jones, D. A., and Kimber, I. 1990. Production of interleukin-1 by draining lymph node cells during the induction phase of contact sensitivity. *Immunology* 71:493–496.

29. Mohler, K. M., and Butler, L. D. 1990. Differential production of IL-2 and IL-4 mRNA in vivo after primary sensitization. *J. Immunol.* 145:1734–1739.

30. Marcinkiewicz, J., and Chain, B. M. 1989. Antigen-specific inhibition of IL-2 and IL-3 production in contact sensitivity to TNP. *Immunology* 68:185–189.

31. Hope, J. C., Dearman, R. J., Debicki, R. J., Kimber, I., and Hopkins, S. J. 1994. Interleukin-6 production by draining lymph node cells following primary contact sensitization of mice: Relationship to the proliferative response. *Int. Arch. Allergy Immunol.* 103:378–383.

32. Dearman, R. J., Ramdin, L. S. P., Basketter, D. A., and Kimber, I. 1994. Inducible interleukin-4-secreting cells provoked in mice during chemical sensitization. *Immunology* 81:551–557.

33. Hope, J. C., Dearman, R. J., Kimber, I., and Hopkins, S. J. 1994. The kinetics of cytokine production by draining lymph node cells following primary exposure of mice to chemical allergens. *Immunology.* 83:250–255.

34. Dearman, R. J., Scholes, E. W., Ramdin, L. S. P., Basketter, D. A., and Kimber, I. 1994. The local lymph node assay: An interlaboratory evaluation of interleukin 6 (IL-6) production by draining lymph node cells. *J. Appl. Toxicol.* 14:287–291.

35. Kimber, I., and Weisenberger, C. 1991. Anamnestic responses to contact allergens: Application in the murine local lymph node assay. *J. Appl. Toxicol.* 11:129–133.

36. Gerberick, G. F., House, R. V., Fletcher, E. R., and Ryan, C. A. 1992. Examination of the local lymph node assay for use in contact sensitization risk assessment. *Fundam. Appl. Toxicol.* 19:438–445.

37. Scholes, E. W., Basketter, D. A., Lovell, W. W., Sarll, A. E., and Pendlington, R. U. 1991. The identification of photoallergic potential in the local lymph node assay. *Photodermatol. Photoimmunol. Photomed.* 8:249–254.

38. Vohr, H.-W., Homey, B., Schuppe, H.-C., and Kind, P. 1993. Detection of photoreactivity demonstrated in a modified local lymph node assay in mice. *Photodermatol. Photoimmunol. Photomed.* 10:57–64.

39. Rodenberger, S. L., Ledger, P. W., and Prevo, M. E. 1993. Murine model for contact sensitization. *Toxicol. Methods* 3:157–168.

40. Basketter, D. A., Roberts, D. W., Cronin, M., and Scholes, E. W. 1992. The value of the local lymph node assay in quantitative structure activity investigations. *Contact Dermatitis* 27:137–142.

41. Kimber, I., and Cumberbatch, M. 1992. Dendritic cells and cutaneous immune responses to chemical allergens. *Toxicol. Appl. Pharmacol.* 117:137–146.

42. Romani, N., Heufler, C., Koch, F., Topar, G., Kampgen, E., and Schuler, G. 1994. Cytokines and Langerhans cells. In *Epidermal growth factors and cytokines,* eds. T. A. Luger and T. Schwarz, pp. 345–363. New York: Marcel Dekker.

43. Bergstresser, P. R. 1994. Cytokine expression by epidermal cell subpopulations in allergic contact dermatitis. In *In vitro skin toxicology,* eds. A. Rougier, A. M. Goldberg, and H. I. Maibach, pp. 303–311. New York: Mary Ann Liebert.

44. Kimber, I. 1993. Epidermal cytokines in contact hypersensitivity: Immunological roles and practical applications. *Toxicol. In Vitro* 7:295–298.

45. Kinnaird, A., Peters, S. W., Foster, J. R., and Kimber, I. 1989. Dendritic cell accumulation in draining lymph nodes during the induction phase of contact allergy in mice. *Int. Arch. Allergy Appl. Immunol.* 89:202–210.

46. Macatonia, S. E., Knight, S. C., Edwards, A. J., Griffiths, S., and Fryer, P. 1987. Localization of antigen on lymph node dendritic cells after exposure to the contact sensitizer fluorescein isothiocyanate. Functional and morphological studies. *J. Exp. Med.* 166:1654–1657.

47. Kripke, M. L., Munn, C. G., Jeevan, A., Tang, J.-M., and Bucana, C. 1990. Evidence that cutaneous antigen presenting cells migrate to regional lymph nodes during contact sensitization. *J. Immunol.* 145:2833–2838.

48. Heufler, C., Koch, F., and Schuler, G. 1988. Granulocyte/macrophage colony-stimulating factor and interleukin 1 mediate the maturation of murine epidermal Langerhans cells into potent immunostimulatory dendritic cells. *J. Exp. Med.* 167:700–705.

49. Cumberbatch, M., and Kimber, I. 1992. Dermal tumour necrosis factor-α induces dendritic cell migration to draining lymph nodes, and possibly provides one stimulus for Langerhans cell migration. *Immunology* 75:257–263.

50. Cumberbatch, M., Fielding, I., and Kimber, I. 1994. Modulation of epidermal Langerhans cell frequency by tumour necrosis factor-α. *Immunology* 81:395–401.

51. Kock, A., Schwarz, T., Kirnbauer, R., Urbanski, A., Perry, P., Ansel, J. C., and Luger, T. A. 1990. Human keratinocytes are a source for tumor necrosis factor α: Evidence for synthesis and release upon stimulation with endotoxin or ultraviolet light. *J. Exp. Med.* 172:1609–1614.

52. Enk, A. H., and Katz, S. I. 1992. Early molecular events in the induction phase of contact sensitivity. *Proc. Natl. Acad. Sci. USA* 89:1398–1402.

53. Enk, A. H., and Katz, S. I. 1992. Identification and induction of keratinocyte-derived IL-10. *J. Immunol.* 149:92–95.

54. Heufler, C., Topar, G., Grasseger, A., Stanzl, U., Koch, F., Romani, N., Namen, A. E., and Schuler, G. 1993. Interleukin 7 is produced by murine and human keratinocytes. *J. Exp. Med.* 178:1109–1114.

55. Shivji, G. M., Gupta, A. K., and Sauder, D. N. 1994. Role of cytokines in irritant contact dermatitis. In *In vitro skin toxicology*, eds. A. Rougier, A. M. Goldberg, and H. I. Maibach, pp. 13–22. New York: Mary Ann Liebert.

56. Schreiber, S., Kilgus, O., Payer, E., Kutil, R., Elbe, A., Mueller, C., and Stingl, G. 1992. Cytokine pattern of Langerhans cells isolated from murine epidermal cell cultures. *J. Immunol.* 149:3525–3534.

57. Matsue, H., Cruz, P. D., Jr., Bergstresser, P. R., and Takashima, A. 1992. Langerhans cells are the major source of mRNA for IL-1β and MIP-1α among unstimulated mouse epidermal cells. *J. Invest. Dermatol.* 99:537–541.

58. Heufler, C., Topar, G., Koch, F., Trockenbacher, B., Kampgen, E., Romani, N., and Schuler, G. 1992. Cytokine gene expression in murine epidermal cell suspensions: Interleukin 1β and macrophage inflammatory protein 1α are selectively expressed in Langerhans cells but are differentially regulated in culture. *J. Exp. Med.* 176:1221–1226.

59. Enk, A. H., and Katz, S. I. 1992. Early events in the induction phase of contact sensitivity. *J. Invest. Dermatol.* 99:39S–41S.

60. Enk, A. H., Angeloni, V. L., Udey, M. C., and Katz, S. I. 1993. An essential role for Langerhans cell-derived IL-1β in the initiation of primary immune responses in the skin. *J. Immunol.* 150:3698–3704.

Chapter Six

THE ALTERNATIVE TO ANIMALS FOR ASSESSING TOPICAL IRRITANTS IS HUMANS

Albert M. Kligman

No animal has skin that closely resembles human skin, either anatomically nor physiologically. Moreover, human skin has a wider range of displays in response to irritating substances, such as abnormal pigmentation, papulo-pustules, vesicles, and petechiae. One can also obtain unique information regarding neurosensory reactions such as itching, burning, and stinging. Humans have a large, mostly naked surface allowing multiple concomitant exposures. The information obtainable from traditional patch tests can be greatly augmented by employing bioengineering technologies that also enable quantification. These include transepidermal water loss, conductance, blood flow, spectrophotometry, high-resolution photography, replicas, and others. Examples are presented.

INTRODUCTION

Those who seek alternatives to animal testing have three sacrosanct goals. In order of achievability these are:

1. Reduction in numbers. Success has greeted this effort. Companies like Procter & Gamble use 90% less animals than a decade earlier, without sacrificing accuracy.
2. Refinement. Progress here has also been substantial. By scrupulous restructuring of technical procedures, the test results have become more reliable.
3. Replacement. Only wild enthusiasts would argue that this goal has yielded to research. Indeed, complete replacement is probably an impossibility. Despite the proliferation of ingenious in vitro models, no combination of these can ever mimic the complex inflammatory reactions provoked by irritants. The declaration by the European Commission that animal testing of topicals must cease by 1996 is irresponsible, if not downright ludicrous.

For inexplicable reasons, it seems to have gone unnoticed that there is an animal at hand that is particularly well suited to replace animals namely the human, the Prince of Primates. There are neither ethical, legal, regulatory, nor technical reasons why humans should not become a surrogate for animals. I deem it "politically correct" to oblige *Homo sapiens,* the chief benefactor of marketed products, to serve as the prototypical model for assessing the safety of topical drugs, cosmetics, and toiletries.

THE UNIQUENESS OF HUMAN SKIN

Despite the assertion of some authorities, the skin of our nearest primate relatives, the great apes and chimpanzees, does not even closely resemble human skin in structural and physiologic properties. The claim that porcine skin shares many anatomical features with human skin is patently ridiculous to the serious student of human anatomy. Space permits only a brief listing of the special features that evolution has conferred on the human integument.

1. **The human is a bloody animal!** The superficial vasculature is extremely dense and elaborate, furnishing thermoregulatory mechanisms that have enabled humans to inhabit every geographic nook on the planet. The complex plexuses of capillaries, venules, and arterioles, which play central roles in all inflammatory processes, make possible the extraordinarily diverse and multitudinous clinical manifestations of chemical injuries. Many of these signs are rarely or never seen in other mammalian skin, for example, vesicles, sweat retention syndromes (miliaria), urticaria (wheals), purpura (hemorrhage), lichenification (enhanced skin markings from rubbing and scratching), infiltrated placques, as in psoriasis, for which there is no animal model, and still others.
2. **The stratum corneum barrier,** which limits the ingress of xenobiotics into skin, is sturdier and thicker in humans. Animal skin is therefore typically more permeable and less protective of underlying structures.
3. **Eccrine sweat glands** are lacking over the body surface of animals.
4. **Pilosebaceous units,** especially the sebaceous follicles of the face, are unique to humans and predispose to common disorders such as acne and seborrhea. Literally thousands of dermatological diseases have been described in human skin. In comparison, the repertoire of skin lesions in animal skin is limited.
5. **Anatomical differences.** To describe the unique morphologic features of human skin would swell this section to textbook size. To cite but one, animal skin lacks the delicately structured papillary dermis made up of fine collagen bundles. This papillary dermis sends forth upward projections (papillae), which indent the epidermis. It is a highly reactive zone in which inflammatory processes are often initiated.

   It cannot be too strongly emphasized that the fabulously varied display of reactions to physiologic and pathologic stimuli is unmatched in any animal species. For this reason alone, human skin should be preferred. It should also be noted that after mechanical, chemical, and physical injuries, healing takes place rapidly and efficiently in human skin, usually with limited scarring. The usual sequel to a variety of superficial injuries is mainly limited to hyperpigmentation, a cosmetic alteration that dependably fades with time.

   Speedy and inconspicuous healing is a great advantage to the cutaneous toxicologist, who can thus comfortably and ethically take 2-mm full-thickness, unsutured punch biopsies for histologic study. With modern histologic techniques, including transmission electronmicroscopy, one can obtain an extraordinary amount of information from a single specimen. It is feasible to biopsy multiple sites on one forearm. In contrast to the wealth of information extractable from histologic sections, the visible signs provoked by modest damage are extremely limited in scope, mainly erythema and scaling. These tell very little of underlying tissue events. Histologically, one can make detailed observations on blood vessels, lymphatics, nerves, keratinocytes, Langerhans cells, melanocytes, a variety of resident dermal cells, diverse inflammatory cells, mast cells (key players in inflammation), and so on. In our laboratory 2-mm punch biopsies are routine and of inestimable value in meticulously delineating the subtlest changes induced by topical substances. By contrast, in animal skin, the histopathologic changes in response to the same chemical stimuli skin are rather diminutive. So, on nearly all counts, animal skin at best has limited value in regard to relevance for human safety testing.
6. **Neurosensory responses.** Animals cannot tell the toxicologist about itching, burning, stinging, tenderness, pain, tightness, and a host of discomforts that go under the general title of "subjective" irritation. It turns out that these varied sensations are the most frequent complaints about skin care formulations, far more so than visible contact dermatitis. A product that otherwise has desirable functional features will not be used if it provokes uncomfortable sensations. It has come to be realized that a sizeable proportion of adult women have "sensitive" skin and experience adverse neurosensory reactions to a variety of topical products in the absence of objective clinical signs. Some feel tightness and dryness from soaps. Fragrances, moisturizers, and sunscreens are often cited as causes of itching, burning, and stinging. Women with "sensitive" skin cannot be identified by physical examination since the skin seems

completely normal, even when itching and burning are intense. Because adverse neurosensory reactions comprise the majority of complaints from skin care products, amounting to as much as 5% of users in some categories, it is imperative that methodologies be developed to detect "subjective irritation" early in product development. Standard tests for irritancy, such as 21-d cumulative irritation patch tests, generally do not screen out formulations that create adverse neurosensory problems when applied to the face. A tactic we employ is to preselect panelists with "sensitive" skin and who will then apply the test products in an exaggerated way, say four times daily. Clearly, animals are useless for this purpose.

7. **Risks to human volunteers.** It would be inappropriate here to describe the multitude of tests that have been developed to determine the irritancy potential of topical drugs, cosmetics and toiletries. On the other hand, it is relevant to discuss ethical issues regarding unacceptable injuries to human volunteers. For the sake of brevity, I shall condense an experience extending over 40 years that shows that it is prudent and safe to expose humans to known irritants, under controlled conditions. The test agents have comprised the entire universe of toxic chemicals such as acids, alkalis, solvents, surfactants, even corrosives, etc., provided that one starts with suitable dilutions using a tiered, phase-in approach. Disturbing reactions such as ulcers, blisters, and painful dermatitis are exceedingly rare, as are infections. The exposure areas are typically small, usually less than a square inch, out of a total surface of 2 square meters! A long-lasting postinflammatory hyperpigmentation is the most frequent problem in test panels, but even that can be avoided by using light-skinned panelists. In summary, human skin is "naked," tough, resilient, and convenient to use for toxicity testing. Dare I say that human testing has still another advantage—it is less expensive! Humans don't have to be housed and fed.

BIOENGINEERING TECHNOLOGY

It is important to realize that substantial tissue changes can occur in the complete absence of clinical signs. I have labeled this dermatologic domain "invisible dermatology." Appropriately stained biopsies commonly reveal cytologic and histologic changes that are not evident at the surface. I have argued that the subclinical, invisible changes are generally more important than what the eye can see. It must be remembered that skin care products are typically used daily for decades. Invisible damage from routine short-term toxicity tests may mislead the toxicologist to underrate cumulative long-term damage. Even minor invisible changes may become permanently harmful after two to three decades. The skin has a long memory and does not easily forget an injury. For example, an intensely sunburned experimental site heals perfectly. Yet, years later the site turns bright every time it is immersed in hot water! Obviously, there is a persistent abnormality despite a normal appearance.

Happily, new tools have become available to identify pathologic changes, no matter how occult. I refer here to the burgeoning field of bioengineering, which utilizes physical devices to detect changes. These are noninvasive assessments that furnish objective quantitative data instead of the traditional clinical readings, which use subjective ordinal, discontinuous grading scales to estimate changes such as redness.

Measurements made by bioengineering techniques have the great advantage of detecting changes that are clinically invisible. For example, an anionic surfactant may induce no visible change, yet measurements of transepidermal water loss may reveal a disrupted horny layer barrier long before clinical signs surface. Similarly, increased blood flow can be detected by laser Doppler velocimetry after doses of ultraviolet radiation that are considerably below those that result in a visible erythema.

There are at least 20 high-powered, purchasable instruments that the modern cutaneous toxicologist can bring to bear to characterize and assess structural and functional alternations induced by injurious substances. These include a variety of imaging techniques, the most wondrous of which are confocal microscopy, ultrasound, magnetic resonance imaging, and scanning electron microscopy. In addition, biophysical measurements can be made of skin elasticity, recovery after deformation, luminescence by Minolta colorimetry, etc. The microtopography of the surface can be captured on Silflo replicas and characterized quantitatively by scanning profilometry. Thus, a new era of precise and accurate measurements is upon us. The well-equipped human toxicologist possesses powerful resources for assessing the potential irritancy of topical agents.

CODA

The Green movement that started in Europe has now become a universal force that is seriously affecting the marketplace and the way products are merchandized. The mantra of the Greens is "cruelty-free," "not tested on animals," statements that are exceedingly appealing to many kind but often uninformed people. Many companies now have to give lip service to the perfervid cries of the animal rights movement, forcing them to entice consumers by advertising that their products have never been tested on animals.

In many respects, this is an artificially generated furor that has irrational, emotional, and political undertones. So, I proffer the Kligman Mantra to reduce the noise level:

Down Animals!
Up Humans!

SUGGESTED READING

1. Hobson, D. W. 1995. General overview of in vitro and other alternatives to skin toxicity evaluation. In *Animal test alternatives,* ed. H. Salem, p. 131. New York: Marcel Dekker.
2. Kligman, A. M. 1991. The invisible dermatoses. *Arch. Dermatol.* 127:1375–1382.
3. Marzulli, F. N., and Maibach, H. I. 1991. *Dermatotoxicology,* 4th ed. New York: Hemisphere.
4. Montagna, W., Kligman, A. M., and Carlise, K. 1992. *Normal human skin.* New York: Springer-Verlag.
5. Rougier, A., Goldberg, A. M., and Maibach, H. I. 1994. In vitro skin toxicology. Irritation, phototoxicity, sensitization. In *Alternative methods in toxicology.* New York: Mary Ann Liebert.
6. Serup, J., and Jemec, G. B. E. 1995. *Handbook of noninvasive methods and the skin.* Boca Raton, FL: CRC Press.

Chapter Seven

HEXOSE MONOPHOSPHATE SHUNT ACTIVITY IN HUMAN EPIDERMAL KERATINOCYTES EXPOSED TO SULFUR MUSTARD

Margaret E. Martens

In their landmark paper, Papirmeister et al.[2] suggested that the mechanism of vesicant injury induced by sulfur mustard (2,2'-dichlorodiethyl sulfide, HD) may involve stimulation of the hexose monophosphate (HMP) shunt resulting from HD-induced inhibition of the glycolytic pathway, and that this stimulation may be linked to vesication via enhancement of protease synthesis and release. Previous studies on the metabolic injury induced by HD from this laboratory by Martens et al.[5] and by others[6] have shown that exposure of cultured human epidermal keratinocytes (HEK) to HD induces a time- and dose-dependent inhibition of anaerobic glycolysis that occurs relatively early after alkylation, preceding the loss of membrane integrity indicative of metabolic cell death. In addition, Smith et al.[8] have demonstrated increased protease activity in HEK exposed to HD. To date, however, there have been no experimental data describing the effects of HD on the activity of the HMP shunt. Therefore, assessment of the HMP shunt activity in control and HD-exposed HEK was undertaken. The activity was measured at 0, 4, 8, and 24 h after HD exposure as the rate of $[^{14}C]O_2$ production from $[1-^{14}C]$glucose (i,e., the oxidative branch of the pathway) corrected for $[^{14}C]O_2$ produced via the Krebs cycle (i.e. from $[6-^{14}C]$-glucose). The results show that the HMP shunt activity of control HEK constituted 1–2% of the total rate of glucose consumption, whereas the rate of glucose oxidation via the Krebs cycle made up less than 0.1%. In these experiments, exposure of HEK to 0.3 mM HD inhibited the overall glucose utilization rate by 53% (± 14) and that of anaerobic glycolysis (measured as lactate production) by 48% (± 9). On the other hand, HD had a much smaller effect on the rates of $[^{14}C]O_2$ production from either $[1-$ or $6-^{14}C]$-glucose: The HMP shunt activity was inhibited by 32% (± 11). No increase in the HMP shunt activity was seen in any of the experiments. We conclude, therefore, that if HD does induce activation of the HMP shunt, it is a transient activation occurring earlier than the first time point measured in these experiments (4 h). Investigation of the HMP shunt activity at very early times after HD exposure is planned and will identify such transients if they occur.

INTRODUCTION

The vesicating chemical warfare agent sulfur mustard (2,2'-dichlorodiethyl sulfide, HD), is a potent alkylating agent,[1] inducing cross-links and strand breaks in DNA, as well as covalent modification of proteins and other cellular components. In their landmark paper, Papirmeister

The author would like to thank Clark L. Gross, SPC James E. Caulfield, SPC Katherine S. Garwood, and Carolyn E. Brenton for their excellent technical assistance.

et al.[2] proposed a mechanism for the cutaneous injury induced by sulfur mustard that involves a cascade of events leading from DNA alkylation to blister formation, or vesication, via perturbations in the metabolism of basal epidermal cells. One tenet of this proposal is that stimulation of the hexose monophosphate (HMP) shunt results from HD-induced inhibition of the glycolytic pathway, and that this stimulation may be linked to blister formation via enhancement of protease synthesis and release. Previous studies in this laboratory[3–5] and others[1,6,7] on the metabolic injury induced by HD have shown that exposure of cultured human epidermal keratinocytes (HEK) to HD induces a time- and dose-dependent inhibition of anaerobic glycolysis that occurs relatively early after alkylation, preceding the loss of membrane integrity indicative of metabolic cell death. In addition, Smith et al.[8] have demonstrated increased protease activity in HEK exposed to HD. To date, however, there have been no experimental data describing the effects of HD on the activity of the HMP shunt. This chapter describes the results of initial studies into the effect of HD on the HMP shunt activity of cultured HEK. These data have been briefly presented elsewhere.[9]

MATERIALS AND METHODS

Materials

Human epidermal keratinocytes, keratinocyte growth medium (KGM), trypsin-EDTA, and trypsin neutralizing solution were purchased from Clonetics Corp. (San Diego, CA). Sulfur mustard was obtained from the U.S. Army Edgewood Research, Development and Engineering Center (Aberdeen Proving Ground, MD). Stock HD (4 mM) was suspended in KGM; all further dilutions were made using KGM. Radiolabeled glucose ([1-^{14}C] and [6-^{14}C]) was purchased from Amersham Corp (Arlington Heights, IL). Enzymes and fine chemicals were from Sigma Chemical Co. (St. Louis, MO). All other chemicals were reagent grade or better and purchased from commercial suppliers.

Methods

HEK purchased as second-passage cells were maintained in KGM at 37°C under 5% CO_2 and subcultured as previously described by Smith et al.[10] Third-passage cells were plated at 20,000–30,000 HEK/well onto 25-mm Falcon tissue culture inserts with a pore size of 0.45 mm (Becton-Dickinson & Co., Lincoln Park, NJ). The supplier's documents indicated these inserts had been precoated with 5μg/cm^2 human plasma fibronectin (Sigma Chemical Co., St. Louis, MO). Cell counts and viabilities were determined on HEK harvested with trypsin-EDTA.[10] Cells were either counted manually using a hemacytometer or in a Coulter counter ZM (Coulter Electronics, Hialeah, FL). Viabilities were determined by propidium iodide dye exclusion using a Coulter EPICS C flow cytometer.[10]

When 50–80% confluence was obtained, (100,000–300,000 HEK/well), each membrane was cut out of the insert and placed in the bottom of a 20-ml scintillation vial containing either [1- or [6-^{14}C] glucose in KGM to give a final specific radioactivity of 0.1–0.2 μCi/μmol glucose. The vial was sealed with a rubber stopper fitted with a center well (Kontes, Vineland, NJ) containing a filter paper soaked with 100 μmol NaOH. Immediately thereafter, ice-cold HD in KGM (to give 300 μM HD) or an equal volume of KGM alone was injected into the vial and the time recorded. The vials were incubated for 0–24 h in a 37°C shaking water bath in the fume hood. Final volume in the vials was 2.0 ml. The reaction was stopped and dissolved CO_2 released by the injection of $HClO_4$ to a final concentration of 0.8 M. The sealed vials were shaken overnight at 37°C. The [^{14}C]O_2 absorbed was determined by liquid scintillation counting of the filter papers and corrected for background levels of [^{14}C]O_2 evolved in the absence of cells.

Glucose and lactate levels in the media were assayed using a YSI model 2700 dual analyzer (Yellow Springs Instruments, Yellow Springs, OH) fitted with glucose- and lactate-selective enzyme membranes. The rates of glucose metabolism in control and exposed vials were measured as the disappearance of glucose and the appearance of lactate as a function of time, and were calculated using linear least-squares regression analysis of the data.

The unpaired Student's t-test was used to assess statistical significance.

Table 1. Effects of HD on Glucose Metabolism by Cultured HEK

	Rate (nmol/h/10^5 HEK)	
	Control	0.3 mM HD
Glucose utilization	245 ± 169	131 ± 107
Anaerobic glycolysis	181 ± 56	87 ± 44
HMP shunt	1.7 ± 0.2	1.2 ± 0.2
Krebs cycle	0.04 ± 0.01	0.04 ± 0.004

Note. Experimental conditions are as described in Materials and Methods. The data are expressed as the mean ± SEM of four experiments.

RESULTS

Glucose utilization, lactate production, and [^{14}C]O$_2$ production were measured at 0, 4, 8, and 24 h after exposure of HEK to 0.3 mM HD. Table 1 shows the rates of overall glucose utilization in control and HD-exposed HEK. In both cases, the rates were linear with time throughout the 24-h experiment. Exposure to HD inhibited the rate of glucose utilization to approximately one half (53 ± 14%) of the control rate, in agreement with the results of our previous studies.[3–5]

The rates of anaerobic glycolysis (measured as lactate production) in control and exposed HEK are shown in Table 1. As can be seen, this pathway constituted a major proportion of the glucose used by these cells, in agreement with our previous findings.[3–5] Like glucose utilization, lactate production was also reduced to about one-half (48 ± 9%) of its control rate by 0.3 mM HD.

The time courses for the production of [^{14}C]O$_2$ by control and HD-exposed HEK are shown in Figure 1, and the HMP shunt and Krebs cycle activities calculated therefrom are shown in Table 1. The activity of the oxidative branch of the HMP shunt was estimated from the rate of [^{14}C]O$_2$ production from [1-^{14}C]glucose corrected for [^{14}C]O$_2$ produced via the Krebs cycle measured with [6-^{14}C]glucose.[11] In control HEK, both activities were very low as compared to either overall glucose utilization or anaerobic glycolysis. The HMP shunt activity constituted only 1–2% of the total rate of glucose consumption, whereas the rate of glucose oxidation via the Krebs cycle made up less than 0.1%. As can be seen, exposure of HEK to 0.3 mM HD caused a 32% (±11) inhibition of the HMP shunt activity, but had no effect on the extremely

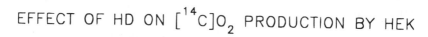

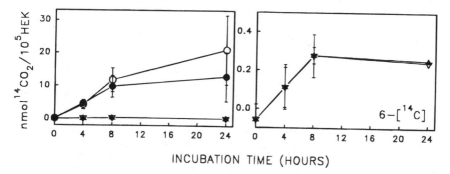

Figure 1. Experimental conditions are as described in Materials and Methods. The data are expressed as the mean ± SEM of four experiments.

low rate of oxidative glucose metabolism via the Krebs cycle. No increase in the HMP shunt activity was seen in these experiments.

DISCUSSION

We conclude from these results that 0.3 mM HD does not activate the HMP shunt in cultured HEK at 4–24 h after exposure. However, the data reported here do not rule out the possibility that HD does induce a transient activation of the HMP shunt at a time earlier than 4 h. Such a transient activation would be more consistent with current understanding of the regulation of cellular metabolic pathways[12] than would be a sustained increase. For example, inhibition of glycolysis by HD could result in buildup of glucose 6-phosphate in the cell. If this compound is not transported out of the cell or dephosphorylated to glucose to any appreciable extent, the increased concentration will drive alternative pathways for its removal, such as the HMP shunt. However, glucose 6-phosphate is also a feedback inhibitor of hexokinase, the enzyme responsible for its own synthesis. Thus, inhibition of glycolysis should also inhibit the net uptake of glucose, maintaining low intracellular levels of glucose 6-phosphate. Another possible mechanism for a transient HD-induced activation of the HMP shunt could be the need of the cell for riboses to repair damaged DNA. However, as DNA repair requires metabolic energy this can only be relevant under mild exposure conditions. In order to determine if there is a transient activation, investigations of the HMP shunt activity at lower levels of HD and earlier times after exposure are planned.

Finally, it should be kept in mind that the methods used in this study only measure the activity of the oxidative branch of the HMP shunt, not the nonoxidative branch. The effects of HD on the flux through the nonoxidative branch also need to be studied. The proportion of glucose 6-phosphate flowing through glycolysis, the oxidative branch, and the nonoxidative branch of the shunt at any particular time depends on the needs of the cell for NADPH, ribose 5-phosphate, and ATP,[12] in addition to the relative V_{max} for each pathway. When one or more pathways are compromised by exposure to HD the relationships among the three may change in interesting and unpredicted ways, depending on the severity of the exposure and/or the time elapsed. Analysis of these changes should provide new insights into the sequence of events initiated by HD which lead to vesication.

REFERENCES

1. Papirmeister, B., Feister, A. J., Robinson, S. I., and Ford, R. D. 1991. *Medical defense against mustard gas: Toxic mechanisms and pharmacological implications.* Boca Raton, FL: CRC Press.
2. Papirmeister, B., Gross, C. L., Meier, H. L., Petrali, J. P., and Johnson, J. B. 1985. Molecular basis for mustard-induced vesication. *Fundam. Appl. Toxicol.* 5:S134–S149.
3. Martens, M. E. 1991. Glucose metabolism and NAD+ content in cultured human epidermal keratinocytes exposed to sulfur mustard (HD). *Proc. 1991 Medical Defense Bioscience Review* (DTIC B158 588)., pp. 101–104. Aberdeen Proving Ground, MD: U.S. Army Medical Research Institute of Chemical Defense.
4. Martens, M. E. 1992. Biochemical studies of sulfur mustard-induced metabolic injury. *Proc. 4th Int. Symp. Protection Against Chemical Warfare Agents,* pp. 325–331. Umeå, Sweden: National Defence Research Establishment.
5. Martens, M. E., and Smith, W. J. 1993. Mechanisms of sulfur mustard-induced metabolic injury. *Proc. 1993 Medical Defense Bioscience Review,* Vol. 1 (DTIC A275 667), pp. 257–264. Aberdeen Proving Ground, MD: U.S. Army Medical Research Institute of Chemical Defense.
6. Mol, M. A. E., van de Ruit, A. M. B. C., and Kluivers, A. W. 1989. NAD+ levels and glucose uptake of cultured human epidermal cells exposed to sulfur mustard. *Toxicol. Appl. Pharmacol.* 98:159–165.
7. Mol, M. A. E., and deVries-van de Ruit, A. M. 1992. Concentration- and time-related effects of sulphur mustard on human epidermal keratinocyte function. *Toxicol. In Vitro* 6:245–251.
8. Smith, W. J., Cowan, F. M., and Broomfield, C. A. 1991. Increased protease activity in human epithelial cells following exposure to sulfur mustard. *FASEB J.* 5:A828. (Abstr.)
9. Martens, M. E. 1994. Hexose monophosphate shunt activity in human epidermal keratinocytes exposed to sulfur mustard. *Proc. NATO Research Study Group,* Panel VIII/RSG-3.
10. Smith, W. J., Gross, C. L., Chan, P., and Meier, H. L. 1990. The use of human epidermal keratinocytes

in culture as a model for studying the biochemical mechanisms of sulfur mustard toxicity. *Cell Biol. Toxicol.* 6:285–291.

11. Larrabee, M. G. 1989. The pentose cycle (hexose monophosphate shunt). Rigorous evaluation of limits to the flux from glucose using $^{14}CO_2$ data, with applications to peripheral ganglia of chicken embryos. *J. Biol. Chem.* 264:15875–15879.
12. Stryer, L. 1988. *Biochemistry,* pp. 427–433. New York: W. H. Freeman.

Chapter Eight

WHAT IS IRRITANT DERMATITIS?
A BIOLOGICAL APPROACH

Sunita Patil, K. Lamintausta, and Howard I. Maibach

Investigators wishing to decrease dermatitis have had a tendency to believe that irritant dermatitis is a monomorphous phenomenon, readily predicted by simply assays. Recently, it has become evident that the opposite case is true: Irritant dermatitis is a complex phenomenon of relatively few phenotypes and many genotypes. This presentation provides the clinical basis of information on the various biological entities of the irritant dermatitis syndrome. Details are provided as to the pantheon of in vitro assays, and how these are related to animal and human assays. QSAR for irritant dermatitis is a relatively new investigative effort, and the limited information on this topic is summarized.

CLINICAL ASPECTS

In 1898, it was first appreciated that contact dermatitis had more than one mechanism: irritant and allergic. Most of this century's investigations have focused on the latter. Recent interest in the former is documented in the 1995 textbooks.[1,2,3] Irritation, or irritant dermatitis, previously considered a monomorphous process, is now understood to be a complex biologic syndrome, with a diverse pathophysiology, natural history, and clinical appearance. Thus, the clinical appearance of irritant contact dermatitis varies depending on multiple external and internal factors. The actual types, with reference to major characteristics in the clinical appearance, are listed in Table 1.

Table 1. Types of Irritation

Irritation	Onset	Prognosis
Acute primary irritant dermatitis	Acute—often single exposure	Good
Irritant reaction	Acute—often multiple exposure	Good
Delayed acute irritant dermatitis	Delayed—12–24 h or longer	Good
Cumulative irritant contact dermatitis	Slowly developing (weeks to years)	Variable
Traumatic irritant dermatitis	Slowly developing after preceding trauma	Acute
Pustcular and acneiform dermatitis	Acute to moderately slowly developing (weeks to months)	Variable
Nonerythematous irritation	Acute to slowly developing	Variable
Friction	Slowly developing	Variable

Acute Irritant Dermatitis (Primary Irritation)

When exposure is sufficient and the offending agent is potent, classic symptoms of acute primary skin irritation are seen. Contact with a strong primary irritant is often accidental, and an acute irritant dermatitis is elicited in almost anyone independent of constitutional susceptibility. This classic, acutely developing dermatitis usually heals soon after exposure. In unusual cases the dermatitis may persist for months after exposure, followed by complete resolution.

The availability of the Material Safety Data Sheet and data from the single-application Draize rabbit test combined with activities of industrial hygienists, toxicologists, dermatologists, and other form, personnel greatly decreased the frequency of such dermatitis in industry. Further educational efforts and appropriate industrial engineering should make this form of irritation a rarity.

Irritant Reaction

Individuals extensively exposed to certain irritants often develop erythematous, chapped skin, in the first months of exposure. This irritant reaction[4-6] may by considered a pre-eczematous expression of acute skin irritation. It is frequently seen in repeatedly exposed hairdressers and variable wet-work-performing employees. Repeated irritant reactions sometimes lead to contact dermatitis, with good prognosis, although chronic contact dermatitis may also develop. We do not understand what separates the pathophysiology of the lower grade irritant reaction from that of cumulative irritant dermatitis (discussed earlier). Once this information becomes available, we may be able to develop interventions to prevent the latter.

Delayed, Acute Irritant Contact Dermatitis

Some chemicals produce acute irritation in a delayed manner so that inflammation is not seen until 8–24 h or more after exposure.[7,8] (Table 2). Except for the delayed onset, the clinical appearance and course resemble those of acute irritant contact dermatitis. The delayed acute irritant contact dermatitis. The delayed acute irritant dermatitis, because of its delayed onset, is often confused with allergic contact dermatitis; appropriately performed and interpreted diagnostic patch tests easily separate the two. Many controls may be required to define those chemicals that are delayed irritants in patch testing (Table 3). If this is not done, the delayed onset in the patch may be misinterpreted as allergy rather than delayed onset of acute irritation.

Cumulative Irritant Dermatitis

When exposure inducing an acute irritant dermatitis is repeated, the dermatitis tends to last longer, and becomes chronic. In cumulative cutaneous irritation, the frequency of exposure is too high in relation to the skin recovery time. Acute irritant skin reaction is not seen in the majority of patients, but mild or moderate invisible skin changes are. Repeated skin exposures and minor reactions lead to a manifest dermatitis when the irritant load exceeds the threshold

Table 2. Effect of Duration of Occlusion on Percutaneous Absorption of Malathion in Humans

Duration (h)	Absorption(%)
0[a]	9.6
0.5	7.3
1	12.7
2	16.6
4	24.2
8	38.8
24	62.8

[a] Immediate wash with soap and water. From Feldmann and Maibach[9] with permission.

Table 3 Chemicals Inducing Delayed Acute Chemical
Irritation

Anthralin
Bis(2-chloroethyl)sulfide
Butanedioldiacrylate
Dichloro(2-chlorovinyl)arsine
Epichlorhydrin
Ethylene oxide
Hydrofluoric acid
Hexanedioldiacrylate
Hydroxypropylacrylate
Podopyllin
Propane Sulfone

for visible effects. The development of a cumulative irritant dermatitis was carefully documented by Malten and den Arend[29] and Malten et al.[7] Cumulative irritant dermatitis was called "traumiterative dermatitis" in the older German literature ("traumiterative" = traumas repeating).[11,12] Classic signs are erythema and increasing dryness, followed by hyperkeratosis with frequent cracking and occasional erythema.

Cumulative irritant dermatitis is the most common type of irritant contact dermatitis. This syndrome may develop after days, weeks, or years of subtle exposure to chemical substances. Variation in individual susceptibility increases the multiplicity of clinical findings. Delayed onset and variable attack lead to confusion with allergic contact dermatitis. To rule out allergic etiology, appropriate diagnostic patch testing is indicated. This should be interpreted with the aid of an operational (multifunctional) definition of allergic contact dermatitis. This also provides additional integrity to the diagnostic process and decreases the opportunity of misinterpretation of this laboratory test.

Traumatic Irritant Dermatitis

Traumatic irritant dermatitis develops after acute skin trauma. The skin does not heal but erythema, vesicles and/or vesicopapules, and scaling appear. The clinical course later resembles nummular (coin-shaped) dermatitis. This may occur after burns or lacerations and after acute irritant dermatitis; it may be compounded by a concurrent allergen exposure. The healing period is generally prolonged.

Often these patients are considered to have a factitial dermatitis because of a healing phase followed by exacerbation. Although factitial (unnatural) aspects may occur in some patients, this peculiar form of irritation appears to be a disease *sui generis*. Its chronicity and recalcitrance to therapy provide a challenge to both patient and physician. We have no information explaining why the occasional patient develops this phenomenon, and how this patient differs from the general population.

Pustular and Acneiform Irritant Dermatitis

Pustular and acneiform irritant dermatitis may develop from exposure to cosmetics, skin care agents, metals, oils and greases, tar asphalt, chlorinated naphthalenes, and polyhalogenated naphthalenes. Certain substances have a capacity to elicit these reactions,[13,14] and even allergic reactions may sometimes be pustular or follicular.[15] In occupational exposure, only a minority of subjects develop pustular or acneiform dermatitis. Thus, the development of this type of irritant contact dermatitis appears to be dependent on both constitutional and chemical factors. This special form of irritant dermatitis has not received adequate investigation.

Nonerythematous Irritation

In the early stages of skin irritation, subtle skin damage may occur without visible inflammation. As a correlate of nonvisible irritation, objectively registered alterations in the damaged epidermis have been reported.[16-18] It is customary in Japan to screen new chemicals, cosmetics, and textiles for subtle signs of stratum corneum damage, employing replicas of stratum corneum (the Kawai method). Consumer dissatisfaction with many chemicals may result from exposure to this low-grade irritation; thus the patient feels more than the physician observes.

Sensory (Subjective) Irritation

Sensory (subjective) irritation is experienced by some individuals ("stingers") in contact with certain chemicals.[18,19] Itching, stinging, or tingling is experienced, for example, from skin contact with lactic acid, a model for nonvisible cutaneous irritation. The threshold for this reaction varies between subjects, independent of susceptibility to other irritation types. The quality as well as the concentration of the exposing agent is also important, and neural pathways may be contributory, but the pathomechanism is unknown. Some sensory irritation may be subclinical contact urticaria. Screening raw ingredients and final formulations in the guinea pig ear swelling test[20] or the human forehead assay allows us to minimize the amount of subclinical contact urticaria.

Although sensory irritation has a neural component (being blocked by local anaesthetics), recent studies by Lammintausta et al.[18,21] suggest that the blood vessel may be more responsive in "stingers" than nonstingers. At least 10% of women complain of stinging with certain facial products; thus, further work is needed to develop a strategy to overcome this type of discomfort. Further investigations on progress of sensory anti-irritants is promising (Hahn, personal communication).

Localization of Irritant Contact Dermatitis

In irritant contact dermatitis the exposed sites are first affected. The dorsal and lateral aspects of the hands and fingers have the greatest contact with chemical irritants. Thick stratum corneum may provide better protection for palms and soles. The degree of protection may be greater than what might be expected from decreases in skin penetration. Some compounds are almost as permeable through the palm as the forearm.[22]

Dermatitis on the anterior thighs, upper back, axillary areas, and feet may be due to an irritant in clothing. When dermatitis is observed on the face, under the collar or belt, or in the flexures, airborne irritants (e.g., dust) may be involved.

EXTERNAL FACTORS

Irritants

Many chemicals qualify as irritant when the exposing dose is high.[23] Molecular size, ionization, polarization, fat solubility, and the other factors important in skin penetration are also important in cutaneous irritation. The threshold of strength and quality of irritation depends on the physio-chemical properties of the substance. Temperature may be important, with warm temperatures generally more damaging than cool[24]—for example, warm citral perfume produced more irritation than citral at lower temperature.

Exposure

The absorbed dose may vary when the substance is suspended in different vehicles.[25-27] The solubility of the irritant in the vehicle and the inherent irritancy of the vehicle have an impact on each reaction.[28] The effective tissue dose depends on concentration, volume, application time, and duration on and in the skin. Long exposure time and large volume may increase penetration. Thus, greater response may be expected. If exposure is repeated, the recovery from previous exposure(s) affects the subsequent response. Sometimes a shorter, repeated exposure leads to a lengthened recovery period.[29] This was demonstrated in experimental studies with dimethyl sulfoxide (DMSO). Intermittent application leads to a different response as compared with one lengthened application.[30] These experimental observations are consistent with the multiple clinical appearances of cumulative irritant dermatitis.

Multiple Simultaneous Exposure

Simultaneous or subsequent exposure may lead to an additive effect and increased reaction, although each chemical alone would elicit only a minor reaction, or none. On the other hand, subsequent exposure may lead to a decreased response. For instance, exposure to a detergent and then to a soap led to a response less than exposure to a detergent alone. The detergent was washed away by the subsequent soap exposure.[31] Recent studies by Patil et al.[32] have revealed that repeated exposure of skin (in vivo) to sodium lauryl sulfate (SLS) leads to a prolonged damage to the skin in that region and the skin does not come back to normal even at 12 d after exposure to the irritant. An "overlap phenomenon" (exaggerated reaction in the adjacent region of the preexposed site) was reported using bioengineering methods. Studies on rat skin[33] have also demonstrated residual levels of SLS in the skin 1 wk after exposure to SLS. SLS tends to accumulate into the epidermis after repeated exposure and is not cleared away by the dermal supply. A radial spread of this compound was observed till ~0.75 cm from the site of application in a classic 24-h study.[34]

The outcome of multiple, subsequent, or simultaneous exposures is sometimes unexpected[35] and rules must be sought.[36]

Other Irritation Sources

Physical trauma from friction often facilitates the harmful effects of a chemical irritant. Repeated microtrauma and friction typically lead to dry, hyperkeratotic, and abraded skin.[37] Although physical irritation alone may produced irritant dermatitis, the additive effect with chemical exposure may lead to irritant contact dermatitis. Corresponding impact is seen with other physical irritants.

Quantification of physical trauma from friction and differences in individual susceptibility to friction are expected to lead to appropriate interventions to decrease such damage.

Environmental Factors

Low environmental humidity enhances irritability: Skin tests with irritants produce more and stronger reactions in winter when the weather is cool, windy, and dry.[38] It also produces variable irritation symptoms: itching and erythema associated with whealing or erythema and scaling.[39,40]

Occlusion often enhances penetration and increases acute irritation (Table 2). Thus, skin reactions frequently become stronger when the chemical is applied under occlusion, providing a humid environment that minimizes evaporation and makes the stratum corneum more permeable. Gloves and clothing increase the susceptibility for irritant dermatitis. Frequent changes of these articles is important, to minimize the humid and occlusive environment.

Airborne Irritation

Airborne irritation dermatitis is located most commonly in exposed skin areas, such as the face, hands, and arms.[41] Volatile chemicals and dusts are common sources of exposure, but even sharp particles in dust may induce lesions (Table 4). Airborne irritation is a type of exposure in which physical sources of irritation frequently exacerbate the response with an additive to chemical exposure. Depending on the occupational situation, multiple environmental and occupational irritants may induce airborne irritation.[14]

PREDISPOSING FACTORS

Methodological Aspects

Although irritant contact dermatitis accounts for most occupational skin diseases, and many nonoccupational eczemas are exclusively or partially induced by irritation, in-depth investigation of irritant contact dermatitis is rare. Epidemiological studies have identified many important irritants, and some information is available about subjects who appear vulnerable to irritant

Table 4. Airborne Irritants

Volatile substances
Acids and alkalis, ammonia
Cleaning products
Formaldehyde
Industrial solvents
Noncarbon required (NCR) paper
Epoxy resins
Foams, e.g., insulation foams in urea–formaldehyde process
Powders
Aluminum
Anhydrous calcium silicate
Cement
Cleaning products
Metallic oxides
Particles
Tree-sawing particles
Wool
Plastics, dry
Particles from plants
Stone particles in mining

dermatitis in occupational circumstances that induce dermatitis. Detergents and soaps are considered principal causes of occupational irritant dermatitis. However, in controlled experimental trials, this implied harmful effect of soap has not always been documented.[42–46] Correspondingly, with evaluation of patch test reactions to detergents by direct visualization, individual differences in irritant reactivity were not documented in healthy skin. Only those subjects with a concurrent eczema reacted more strongly.[18,47] Bioengineering methods now make it possible to quantitate minor differences in cutaneous reactivity; it is expected that the development of methods is still proceeding.

Nonvisible cutaneous changes are measurable with various methods in which different aspects of skin function are quantitated. Table 5 lists the available and most useful instrumentation with reference to the measured physicochemical parameters. Documented are alterations in skin impedance,[48] in the amount of transepidermal water loss (TEWL), in dielectric characteristics,[49] and in conductance and resistance,[50] and alterations in blood flow velocity[51] and skin thickness.[52] Skin pH[53] and O_2 resistance and CO_2 effusion rate[54,55] are further measurable changes in skin irritation.

Measurements of these variables often show poor correlation with each other, probably because these methods give information about different aspects of cutaneous irritation and skin function. Three recent textbooks provide in-depth overview of utilization of these methods in dermatopharmacology, toxicology, and physiology.[3,56,57]

In addition to patch testing with irritants accompanied by visual scoring, alkali resistance and alkali neutralization capacity have been evaluated in some European countries by using ammonium hydroxide applications. Their capacity to reflect individual susceptibility appears to be limited or minimal[58] and their value is questioned.

Recently K. Wilhelm[59] utilized sodium hydroxide to produce transepidermal water loss as a measure of skin damage. This assay shows a high correlation between subjects developing increased water loss after application of sodium hydroxide and a propensity for SLS damage. This simple approach may provide a first step toward a preemployment test for irritant dermatitis potential.

Individual susceptibility to chemicals has been studied by documenting skin reactivity to model irritants. The intensity of the wheal created by DMSO, the time required to raise a blister (MBT) after cutaneous application of aluminum hydroxide solution, and the reactivity to SLS are some examples of objective methods that have been used.[60] Stinging (sensory irritation) occurs with certain test substances (e.g., lactic acid), and clinical experiments provide some information about individual susceptibility.[19]

Table 5. Bioengineering Techniques Used in the Evaluation of Cutaneous Irritation

Technique	Measured skin function	Advantages	Disadvantage
Laser Doppler velocimetry	Velocity of the moving erythrocytes with blood flow	Slight, preerythema	Does not measure nonerythematous irritation
Evaporimeter	Transepidermal water exchange evaluated	Epidermal damage evaluated Easy to use	Visible erythema Inflammation contributes but does not directly correlate Standardized environmental circumstances important
Ultrasound	Skin thickness	Edematous inflammation measured	Minimal correlation with visible erythema or epidermal damage
Impedence, conductance, and capacitance	Skin hydration	Correlation with epidermal damage	
Colorimeter	Skin colors	Correlation with erythema, inflammation	Correlates with the amount of pigment, too Minimal correlation with epidermal damage and other nonerythematous inflammation

Despite important steps taken in the investigation of the pathogenesis of irritant contact dermatitis, no experimental design has proved entirely successful for the clinical evaluation of individual susceptibility. Hopefully, the Wilhelm studies[59] will lead toward objective test(s).

Regional Anatomic Differences

Anatomic differences in the exposure site are important. Because skin permeability is variable in different skin sites, being generally greatest in thin skin areas,[22,61–64] corresponding association between permeability, skin thickness, and skin irritation is expected, but direct correlation is lacking (Figure 1). Regional variation has been studied comparing the whealing response—a variation of immediate irritation—to DMSO and measuring differences in minimal blistering time (MBT) after topical ammonium hydroxide application in different skin sites.[19] Both tests showed the mandibular area to be most reactive, followed by the upper back, forearm, lower leg, and palm. With DMSO whealing, the forehead was more sensitive than the back, the antecubital area reaction preceded that of the rest of the upper extremity, and the wrist was more sensitive than the leg.

In patch testing, the irritant benzalkonium chloride and several allergens produced maximal reactivity in the upper back,[65] an observation recently extended to the middle scapula.[66] The greater reactivity may be related to pressure in this area when sleeping.[67,68] Certain "inherent" differences between different skin sites in irritation reactivity may also exist. Vulvar skin may be more sensitive than forearm skin[10,69] (Figure 2). On the other hand, it is often noted in clinical occupational dermatology that male genitalia are affected in occupational irritant dermatitis.

The threshold for skin irritation is decreased in babies, who develop dermatitis from irritation that does not occur in adult skin.[70] Except for structural and functional immaturity of infant's skin, other factors (intestinal *Candida albicans,* completed breast feeding, low frequency of diaper changes) are contributory.[71] Children below the age of 8 years are generally believed to

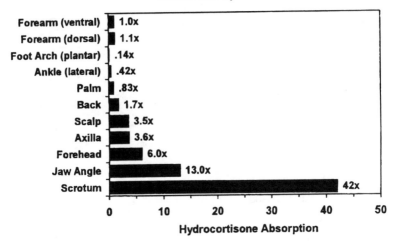

Figure 1. Anatomic regional variation of percutaneous absorption in humans. Adapted from Feldmann and Maibach[22] with permission.

be more susceptible to skin irritation.[72-74] Irritation susceptibility gradually decreases after this age. Maibach and Boisits[75] define this database; unfortunately, despite extensive chemical exposure of infants and children, our experimental evidence is lacking because of methodologic problems and limited data.

Skin problems commonly occur in the elderly,[76] who do not routinely seek help from physicians. In a majority of cutaneous symptoms, cutaneous irritation is contributory. Elderly subjects may develop reactions to skin irritants less sharply and more slowly than younger individuals.[77,78] A corresponding alteration occurs with regard to cutaneous reactivity to allergens. With ammonium hydroxide skin tests, older subjects had a shorter reaction time (MBT, minimal blistering time), whereas the time needed to develop a tense blister was longer,[79] and a longer time was needed

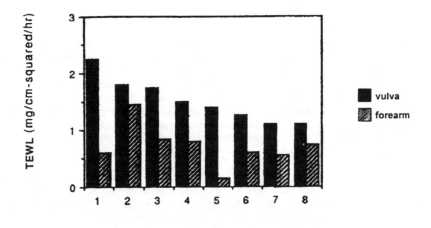

Figure 2. Transepidermal water loss from vulva and forearm. From Oriba et al.[69] by permission of W. B. Saunders.

for the resorption of a wheal elicited by saline injection.[80] That aspect of responsiveness related to percutaneous penetration has been reviewed by Roskos.[81]

Age-associated alterations in skin reactivity may be related to altered cutaneous permeation, although contradictory results have been reported.[82–85] Alterations in structural lipids[86] and in cell composition[87] and renewal[88,89] are reported in association with structural alteration.[90,91] Thus, age-associated alterations in cutaneous reactivity are expected; however, more investigation of this subject is required.

Race

It is difficult to compare irritant reactions in white and black skin, although black skin less frequently seems (to the naked eye) to develop irritation from chemicals eliciting irritant reactions in white skin.[92,93] When blood flow velocity is altered in an irritant reaction, the reaction is measurable with laser Doppler velocimetry (LDV). Observations in experimental studies using LDV support increased reactivity to a detergent in black subjects[16] (Table 6).

Negroid skin has higher electrical resistance than does Caucasoid skin.[94] Owing to this characteristic it may have increased resistance to irritants that themselves often lower electrical skin resistance. Structural differences are reported, too, such as difference in skin reactivity to irritants when minimal perceptible erythema was registered.[92] Negroid skin, however, needs more stripping for the removal of stratum corneum.[95] With methacholine-induced erythema and flare response, blacks appear to be less reactive than whites.[96]

Clinical experiments suggest that Negroid skin has differences in the modulation of irritation reactivity as compared with Caucasoid skin.[16] It may be reflected in certain aspects of the multifactoral development of skin irritation, which is, however, still poorly understood. Cutaneous erythema induced by methacholine injections was compared in Warain Indians, Tibetans, and Caucasians. Caucasians reacted to the greatest degree,[97] and associations between skin irritation and cholinergic reactivity may exist.[16]

Gender

The incidence of irritant contact dermatitis—most often located in the hands—is higher in females than in males.[12,98,99] Because of the clinical observation, susceptibility to skin irritation has been related to female skin, which also seems to elicit more tape irritation.[100,101] Skin tests with surfactants, however, have not experimentally documented a difference.[102,103] The increased occurrence of irritant contact dermatitis may be related to the more extensive exposure to irritants and wet work. A minimal relationship between gender and constitutional skin irritability is supported by the fact that the female preponderance in the irritant contact dermatitis populations does not hold true for all geographic areas.[104] Socioeconomic factors may be responsible.

Genetics

Interindividual variation based on genetic constitutional differences has been demonstrated.[47,60] When patch-test reactivity to common irritants was compared between monozygotic and dizygotic twins with control subjects, the highest degree of concordance was demonstrated for the monozygotic twin pairs.[105]

Susceptibility to sunlight has been associated with vulnerability to chemical irritants. Sun-sensitive skin and low minimal erythema dose (MED) seem to be correlated with high cutaneous

Table 6. Laser Doppler Velocimetry (LDV) Values in Blacks and Whites

LDV (mV)	0.5%[a]	Preoccluded	2.0%
Whites	73.6 ± 34	$p < .01$	179 ± 128
Blacks	58 ± 25	$p < .01$	234 ± 194

Note. p Values refer to the comparison between 0.5% and 2% sodium lauryl sulfate (SLS) concentration.
[a] Significant difference at $p < .04$ for blacks versus whites.

irritability.[106,107] Marked interindividual variation in skin reactivity has been demonstrated with the alkali resistance test, although the relevance to clinical irritant reactivity is minor.[58]

In a large series, individual skin irritability varied for different chemical irritants when reactions were evaluated with visual scoring.[47] These results were confirmed by Cerwinska-Ditram and Rudzki.[108] Both sets of data support the simultaneous influence of the quality of irritant, individual susceptibility, and multiple environmental factors. For experimental studies, certain model irritants are needed; however, the results may not be generalizable.

A test battery consisting of DMSO reactivity, blistering susceptibility to ammonium hydroxide, and SLS reactivity was found to be useful.[60] Unfortunately, it is too complicated to be used in clinical practice for preemployment testing.

Newer bioengineering test methods show great interindividual variation. For example, TEWL, which is easy to measure, reflects important components of detergent-induced irritation. In the evaluation of individual irritant reactivity, however, repeated follow-up measurements are needed, because baseline values do not necessarily reflect the reactivity when irritation is produced.

Previous and Preexisting Skin Diseases

Subjects with a previous or present atopic dermatitis have an increased susceptibility to develop irritant dermatitis.[98,109] Ichthyosis vulgaris is sometimes seen in association with atopic dermatitis; in ichthyosis vulgaris, patients' irritant reactivity has been shown to be increased to alkali irritants.[110] The increased general cutaneous irritability related to atopic dermatitis[111] could not be demonstrated with regular patch tests when skin irritants were used.[112,113]

Reduced capacity to bind water has been related to atopic skin,[114] which in noneczematous sites demonstrates greater transepidermal water loss than does nonatopic skin. Stratum corneum water content may even be increased.[11,115,116] An increased water loss was induced with detergent patch tests in atopic skin.[117] Itchy and dry atopic skin has been connected with an increased risk for developing hand dermatitis.[98,118] However, certain atopic subjects with rhinitis or asthma have normal, nonirritable skin, and an itchy and dryness-prone skin may be seen in some nonatopic subjects. Accurate objective tools are not available to evaluate the atopic cutaneous characteristics or atopic skin diathesis.

Seborrheic skin has not been shown to possess increased susceptibility to skin irritants; reports and interpretations are contradictory.[119–121] Clinical experience suggests that some increased irritability is associated with a seborrheic constitution in certain subjects. This may be true in certain geographic areas, where environmental humidity is low in the winter in relation to the cold temperatures. Different methods have been used in studies on skin irritability in psoriatic individuals. Those studies revealed decreased and increased irritant reactivity[107,122–124] when anthralin (dithranol) irritancy was the main interest. Psoriatic skin is particularly irritable in certain individuals,[125] and the development of psoriatic lesions in irritation sites (Koebner phenomenon) is often seen.

In the presence of eczema, the threshold for skin irritation is decreased.[47,126–128] A whole-body examination of employees sometimes reveals nummular lesions or other constitutional eczema symptoms. Such a clinical finding may suggest an increased skin irritability in different locations. Pompholyx (dyshidrosis) type dermatitis is harmful. As a constitutional eczema, it probably increases skin irritability in general. These patients often have difficulty wearing gloves, since pompholyx is made worse by occlusion.

A history of contact dermatitis may be important when susceptibility to irritant contact dermatitis is evaluated.[30,129] Although increased irritability has been hard to demonstrate,[30,47] further improvement of methodological equipment in the bioengineering industry should make this possible.

Systemic Skin Disease

Atopic Dermatitis

On the basis of dermatologic clinical experience, atopic dermatitis patients have irritable skin manifested by reactivity to all types of irritants.[109] Since facial dermatitis and hand dermatitis are common in atopic dermatitis, it appears that irritation is an important factor. In wet work, for example, in which exposure to water, detergents, or other chemicals is frequent or continuous, the subjects with a history of atopic dermatitis develop hand dermatitis more often than those without a history of atopic symptoms.[17,118,129] The studies also suggest that atopic subjects with dry, itchy skin have skin problems more often than nonatopic subjects in environments where exposure to irritants is extensive, although they would not have histories of manifest skin effects.[118] In these subjects, the threshold level for cutaneous irritation from repeated irritant attacks appears intermediate between those with atopic dermatitis and those with a nonatopic constitution. Cutaneous irritability in atopic subjects shows considerable clinical variation. The degree is dependent on the number of characteristics in the skin that make the skin particularly prone to develop cutaneous irritation. The scale is wide. Simultaneously, many atopic subjects— some 30–40% of those with only mucosal symptoms—have normal skin without any demonstrable susceptibilities. The importance of motivated protection and self care for vulnerable groups appears evident. Although many atopic subjects learn to handle difficulties, despite some skin effects appearing intermittently, problems may arise in occupations with repeated irritation exposure. A subject with a history of severe atopic dermatitis, with atopic hand problems as a child, or with relapsing atopic skin effects in adulthood should not start work in conditions where irritation exposure is extensive until both the individual and the employer have been apprised of the risk.

STUDIES IN IRRITANT DERMATITIS SYNDROME

Experimental Irritant Dermatitis

Irritant dermatitis is induced with patch-test technique and read on the basis of visual scoring of elicited irritant reactions of variable degree. The strength of one reaction does not usually predict reactivity to other irritants.[47] The alkali resistance test as a predictive test for irritability has not proven reliable.[58]

In human experiments, visible reactions to different irritants—whealing from dimethyl sulfoxide contact, blister formation from ammonium hydroxide, and eczematous reaction—after contact with SLS, alkyldimethyl benzyl ammonium chloride, croton oil, or kerosene, have suggested that some part of individual variation in cutaneous irritant reactivity may be predictable.[60] Hyper- and hyporeacting groups may be recognizable to some extent.

Investigators have worked on methodologic improvements in irritant dermatitis studies, because visual assessment measures mainly erythema and edema and is subjective.

Besides the limitations in qualitative aspects, the reliability of observed and visually quantitated results may be limited. Tools employed in clinical experiments are the laser Doppler flowmeter, evaporimeter, micrometers, and ultrasonography. Skin impedance and water content have been measured and replica systems developed to qualify and quantify reactions.[49] In experimental irritant dermatitis studies, certain model irritants, usually detergents, were used. SLS is the model surfactant that has been used most frequently.[130] It induces epidermal damage as well as visible erythematous irritation and thus is a useful model irritant for such experiments.

The laser Doppler flowmeter gives information about cutaneous circulatory changes associated with erythematous irritation. Results obtained with laser Doppler generally correlate with visible changes.[51,131,132] This method appears slightly more sensitive than the naked eye in evaluating erythema, which is often correlated with the amount of epidermal damage.[18,30]

Edema may sometimes interfere with measurements, and thus reactions with associated edema yield lower flowmeter values, although irritation-induced reaction in skin vasculature is apparent.[18] Nonerythematous irritation cannot be detected with this method.

The evaporimeter is a practical tool for the measurement of transepidermal loss.[132] Cumulative irritation leads to increased transepidermal water loss.[30] Increased irritation from more concentrated irritants leads to greater increase in transepidermal water loss, although no erythema is seen. These alterations can be demonstrated before visible changes appear. Transepidermal water loss often increases in association with erythematous irritation,[30,133] which makes this method useful in studies of more acute irritant responses. The recovery of epidermis after irritant attacks has been demonstrated with gradually normalizing transepidermal water loss values. Evaporimeter measurements are quick: Measurement can be registered in minutes. However, resting time is needed before values are obtained. Environmental circumstances (temperature and humidity) must be standardized. For evaluations of individual reactivity, repeated values have to be followed up, since individual baseline values are different. On the other hand, baseline values for an individual subject show day-to-day variation. Transepidermal water loss measurements still need standardization and improvement before this tool is useful for routine clinical purposes.

The measurement of skin electrical impedance and measurement of skin water content provide further approaches to studying cutaneous hydration.[48–50] Impedance measurement is based on the facilitated current conduction in stratum corneum related to the ionic movements of hydrates. Stratum corneum water content is assessed by means of a microwave dielectric probe.

Future efforts will be directed to developing these methods for practical purposes. Studies of the mechanisms of irritant contact dermatitis on the cellular and biochemical level will reveal new aspects to this syndrome. Increasing knowledge about mediators[134,135] and cell interactions[136,137] will also help us to understand this multifactorial clinical problem.

Concomitant Disease

Generalized wasting and debilitation in patients with advanced carcinoma have been associated with decreased skin reactivity to croton oil and DNCB.[138] Decreased reactivity to croton oil[139] and increased susceptibility to alkali[110] were reported in patients with ichthyosis vulgaris. Other investigators noted increased reactivity to phenol[140] but decreased reactivity to croton oil[141] on the depigmented skin in patients with vitiligo. The literature on patch-test reactions to irritants in the presence of eczema is conflicting. This subject has been partly clarified by Bjornberg,[47] who showed that an increased susceptibility to irritants may be demonstrated in eczematous patients with some but not all irritants. Susceptibility to irritation has also been correlated with the extent of the eczema. Patients with localized hand eczema had increased reactivity to SLS; patients with generalized eczema had increased reactivity to four additional irritants (croton oil, trichloroacetic acid, mercury bichloride, and sapo kalinus). Bjornberg[142] further demonstrated that patients with healed hand eczema have no greater susceptibility to irritants than noneczematous controls. The type of eczema may also influence the response to irritants. Skog[112] showed an increased incidence of primary irritant reactions to pentadecylcatechol in patients with preexisting allergic contact eczema but not in patients with preexisting irritant eczema or atopic dermatitis. Although clinical observations have suggested that individuals with atopic dermatitis or atopic diathesis are more susceptible to skin irritation, experimental proof is lacking.

Neurologic Influence

Neurologic factors may influence cutaneous reactivity. Biberstein[143] reported an increased inflammatory response to mustard oil on sympathectomized ears in rabbits, compared with nonsympathectomized contralateral control ears. Others reported decreased reactivity to phenol in areas of peripheral paralysis but increased reactivity to phenol in areas of central paralysis,[144] decreased reactivity to tincture of iodine in areas of peripheral anesthesia,[145] and a generalized increase in reactivity in areas of peripheral neuritis.[141]

The nervous system is obviously involved in the subjective response to irritants. A specific somatosensory receptor, selectively stimulated by certain irritants (e.g., lacrimators), has been identified in cat skin.[146]

Medication

Corticosteriods in sufficient dose administered either topically or systemically may suppress subsequent irritant responses to croton oil,[147] but not to turpentine or cantharidin.[148] In general, there appears to be a limiting dose of systemically administered corticosteriod below which the inflammatory response is not inhibited. Although there is not universal agreement, the limiting dose appears to be in the range of 15 mg prednisone or equivalent.[149] Antihistamines in any dose probably do not impair responses to irritants. No data exist on the cutaneous response to irritants in patients with Addison's or Cushing's disease. Funk[150] has reviewed this area in depth.

PREDICTIVE IRRITANCY TESTING

Predictive irritancy testing involved specific tests for the irritant potential of individual chemicals as well as tests for individual susceptibility to irritation.

Predictive Testing for Chemical Irritant Potential

Predictive testing is widely performed to determine the irritant potential of various chemicals. The most popular methods are bioassays with human or animal subjects. Most procedures employ a single application of a test substance, with evaluation of the response in 24–48 h. The oldest of these assays is the Draize rabbit test, in which test substances are applied for 24 h under occlusion to abraded and nonabraded skin. While this procedure detects severe irritants for human skin, it is unsatisfactory for mild to moderate irritants.[151] Numerous modifications adaptable to special situations have been developed. The reader is referred to the National Research Council[152] special publication that discusses the principles and practices involved.

Because of species variability, correlation of irritancy studies of animal skin with human skin has not been entirely satisfactory. A rabbit cumulative irritancy test has been described that compared favorably with a cumulative human irritancy assay.[153,154]

Bioassays involving human subjects are patterned after those involving animal models. Frosch and Kligman[155] introduced a chamber scarification test, which enhanced the capacity to detect mild irritants. The forearm is scarified in a crisscross pattern; the suspected irritant is applied to this area in a large aluminum chamber once daily for 3 d.

To date, bioassays have utilized visible degrees of erythema and edema as indices of irritancy; this method is simple and convenient. The development of physical techniques for measuring subtle degrees of noninflammatory skin damage has improved our understanding of this area. Skin permeability to water vapor (transepidermal water loss) was the first physical measurement to be used for this purpose. Early investigations clearly established that chemicals that provoked inflammation increased transepidermal water loss.[156–158] Malten and Thiele[159] subsequently showed that increases in transepidermal water loss occurred before visible inflammation when ionic, polar, water-soluble substances (e.g., sodium hydroxide, soaps, detergents) were used as irritants. Malten and den Arend[29] showed that an unionized, polar irritant (DMSO) did not provoke increased water vapor loss until visible inflammation had already occurred. Similarly, two unionized nonpolar (water-insoluble) irritants, hexanediol diacrylate and butanediol diacrylate, did not provoke increased skin water vapor loss until visible inflammation occurred.[7] Thus, transpidermal water loss measurements may detect the irritant capacity of certain chemicals in the absence of visible inflammation, but possibly only for ionizable, polar, water-soluble substances.

Measurements of the electrical impedance (resistance) of human skin also detect subtle degrees of skin damage before skin inflammation occurs.[48] This method has an advantage over water loss measurements in that it is capable of detecting subtle changes produced by unionizable or nonpolar substances as well as ionizable, polar ones.[7]

Measurements of carbon dioxide emission from human skin have been developed.[159] Rates of carbon dioxide emission from irritated skin increase roughly in proportion to the degree of irritation.[160]

Electrolyte flux through the skin barrier may be measured with the aid of ion-specific skin electrodes.[55,161] Measurements of chloride ion flux through psoriatic or eczematous skin indicate that, despite the dramatic increases in permeability to water vapor, the electrolyte barrier remains relatively intact.[55] Chloride ion flux may provide another noninflammatory index of cutaneous irritation. A potassium ion electron has been of value in quantifying potassium flux post damage.[162]

Predictive Testing for Susceptibility to Irritation

The ability to predict which individuals are more prone to irritant skin reactions has practical significance as a preemployment screening test. The ability of the skin to neutralize solutions of sodium hydroxide was first proposed as a screening test for susceptibility to irritation by Gross et al.[163] Bjornberg[47] reviewed previous attempts to predict general susceptibility by determining irritant responses to selected irritants. He was unable to corroborate early claims that inability to neutralize alkaline solutions would decrease resistance to alkaline irritation, or that increased susceptibility to common experimental irritants could be used to predict susceptibility to irritations in a preemployment setting.

Frosch and Kligman[79] used the length of time to slight blister formation after experimental exposure to ammonium hydroxide as a predictive index. They found that short times were highly correlated with the intensity of inflammation produced by irritating concentrations of SLS. They also found that patients with atopic dermatitis (who were presumably more susceptible to irritation) had shorter times to blister formation than controls.[164]

IN VITRO ASSAYS

This rapidly developing areas has been reviewed by Rougier et al.[165]

HISTOLOGY, HISTOPATHOLOGY, AND PATHOLOGY

Contact dermatitis, eczema, and eczematous lesions are imprecise terms in dermatologic history. Irritant contact dermatitis cannot be characterized on the basis of histologic finding. The histology is different in acute and chronic contact dermatitis. The degree and severity of the dermatitis and the interval between the onset and the actual time of biopsy influence the histological findings. If the acute irritant or toxic skin reaction is strong, vesicles may be seen. In the vesicle, a mixture of neutrophils and lymphocytes is seen. In initial acute irritant contact dermatitis, dermal changes may be absent or minimal. Dermal infiltrates appear and increase during the first day of the developing dermatitis. The cell infiltrates in irritant and allergic contact dermatitis are not significantly or diagnostically different. In chronic irritant contact dermatitis, scaling, hyperkeratosis, and lichenification are apparent in older skin lesions, often resembling neurodermatitis.

In immunohistologic studies, identical composition of peripheral T lymphocytes, associated with peripheral HLA-DR (histocompatibility locus A) positive macrophages and Langerhans cells, is seen in irritant and allergic contact dermatitis.[166,167] In the lymphocyte population, helper/inducer lymphocytes exceed the number of T-suppression/cytotoxic cells.[166,168] In irritant contact dermatitis, keratinocytes have been demonstrated to express major histocompatibility complex (MHC) class II antigens concerned with the antigen presentation and the elicitaiton of the T-lymphocyte-dependent immune response.[137] These antigens were expressed by the keratinocytes in both allergic and irritant contact dermatitis.

The inflammatory cell response has also been characterized in guinea pigs treated with toxic croton oil application or repeated SLS applications. In both reactions monocyte counts were increased, even as compared with an allergic reaction. The heterogeneous monocyte group, however, consisted of lymphocytes, fibroblasts, and monocytes. Only a minority of basophils was seen, less than in allergic contact reactions. Mast cells were also slightly increased, suggesting some association between nonimmunologic contact urticaria and an acute irritant contact reaction.[169]

Irritants, such as surfactants, removed skin lipids and keratins. The mechanisms of inflammation in the development of irritant contact dermatitis are still poorly understood. In laboratory animals, the importance of the function and inflammation mediators of different cell types is appreciated, and certain preliminary observations have been reported in constructed experimental designs. For example, SLS and alkyl dimethyl benzammonium chloride (ADBC) were shown to enhance the migration of polymorphonuclear leukocytes. A corresponding inhibition was induced by leukotriene B4; that is, SLS and ADBC also induced the secretion of preformed mediators, such as histamine and lysozymal and enzyme beta-G from the cells.[136] Wide variation in the inhibitory response was documented for cutaneous inflammation elicited by different irritants, whether induction was by histamine antagonists, prostaglandin and kinin synthesis inhibitors, or by neutropenia-inducing agents.[170]

The importance of leukotrienes in irritant contact dermatitis appears evident,[135] and a peptido-leukotriene antagonist and an antagonist of platelet-activating factor (PAF) were documented to be less effective in irritant contact dermatitis than in the allergic type, suggesting that cytotoxic effects predominate in irritant contact dermatitis.[134]

A corresponding interpretation was made based on the observation that lipoxygenesis pathway is enhanced in irritant contact dermatitis, being inhibited in allergic contact dermatitis.[171]

Ulcerations

Ulcerative lesions can develop from skin contact with strong acids or strong alkalies. Calcium oxide and calcium hydroxide, sodium hydroxide, sodium metasilicate and sodium silicate, potassium cyanide, and trisodium phosphate may induce strong cutaneous irritation with ulcerations. Chrome ulcers are the most common type of cutaneous ulcers induced by irritant action of dichromates. Compounds of beryllium, arsenic, or cadmium are also capable of inducing strong irritation and ulcers.

Solvents such as acrylonitrile and carbon bisulfide as well as gaseous ethylene oxide are examples of contactants that may induce ulceration in certain occupations. Cutaneous ulcerations develop from the direct corrosive and necrotizing effect of the chemical on the living tissue. Exposed areas, where both friction and chemical irritation are associated, are most susceptible for ulcers; minor preceding trauma in the exposed skin increases the risk. The ulcerations tend to be deeper, with an undermined thickened border, and the exudate under the covering crusts predisposes to infection. The treatment for ulcers is usually conservation, with dressings, powders, and different coverings according to the phase of healing. In some cases, such as beryllium ulcerations, excision has been recommended.

Granulomas

Cutaneous granulomas are considered a variant of irritant contact dermatitis when caused by a biologically inactive substance inoculated into the skin. A granuloma appears as a focal, tumid lesion persisting chronically in its primary site. It is subjectively symptomless. Macrophages respond with phagocytosis to the foreign body inoculation, and even giant cells may be seen.[172]

In clinical occupational dermatitis, the development is generally due to an accidental foreign body inoculation of hard and sharp plant parts, hairs, or different hard keratin animal parts into the skin of the employee. Powders, lead, and metal such as metallic mercury, beryllium, and silica are examples of substances that elicit toxic skin granulomas.[173] Infectious granulomas may be caused by deep fungi, bacteria, or parasites. In these cases, inflammation and macrophage response, with phagocytic secretory and mixed function macrophages, are seen.

The examining occupational dermatologist should keep the possibility of irritation granuloma in mind when studying and performing biopsy on this type of lesion; the dermatologist should remind the histopathologist to utilize the special maneuvers needed to demonstrate possible foreign bodies. Special stains, electron microscopy, and the use of polarized light are often useful.[174]

Hardening

Extensive and repeated exposure often produces an increased resistance to further irritation in the course of weeks or months. The importance of interindividual variation in the development of hardening may be even greater than the threshold level for cutaneous irritation, since the individual capacity to recover from previous attacks is a factor. The developed resistance or hardening is specific to the substance inducing it. It is restricted to the affected skin area; also, certain subjects appear to be unable to develop hardening. Relatively short periods away from work decrease the resistance, again increasing the vulnerability for irritant contact dermatitis after holidays. The "hardened" skin appears coarse, thickened, and somewhat lichenified. Increased skin thickness may play a role in the development of hardening. Skin thickening was evident in the experimental "hardening" state in guinea pigs.[175] Unfortunately, the main biologic mechanisms are unknown.

Repeated UV exposures also increase the capacity to resist irritation in the skin. This effect appears to be nonspecific.[176] Repeated UV exposures are therapeutic, followed by a period of "hardening" in the treatment of subacute or chronic irritant contact dermatitis. When the acute phase of an irritant contact dermatitis is over and relapses are expected, repeated UV exposures

Table 7. Clinical Features That May Suggest the Etiology of Irritant Contact Dermatitis

Ulcerations
  Strong acids, especially chromic, hydrofluoric, nitric, hydrochloric, sulfuric
  Strong alkalis, especially calcium oxide, sodium hydroxide, potassium hydroxide, ammonium hydroxide,
    calcium hydroxide, sodium metasilicate, sodium silicate, potassium cyanide, trisodium phosphate
  Salts, especially arsenic trioxide, dichromates
  Solvents, especially acrylonitrile, carbon disulfide
  Gases, especially ethylene oxide, acrylonitrile
Folliculitis and acneiform
  Arsenic trioxide
  Glass fibers
  Oils and greases
  Tar
  Asphalt
  Chlorinated naphthalenes
  Polyhalogenated biphenyls and others
Miliaria
  Occlusive clothing and dressing
  Adhesive tape
  Ultraviolet
  Infrared
  Aluminum chloride
Pigmentary alterations
  Hyperpigmentation
  Any irritant or allergen, especially phototoxic agents such as psoralens, tar, asphalt, phototoxic plants, others
  Metals, such as inorganic arsenic (systemically), silver, gold, bismuth, mercury
  Radiation: ultraviolet, infrared, microwave, ionizing
  Hypopigmentation
  p-tert-Amylphenol
  p-tert-Butylphenol
  Hydroquinone
  Monobenzyl ethyl hydroquinone
  Monomethyl hydroquinone ether
  p-tert-Catechol
  p-Cresol 3-hydroxyanisole
  Butylated hydroxyanisole
  1-tert-Butyl-3,4-catechol
  1-Isopropyl-3,4-catechol
  4-Hydroxypropriophenone
Alopecia
  Borax
  Chloroprene dimers
Urticaria
  Numerous chemicals, cosmetics, animal products, foods, plants, textile, woods
Granulomas
  Keratin
  Silica
  Beryllium
  Talc
  Cotton fibers
  Bacteria
  Fungi
  Parasites and parasite parts

Table 8. Major Industrial Uses for Fibrous Glass

Insulation
Weatherproofing
Plastic reinforcement: laminates with polyesters, epoxy, polyurethanes, and other resins
Filtration media
Structural materials
Textiles

may elicit nonspecific "desensitization" in the skin, increasing the capacity to avoid relapses. Alterations at the cellular level, in cell surface proteins, and in the releasability of inflammatory mediators probably are important in the therapeutic benefit achieved by UV therapies of irritant contact dermatitis.

SUMMARY OF CLINICAL ASPECTS

The clinical appearance of irritant contact dermatitis is dependent on multiple factors. Some clinical features that may suggest the etiology are listed in Table 7. Fibrous glass is one of the most common causes of occupational contact dermatitis, and dermatitis elicited by fibrous glass appears variable depending on individual characteristics, exposure, and mechanisms. Table 8 showed the major industrial uses for fibrous glass.

The diagnosis of irritant contact dermatitis is always clinical, and patch testing is done to exclude allergic contact dermatitis. Hardening against certain irritants may sometimes develop.

GENERAL READING

Elsner, P., and Maibach, H. I., eds. 1995. *Irritant dermatitis syndrome.* New York: Karger.
Menne, T., and Maibach, H. I., eds. 1994. *Hand eczema.* Boca Raton, FL: CRC Press.
Van der Valk, P., and Maibach, H. I. eds. 1995. *Irritant dermatitis.* Boca Raton, FL: CRC Press.

REFERENCES

1. Bason, M., Lammintausta, K., and Maibach, H. 1991. Irritant dermatitis (irritation). In *Dermatotoxicology,* eds. F. Marzulli and H. I. Maibach, Chap. 11. New York: Hemisphere.
2. Elsner, P., Berardesca, E., and Maibach, H., eds. *Bioengineering of the skin: Water and the stratum corneum.* Boca Raton, FL: CRC Press.
3. van der Valk, P. G. M., and Maibach, H. I., eds. 1995. *Irritant dermatitis.* Boca Raton, FL: CRC Press.
4. Fregert, S. F. 1981. Irritant contact dermatitis. In *Manual of contact dermatitis,* 2nd ed., ed. S. F. Fregert, pp. 55–62. Copenhagen: Munksgaard.
5. Griffiths, W. A. D., and Wilkinson, D. S. 1985. Primary irritants and solvents. In *Essentials of industrial dermatology,* eds. W. D. Griffiths and D. S. Wilkinson, pp. 58–72. Oxford: Blackwell Scientific.
6. Hjorth, N., and Avnstorp, C. 1986. Rehabilitation in hand eczema. *Derm. Beruf. Unwelt.* 34:74–76.
7. Malten, K. E., den Arend, J., and Wiggers, R. E. 1979. Delayed irritation: Hexanediol diacrylate and butanediol diacrylate. *Contact Dermatitis* 5:178–184.
8. Lovell, C. R., Rycroft, R. C. G., Williams, D. M. J. 1985. Contact dermatitis from the irritancy (immediate and delayed) and allergenicity of hydroxy acrylate. *Contact Dermatitis* 12:117–118.
9. Feldmann, R. J., and Maibach, H. I. 1974. Systemic absorption of pesticides through the skin of man. Occupational Exposure to Pesticides: Report to the Federal Working Group on Pest Management from the Task Group on Occupational Exposure to Pesticides, Appendix B, pp. 120–127 Washington, DC: U.S. Government Printing Office.
10. Britz, M. B., and Maibach, H. I. 1979. Human cutaneous vulvar reactivity to irritants. *Contact Dermatitis* 5:375–377.
11. von Hagerman, G. 1975. Uber das "traumiterative" (toxische) Ekzem. *Dermatologica* 115:525–529.
12. Agrup, G. 1969. Hand eczema and other dermatoses in South Sweden. (Thesis.) *Acta Dermatol. Venereol. I Suppl. (Stockh.)* 49:61.
13. Wahlberg, J. E., and Maibach, H. I. 1982. Identification of contact pustulogens. In *Dermatotoxicology,* 2nd ed., eds. F. N. Marzulli and H. I. Maibach, pp. 627–635. New York: Hemisphere.
14. Dooms-Goossens, E., Delusschene, K. M., Gevers, D. M. 1986. Contact dermatitis caused by airborne irritant. *J. Am. Acad. Dermatol.* 15:1–10.

15. Fischer, T., and Rystedt, I. 1985. False positive, follicular and irritants patch test reactions to metal salts. *Contact Dermatitis* 12:93–98.
16. Berardesca, E., and Maibach, H. I., Racial differences in sodium lauryl sulphate induced cutaneous irritation: Black and white. *Contact Dermatitis* 18:65–70.
17. van der Valk, P. G. M., Nater, J. P. K., and Bleumink, E. Vulnerability of the skin to surfactants in different groups in eczema patients and controls as measured by water vapour loss. *Clin. Exp. Dermatol.* 101:98.
18. Lammintausta, K., Maibach, H. I., and Wilson, D. 1988. Mechanisms of subjective (sensory) irritation propensity to nonimmunologic contact urticaria and objective irritation in stingers. *Dermatosen Beruf. Umwelt.* 36:45–49.
19. Frosch, P. J., and Kligman, A. M. 1982. Recognition of chemically vulnerable and delicate skin. In *Principles of cosmetics for dermatologists,* pp. 287–296. St. Louis, MO: C. V. Mosby.
20. Lahti, A., and Maibach, H. I. 1985. Guinea pig ear swelling test as an animal model for nonimmunologic contact urticaria. In *Models in dermatology,* vol. II, eds. H. I. Maibach and N. I. Lowe, pp. 356–259. New York: Karger.
21. Berardesca, E., Cespa, M., Farinelli, N., Rabbiosi, G., and Maibach, H. 1991. In vivo transcutaneous penetration of nicotinates and sensitive skin. *Contact Dermatitis* 25(1):35–38.
22. Feldmann, R. J., and Maibach, H. I. 1967. Regional variations in percutaneous absorption of C-cortisol in man. *J. Invest. Dermatol.* 48:181–183.
23. Kligman, A. M., and Wooding, W. A. 1967. A method for the measurement and evaluation of irritants on human skin. *J. Invest. Dermatol.* 49:78–94.
24. Rothenborg, H. W., Menne, T., and Sjolin, K. E. 1977. Temperature dependent primary irritant dermatitis from lemon perfume. *Contact Dermatitis* 1:37–48.
25. Cooper, E. R. 1985. Vehicle effects on skin penetration. In *Percutaneous absorption,* eds. H. I. Maibach and R. L. Bronaugh, pp. 525–530. New York: Marcel Dekker.
26. Gummer, C. L. 1985. Vehicles as penetration enhancers. In *Percutaneous absorption,* eds. H. I. Maibach and R. L. Bronaugh, pp. 561–570. New York: Marcel Dekker.
27. Smith, E., and Maibach, H. 1995. *Percutaneous penetration enhancers.* Boca Raton, FL: CRC Press.
28. Flannigan, S. A., and Tucker, S. B. 1985. Influence of the vehicle on irritant contact dermatitis. *Contact Dermatitis* 12:177–178.
29. Malten, K. E., and den Arend, J. 1978. Topical toxicity of various concentrations of DMSO recorded with impedance measurements and water vapour loss measurements. *Contact Dermatitis* 4:80–92.
30. Lammintausta, K., Maibach, H. I., and Wilson, D. 1988. Susceptibility to cumulative and acute irritant dermatitis. An experimental approach in human volunteers. *Contact Dermatitis* 19:84–90.
31. Malten, K. E. 1981. Thoughts on irritant contact dermatitis. *Contact Dermatitis* 7:238–247.
32. Patil, S. M., Singh, P., and Maibach, H. I. 1994. Cumulative irritancy to sodium lauryl sulfate: The overlap phenomenon. *Int. J. Pharm.* 110:147–154.
33. Patil, S. M., Singh, P., and Maibach, H. I. 1995. Quantification of sodium lauryl sulfate (SLS) penetration into the skin and underlying tissues after topical application—Pharmacological and toxicological implications. *J. Pharm. Science* 84:1240–1244.
34. Patil, S. M., Singh, P., and Maibach, H. I. 1995. Radical spread of sodium lauryl sulfate below a topically applied site. *Pharmaceutical Research* 12:2018–2023.
35. Lammintausta, K., Maibach, H. I. and Wilson, D. 1987. Human cutaneous irritation: Induced hyperreactivity. *Contact Dermatitis* 17:193–198.
36. Pittz, E. P., Smorbeck, R. V., and Rieger, M. M. 1985. An animal test procedure for the simultaneous assessment of irritancy and efficacy of skin care products. In *Models in dermatology,* eds. H. I. Maibach and N. J. Lowe, vol. II, pp. 209–224. New York: Karger.
37. Susten, A. S. 1985. The chronic effects of mechanical trauma to the skin: A review of the literature. *Am. J. Intern. Med.* 18:281–288.
38. Hannuksela, M., Pirila, V., and Salo, O. P. 1975. Skin reactions to propylene glycol. *Contact Dermatitis* 1:112–116.
39. Rycroft, R. J. G. 1981. Occupational dermatoses from warm dry air. *Br. J. Dermatol.* 105(Suppl.)(21):29–34.
40. Agner, T., and Serup, J. 1989. Seasonal variation of skin resistance to irritants. *Br. J. Dermatol.* 121:323–328.
41. Lachapelle, J. M. 1986. Industrial airborne irritant or allergic contact dermatitis. *Contact Dermatitis* 14:137–145.
42. Jambor, J. J. 1955. Etiologic appraisal of hand dermatitis. *J. Invest. Dermatol.* 24:387–392.
43. Bettley, F. R. 1960. Some effects of soap on the skin. *Br. Med. J.* 1:1675–1679.
44. Suskind, R. R. Meister, M. M., Scheen, S. R. 1963. Cutaneous effects of household synthetic detergents and soaps. *Arch. Dermatol.* 88:117–124.

45. Stoughton, R. B., Potts, L. W., Clendenning, W. 1969. Management of patients with eczematous diseases: Use of soap vs. no soap. *J. Am. Med. Assoc.* 175:1196–1198.
46. White, M. I., Jenkinson, D. M., and Lloyd, D. H. 1987. The effect of washing on the thickness of the stratum corneum in normal and atopic individuals. *Br. J. Dermatol.* 116:525–530.
47. Bjornberg, A. 1968. Skin Reactions to Primary Irritants in Patients with Hand Eczema. Thesis. Gothenburg, Sweden: Oscar Isacsons Tryckeri AB.
48. Thiele, F. A. J., and Malten, K. E. 1973. Evaluation of skin damage I. Skin resistance measurements with alternative current impedance measurements. *Br. J. Dermatol.* 89:373–382.
49. Maibach, H. I., Bronaugh, R., Guy, R. 1984. Noninvasive techniques for determining skin function. In *Cutaneous Toxicity,* eds. V. A. Drill and P. Lazar, pp. 63–97. New York: Raven Press.
50. Tagami, H., Masatoshi, O., Iwatsuki, K. 1980. Evaluation of the skin surface hydration in vivo by electrical measurements. *J. Invest. Dermatol.* 75:500–507.
51. Guy, R. H., Tur, E., and Maibach, H. I. 1985. Optical techniques for monitoring cutaneous microcirculation. *Int. J. Dermatol.* 2:88–94.
52. Maibach, H. I., Feldmann, R. J., Millby, T. H. 1971. Regional variation in percutaneous penetration in man. Pesticides. *Arch Environ. Health* 23:208–294.
53. Grice, K., Sattar, H., and Baker, H. 1973. The cutaneous barrier to salts and water in psoriasis and in normal skin. *Br. J. Dermatol.* 88:459–463.
54. Frame, G. W., Strauss, W. G., and Maibach, H. I. 1972. Carbon dioxide emission of the human arm and hand. *J. Invest. Dermatol.* 59:155–158.
55. Grice, K., Sattar, H., Casey, T., and Baker, H. 1975. An evaluation of Na^+, Cl, and pH ion-specific electrodes in the study of the electrolyte contents of epidermal transudate and sweat. *Br. J. Dermatol.* 92:511–518.
56. Berardesca, E., Elsner, P., and Maibach, H., eds. 1994. *Bioengineering of the skin. Cutaneous blood flow and erythema.* Boca Raton, FL: CRC Press.
57. Serup, J., and Jemec, G. B. E. 1995. Noninvasive techniques for assessments of skin penetration and bioavailability. In *Handbook of non-invasive methods and the skin,* pp. 201–205. Boca Raton, FL: CRC Press.
58. Ummenhofer, B. 1980. Zum Methodik der Alkaliresistenzprufung. *Dermatosen Beruf. Umwelt.* 28:104.
59. Wilhelm, K. P., Pasche, F., Surber, C., and Maibach, H. 1990. Sodium hydroxide-induced subclinical irritation—A test for evaluating stratum corneum barrier function. *Acta Dermato-Venereol.* 70:463–467.
60. Frosche, P. J. 1985. Hautirritation und empfindliche Haut, pp. 1–118. Thesis. Grosse Scripta 7. Berlin: Grosse Verlag.
61. Cronin, E., and Stroughton, R. B. L. 1962. Percutaneous absorption: Regional variations and the effect of hydration and epidermal stripping. *Br. J. Dermatol.* 74:7265–7272.
62. Wester, R. C., and Maibach, H. I. 1985. Dermatopharmocokinetics. In *Clinical dermatology in percutaneous absorption,* eds. H. I. Maibach and R. L. Bronaugh, pp. 525–530. New York: Marcel Dekker.
63. Wester, R. C., and Maibach, H. I. 1989. Regional variation in percutaneous absorption. In *Percutaneous absorption,* eds. R. L. Bronaugh and H. I. Maibach, pp. 111–119. New York: Marcel Dekker.
64. Tur, E., Maibach, H. I., and Guy, R. H. 1985. Spatial variability of vasodilatation in human forearm skin. *Br. J. Dermatol.* 113:197–303.
65. Magnusson, B., and Hersle, K. 1965. Patch test methods: II. Regional variation of patch test responses. *Acta Derm. Venereol. (Stockh.)* 45:226–257.
66. Flannigan, S. A., Smith, R. E., and McGovern, J. P. 1984. Intraregional variation between contact irritant patch test sites. *Contact Dermatitis* 10:123–124.
67. von Hornstein, O. P., and Kienlein-Kletschka, B. M. 1982. Improvement of patch test allergen exposure by short-term local pressure. *Dermatologica* 165:607–611.
68. Gollhausen, R., and Kligman, A. M. 1985. Effects of pressure on contact dermatitis. *Am. J. Ind. Med.* 8:223–328.
69. Oriba, H. A., Elsner, P., and Maibach, H. I. 1989. Vulvar physiology. *Semin. Dermatol.* 8:2–6.
70. Jordan, W. E., and Blaney, T. L. 1982. Factors influencing infant diaper dermatitis. In *Neonatal skin,* eds. H. I. Maibach and E. K. Boisits, pp. 205–221. New York: Marcel Dekker.
71. Seymour, J. L., Keswich, B. H., Hanifin, J. M., et al. 1987. Clinical effects of diaper types on the skin of normal infants and infants with atopic dermatitis. *J. Am. Acad. Dermatol.* 17:988–997.
72. Mobly, S. L., and Mansmann, H. C. 1974. Current status of skin testing in children with contact dermatitis. *Cutis* 13:995–1000.
73. Epstein, E. 1971. Contact dermatitis in children. *Pediatr. Clin. North Am.* 18:839–852.
74. Fisher, A. A. 1975. Childhood allergic contact dermatitis. *Cutis* 15:635–645.
75. Maibach, H. I., and Boisits, E. K., eds. 1982. *Neonatal skin: Structure and function:* New York: Marcel Dekker.
76. Beauregaard, S., and Gilchrest, B. A. 1987. A survey of skin problems and skin care regimens in the elderly. *Arch. Dermatol.* 123:1638–1643.

77. Lehman, E., Stoudemayer, T., Grove, G. 1984. Age differences in poison ivy dermatitis. *Contact Dermatitis* 11:163–167.

78. Grove, G. L., Lavker, R. M., Hoelzle, E.1981. Use of nonintrusive tests to monitor age-associated changes in human skin. *J. Soc. Cosmet. Chem.* 32:15–26.

79. Frosche, P. J., and Kligman, A. M. 1977. Rapid blister formation in human skin with ammonium hydroxide. *Br. J. Dermatol.* 96:461–473.

80. Kligman, A. M. 1976. Perspectives and problems in cutaneous gerontology. *J. Invest. Dermatol.* 73:39–46.

81. Roskos, K. V., and Maibach, H. 1992. percutaneous absorption and age: Implications for therapy. *Drugs Aging 2* 5:432–449.

82. Christophers, E., and Kligman, A. M. 1965. Percutaneous absorption in age skin. In *Advances in the biology of the skin,* ed. E. Montagna, pp. 160–179. Oxford: Pergamon Press.

83. Tanami, H. 1971. Functional characteristics of aged skin. *Acta Derm. Venereol. (Stockh.)* 66:19–21.

84. DeSalva, S. J., and Thompson, G. 1965. $Na^{22}Cl$ skin clearance in humans and its relation to skin age. *J. Invest. Dermatol.* 45:315–318.

85. Guy, R. H., Tur, E., Bjerke, S. 1985. Are there age and racial differences in methyl nicotinate-induced vasodilatation in human skin? *J. Am. Acad. Dermatol.* 12:1001–1006.

86. Elias, P. M. 1981. Lipids and the epidermal permeability barrier. *Arch. Dermatol. Res.* 270:95–117.

87. Gilchrest, B. A., Murphy, G. F., and Sotter, N. A. 1982. Effects of chronologic aging and ultraviolet irradiation on Langerhans cells in human skin. *J. Invest. Dermatol.* 79:85–88.

88. Roberts, D., and Marks, R. 1980. The determination of regional and age variations in the rate of desquamation: A comparison of four techniques. *J. Invest. Dermatol.* 74:13–16.

89. Baker, H., and Blair, C. P. 1968. Cell replacement in the human stratum corneum in old age. *Br. J. Dermatol.* 80:367–372.

90. Montaga, W., and Carlisle, K. 1979. Structural changes in aging human skin. *J. Invest. Dermatol.* 73:47–53.

91. Holzle, E., Plewig, G., and Ledolter, A. 1986. Corneocyte exfoliative cytology: A model to study normal and diseased stratum corneum. In *Skin models,* eds. R. Marks and G. Plewig, pp. 183–193. New York: Springer Verlag.

92. Weigand, D. A., and Gaylor, J. R. 1974. Irritant reaction Negro and Caucasian skin. *South. Med. J.* 67:548–551.

93. Anderson, K. E., and Maibach, H. I. 1979. Black and white human skin differences. *J. Am. Acad. Dermatol.* 1:276–282.

94. Johnson, L. C., and Corah, N. L. 1960. Racial skin differences in skin resistance. *Science* 139:776–767.

95. Weigand, D. A., Haygood, C., and Gaylor, J. R. 1974. Cell layers and density in Negro and Caucasian stratum corneum. *J. Invest. Dermatol.* 62:563–568.

96. Buckley, C. E. III, Lee, K. L., and Burdick, D. S. 1982. Metacholine-induced cutaneous flare response: Bivariate analysis of responsiveness and sensitivity. *J. Allergy Clin. Immunol.* 69:25–64.

97. Buckley, C. E. III, Larrick, J. W., and Kaplan, J. E. 1985. Population differences in cutaneous metacholine reactivity and circulating IgE concentrations. *J. Allergy Clin. Immunol.* 76:847–854.

98. Rystedt, I. 1985. Factors influencing the occurrence of hand eczema in adults with a history of atopic dermatitis in childhood. *Contact Dermatitis* 12:247–254.

99. Lantinga, H., Nater, J. P., and Coenraads, P. J. 1984. Prevalence, incidence and course of eczema on the hand and forearm in a sample of the general population. *Contact Dermatitis* 10:135–139.

100. Wagner, G., and Porschel, W. 1962. Klinisch-analytische studie zum neurodermatitisproblem. *Dermatologica* 125:1–32.

101. Magnusson, B., and Hillgren, L. 1962. Skin irritating and adhesive characteristics of some different adhesive tapes. *Acta Derm. Venereol. (Stockh.)* 42:463–472.

102. Bjornberg, A. 1975. Skin reactions to primary irritants in men and women. *Acta. Derm. Venereol. (Stockh.)* 55:191–194.

103. Lammintausta, K., Maibach, H. I., and Wilson, D. 1987b. Irritant reactivity in males and females. *Contact Dermatitis* 17:276–280.

104. Olumide, G. 1987. Contact dermatitis in Nigeria. II. Hand dermatitis in men. *Contact Dermatitis* 17:136–138.

105. Holst, R., and Moller, H. 1975. One hundred twin pairs tested with primary irritants. *Br. J. Dermatol. Res.* 93:145–149.

106. Frosche, P. J., and Wissing, C. 1982. Cutaneous sensitivity to ultraviolet light and chemical irritants. *Arch. Dermatol. Res.* 272:269–278.

107. Maurice, P. D. L., and Greaves, M. W. 1983. Relationship between skin type and erythema response to anthralin. *Br. J. Dermatol.* 109:337–341.

108. Cerwinska-Ditram, I., and Rudzki, E. 1986. Skin reactions to primary irritants. *Contact Dermatitis.* 7:315–319.

109. Hanifin, J. M., and Rajka, G. 1980. Diagnostic features of atopic dermatitis. *Acta Derm. Venereol. Suppl. (Stockh.)* 92:44–47.

110. Ziierz, P., Kiessling, W., and Berg, A. 1960. Experimentelle Prufung der Hautfunktion bei Ichthyosis Vulgaris. *Arch. Klin. Exp. Dermatol.* 209:592.

111. Hanifin, J. M., and Lobitz, W. C. 1977. Newer concepts of atopic dermatitis. *Arch. Dermatol.* 113:663–670.

112. Skog, E. 1960. Primary irritant and allergic eczematous reactions in patients with different dermatoses. *Acta Derm. Venereol. (Stockh.)* 40:307.

113. Rajka, G. 1975. The aetiology of atopic dermatitis. In *Atopic dermatitis,* ed. G. Rajka, pp. 43–104. Philadelphia: W. B. Saunders.

114. Werner, Y., Lindberg, M., and Forslind, B. 1982. The water binding capacity of stratum corneum in dry non-eczematous skin of atopic eczema. *Acta Derm. Venereol. (Stockh.)* 62:334–336.

115. Finlay, A. Y., Nocholls, S., King, C. S. 1980. The "dry" non-eczematous skin associated with atopic eczema. *Br. J. Dermatol.* 102:249–256.

116. Al Jaber, H., and Marks, R. 1984. Studies of the clinically uninvolved skin in patients with dermatitis. *Br. J. Dermatol.* 111:437–443.

117. Gloor, M., Heyman, B., and Stuhlert, T. 1981. Infrared spectroscopic determination of water content of the horny layer in healthy subjects and in patients suffering from atopic dermatitis. *Arch. Dermatol. Res.* 271:429–458.

118. Lammintaussta, K., and Kalimo, K. 1981. Atopy and hand dermatitis in hospital wet work. *Contact Dermatitis.* 7:301–308.

119. Vickers, H. R. 1962. The influence of age on the onset of dermatitis in industry. *Prague, Symp. Dermatologorum de Morbis Cutaneis,* pp. 145–148.

120. Holland, B. D. 1958. Occupational dermatoses—Predisposing and direct causes. *J. Am. Med. Assoc.* 167:2203–2205.

121. von Hornstein, O. P., Baurle, G., and Kienlein-Kletschka, B. M. 1986. Prospektiv-Studie zur bedeutung konstitutioneller Parameter fur die Ekzemgenese im Friseur und Baugewerbe. *Dermatosen Beruf. Umwelt.* 33:43–498.

122. Kingston, T., and Marks, R. 1983. Irritant reactions to dithranol in normal subjects and in psoriatic patients. *Br. J. Dermatol.* 108:307–313.

123. Lawrence, C. M., Howel, C., and Schester, S. 1984. The inflammatory response to anthralin. *Clin. Exp. Dermatol.* 9:336.

124. MacDonalds, K. J. S., and Marks, J. 1986. Short contact anthralin in the treatment of psoriasis: A study of different contact times. *Br. J. Dermatol.* 114:235–239.

125. Epstein, E., and Maibach, H. I. 1985. Eczematous psoriasis: What is it? In *Psoriasis,* eds. H. H. Roenigk, Jr., and H. I. Maibach, pp. 9–14. New York: Marcel Dekker.

126. Mitchell, J. C. 1981. Angry back syndrome. *Contact Dermatitis* 7:359–360.

127. Bruynzeel, D. P., van Ketel, W. G., and Scheper, R. J. 1983. Angry back or the excited skin syndrome: A prospective study. *J. Am. Acad. Dermatol.* 8:392–397.

128. Bruynzeel, D. P., and Maibach, H. I. 1986. Excited skin syndrome (angry back). *Arch. Dermatol.* 12:323–328.

129. Nilsson, E., Mikaelsson, B., and Andersson, S. 1985. Atopy, occupation and domestic work as risk factors for hand eczema in hospital workers. *Contact Dermatitis* 13:216–223.

130. Lee, C. H., and Maibach, H. I. 1995. SLS—An overview. *Contact Dermatitis* 33:1–71.

131. van der Valk, P. G. M., Nater, J. P., and Bleumink, E. 1984. Skin irritancy of surfactants as assessed by water vapour loss measurements. *J. Invest. Dermatol.* 89:291.

132. Elsner, P., and Maibach, H. I., eds. 1995. *Irritant dermatitis syndrome.* New York: Kargen.

133. Blanker, R., van der Valk, P. G. M., and Nater, J. P. 1986. Laser Doppler flowmetry in the investigation of irritant compounds on human skin. *Dermatosen* 34:5.

134. Csato, M., and Czarnetzki, B. M. 1988. Effect of BN 52021, a platelet activating factor antagonist, on experimental murine contact dermatitis. *Br. J. Dermatol.* 118:475–480.

135. Rosenbach, T., Csato, M., and Czarnetzki, B. M. 1988. Studies on the role of leukotrienes in murine allergic and irritant contact dermatitis. *Br. J. Dermatol.* 18:1–6.

136. Frosch, P. J., and Czarnetzki, B. M. 1987. Surfactants cause in vitro chemotaxis and chemokinesis of human neutrophils. *J. Invest. Dermatol.* 88:525–555.

137. Gawkrodger, D. J., Carr, M. M., McVittie, E. 1987. Keratinocyte expression of MCH class III antigens in allergic sensitization and challenge reactions and in irritant contact dermatitis. *J. Invest. Dermatol.* 88:11–20.

138. Johnson, M. A., Maibach, H. I. and Salmon, S. E. 1971. Skin reactivity in patients with cancer-impaired delayed hypersensitivity of faulty inflammatory response. *N. Engl. J. Med.* 284:1255.

139. Weidenfeld, S. 1912. Beitrage zur Pathogenese des Ekzems. *Arch. Dermatol. Syph. II* 1:891. Cited on p. 21 in Bjornberg.[47]

140. Schultz, I. H. 1912. Beitrag zum klinischen Studium und der quantatitiven Pruefung der Hautreaktion auf chemische Reize. I. Mitteilung: Ueber das Verhalten normaler und leukopathischer Hautstellen Hautkranker und Hautreaktion bei peripheren und zentralen Lahmungen. *Arch. Dermatol. Syph.* 13:987. Cited on p. 21 in Bjornberg.[47]

141. Halter, K. 1941. Zur Pathogenese des Ekzems. *Arch. Dermatol. Syph.* 181:593. Cited on p. 21 in Bjornberg.[47]

142. Bjornberg, Al 1974. Skin reactions to primary irritants and predisposition to eczema. *Br. J. Dermatol.* 91:425.

143. Biberstein, H. 1940. The effects of unilateral cervical sympathectomy on reactions of the skin. *J. Invest. Dermatol.* 3:201.

144. Schaefer, W. 1921. Beitrage zum klinischen Studium und der quantatitiven Prufung der Hautreaktion auf chemische Reize. II. Uberdie chemische Hautreaktion bei Peripheren und zentralen Lahmungen. *Arch. Dermatol. Syph.* 132:87. Cited in Bjornberg.[47]

145. Kaufman, A. M., and Winkel, M. 1922. Entzuendung und Nervensystem. *Klin. Wochenschr.* 1:12.

146. Foster, R. W., and Ramaze, A. G. 1976. Evidence for a specific somatosensory receptor in the cat skin that responds to irritant chemicals. *Br. J. Pharmacol.* 57:436.

147. Nilzen, A., and Wikstrom, K. 1955. Factors influencing the skin reaction in guinea pigs sensitized with 2,4-dinitrochlorobenzene. *Acta Derm. Venereol. (Stockh.)* 35:415.

148. Goldman, L., Preston, R., and Rockwell, E. 1952. The local effect of 17-hydroxycorticosterone-21-acetate (compound F) on the diagnostic patch test reaction. *J. Invest. Dermatol.* 18:89.

149. Feuerman, E., and Levy, A. 1972. A study of the effect of prednisone and an antihistamine on patch test reactions. *Br. J. Dermatol.* 86:68.

150. Funk, J. O., and Maibach, H. I. 1994. Horizons in pharmacologic intervention in allergic contact dermatitis. *J. Am. Acad. Dermatol.* 31:999–1014.

151. Phillips, L., Steinberg, M., Maibach, H. I., and Akers, W. A. 1972. A comparison of rabbit and human skin responses to certain irritants. *Toxicol. Appl. Pharmacol.* 21:369.

152. National Research Council. 1977. *Principles and procedures for evaluating the toxicity of household substances.* Washington, DC: National Academy of Sciences.

153. Marzulli, F. N., and Maibach, H. I. 1975. The rabbit as a model for evaluating skin irritants: A comparison of results in animals and man using repeated skin exposures. *Food Cosmet. Toxicol.* 13:533.

154. Steinberg, M., Akers, W. A., Weeks, M., McCreesh, A. H., and Maibach, H. I. 1975. A comparison of test techniques based on rabbit and human skin responses to irritants with recommendations regarding the evaluation of mildly or moderately irritating compounds. In *Animal models in dermatology,* ed. H. I. Maibach, pp. 1–11. New York: Churchill Livingstone.

155. Frosche, P. J., and Kligman, A. M. 1977. The chamber scarification test for assessing irritancy of topically applied substances. In *Cutaneous toxicity,* eds. V. A. Drill and P. Lazar, p. 150. New York: Academic Press.

156. Rollins, T. G. 1978. From xerosis to nummular dermatitis: The dehydration dermatosis. *J. Am. Med. Assoc.* 206:637.

157. Spruit, D. 1970. Evaluation of skin function by the alkali application technique. *Curr. Probl. Dermatol.* 3:148.

158. Spruit, D. 1971. Interference of some substances with water vapor loss of human skin. *Am. Perfum. Cosmet.* 8:27.

159. Malten, K. E., and Thiele, F. A. J. 1973. Evaluation of skin damage. II. Water loss and carbon dioxide release measurements related to skin resistance measurements. *Br. J. Dermatol.* 89:565.

160. Thiele, F. A. J. 1974. *Measurements on the surface of the skin,* p. 81. Nijmegen, the Netherlands: Drukkeij van Mammeren BV.

161. Anjo, D. M., Cunico, R. L., and Maibach, H. I. 1978. Transepidermal chloride diffusion in man. *Clin. Res.* 26:208A.

162. Lo, J. S., Oriba, H. A., Maibach, H. I., and Bailin, P. L. 1990. Transepidermal potassium ion, chloride ion, water flux across delipidized and cellophane tapestripped skin. *Dermatologica* 180:66–68.

163. Gross, P., Blade, M. O., Chester, J., and Sloane, M. B. 1954. Dermatitis of housewives as a variation of nummular eczema. A study of pH of the skin and alkali neutralization by the Burckhart technique. Further advances in therapy and prophylaxis. *Arch. Dermatol.* 70:94.

164. Frosch, P. J. 1978. Rapid blister formation in human skin with ammonium hydroxide. Presented to the Society of Investigative Dermatology, San Francisco.

165. Rougier, A., Goldberg, A. M., and Maibach, H. I., eds. *In vitro skin toxicology: Irritation, photoxicity, sensitization.* Alternative Methods in Toxicology Series, vol. 10. New York: Mary Ann Liebert.

166. Scheynius, A., Fischer, T., Forsum, U. 1984. Phenotypic characterization in situ of inflammatory cells in allergic and irritant contact dermatitis in man. *Clin. Exp. Immunol.* 55:81–90.

167. Ferguson, J., Gibbs, J. H., and Swanson Beck, J. 1985. Lymphocyte subsets and Langerhans cells in allergic and irritant patch test reactions: Histometric studies. *Contact Dermatitis* 13:166–174.

168. Avnstorp, C., Ralflkiaer, E., Jorgensen, J. 1987. Sequential immunophenotypic study of lymphoid infiltrate in allergic and irritant reactions. *Contact Dermatitis* 16:239–245.
169. Anderson, K. E., Sjolin, K. E., and Soelgaard, P. 1988. Acute irritant contact folliculitis in a galvanizer. *Eur. Symp. Contact Dermatitis,* Heidelberg, May 27–29, p. 62.
170. Patrick E., Burkhalter, A., and Maibach, H. I. 1987. Recent investigations of mechanisms of chemically induced skin irritation in laboratory mice. *J. Invest. Dermatol.* 88:245–315.
171. Ruzicka, T., and Printz, M. P. 1982. Arachidonic acid metabolism in skin: Experimental contact dermatitis in guinea pigs. *Int. Arch. Allergy Appl. Immunol.* 69:347–353.
172. Epstein, W. L. 1983. Cutaneous granulomas as a toxicologic problem. In *Dermatotoxicology,* 2nd ed., eds. F. M. Marzulli and H. I. Maibach, pp. 533–545. New York: Hemisphere.
173. Kresbach, H., Karl, H., and Wawschink, O. 1971. Cutaneous mercury granuloma. *Berufsderma-toisen* 18:173–186.
174. Andreas, T. L., Flallyathan, N. V., and Madison, J. F. 1981. Electron probe microanalysis: Aid in the study of skin granulomas. *Arch. Dermatol.* 116:1272–1276.
175. McOsker, D. E., and Beck, L. W. 1967. Characteristics of accommodated (hardened) skin. *J. Invest. Dermatol.* 48:372–383.
176. Thorvaldsen, J., and Volden, G. 1980. PUVA-induced diminution of contact allergic and irritant skin reactions. *Clin. Exp. Dermatol.* 5:43–46.

Chapter Nine

SKIN²: AN IN VITRO TISSUE MODEL FOR ASSESSMENT OF CUTANEOUS SAFETY AND EFFICACY NEEDS

Lawrence A. Rheins, Tracy A. Donnelly, and Susan M. Edwards

As new ingredients and products are developed and marketed, industry must continue to develop and refine dermal safety assessments, especially new, nonanimal testing methods. The use of animals, and even humans, for testing skin reactions is partly the result of the complexity of the human skin, which is not only the body's highly organized, heterogeneous, and multilayered barrier but also a dynamic, living tissue with many different physiological and metabolic functions. The composition of human skin includes the epidermis (10–20 layers of cells); the dermis (cells, fibers, and an amorphous ground substance); and the boundary between the epidermis and dermis (a complex interdigitation basement membrane network). To reliably assess cutaneous safety and efficacy of products without using animals, Advanced Tissue Sciences (La Jolla, CA) has developed Skin². Grown from tested cells from human neonatal foreskin, the "Barrier Function Model" (Skin² ZK1300) is a living, three-dimensional, human skin substrate; it is composed entirely of metabolically and mitotically active dermal and epidermal cell layers. Its characteristics and functions are similar to those of in vivo human skin; studies have shown this model to be effective in assessing products for irritancy, phototoxicity, and sun protection factor (SPF) classification. Moreover, it is uniquely helpful in achieving a mechanistic understanding of skin processes. Studies indicate that Skin² can accurately assess in vitro cutaneous safety and efficacy of new products.

INTRODUCTION

The consumer products, personal care, and chemical manufacturers industry of the 1990s will continue to evolve with technological advances that provide consumers with innovative products and, ultimately, exposure to new ingredients. As exposure to and experience with new ingredients and products occur, it will become increasingly important for the industry to respond with continued development and refinement of preclinical and clinical dermal safety assessments, especially new testing methods that replace or reduce use of animals. The challenge of providing an effective, reliable in vitro method for testing cutaneous safety and efficacy derives from the complex nature and function of the human skin (which involves elaborate interactions among the cells and other components of the dermis, epidermis, and epidermal–dermal interface).

Skin² is a registered trademark of Advanced Tissue Sciences, Inc., a Delaware corporation.
The authors thank Bart DeWever, Elizabeth Whalen, and Janice Medina for critically evaluating and preparing this chapter.

Skin[2] (Advanced Tissue Sciences, La Jolla, CA), a unique, three-dimensional, in vitro human skin analog, faces this challenge and now provides investigators with metabolically and mitotically viable skin constructs to conduct preclinical safety/hazard dermal assessments. Biochemical endpoints indicative of inflammatory and/or extracellular matrix changes allow more precise and quantitative evaluation of ingredients and/or finished products under "modeled real world" exposure conditions. The Skin[2] model, which consists of a functional dermis, epidermis, and stratum corneum, can be used to evaluate a variety of potential safety concerns (e.g., skin irritation, phytotoxicity), as well as efficacy issues (e.g., sun-protection-factor claims). Moreover, the benefits of using Skin[2] include a remarkably small amount of biological variance, especially when that variance is compared with that of in vivo surgical and/or cadaveric skin specimens.

THE STRUCTURE AND FUNCTION OF THE HUMAN SKIN

The human skin consists of three associated tissues (the stratum corneum/epidermis, underlying dermis, and hypodermis), as well as extracutaneous appendices, hairs, glands, and nails. Not only the outermost covering of the human body and thus a protective barrier, the skin is also a dynamic, living tissue involved in a variety of physiological and metabolic functions. The skin is a highly organized, heterogeneous, and multilayered barrier; it effectively separates the internal milieu from the external environment, and it helps constitute effective immunological, toxicological and mechanical protection for the body against external insults.[1] Its other roles include providing important thermoregulatory controls, such as maintaining fluid balance by limiting the excessive loss of body water.[2]

The major cell types present in the dermis and epidermis must function together in a dynamic and integrated fashion in order for the skin to provide the optimal protection against hazardous environmental agents and organisms. Additionally, cells of the connective tissue assist in modulating epidermal growth and differentiation, thereby providing a homeostatic biochemical signal transduction between the two tissue compartments to ensure the skin's integrity.

The Epidermis

In humans, the epidermis comprises 10–20 layers of cells (the number of cell layers differs in various locations on the body). Five main cell types are found in the epidermis: keratinocytes (making up approximately 95% of the entire epidermal cell population), Langerhans cells, melanocytes (pigment cells), Merkel cells, and various dendritic epidermal T lymphocytes (DETCs).

Primarily, the epidermis provides the body's first defense against cutaneous environmental insults. Besides this defensive role, the epidermis can also metabolize xenobiotics by using a variety of enzymes and may also be involved in the biotransformation of many different chemicals, including drugs, hormones, and carcinogens.[3]

Keratinocytes

Under exquisite cell–cell signaling control, the keratinocytes of the basal epidermal layer start to differentiate and move up in the epidermis to form a horny layer called the stratum corneum. This layer acts as a first-line defense against the invasion of microorganisms, environmental toxins, and ultraviolet (UV) radiation; thus it provides a protective envelope that surrounds the human body.

Langerhans Cells

Together with keratinocytes, the Langerhans cells and resident CD4 lymphocytes are involved in many immune reactions of the skin.[4] When an external antigen is recognized, the Langerhans cells introduce the antigen to lymphocytes either at local skin sites or at regional lymph nodes. These factors, along with the keratinocytes, induce a series of distinct T-cell-activating and growth-stimulating cytokines (e.g., the interleukins IL-1, IL-6, and IL-8, and GM-CSF); thus they modulate cellular immune functions, both locally and distally.[5]

Melanocytes

The melanocytes originate in the neural crest and participate in dynamic interactions with surrounding keratinocytes to synthesize melanin. Organized in spherical bodies, melanosomes are transferred through dendritic processes to keratinocytes.[6] Recent studies have shown that pigment cells also produce a variety of inflammatory and immunologic cytokines.[7] Therefore, melanocytes not only provide protection via melanin in response to UV radiation but may also amplify cutaneous inflammatory reactions.

Merkel Cells

Merkel cells, located near the basal keratinocyte layer, are often seen in association with the underlying nerve endings; therefore, these cells are thought to be important in epidermal enervation. Nociceptive responses (such as itching, stinging, and tingling) are believed to be associated with these cell types and their reservoir of neuropeptides (e.g., substance P, VIP).

The Dermis

Under the epidermis and firmly attached to it lies the dermis, the connective tissue of the skin. Like all connective tissues, it includes cells, fibers, and an amorphous ground substance. The cellular fraction of the dermis consists mainly of fibroblasts that secrete different macromolecules, like collagen, elastic fibers, and reticular fibers embedded in a matrix of glycosaminoglycans. The many collagenous fibers are arranged in bundles that form an irregular lattice with other elastic fibers and thereby provide the skin with a high tensile strength.

The ground substance of the dermis mainly consists of two different glycosaminoglycans, dermatan sulfate and hyaluronic acid. Both glycosaminoglycans bind large quantities of interstitial fluid; by this means, they mediate transport of nutrients and waste products between the dermal blood capillaries and the cells of the dermis and the avascular epidermis. Moreover, the extracellular matrix (ECM) is actively involved in collagen fiber formation; its proteoglycans can modulate cell behavior by mediating the interaction of cells with the ECM, sequestering extracellular growth factors, and modulating their activities.[8]

The dermis is also actively involved in local and systemic immune/inflammatory reactions: fibroblasts can be stimulated by epidermal IL-1 release to produce specific prostaglandins, which are important in inflammatory reactions.[9] Preliminary data have shown that fibroblasts can modify the expression of IL-6 by keratinocytes.[10] Furthermore, in reactions with dermal mast cells, dermal dendritic cells serve as a reservoir for inflammatory cytokines. These cytokines (along with the various dermal cell types and their associated receptors) provide autocrine, paracrine, and endocrine signals; these signals upregulate and downregulate the dermal/epidermal inflammatory responses.

The Dermal–Epidermal Interface

The important basement membrane, the boundary between the epidermis and dermis, maintains the attachment between dermis and epidermis by a complex interdigitated network of hemidesmosomes, anchoring filaments and fibrils, and tonofilaments. Composed of a basal lamina produced by basal epidermal keratinocytes and reticular fibers that may be partially dermal in origin, the basement membrane serves as an active filter controlling the exchange between dermis and epidermis and seems to be involved in regenerative processes in the epidermis.[11]

SKIN^2: A HUMAN, THREE-DIMENSIONAL, SKIN-EQUIVALENT TISSUE

The Development of Skin^2

In the last decade, industry has seen a rapid development and improvement in reliable and well-standardized in vitro methods for assessing human cutaneous toxicity. The continuing and pressing need to reduce or replace the use of animals, as well as economic considerations, has hastened progress and discovery in this area. Seeing the need for a reliable product and using its patented core technology, Advanced Tissue Sciences, Inc. (La Jolla, CA) has successfully developed a three-dimensional human skin tissue model called Skin[2]. This in vitro model was tissue-engineered to mimic the human skin both biochemically and morphologically (Figure 1).

Composed entirely of metabolically and mitotically active dermal and epidermal cell layers, the "Barrier Function Model" (Skin[2] ZK1300) is a living, three-dimensional, human skin substrate. The coculture system is seeded onto a nylon mesh and is comprised of fibroblasts from pathogen tested neonatal foreskin; these fibroblasts secrete a functional extracellular matrix.[12] After 4 wk

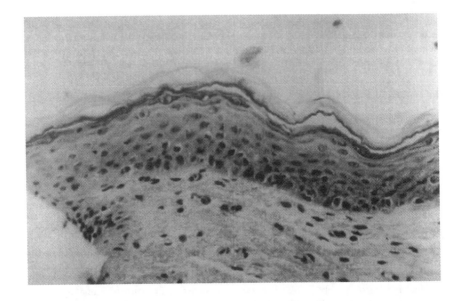

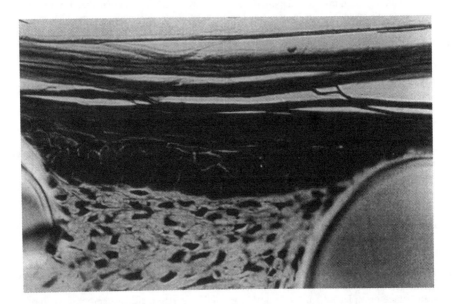

Figure 1. Cross section of human skin vs. Skin[2] ZK1300 model, hematoxylin–eosin staining.

in culture, epidermal keratinocytes are seeded onto the three-dimensional dermi. This dermal tissue provides a physiological support structure for the growth and differentiation of a functional, multilayered epidermis including stratum corneum.[13]

The Structure of Skin^2 Model ZK 1300

The epidermis of this model consists of keratinocytes differentiated into distinct basal, spinous, and granular layers. Differentiation markers include cytokeratins 1, 5, 10, and 14; fillagrin; trichohyalin; and involucrin. These markers show quantitative correlation with human in vivo skin biopsies.[14,15] At the ultrastructural level, electron microscopy studies reveal that this model displays a well-developed basement membrane structure consisting of lamina densa, lamina lucida, anchoring filaments, hemidesmosomes, tonofilaments, and elastin-associated microfibrils.[16,17] Moreover, immunocytochemistry results have shown that the basal lamina contains collagen type IV, laminin, nidogen, and heparin sulfate.[15]

The dermal compartment of this model consists of fibroblasts that deposit an ECM rich in collagen types I, III, and V; fibronectin; decorin; tenascin; and glycosaminoglycans (Table 1).

The Function of Skin^2 Model 1300

Studies have shown the remarkable similarity in the functioning of Skin^2 and in vivo human skin. Recently, antibodies against aminopropeptides of types I and III procollagen were found to bind to small microfibrils, suggesting collagen fibrillogenesis in Skin^2 tissue.[18] A study by Slivka[19] indicates that this model can be used to evaluate skin metabolism. This data demonstrated the breakdown of testosterone to dihydrotestosterone (catalyzed by 5-alpha-reductase) and the accompanying polar metabolites (catalyzed by cytochrome P-450).

A close comparative study on the capability of the Skin^2 model to synthesize lipids from [^{14}C]acetate obtained lipid fractions qualitatively and quantitatively comparable to those of normal human skin samples (Table 2).[20]

Preliminary results indicate that this model can metabolize retinoic acid at the same rate as human epidermis (Vanden Bossche et al., personal communications). Moreover, enzyme

Table 1. Comparison of Immunofluorescent Patterns of Skin^2 versus Embryonic and Adult Skin

Epidermis	Skin^2 ZK1300	Human embryonic cells	Human adult cells
K-10 keratin	Suprabasal	Suprabasal	Suprabasal
Fillagrin	Granular layer	Granular layer	Granular layer
Trichohyalin	Granular layer	Granular layer	Granular layer
		Dermis	
Type IV collagen	Basal lamina–dermis	Basal lamina	Basal lamina
Laminin	Basal lamina	Basal lamina	Basal lamina
Heparan sulfate	Basal lamina	Basal lamina	Basal lamina
	Fibroblasts (?)		
Nidogen	Basal lamina	Basal lamina	Basal lamina
	Fibroblasts		
Fibronectin	Dermis	Dermis	Dermis
Tenascin	Dermis	Upper dermis	Upper dermis
Type VI collagen	Dermis network	Dermis network	Dermis
Type VII collagen	Epidermo–dermal junction	Epidermo–dermal junction	Epidermo–dermal junction
Type I collagen	Dermis	Dermis	Dermis
N-pro I collagen	Dermis	Dermis	Epidermo–dermal junction
Type III collagen	Dermis	Dermis	Dermis
N-pro III collagen	Dermis	Dermis	Epidermo–dermal junction
Fibrillin	Dermis network	Elastic fibers	Elastic fibers
Elastin			Elastic fibers
Vitronectin			Elastic fibers
Decorin	Dermis	Dermis	Dermis

Table 2. Lipid Synthesis from [^{14}C]Acetate

Lipid fractions[a]	Radioactivity incorporated as % of total found in the lipid extracts[b]		
	Human skin, 3 d (19)	Human skin epidermis, 2 d (6)	Human skin equivalents, 2 d (7)
Phospholipids	34.5 ± 6.0	20.7 ± 2.6	42.4 ± 14.4
"Ceramides"	7.2 ± 2.1	12.6 ± 1.1	4.4 ± 1.1
Cholesterol	12.9 ± 2.6	21.5 ± 2.9	23.5 ± 9.4
Lanosterol	1.3 ± 1.1	2.1 ± 0.7	1.5 ± 0.6
Fatty acids (free)	1.7 ± 0.6	3.1 ± 0.7	1.0 ± 0.4
Triglycerides	24.2 ± 6.1	5.8 ± 0.8	18.4 ± 3.5
Sterol esters	2.1 ± 2.2	1.5 ± 0.2	1.1 ± 0.5
Others	15.9 ± 5.6	32.7 ± 3.0	7.7 ± 2.6

[a] Tentative identification on R_f values of standards. Standards used were phospholipids (dipalmitoylphosphatidylcholine, dilauroylphosphatidylcholine, dipalmitolyphosphatidyl-N, N-dimethylethanolamine, dipalmitoylphosphatidyl-N-methylethanolamine, and phosphatidylethanolamine); ceramides (ceramide III and IV); fatty acid (oleic acid); triglyceride (triolein); sterol ester (cholesterol stearate). Others are unidentified compounds.

[b] Results are mean values ± SD of (n) experiments. From Vanden Bossche et al.[20]

immunocytochemistry with antibodies raised against cytochrome P-450 1a and 2b showed that the distribution of these enzymes in Skin^2 was comparable to that of whole human skin.[21]

Selected Uses for Skin^2 Model ZK 1300

A variety of environmental insults, microorganisms, chemicals, UV light, cosmetics, drugs, and even mechanical perturbations can alter the various skin cell types and biochemical signals, leading to symptoms and diseases ranging from irritant or allergic reactions to potentially life-threatening forms of skin cancer.[22]

An in vitro skin model such as Skin^2, which is metabolically equivalent to normal human skin, provides not only the capability to evaluate the potential for skin damage but also a mechanistic understanding of the events leading to irritancy after topical exposure of several different types of chemical insults.

Cutaneous Irritation Testing

In early studies to evaluate the potential for using this in vitro model to assess skin irritation and cytotoxic effects, we topically applied 12 reference test chemicals (from the list of the Commission of the European Communities, CEC). Tissues were exposed to each test material for 5 min; 24 h after exposure, cell viability was determined by using the Thiazolyl Blue (MTT) assay. The in vitro data obtained with this model yielded a high correlation to the historical in vivo data published in the CEC's database of Draize Primary Dermal Irritation (PDII) scores.[23] No false-negative or false-positive results were found.[24]

The relative response of epidermal and dermal cells to a known irritant was also identified by use of Skin^2. Slivka et al.[25] demonstrated that exposure of the skin model to phorbol myristate acetate, a known skin irritant, resulted in a concentration-dependent increase of IL-1 alpha, tissue type plasminogen activator (TPA), and specific gelatinases.

Phototoxicity Testing

Recently we developed a method to assess the phototoxic potential of several known phototoxicants and nonphototoxicants. This protocol mimics the human in vivo phototoxicity test. After we applied various concentrations of test agents topically on the epidermal side of the tissue, the tissue was exposed to UVA (1.6 mW/cm^2) for 30 min. After exposure, the tissue was incubated for an additional 16–24 h at 37°C. Cytotoxicity was determined using an MTT assay. Some test materials (e.g., *para*-aminobenzoic acid, thiourea, uvinul MS40, and penicillin G) were identified as nonphototoxic after UVA exposure, while known phototoxic chemicals (e.g., chlorpromazine

HCl, promethazine HCl, 8-MOP) demonstrated predictable cytotoxicity after UVA exposure. The correlation between our in vitro data and existing in vivo data was 98%.[26]

Exposure of skin to UV light can also alter epidermal immune functions, including epidermal cytokine levels of IL-1, IL-6, IL-10, and TNF alpha.[27,28] We reported a significant increase in cytokine IL-1 alpha and TNF alpha activity versus control non-UV-irradiated Skin^2 tissues. Moreover, topical administration of indomethacin, a well-known nonsteroidal anti-inflammatory drug (NSAID), blocked the release of these cytokines after UV radiation. As expected, the UV-treated Skin^2 tissues demonstrated a significant amount of prostaglandin E_2 (PGE$_2$) release, while the topically applied indomethacin completely abolished this response.[28] Other studies have demonstrated that PGE$_2$ synthesis is required for IL-1 alpha and IL-1 beta activity. The recent Skin^2 experiments with this common NSAID might explain the observed decrease of IL-1 after UV exposure (Figures 2 and 3).

Sun Protection Factor Classification

The currently accepted method for sunscreen testing uses human panelists to determine the sun protection factor (SPF). Panelists receive doses of UVB radiation until an erythema reaction is observed. This dose at which the reaction occurs is called the mean erthyemal dose (MED). The sunscreen to be tested is then placed onto the panelist, who once again receives UVB radiation at the site of sunscreen application until an erythema reaction is perceived. The SPF is determined by how many MEDs are required to produce the reaction when the area was protected by the sunscreen. For example, if 4 MEDs produce a reaction in the protected area, the product is classified and labeled as an "SPF 4" sunscreen. The disadvantages of these tests include the necessity to subject panelists twice to UVB radiation, the effects of which could include photodamage, photoaging, and cancer. Another problem associated with human testing is the innate differences among skin types in humans. SPF testing must be well controlled for accurate results with these tests. Finally, tests on human panelists tend to be expensive.

The Skin^2 model ZK1351 has been evaluated recently in a protocol that closely follows the human protocol to test sunscreen products for SPF labeling. The sunscreen to be classified is applied onto the stratum corneum of the Skin^2 tissue, and the tissue is exposed to UVB radiation. Then the MTT assay is used to assess the tissue quantitatively for viability. Preliminary data indicate excellent correlation ($r = .917$) with the known SPF of tested products (Figure 4). Further studies will be required to confirm this correclation.

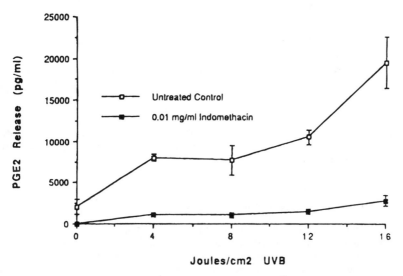

Figure 2. PGE$_2$ release $\pm$ indomethacin. From Rheins et al.[28] with permission.

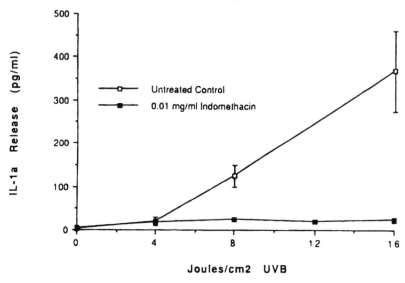

Figure 3. IL-1 alpha release $\pm$ indomethacin. From Rheins et al.[28] with permission.

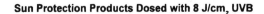

Sun Protection Products Dosed with 8 J/cm$_2$ UVB

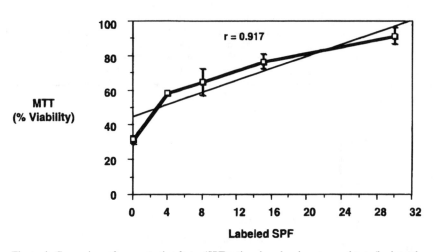

Figure 4. Comparison of sun protection factor (SPF) ratings based on human-panel tests (horizontal axis) and tests with Skin^2 model ZK1351 (boxes). For these studies, sun protection products were dosed with 8 J/cm^2 UVB.

Mechanistic Understanding of Skin Injury Processes

Because it is manufactured from human skin cells, Skin^2 can help evaluate various inflammatory and immunotoxicological events that may occur to the skin after exposure to ingredients and finished products.[22] The Skin^2 tests can be conducted with an approach that includes multiple biochemical and inflammatory endpoints. With such tests, we can begin to define the mechanisms involved in cytotoxic and irritant responses observed in vivo after topical exposures.

CONCLUSION

Despite the complexity of cellular interactions that take place in the human skin, studies have shown that the Skin^2 ZK1300 Barrier Function Model is equivalent to human skin in substance and function. As an in vitro model used to reduce or replace the number of animals used in testing, Skin^2 can help assess both the cutaneous risks and the efficacy of chemicals and skin-care products.

REFERENCES

1. Odland, G. F. 1983. In *Biochemistry and physiology of the skin,* vol. 1, ed. L. A. Goldsmith, pp. 3–63. New York: Oxford University Press.
2. Scheuplein, R. J., and Bronaugh, R. L. 1983. In *Biochemistry and physiology of the skin,* vol. 1, ed. L. A. Goldsmith, pp. 1255–1295. New York: Oxford University Press.
3. Kirnbauer, R., Schauer, E., Charvat, B., Urbanski, A., Forster, E., Neuner, P., Mickache, M. S., Schwartz, T., and Luger, T. A. 1991. Regulation of ICAM-1 expression on human melanocytes and melanoma cells by cytokines and UV-light. *J. Invest. Dermatol.* 96:609.
4. Baadsgaard, O., and Wang, T. 1991. Immune regulation in allergic and irritant skin reactions. *Int. J. Dermatol.* 30:161–172.
5. Rheins, L. A. 1992. What's new in cutaneous toxicology. *J. Toxicol. Cutaneous Ocul. Toxicol.* 11(3):225–238.
6. Yaar, M., and Gilchrest, A. 1991. Human melanocyte growth and differentiation: A decade of new data. *J. Invest. Dermatol.* 97:611–617.
7. Kao, J., and Carver, P. 1991. Cutaneous metabolism of xenobiotics. *Drug Metab. Rev.* 22(4):363–410.
8. Humphries, M. J. 1990. The molecular basis and specificity of integrin-ligand interactions. *J. Cell Sci.* 97:585–592.
9. Ras, A., Wyche, A., and Siegel, N. 1988. Regulation of fibroblast cyclooxygenase synthesis by interleukin-1. *J. Biol. Chem.* 263:3022–3028.
10. Mitsuhashi, Y., Ishikawa, H., Takagi, Y., and Hashimoto, I. 1993. Bi-phase separated cell culture: A good tool for studies of fibroblast–keratinocyte interaction. Abstr. 483. *Dermatology* 2000:213.
11. Goldsmith, L. A. 1983. *Biochemistry and physiology of the skin.* New York: Oxford University Press.
12. Slivka, S. R., Landeen, L. K., Naughton, G. K., and Bartel, R. L. 1993. Regulation of collagen deposition by human fibroblasts grown in a three-dimensional skin culture system. In *Alternative methods in toxicology,* vol. 8, ed. A. M. Goldberg, pp. 335–343. New York: Mary Ann Leibert.
13. Slivka, S. R., Landeen, L. K., Ziegler, F., and Zimber, M. P. 1993. Characterization, barrier function, and drug metabolism of an in vitro skin model. *J. Invest. Dermatol.* 100:40–46.
14. Borghgraef, P., De Wever, B., Stoppie, P., Geysen, J., Ramaekers, F., and Borgers, M. 1993. Evaluation of an organotypic human skin equivalent. Abstr. *Dermatology* 2000:214, 488.
15. Fleischmajer, R., MacDonald, E. D. II, Contard, P., and Perlish, J. S. 1993. Immunochemistry of a keratinocyte-fibroblast co-culture model for reconstruction of human skin. *J. Histochem. Cytochem.* 9:1359–1366.
16. Stoppie, P., Borghgraef, P., De Wever, B., Geysen, J., and Borgers, M. 1993. The epidermal architecture of an in vitro reconstructed human skin equivalent. *Eur. J. Morphol.* 31:26–29.
17. Contard, P., Bartel, R., Jacob, L. II, Perlish, J. S., MacDonald, E. D. II, Handler, L., Cone, D., and Fleischmajer, R. 1993. Culturing keratinocytes and fibroblasts in a three dimensional mesh results in epidermal differentiation and formation of a basal lamina anchoring zone. *J. Invest. Dermatol.* 100:35–39.
18. Contard, P., Jacob, L. II, Perlish, J. S., and Fleischmajer, R. 1993. Collagen fibrillogenesis in a three-dimensional fibroblast cell culture system. *Cell Tissue Res.* 273:571–575.
19. Slivka, S. R. 1993. Testosterone metabolism in an in vitro skin model. *Cell Biol. Toxicol.* 8:267–276.
20. Vanden Bossche, H., Willemsens, G., Schrueders, H., Cone, M. C., Vanhove, C., and Cools, W. 1993. Use of human skin models in the study of retinoic acid metabolism and lipid synthesis, effects of liarozole. In *Human cells in in vitro pharmatoxicology,* pp. 61–76. Brussels: VUB Press.
21. Pendlington, R. U., Williams, D. L., Naik, J. T., and Sharma, R. K. 1993. Localization, distribution and induction of specific xenobiotic metabolizing enzymes in rodent and human skin. Abstr. *Practical In Vitro Toxicology III,* Nottingham.
22. Stark, N. J. 1991. A chemist's view of biocompatibility. *Med. Device Diag. Ind.* 86:88–93.
23. CEC Report. 1989. Collaborative Study on Relationship Between In Vivo Primary Irritation and In Vitro Experimental Models, Rev. 1, CEC/V/E/3/LUX/157/88.
24. Donnelly, T. A., and Naughton, G. K. 1993. Toxicity and penetration prediction using a human three-dimensional skin model. Presented at the annual meeting of the Society of Toxicology, New Orleans.
25. Slivka, S. R., and Ziegler, F. 1993. Use of an in vitro skin model for determining epidermal and dermal contributions to irritant responses. *J. Toxicol. Cutaneous Ocul. Toxicol.* 12(1):49–57.

26. Edwards, S. M., Donnelly, T. A., Sayer, R. M., and Rheins, L. A. 1993. Quantitative in vitro assessment of phototoxicity using a human skin model, Skin². *J. Photoderm. Photoimmunol. Photoirrit.* 10:111–117.
27. Dahl, M. W. 1988. The skin as an immunologic organ. In *Clinical immunodermatology,* ed. M. Dahl, pp. 364–371. Chicago: Year Book Medical.
28. Rheins L. A., Edwards, S. M., Miao, O., and Donnelly, T. A. 1993. Skin²: An in vitro model to assess cutaneous immunotoxicology, *In Vitro. Toxicol.* 8:1007–1014.
29. DeWever, B., and Rheins, L. A. 1994. Skin²: An in vitro human skin analog. In *Alternative methods in toxicology,* vol. 10, eds. A. Rougier, A. M. Goldberg, and H. I. Maibach, pp. 121–131.

Chapter Ten

BIOCHEMICAL AND FLOW CYTOMETRIC STUDIES OF THE MECHANISM OF ACTION OF SULFUR MUSTARD USING HUMAN CELLS IN CULTURE

William J. Smith, Margaret E. Martens, Clark L. Gross, Offie E. Clark, and Fred M. Cowan

Over the past few years, our laboratory has studied the biochemical sequelae resulting from exposure to the vesicating agent sulfur mustard (2,2'-dichlorodiethylsulfide, HD). We have utilized isolated human peripheral blood lymphocytes (PBL), human epidermal keratinocytes (HEK), human epithelial tumor cells (HeLa), and a human skin equivalent, TESTSKIN. We have determined that HD causes depletion of cellular glutathione levels, disruption of cell cycle kinetics and DNA structure, activation of the nuclear enzyme poly(ADP-ribose) polymerase (PADPRP), concentration- and time-dependent decrease of cellular NAD^+, alterations in glucose metabolism, and increased proteolysis. Since there is no current prophylactic or therapeutic intervention available to prevent blister formation after contact with HD, we have evaluated compounds that might ameliorate HD pathology.

INTRODUCTION

This chapter summarizes research done at the U.S. Army Medical Research Institute of Chemical Defense (USAMRICD) in defining the biochemical mechanism of cutaneous vesication by sulfur mustard (HD) and approaches to therapy of the skin injury. Most of the work was accomplished using in vitro techniques with cultures of human peripheral blood lymphocytes (PBL), normal human epidermal keratinocytes (HEK), and the human epithelial tumor cell line, HeLa, and was supported by limited in vivo studies using the hairless guinea pig.

DNA STUDIES

Historic data on the cutaneous injury following exposure of humans to HD suggest that degenerative changes at the basal epidermal layer of the skin eventually lead to blister formation.[1] Since this layer of the skin contains the most proliferative cells of the skin and alkylating agents such as HD are known to have genotoxic effects,[2] the DNA damaging effects of HD on cells in culture have been extensively studied. Human PBL were stimulated to enter cell division by the lectin concanavalin A, and then were exposed to HD at various stages of the cell cycle. Cells in the S phase were the most sensitive to the cytotoxic effects of HD.[3] Utilizing flow cytometric analyses of cell cycle kinetics following exposure to HD, we showed that vesicating equivalent concentrations (50 μM or higher) resulted in a blockage of cell cycle progression at the G1/S interface. Subvesicating equivalent concentrations resulted in a blockage in the G2 phase.[4] The most recent data suggest that the cells blocked at G1/S are irreversibly blocked and the DNA becomes terminally fragmented. Those populations blocked at G2 suffer some cell loss but can recover from this blockage after 4 or 5 d. The observation that cell cycle kinetics are intimately involved in cytotoxic processes following HD led to a study of reversible inhibitors of the cell cycle. These compounds might be used to hold the cells in a selected phase in order to permit DNA repair processes to correct the damaged DNA before normal proliferative events are allowed to proceed. One such inhibitor, mimosine, was shown to provide a limited protection against the cytotoxicity of vesicating equivalent concentrations of HD in HeLa and HEK.[4]

In addition to cell cycle kinetic analysis, flow cytometric studies have demonstrated an altered intercalating dye response in HD-exposed cells.[4] This alteration is thought to be related to HD-induced structural changes in cellular DNA. Reduction of the DNA structural changes may be possible by the use of compounds that react with or "scavenge" HD and lower DNA alkylation levels. Cellular glutathione is an endogenous scavenger that provides cells protection against xenobiotic attack. Several approaches are being investigated to pharmacologically enhance cellular glutathione levels to protect against HD exposure.[5] One such approach, use of the prodrug N-acetyl-L-cysteine (NAC), has shown that pretreatment of PBL with NAC can reduce the amount of DNA damage induced by HD as detected by altered dye uptake.[4]

PADPRP STUDIES

It is well documented that DNA damage is usually accompanied by activation of a nuclear enzyme, poly(ADP-ribose) polymerase (PADPRP), which utilizes the metabolic cofactor NAD^+ as a substrate. Activation of PADPRP can result in a significant depletion of NAD^+ and is believed to contribute to metabolic disruptions that may lead to cellular pathology following alkylation.[6] Using HeLa cells in culture, we showed that PADPRP activation following HD exposure occurred in time- and concentration-dependent patterns.[7] Following 100 μM HD, the PADPRP activity increased to maximum values by 1 h, then declined to normal values over the next 6 h. When cells were exposed to 10 μM HD, the maximal PADPRP activity was reached by 3–4 h, then declined to normal levels. A secondary peak activity was noted at 24 h after HD. This finding could account for the biphasic decrease of cellular NAD^+ following HD. Experiments show that NAD^+ decreases over the first 4 h, plateaus from 4 to 8 h, then undergoes another significant decrease between 8 and 24 h after exposure.

The probable role of PADPRP in HD injury led investigators to evaluate inhibitors of the enzyme, particularly niacinamide, as a potential therapy.[8] While providing significant protection against the cytotoxicity of HD in resting cells, niacinamide's protection in actively proliferating cells is limited.[9] Niacinamide, however, is the only drug which has demonstrated protection against microblister formation in the hairless guinea pig.[10] While the incidence of microblisters was lowered, numerous degenerative changes were not affected by niacinamide treatment.[11]

METABOLIC DISRUPTION

Loss of cellular NAD^+ has been postulated to generate an extensive disruption of metabolic activity in HD-exposed cells.[6] It has been known that HD-exposed cells have a disturbance in their glycolytic capacity.[12] Studies of glucose utilization have demonstrated that while NAD^+ depletion and decreased glucose utilization are correlated, the correlation is not one to one.[13] This finding suggests that other alterations are taking place that require considerable study. Even though niacinamide can preserve NAD^+ levels in many cells following HD exposure, it has no protective effect against decreased glucose utilization, decreased lactate production, or loss of cellular ATP.[13]

PROTEASE STUDIES

Histopathologic studies of the HD injury suggest that proteolytic activity at the basilar surface of the basal epidermal cells is an early step in the separation at the epidermal–dermal junction.[14]

Spectrophotometric studies of proteolytic activation following HD exposure of human PBL in culture demonstrated an increase in serine protease activity.[15] This activity was detected against a panel of protease substrates and was shown to occur in a time period consistent with pathology following HD exposure in vivo.[15] The proteolysis could be inhibited by selected protease inhibitors and by treatment of the HD-exposed cells with niacinamide, dexamethasone, or *N*-acetyl-L-cysteine.[16] These chromogenic studies were also conducted in skin punch biopsies from the hairless guinea pig, and proteolytic activities similar to those seen in vitro were detected.[17]

The use of cells in culture has provided a strong biochemical background to the histopathologic and in vivo studies of HD toxicity. Further amplification of the biochemical mechanisms of cell and tissue injury will provide a means for designing and evaluating pharmacologic approaches against HD-induced pathology.

REFERENCES

1. Papirmeister, B., Feister, A. J., Robinson, S. I., and Ford, R. D. 1991. *Medical defense against mustard gas: Toxic mechanisms and pharmacological implications.* Boca Raton, FL: CRC Press.
2. Fox, M., and Scott, D. 1980. The genetic toxicology of nitrogen and sulfur mustard. *Mutat. Res.* 75:131–168.
3. Smith, W. J., Sanders, K. M., Gales, Y. A., and Gross, C. L. 1991. Flow cytometric analysis of toxicity by vesicating agents in human cells *in vitro. J. Toxicol. Cutaneous Ocul. Toxicol.* 10(1):33–42.
4. Smith, W. J., Sanders, K. M., Ruddle, S. E., and Gross, C. L. 1993. Cytometric analysis of DNA changes induced by sulfur mustard. *J. Toxicol. Cutaneous Ocul. Toxicol.* 12:343–353.
5. Gross, C. L., Innace, J. K., Hovatter, R. C., Meier, H. L., and Smith, W. J. 1993. Biochemical manipulation of intracellular glutathione levels influences cytotoxicity to isolated human lymphocytes by sulfur mustard. *Cell Biol. Toxicol.* 9:259–268.
6. Papirmeister, B., Gross, C. L., Meier, H. L., Petrali, J. P., and Johnson, J. B. 1985. Molecular basis for mustard-induced vesication. *Fundam. Appl. Toxicol.* 5:S134–S149.
7. Clark, O. E., and Smith, W. J. 1993. Activation of poly(ADP-ribose) polymerase by sulfur mustard in HeLa cell cultures. *Proc. 1993 Medical Chemical Defense Bioscience Rev.* 1:199–205. (DTIC Accession number A275667.)
8. Meier, H. L., Gross, C. L., and Papirmeister, B. 1987. 2,2′-Dichlorodiethyl sulfide (sulfur mustard) decreases NAD$^+$ levels in human leukocytes. *Toxicol. Lett.* 39:109–122.
9. Smith, W. J., Sanders, K. M., Caulfield, J. E., and Gross, C. L. 1992. Sulfur mustard induced biochemical alterations in proliferating human cells in culture. *J. Toxicol. Cutaneous Ocul. Toxicol.* 11(4):293–304.
10. Yourick, J. J., Clark, C. R., and Mitcheltree, L. W. 1991. Niacinamide pretreatment reduces microvesicle formation in hairless guinea pigs cutaneously exposed to sulfur mustard. *Fundam. Appl. Toxicol.* 17:533–542.
11. Yourick, J. J., Dawson, J. S., Benton, C. D., Craig, M. E., and Mitcheltree, L. W. 1993. Pathogenesis of 2,2′-dichlorodiethyl sulfide in hairless guinea pigs. *Toxicology* 84:184–197.
12. Dixon, M., and Needham, D. M. 1946. Biochemical research on chemical warfare agents. *Nature* 158:432–438.
13. Martens, M. E., and Smith, W. J. 1993. Mechanisms of sulfur mustard-induced metabolic injury. *Proc. 1993 Medical Chemical Defense Bioscience Rev.* 1:257–263. (DTIC Accession number A275667.)
14. Papirmeister, B., Gross, C. L., Petrali, J. P., and Meier, H. L. 1984. Pathology produced by sulfur mustard in human skin grafts on athymic nude mice. II. Ultrastructural changes. *J. Toxicol. Cutaneous Ocul. Toxicol.* 3:393–408.
15. Cowan, F. M., Broomfield, C. A., and Smith, W. J. 1991. Effect of sulfur mustard exposure on protease activity in human peripheral blood lymphocytes. *Cell Biol. Toxicol.* 7:239–248.
16. Cowan, F. M., Broomfield, C. A., and Smith, W. J. 1992. Inhibition of sulfur mustard-increased protease activity by niacinamide, *N*-acetyl cysteine, or dexamethasone. *Cell Biol. Toxicol.* 8(2):129–138.
17. Cowan, F. M., Yourick, J. J., Hurst, C. G., Broomfield, C. A., and Smith, W. J. 1993. Sulfur mustard-increased proteolysis following in vitro and in vivo exposures. *Cell Biol. Toxicol.* 9:253–262.

Chapter Eleven

A MULTIPHASE SCREEN FOR THE EVALUATION OF TOPICAL SKIN PROTECTANTS AGAINST CHEMICAL WARFARE AGENTS

T. H. Snider, Ronald G. Menton, D. W. Hobson, and D. W. Korte, Jr.

A multiphased screen using a physicochemical (p-chem) model was validated and used in a tiered approach to evaluate topical skin protectants (TSPs) against dermal chemical warfare agent (CWA) exposure. The p-chem model used in the first tier measured the time of CWA penetration of each TSP layered on M-8 chemical detection paper. The second tier consisted of an in vivo test that validated the p-chem model and evaluated TSPs determined to be more effective than the benchmark standard. This tiered approach has enhanced the screening process by eliminating the least effective TSPs from expensive in vivo testing, and has significantly reduced animal usage.

INTRODUCTION

Percutaneous exposure to small quantities of chemical warfare agents can result in deleterious or even lethal effects. Studies have shown that significant protection from such exposures is practical and achievable with the application of topical skin protectants (TSPs). The cost in terms of animal usage and laboratory resources prohibits a complete in vivo evaluation of the relative effectiveness of every new candidate TSP. Therefore, a multitiered screening procedure was developed and used to identify candidate TSP compounds that would be efficacious against topical challenges with GD, TGD, VX, and HD.

METHODS

Candidate TSP screening was conducted in two sequential tests. Initial efficacy was assessed by a physicochemical test that involved spreading a 0.15-mm layer of TSP on U.S. Army M-8 chemical detection paper and applying an 8-μl volume of either GD, TGD, VX, or HD onto the TSP. The index of TSP performance was the time period from CWA application to a color change observed on the underside of the M-8 paper, indicating TSP penetration by the agent. Longer "breakthrough times" (up to a maximum 1 h observation for HD and 6 h for the nerve agents) indicated more effective protection.

The in vivo test was performed by applying a 0.1-mm-thick layer of TSP on the shaved dorsa of New Zealand White rabbits followed by application of either GD (1.35 mg/kg), TGD (3.35 mg/kg), VX (0.5 mg/kg), or HD (1.0 μl doses at multiple test sites per rabbit). The endpoint for in vivo screening with nerve agent challenges was the timed measurement (30, 60, and 120 min of erythrocyte acetylcholinesterase (AChE) activity expressed as a percentage of preexposure baseline values. Nerve agent doses were selected to produce between 10 and 30% AChE relative activity (RA) in the 120-min blood samples from rabbits protected by polyethylene glycol with a mean molecular mass of 540 daltons (PEG 540). TSP efficacy was expressed as an "RA score" value, the average of AChE RA levels across sample times for each animal. The measure in all screens with HD challenges was the dermal lesion area ratio (LAR), the lesion area at a TSP-pretreated site divided by the lesion area at an unprotected, challenged site on the same rabbit. A composite endpoint variable, "LAR score," was calculated as the mean LAR for the 1-, 2-, and 4-h exposures for each rabbit. Thus, high TSP efficacy against nerve agents was indicated by a high mean RA score, but against HD by a low mean LAR score.

Nominal sample sizes were 12 penetration cells per TSP in the M-8 paper method and 24 rabbits (8 rabbits on each of 3 test days) per TSP in each in vivo screen. In all tests, the control TSP was PEG 540. The number of TSPs, including PEG 540, examined was 17 in HD testing and 7 for each nerve agent tested.

Univariate analysis indicated that M-8 paper breakthrough times were lognormally distributed. For each challenge agent, the mean log-transformed breakthrough times were plotted against mean in vivo scores determined for a TSP, and a Pearson correlation analysis was performed at $\alpha = .05$ to determine an association between the M-8 paper and in vivo results.

RESULTS

The correlation between the M-8 paper and in vivo tests is summarized for each agent in Table 1. Means of log-transformed M-8 chemical detection paper breakthrough times were negatively correlated ($p < .05$) with in vivo LAR scores for an HD challenge (Figure 1), and were positively correlated with in vivo AChE RA scores for GD and TGD (Figures 2 and 3, respectively). Based on the current limited data, the linear relationship between the results for VX was not strong enough to indicate a significant correlation (Figure 4). Further investigations using more TSPs may improve the correlation. Nevertheless, data on hand show that the M-8 paper test with a VX challenge can probably be used to predict efficacy and eliminate TSPs of the lowest efficacy from the evaluation process. When used as a first-level test for TSP evaluation in our facility,

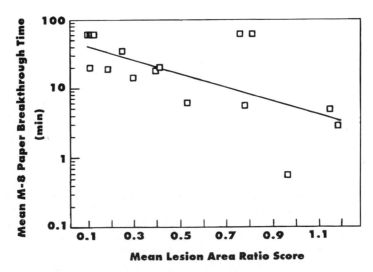

Figure 1. Correlation of topical skin protectant test results following HD challenge: mean log breakthrough times on M-8 paper versus mean lesion area ratio scores in rabbits.

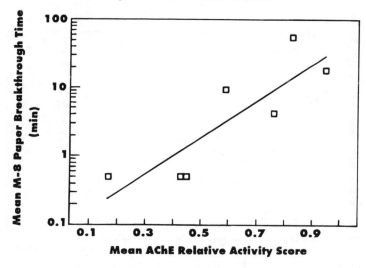

Figure 2. Correlation of topical skin protectant test results following GD challenge: mean log breakthrough times on M-8 paper versus mean erythrocyte AChE relative activity scores in rabbits.

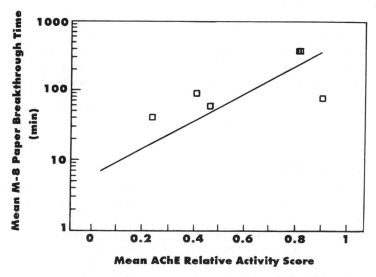

Figure 3. Correlation of topical skin protectant test results following TGD challenge: mean log breakthrough times on M-8 paper versus mean erythrocyte AChE relative activity scores in rabbits.

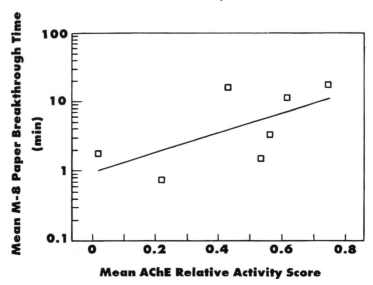

Figure 4. Correlation of topical skin protectant test results following VX challenge: mean log breakthrough times on M-8 paper versus mean erythrocyte AChE relative activity scores in rabbits.

the M-8 paper method has been used to reduce the number of candidates for in vivo testing from an initial 108 to approximately 40. Over the course of this work, the use of the multitiered approach has saved approximately 2000 rabbits. Due to the multiplicity of experimental factors that can affect in vivo results, almost half of these rabbits would have been required for process quality control. Thus, in terms of animal usage, time, and laboratory resources, the M-8 paper test was very cost-effective.

CONCLUSIONS

The U.S. Army M-8 chemical detection paper test is a rapid, inexpensive method for reliably predicting the in vivo efficacy of topical skin protectants and assigning them preliminary relative ranking against chemical warfare agents. The M-8 paper test can be employed to enhance topical skin protectant development.

Including the M-8 paper test in one series of studies conserved approximately 2000 rabbits, a 90% reduction in the number of animals that would have been required to perform in vivo evaluations for all TSPs examined.

FUTURE DIRECTIONS

Related studies have shown that the correlation between in vitro and in vivo results may be improved if a skin substitute preparation is included in the in vitro model, providing for the

Table 1. Summary of Correlation Analyses Between M-8 Paper Physicochemical and In Vivo Tests for Topical Skin Protectant Efficacy

Agent	Correlation coefficient, R	Degree of freedom	$p : \lvert R \rvert = 0$
HD	−.64	14	0.0071
GD	.86	5	0.0142
TGD	.82	5	0.0225
VX	.64	5	0.1219

interaction of TSPs with skin (e.g., the transfer of water or oils). This has led to investigations using the TSP films applied to a cultured human skin equivalent (HSE) preparation in an in vitro flow cell model. The initial results using topical applications of paraoxon and pyridostigmine bromide indicated an efficacy ranking of three pretreatment conditions as: a suspension of polytetrafluoroethylene particles in perfluorinated polyethylene oil > PEG 540 = no TSP. This HSE model requires further study in order to fully evaluate its potential as a replacement for in vivo tests.

PART II

DEVELOPMENTAL/REPRODUCTIVE TOXICITY

Chapter Twelve

INDUCTION OF LOW-MOLECULAR-WEIGHT HEAT-SHOCK PROTEINS IN *DROSOPHILA* AND HUMAN EMBRYONIC LINEAGE CELLS AFTER TERATOGEN EXPOSURE

Nicole Bournias-Vardiabasis, Kuyng-Won Huh, Keri Hopkins, and Tae-Wook Chun

Drosophila *embryonic cells exposed to a wide range of teratogens respond to this type of environmental perturbation by dramatically increasing the levels of two low-molecular-weight heat-shock (stress) proteins (hsp 22 and hsp 23). Similar response was observed in teratogen-treated human amniotic fluid and chorionic villi cells (hsp 27 induction). Here we report the expression pattern and induction levels of an hsp 23 heterologous promoter (hsp 23-β-galactosidase) construct in teratogen-treated* Drosophila *embryonic cells. The levels of fusion protein expression vary according to the teratogen used, but the staining pattern (X-gal in situ protocol) is seemingly restricted to the cytoplasmic area of embryonic neuronal cells. Teratogen-exposed human embryonic lineage cells (amniotic fluid and chorionic cells) were also examined and shown to exhibit dramatically increased levels of the low-molecular-weight hsp 27. Hsp 27 induction was investigated, utilizing a biotinylated hsp 27 cDNA probe, and immunocytochemistry was performed, using an antibody that binds to human hsp 27. The teratogen-induced hsp 27 localization was mostly cytoplasmic, with some perinuclear staining also being present. The developmental or thermoprotectant role of the low-molecular-weight hsp has yet to be ascertained in this or any other organism. The observed spatial restriction to* Drosophila *neuronal cells of hsp 23 points to a possible protective role, since these types of cells are thought to be rather sensitive and could be easily damaged. Several hypotheses are put forth regarding the possible function of these hsp, although it is unlikely that their induction, per se, leads to developmental malformations. At this point, teratogen induction of both* Drosophila *hsp 23 and 22 and human hsp 27 allows them to be used as accurate biomarkers of a teratogenic insult.*

INTRODUCTION

Organisms most often carry out their developmental program and respond to a variety of environmental changes by modifying their set of transcriptionally active genes. Molecular biology advances, such as solution and solid support hybridization, reporter gene constructs, in situ

We thank Lynn Douglass for her excellent word processing skills. This research was partially funded by a Johns Hopkins CAAT grant and a Demeter Fund grant to N. Bournias-Vardiabasis.

transcription, and PCR, have allowed developmental biologists to investigate the temporal and spatial regulation of such events.

Recent teratology studies have centered both in elucidating mechanisms of normal development and the possible genetic and epigenetic contributions that can lead to the alteration of the normal developmental program. Cell proliferation, cell migration, cell death, cell differentiation, and general cell–cell interactions have all been suggested to be possible targets for teratogens.[1] Disturbances of any of these processes, especially during early development, have been shown in a variety of animal models to lead to specific congenital malformations. More recently, several in vitro models have been proposed and utilized in an effort to identify putative teratogens and the mechanisms, involved in the teratogenic response (developmental malformations).[2–7]

Our laboratory has concentrated on utilizing *Drosophila melanogaster* embryonic cells in an effort to investigate such mechanisms, and also to develop an in vitro assay capable of identifying teratogenic agents.[8] The use of *Drosophila melanogaster* embryos as a model certainly allows exploitation of the wealth of genetic and developmental information already available. A large number of developmentally important genes have been identified and their temporal and spatial expression defined. Similar studies have been more recently extended to higher eukaryotes, with many of these developmentally important genes, such as homeotic genes, being found playing similar roles from *Drosophila* to humans. *Drosophila* embryonic cells are capable of differentiating in vitro to a variety of representative cell types (neurons, myotubes, fat cells, etc.), and many of the developmental processes that have been previously shown to be disrupted by teratogens are easily investigated.[9,10] Previous studies by us have established the *Drosophila* embryonic cell culture system as an excellent choice for identifying teratogens (physical and chemical agents) by utilizing morphological (cell differentiation), biochemical (neurotransmitter) and molecular (gene expression) endpoints.[8,11–15] Teratogen-treated *Drosophila* embryonic cell cultures exhibit a variety of responses, including inhibition of neuron and muscle differentiation,[11,12,16] neurotransmitter decline[15] (also see unpublished observations), and induction of a subset of heat-shock proteins (hsp) (stress proteins), namely, hsp 22 and 23.[13,14] The induction levels for these two small (or low-molecular-weight) hsp vary according to the treatment with heat shock, ether, and heavy metals—exposure resulting in the highest levels of hsp 23 and hsp 22 expression.[13] The molecular basis of hsp induction has been extensively investigated and the function(s) of many of these hsp have been proposed.[17–19] Elevated levels of all or some of these hsp are thought to help cells survive deleterious effects of subsequent environmental stress. Mitchell et al.[20] and Berger and Woodward[21] have suggested that synthesis of low-molecular-weight hsp leads to heat resistance in pupae. Admittedly, the small heat-shock proteins have not been as thoroughly investigated, although such heat-shock genes have been found in a large spectrum of organisms.[19] The small hsp are of particular interest, since, at least in *Drosophila* and in a limited number of other higher organisms investigated such as mice and rabbits, they have been shown to be developmentally regulated.[22–24]

Our current studies center not on the normal expression pattern of these small hsp, but rather, at their out-of-phase (ectopic) expression, due to exposure to teratogens. One of the most interesting and yet unanswered questions in teratology has been regarding their function(s) as it relates to developmental malformations.[18] Does this out-of-phase expression of hsp 22 and 23 serve as a mere biomarker of stress? Do the cells benefit from increased expression (teratogen protective response)? Or does this unscheduled expression alter a cascade of developmentally important genes (i.e., homeotic genes or patterning)? Our earlier studies have shown that induction of the whole set of hsp leads to partial protection from a subsequent teratogenic exposure.[25] Due to the induction kinetics of teratogen-induced hsp, the reverse experiment cannot be carried out; that is, diphenylhydantoin exposure results in hsp 23 and hsp 22 induction only after 6–8 h of incubation.[14] Since, thus far, we and other workers have been unable to experimentally support any of these hypotheses, we have presently concentrated on utilizing the induction of hsp 23 as a biomarker of cellular response to teratogens and extended these studies to utilizing human embryonic cells (amniotic fluid and chorionic villi). The rationale for extending the studies to some type of human embryonic cell or tissue stems from the need to develop a model that directly yet noninvasively assesses teratogenic response (possible developmental malformation) of the human fetus. To our knowledge such cells have not been used to carry out teratogen studies, although they are very much routinely utilized for assessing the genome status of the developing fetus. Earlier preliminary studies[26] and data presented here indicate that exposure to a number of different teratogens results in the induction of hsp 27. Exposure to nonteratogens elicits no such response. Induction of human hsp 27 after teratogen exposure has not been reported by others, although several reports have been published on the teratogen and hyperthermia-induced hsp response in developing rat and mouse embryos.[27–31] In mammalian embryos, exposure to heat shock or to a variety of other chemical and physical stresses leads to induction of specific set of heat-shock proteins, hsp 27, 71, and 88 (these numbers tend to vary according to the investigator and the species used).[32]

For the *Drosophila* studies, we have used an hsp 23–β-galactosidase reporter gene construct inserted into the germline of an SOR strain. Induction of hsp 23 promoter (i.e., teratogenic response) was assessed by processing the teratogen treated cells for β-galactosidase expression (X-gal in situ assay) and comparing the induction pattern and level of the fusion protein to control cultures. For the human embryonic cell studies, we originally carried out standard two-dimensional gel electrophoresis analysis, and ultimately utilized a human hsp 27 cDNA to assess expression of hsp 27 mRNA after teratogen exposure. We also have preliminary trials with a human hsp 27 antibody for in situ analysis of hsp 27 induction in human embryonic lineage cells after exposure to a number of different teratogens.

These studies are aimed at first establishing conditions for relatively easy assessment of *Drosophila* hsp 23 and human hsp 27 induction. Such development will allow use of these two hsp as biomarkers of teratogenic response. When this is accomplished, we hope to extend our studies to investigate the possible developmental role these proteins, have once they are extrinsically induced by teratogens or other agents. With the large number of developmentally important genes currently under investigation, it should be relatively easy to obtain DNA probes for such a fascinating and inherently important project.

MATERIALS AND METHODS

Drosophila Studies

***Drosophila* embryonic cultures.** Embryos were collected for 2 h from population cages containing an hsp 23-β-galactosidase construct trangenic *Drosophila melanogaster* adults (strain 700.2 kindly provided by Dr. Voellmy, University of Miami, Miami, FL). The eggs were allowed to age undisturbed for 3.5 h at room temperature (RT). This procedure assured that less than 95% of the embryos were in the early gastrula stage (pregastrula cells are unable to differentiate in vitro). The embryos were then dechorionated, surface sterilized, and mechanically dissociated into single cells, pelleted by centrifugation, and plated out in 35-mm tissue culture dishes, containing sterile glass coverslips, at 1.6×10^6 cells per dish in modified *Drosophila* medium supplemented with 18% fetal calf serum. Approximately 15 min was required for the cells to attach to the bottom of the dish or to the surface of the coverslips. At that time, the teratogen (or other agent) to be tested, dissolved in medium at the appropriate concentration, was added to several dishes. Teratogen concentrations have been established from previous studies.[8] Control cultures received only a change of medium. Scoring of the culture was carried out 18 h later (equivalent to a 24-h-old embryo). A total of four dishes (12 coverslips) per trial was scored, and the number of myotubes and ganglia were ranked to the cell numbers obtained in parallel control cultures (Wilcoxon's signed rank test). A 50% reduction in the number of either myotubes and/or neuronal clusters (ganglia) was taken as a teratogenic response. These counts are reported here, since they have already been reported previously.[8] For more details regarding the cell cultures procedure, see Refs. 8 and 33.

β-Galactosidase in situ assay (X-gal). *Drosophila* embryonic cells, cultured on coverslips for 18 h were rinsed with *Drosophila* saline and incubated for 15 min at RT in Buffer A (10 mM phosphate, 150 mM NaCl, 1 mM MgCl$_2$) containing 1% glutaraldehyde. The cells were then rinsed in Buffer A and incubated for 5 min at RT in Buffer A containing 3.1 mM K$_4$Fe(II)(CN$_6$) and 3.1 mM K$_3$Fe(III)(CN$_6$). The cells were then rinsed again in Buffer A and incubated in the same Fe/NaP solution containing 0.2% X-gal (substrate for β-galactosidase) at 37°C in a dark humid box for 4 h.[34] They were then rinsed in Buffer A and the coverslips were mounted on slides with glycerol and stored in the dark at 4°C.

Scoring of X-gal-positive cells. Coverslips processed for the X-gal assay were scored as follows: Cells on each coverslip were counted, using a phase/bright-field Olympus microscope. Neuron clusters and myotubes were scored for each treatment group, and the numbers from the four dishes were averaged and computed as percentage of the control average (for details on scoring, see Ref. 8). Then the coverslip was viewed under bright field and the number of X-gal positive cells was counted. After preliminary trials, it became evident that only neuronal cells expressed the fusion protein (only rarely would an occasional myotube be stained blue). To simplify the scoring process, hsp-23-expressing cells (X-gal positive) were calculated at a percent of the total number of neuronal clusters. Thus if one or more neuronal cells within the cluster was X-gal positive, that was scored as a positive cluster. This scoring was necessitated by the limitations of resolution using the X-gal assay and the difficulty of ascertaining the total number of neurons per cluster. Teratogen-treated groups were then compared to control cultures, and the degree of teratogen-induced expression of the fusion protein was calculated as fold induction over the control. For example, the average number of neuronal clusters expressing the β-galactosidase protein in the control cultures was 11%, while a teratogen treatment (i.e. arsenate) resulted in 33% of the neuronal clusters being X-gal positive. This increase would be expressed as a threefold induction of the hsp 23 gene. Our present study was not concerned with ranking the levels of induction or deciding on statistical significance limits. We do not feel there can be a correlation between malformation rates in humans after prenatal teratogen exposure and levels of induction of *Drosophila* hsp 23.

Amniotic Fluid and Chorionic Villi Cell Studies

Preparation of amniotic or chorionic villi cell lines. Amniotic fluid or chorionic villi primary cell cultures were provided to us by Dr. B. Wang of the Prenatal Diagnosis Center, Beverly Hills, CA. The cells were established in RPMI-1640 medium or Chang's medium supplemented with 10% fetal calf serum (FCS) and antibiotics. Cells were incubated in 75-mm flasks in a humidified atmosphere (CO_2/air, 5/95 by volume) at 37°C for 24 or 48 h.

Teratogen treatments. Each teratogen to be tested was added to the cells diluted to the appropriate concentration. Cells were examined at 24 h for cell death (trypan blue assay) and processed for protein analysis or RNA isolation at either 24 or 48 h. Each teratogen was tested a total of three times. Each run included a heat-shock treatment group that served as a positive control (45°C for 20 min). Four 75-mm flasks were used for each teratogen treatment.

Labeling and two-dimensional gel analysis of teratogen-treated human cells. After cells were exposed to a particular teratogen, they were labeled in the presence of agent for 1 h with 200 Ci of [³H]leucine (ICN Biomedicals, Costa Mesa, CA). Heat-shock treatments were given either 90 min or 16 h prior to labeling. Cells were incubated for 20 min at 45°C and labeled with 200 μ Ci of ³H. After labeling the heat or drug, treated cells were washed 3 times in cold phosphate-buffered saline (PBS) containing 300 μg/ml phenylmethyl sulfonate (PMSF). Cells were then scraped off the dish, pelleted, resuspended, and dried on a Savant vacuum centrifuge. Samples were solubilized in 20 ml of sonication buffer boiled for 3 min. Solid urea was added to a final concentration of 9 *M* and samples were diluted 1:1 with O'Farrell's lysis buffer. Samples were separated by two-dimensional polyacrylamide gel electrophoresis (PAGE), using a pH 5–7 gradient for isoelectric focusing and a 9–15% gradient acrylamide slab for sodium dodecyl sulfate (SDS) electrophoresis. Gels were stained with Coomassie blue, fluorographed, dried, and exposed to Kodak XAR film.

RNA isolation and northern blot assay. Total RNA from either amniotic or chorionic villi cells was prepared by a modified guanidinium thiocyanate procedure. Briefly, the procedure is as follows: Cells were lysed in 1 ml of denaturing solution (guanidinium thiocyanate plus mercaptoethanol). After denaturation, the lysate was treated with a 2 *M* sodium acetate, saturated phenol, and chloroform:isoamyl alcohol solution. It was then microcentrifuged for 20 min at 4°C. The RNA was then cleaned with isopropanol, and the RNA pellet after a −20°C, 20 min incubation was dried using a speed vac. The pellet was then resuspended in DEPC-treated Diethyl pyrocarbonate water. The yields of total RNA range between 30 and 200 μg of RNA per four 75-mm flasks of confluent chorionic or amniotic fluid cells. The purity of RNA was determined by standard optical density (OD) analysis. The RNA was aliquoted in 20-μg portions and stored at $-70°C$. Depending on the detection method (chemiluminescence or colorimetric), nylon or nitrocellulose membrane was utilized for the dot blot apparatus. The rationale for using nonradioactive labeling for the cDNA probe comes from the ultimate utilization of such developed protocol. It is hoped that Northern dot blot detection of hsp 27 mRNA can be used as a biomarker for assessing teratogenic response in human embryonic lineage cells. Such clinical setting development favors a nonradioactive labeling protocol.

The RNA samples were loaded into individual wells, and 20μg of RNA was applied to each well. The filters were hybridized (as recommended by probe provider) in a solution including random-primed (Random Primed Images-Biotin Labeling Kit, United States Biochemical, Cleveland, OH) biotinylated human hsp 27 cDNA probe (StressGen, Victoria, British Columbia, Canada). Duplicate samples were probed with a biotinylated β-actin probe (Oncor, Gaithersburg, MD). The blot was then taken through a series of washes, as recommended by the hsp 27 cDNA probe provider before visualization of cDNA-mRNA hybrids. Visualization was accomplished either by using an alkaline phosphatase-strepavidin kit (BRL Detection System, Bethesda Research Laboratories, Bethesda, MD) or a chemilluminescent detection kit (Plex-luminescent, Millipore, Bedford, MA).

Immunocytochemistry. Anti-hsp 27 antibody binding was determined by utilizing a biotin-strepavidin labeling complex kit (Bio Genex Laboratories, San Ramon, CA). Amniotic fluid or chorionic villi cells were cultured on gas-sterilized glass coverslips placed on the bottom of a 35-mm culture dish. The teratogens tested were from the original list used for the two-dimensional gel electrophoresis analysis. The coverslips were rinsed with PBS containing 1 μg/ml bovine serum albumin (BSA) and fixed for 30 min in 4% paraformaldehyde in PBS. Following 2 rinses with PBS-BSA (1 μg/ml), cells were incubated for 30 min at RT with a mouse anti-hsp 27 monoclonal antibody (BioGenex Laboratories, San Ramon, CA). Antigen antibody complexes were revealed with a biotinylated anti-immunoglobulin and subsequent horseradish peroxidase labeling (20 min RT) (BioGenex Laboratories, San Ramon, CA). 3.3'-Diaminobenzidine (DAB) was used as a chromogen (10 min RT). Brown precipitate formation indicated cells expressing hsp 27. Comparisons were made to heat-shocked and control cultures.

RESULTS

Drosophila Studies

Exposure of hsp-23 β-galactosidase-transformed *Drosophila* embryonic cells to a number of different teratogens resulted in the significant increase of β-galactosidase (i.e., hsp 23 promoter activation) over control cultures. The induction levels varied according to the treatment with heat shock (37°C for 30 min) and exposure to heavy metals, giving the highest increase in the expression of the fusion protein. The levels of increase followed closely those reported by us using two-dimensional gel protein analysis.[13,14] Table 1 summarizes the teratogens tested and the levels of hsp 23–β-galactosidase induction. Figure 1 compares the X-gal staining patterns for control and teratogen-treated embryonic cell cultures. What is quite apparent in both the heat-shocked and teratogen-treated cells is that only neuronal cells express the fusion protein (i.e., hsp 23 promoter is induced) (Figure 1). The X-gal assay does not allow for accurate determination of where within the cell this fusion protein is expressed. We plan to repeat these experiments using a monoclonal antibody against β-galactosidase; preliminary trials indicate a very discrete staining pattern can be attained. Duband et al.[35] have shown that after the cell recovers from the environmental stress, the hsp are restricted to the perinuclear region. Ireland et al.[36] have also demonstrated cytoplasmic localization in ecdysone-treated *Drosophila* larvae. Our findings are in agreement with earlier studies carried out by Arrigo[37] and Haass et al.[38] who reported that neuronal lineage cells express hsp 23 (under hyperthermia conditions). There have been no similar reports on the ectopic expression of a hsp 23 construct in *Drosophila* embryos, larvae, adults, or cell lines. Our findings constitute the first demonstration of spatial restrictions (embryonic cell type specificity) on the expression of hsp 23 reporter gene construct.

Human Embryonic Cell Studies

Earlier and current two-dimensional gel electrophoresis studies indicate that teratogen-exposed amniotic fluid and chorionic cells respond to these extrinsic factors by expressing increased

Table 1. Hsp 23 Induction in Teratogen-Treated *Drosophila* Embryonic Cells:
β-Galactosidase Localization

Treatment	Concentration (m*M*)	T/NT[b]	Fold induction of X-gal-positive neuronal clusters[a]
Heat shock	37°C, 30 min	T	4.39
Arsenate	0.10	T	4.90
	0.05		4.26
Caffeine	1.00	NT	0.83
Cadmium chloride	1.00	T	Cell death
	0.20		3.50
	0.10		2.56
	0.01		1.07
Coumarin	0.50	T	Cell death
	0.01		1.28
Diethylstilbestrol	0.01	T	1.35
Diphenylhydantoin	0.10	T	1.31
Ethyl alcohol	3%	T	2.10
Mercuric chloride	0.005	T	1.29
	0.001		1.31
Retinoic acid	0.1	T	1.85
	0.05		1.53
	0.01		1.09
Thalidomide	0.5	T	1.20

[a] Calculation of fold induction is explained in text.
[b] T/NT, teratogen/nonteratogen classification as reported in the literature.

levels of hsp 27. None of the teratogens tested in this trial resulted in hsp 70 induction (Figure 2). Heat-shock treatment (45°C for 20 min) results in the induction of hsp 70 and hsp 27 among other not presently analyzed heat shock proteins. The hsp 27 levels vary according to the teratogen used (Figure 2 and Table 2).

Densitometric analysis was carried out on hsp 27 induction. The Northern dot blot analysis utilizing an hsp 27 cDNA also resulted in ascertaining that teratogen treatment leads to increased levels of hsp 27 mRNA (Figure 3). The levels of induction vary according to the teratogen used with 5-azacytidine, heavy metals, and heat-shock treatments resulting in the highest degree of induction. Use of nonradioactive labeled cDNA probe obviously results in several compromises, including degree of sensitivity, reprobing of the mRNA, and irreproducibility problems, but since one of our aims has been to avoid radioactive labeling of the probes, we had to settle for these disadvantages in hope of ultimately developing this assay for a clinical setting. Similar levels of hsp 27 mRNA and heat-shock protein 27 induction were observed. Immunocytochemistry studies also confirmed the protein and mRNA studies (Table 3). The distribution of hsp 27 protein seems to be confined to the cytoplasm with very little, if any, nuclear staining. The level of staining varies according to the teratogen used. Control cultures show a faint staining pattern indicating constitutive expression of hsp 27 in human embryonic lineage cells. This constitutive expression is not restricted to the cytoplasm (Figure 4). Our current studies do not have the level of resolution required to definitely ascertain patterns of intracellular localization of hsp 27. We also did not carry out any heat shock or teratogen recovery studies to ascertain if any protein shuttling was taking place. Arrigo et al.[39] have also reported on the distribution of hsp 28 (hsp 27 in our system) in HeLa cell cultures. In their case, hsp 28/27 protein was shown to be localized in the perinuclear region, but after heat shock the protein relocalized within the nucleus.

DISCUSSION

During embryogenesis, varied developmental events occur in rapid procession. Any point during the transition from zygote to embryo to fetus is highly vulnerable to environmental disturbances. Disruption of any normally occurring developmental sequences can result in a structural or

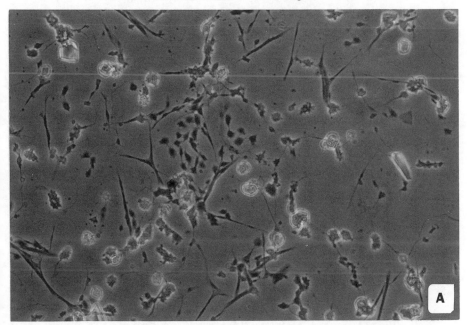

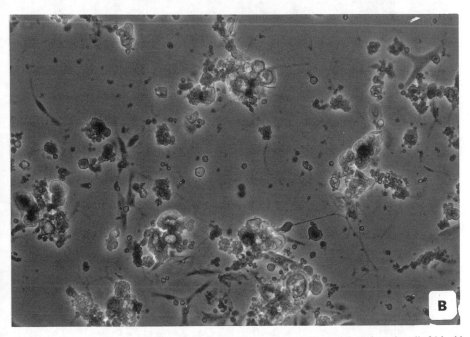

Figure 1. Pattern of β-galactosidase activity in hsp-23 transformant. *Drosophila* embryonic cells 24 h old were assayed for the teratogen-induced expression of integrated hsp 23-β-galactosidase fusion genes by incubation in a buffer containing X-gal. A, control; B, teratogen (transretinoic acid; 0.01 mM). In control cultures the number of X-gal positive neuronal cells (blue stain) is dramatically smaller than in teratogen treated ones ×320.

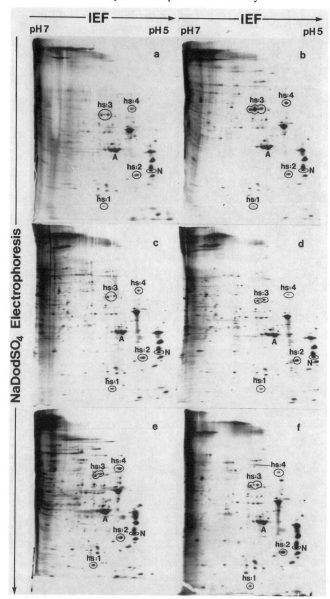

Figure 2. Two-dimensional gel electrophoresis patterns from heat-shocked, teratogen-treated, and control amniotic fluid cells. The indicated drug was added 18–20 h before labeling. Cells were labeled for 1 h with [³H]leucine at 37°C.

Heat-shocked cells (45°C for 20 min) were labeled 90 min after heat shock. (a) Control; (b) heat shock; (c) diphenylhydantoin (0.1 m*M*); (d) diethylstilbestrol (0.01 m*M*); (e) alcohol (3%); (f) coumarin (0.01 m*M*). Exposures (cpm × days) were as follows: (a) 506,059; (b) 511,582; (c) 492,000; (d) 509,059; (e) 512,190; (f) 492,234. A, actins; N, control; hs:2, hsp 27; hs:3, hsp 70

Table 2. Induction Levels of hsp 27 in Teratogen-Treated Human Amniotic Fluid Cells: Two-Dimensional Gel Electrophoresis

Treatment	Concentration (mM)	T/NT	Relative increase over control[a]
Control	—	—	—
Alcohol	3%	T	3.42
5-Azacytidine	0.03	T	40
Caffeine	1.00	NT	0[b]
Coumarin	0.10	T	20
Diphenylhydantoin	0.10	T	8
Diethylstilbestrol	0.01	T	4
DMSO (dimethyl sulfoxide)	160	NT	0
Heat shock	45°C, 20 min	T	30
Saccharin	1.00	NT	0

[a] Integrated optical densities for hsp 27 were determined from fluorographs, using a Bausch & Lomb automated image analysis system. Values were normalized to the integrated optical density of action on the same film. The normalized values were averaged, and the results are expressed as relative increases over normalized untreated control values.

[b] Designation for relative increase over control of less than 1.

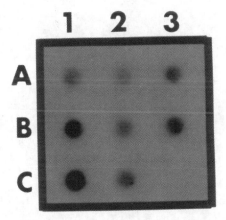

Figure 3. Northern dot blot analysis of teratogen treated human chorionic cells utilizing a biotinylated hsp 27 cDNA probe. Visualization of mRNA–cDNA hybrids was accomplished using a chemiluminescent kit (Plex-luminescent, Millipore, Bedford, MA) (see Materials and Methods). A1, alcohol; A2, diethylstilbestrol; A3, coumarin; B1, heat shock; B2, coumarin; B3, cadmium; C1, heat shock; C2, retinoic acid; C3, control. For concentrations used, see Table 1.

functional deficit (teratogenesis). Elucidating the mechanisms responsible for this abnormal pathway will ultimately have to come from a gene-level approach (i.e., which are the embryonic genes that get turned on or off by an environmental change). This hunt for genes involved in the teratogenesis process has led us to identifying the teratogen-induced transcriptional enhancement of a subset of the *Drosophila* heat-shock protein genes (hsp 23 and hsp 22.)[14,25] When those proteins were identified as being teratogen responsive, questions of function and of spatial and temporal expression presented themselves for investigation. Utilizing reporter gene technology (hsp 23–β-galactosidase construct) allowed us to investigate the cell specificity of the

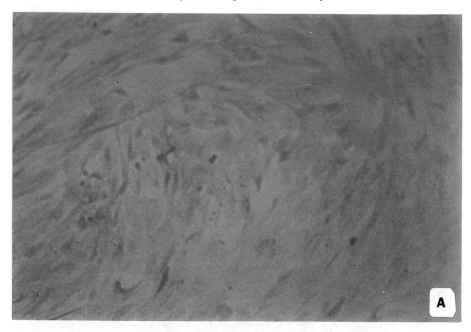

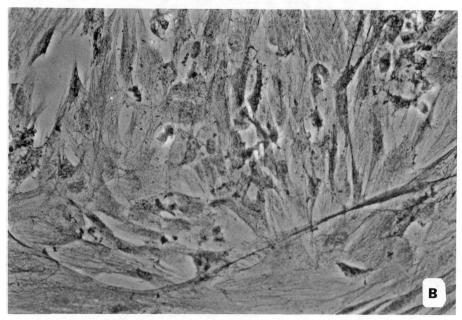

Figure 4. Immunolocalization of teratogen-induced hsp 27 in human chorionic villi cells with hsp 27 antibody. (A) control; (B) arsenate (0.05 m*M*) (24-h treatment). Visualization of antigen–antibody complex was made using biotinylated anti-immunoglobulin and subsequent horseradish peroxidase. DAB was used as a chromogen. ×160.

induction process. Our results from ectopic expression of the hsp 23 promoter after teratogen exposure agree with those of Haass et al.,[38] who recently reported on the developmental expression pattern of hsp 22, 23, 26, and 27. Utilizing *in situ* immunocytochemistry, they reported that low-molecular-weight hsp expression can be observed after 6 h of development in large neuroblast-like cells. They also examined the adult expression pattern for these hsp, which included expression in the nervous system and ovary. This change in expression pattern could suggest a protection function for these low-molecular-weight hsp. Embryonic and adult neuronal cells are thought to be much more sensitive to extracellular perturbations than muscle cells. In the *Drosophila* embryonic cultures we have enhanced muscle and neuron differentiation and, as such, these 2 cell types represent approximately 80% of the total cell population. We cannot ascertain if other underrepresented cell types, such as chitin-producing cells and imaginal disc predecessor cells, are expressing hsp 23. Nevertheless, what makes this suggestion of protective function even stronger is that a strikingly similar expression pattern is observed with our X-gal assay, utilizing an *in vitro* system, and the pattern observed by Haass et al.,[38] using intact wild-type *Drosophila* embryos.

Extending our hsp studies to human embryonic lineage cells was a natural progression, since we were very much interested in establishing a universality for teratogen-induced transcriptional activation of hsp genes and their contributions to both the normal and abnormal developmental pathways. Since our original studies with *Drosophila*, several investigators have linked the induction of a heat-shock response to exposures involving drugs and chemicals, with the majority utilizing cell lines or adult organisms (for a review, see Ref. 19). A limited number of recent studies have also reported on the induction of hsp in mammalian embryos after exposure to teratogens.[19,23,31,40,41] Regarding tissue specificity of the hsp induction pattern, several workers have reported such spatial restrictions. Anson et al.,[30] have shown that retinoic acid-exposed rat embryos responded to the teratogenic insult by a concomitant induction of a subset of hsp. Furthermore, the induction was target tissue specific (tissue that exhibited malformations was also the one capable of mounting a hsp response). Similar results (specific induction of hsp at the tissue targeted by the teratogen) have been reported by Hansen et al.[42] Higo et al.[43] reported on tissue-specific induction of hsp in embryonic rat hearts after teratogen exposure (specific induction of hsp at the tissue targeted by teratogen). Walsh and Morris[44] have also reported that heat shock affects cell cycling of the neuroectoderm of developing mouse embryos with the hsp 71/72 being induced. No mention was made of induction pattern of hsp 27.[44,45] This tissue response specificity again points to a possible functional link between hsp induction and teratogenic response of the developing embryo. Hsp induction by heat shock has been linked to thermotolerance in studies involving mice and rat embryos.[27–29] Studies involving a Chinese hamster lung fibroblast cell line have provided direct evidence that heat-induced hsp 27 expression directly confers thermotolerance by possibly stabilizing heat-induced perturbation.[46] This thermotolerance has also been demonstrated, in the same system, by a variety of other agents, such as ionophores, arsenite, mitogens, and cycloheximide.[46] Further studies by the same group implicate hsp 27 phosphorylation as contributing to the thermoresistance.[47] Human cell studies (HeLa cells) have also implicated hsp 27/28 induction as conferring thermoprotection.[39] Since our human cell studies involve the use of a single cell type, we cannot address the issue of tissue specificity but can only report on the relative levels of hsp 27 induction. In the present studies, we did not carry out protection studies. Such studies are currently in the planning stage.

Studies completed so far, including this one, indicate that the genes for the various hsp can be and are expressed independently of each other, and the profile of protein expression shown after teratogen exposure follows this variable pattern. Thus, although each teratogen certainly differs in the pattern of malformation that it elicits and the biochemical mechanism(s) involved could be not the same, hsp expression is always enhanced. If hsp activation relates to a switch in the developmental pathway, then identification of teratogen-responsive elements (TRE) and other gene activations must be investigated. Such promoter activation sites have been identified in the case of ecdysone activation of hsp 22, 23, 26, and 27 in *Drosophila* larvae.[48] Several hypotheses have been put forth regarding the modus operandi of teratogen-induced heat-shock proteins and the general induction of all the hsp. A developing cell's encounter with heat shock or a teratogen could be resulting in posttranscriptional alterations, denaturation of mRNA of developmentally important genes. Heat shock has been suggested to denature mRNAs of other

Table 3. Hsp 27 Induction in Teratogen-Treated Chorionic Villi Cells: Immunocytochemical Detection

Treatment	Concentration (mM)	Relative intensity[a]
Control	+	
Heat shock	45°C, 20 min	+ + + +
5-Azacytidine	0.03	+ + +
CdCl$_2$ 0.01	+ + + +	
Cortisone	0.01	+ + + +
Arsenate 0.05	+ + + +	

[a] Relative intensity of hsp 27 induction is scored by intensity of brown precipitate (antigen–antibody complexes) formed. Formal density values were not obtained; only the attached camera photometer was used to roughly rank hsp 27 induction levels.

transcriptionally active genes.[49] It is also possible that enhanced levels of hsp hinder promoter sites; thus, no transcription takes place or a suboptimal amount of that mRNA is expressed. If, on the other hand, hsp are stabilizing critical mRNAs, thus preventing developmental abnormalities, then what we observe in the teratogenic response are the survivors (cells capable of rescuing gene expression). Cells of different lineages that did not survive were incapable of responding appropriately. Many teratologists have implicated activation of programmed cell death as being responsible for several types of malformations observed; certainly such activation requires some type of transcription factor(s) to be present (heat-shock transcription factor?).

In summary, we have demonstrated that teratogens induce a subset of hsp and that the subset, at least in the case of hsp 23 induction, is spatially and temporally limited. Furthermore, the X-gal assay can be easily adapted to be utilized as a Tier I teratogen screen to deal with the large number of untested chemicals and environmental pollutants. Preliminary trials have indicated that we can also test for the presence of teratogens in polluted water sites (unpublished observations). The X-gal in situ assay can be used in conjunction with neurotransmitter-antibody probes, such as ChaT and histamine, so that we can further investigate the population of neuronal cells mounting the teratogen-induced hsp 23 response. Neurotransmitters have recently been implicated as being very important in the early neuronal development of the embryo, and there is considerable interest in developing models for identifying neuroteratogens. With the number of homeotic gene probes currently available, we do plan to carry out studies investigating the spatial and temporal expression patterns of such genes after heat shock or teratogen treatment.

Our human cell studies, obviously, do not lend themselves yet to any mechanistic type of studies, but we certainly can use the Northern dot blot analysis to investigate hsp 27 induction patterns in other available embryonic cell lineage cells. For the moment we are planning to validate this assay for possible use in future clinical studies. It is anticipated that such an assay could be used to inform a pregnant woman of the developmental status of her unborn baby very much the way she is currently informed of its karyotype and genome status utilizing amniocentesis or chorionic villi sampling technology.

REFERENCES

1. Wilson, J. G. 1977. Current status of teratology. In *Handbook of teratology*, eds. J. G. Wilson and F. C. Fraser, p. 309. New York: Plenum Press.
2. Brown, N. A., and Freeman, S. J. 1984. Alternative tests for teratogenicity. *Alternatives to Laboratory Animals* 12:7–23.
3. Faustman, E. M. 1988. Short-term tests for teratogens. *Mutat. Res.* 205:355–384.
4. Johnson, E. M., and Kochhar, D. M. 1983. *Teratogenesis and reproductive toxicology handbook. Experimental pharmacology*, vol. LXV. Berlin: Springer-Verlag.
5. Kimmel G. L., Smith, K., Kochhar, D. M., and Pratt, R. M. 1982. Overview of *in vitro* teratogenicity testing: Aspects of validation and application to screening. *Teratogen. Carcinogen. Mutagen.* 2:221–229.
6. Neubert, D. 1989. *In vitro* techniques for assessing teratogenic potential. In *Advances in applied toxicology*, eds. A. D. Dayan and A. J. Paine, pp. 191–211. London: Taylor & Francis.
7. Welsh, F. 1990. Short-term methods of assessing developmental toxicity hazard: Status and critical evaluation. *Issues Rev. Teratol.* 5:115–153.
8. Bournias-Vardiabasis, N., Teplitz, R. L., Chernoff, G. P., and Seecof, R. L. 1983. Detection of teratogens in the *Drosophila in vitro* test: Assay of 100 chemicals. *Teratology* 28:109–122.

9. Seecof, R. L., Donady, J. T., and Teplitc, R. L. 1973. Differentiation of *Drosophila* neuroblasts to form ganglion like clusters of neurons *in vitro*. *Cell Differ.* 2:143–149.

10. Seecof, R. L., Gerson, I., Donady, J. T., and Teplitc, R. L. 1973. *Drosophila* myogenesis *in vitro*. The genesis of small myocytes and myotubes. *Dev. Biol.* 35:250–261.

11. Bournias-Vardiabasis, N., and Flores, J. 1983. Drug metabolising enzymes in *Drosophila melanogaster*: Teratogenicity of cyclophosphamide *in vitro*. *Teratogen. Carcinogen. Mutagen.* 3:255–262.

12. Bournias-Vardiabasis, N., Buzin, C. H., and Reilly, J. G. 1983. The effect of 5-azacytidine and cytidine analogs on *Drosophila melanogaster* cells in culture. *Wilhelm Roux' Arch. Dev. Biol.* 192:299–302.

13. Bournias-Vardiabasis, N., Buzin, C. H., and Flores, J. 1990. Differential expression of heat shock proteins in *Drosophila* embryonic cells following metal ion exposure. *Exp. Cell Res.* 189:177–182.

14. Buzin, C. H., and Bournias-Vardiabasis, N. 1984. Teratogens induce a subset of small heat shock proteins in *Drosophila* primary embryonic cell cultures. *Proc. Natl. Acad. Sci. USA* 81:4075–4079.

15. Salvaterra, P. M., Bournias-Vardiabasis, N., Nair, T., Hou, G., and Lieu, C. 1987. *In vitro* neuronal differentiation of *Drosophila* embryo cells. *J. Neurosci.* 7:10–22.

16. Bournias-Vardiabasis, N., and Flores, J. 1986. Response of *Drosophila melanogaster* embryonic cells to tumor promoters: carcinogens as teratogens. *Toxicol. and Appl. Pharmacol.* 85:196–206.

17. Bond, U., and Schlesinger, M. L. 1987. Heat-shock proteins and development. *Adv. Genet.* 24:1–29.

18. Petersen, N. S. 1990. Effects of heat and chemical stress on development. *Adv. Genet.* 28:275–295.

19. Nover, L. 1991. *Heat shock response*. Boca Raton, FL: CRC Press.

20. Mitchell, H. K., Moller, G., Petersen, N. S., and Lipps-Sarmiento, L. 1979. Specific protection from phenocopy induction by heat shock. *Dev. Genet.* 1:181–192.

21. Berger, E. M., and Woodward, M. P. 1983. Small heat shock proteins in *Drosophila* may confer thermal tolerance. *Exp. Cell Res.* 147:437–442.

22. Bensaude, O., Babinet, C., Morange, M., and Jacob, F. 1983. Heat shock proteins, the first major products of zygotic gene activity in mouse embryos. *Nature* 305:331–332.

23. Heikkila, J. J., and Schultz, G. A. 1984. Differential environmental stresses can activate the expression of a heat shock gene in rabbit blastocysts. *Gamete Res.* 10:45–56.

24. Marin, R., Valet, J. P., and Tanguay, R. M. 1993. Hsp23 and hsp26 exhibit district spatial and temporal patterns of constitutive expression in *Drosophila* adults. *Dev. Genet.* 14:69–77.

25. Buzin, C. H., and Bournias-Vardiabasis, N. 1982. Teratogens induce small heat-shock proteins. In *Heat shock: From bacteria to man*, eds. M. J. Schlesinger, M. Ashburner, and A. Tissières p. 387. Cold Spring Harbor, NY: Cold Spring Harbor Laboratory.

26. Bournias-Vardiabasis, N. 1985. Use of amniotic fluid cells for testing teratogens. *In Vitro Toxicol.* 3:317–331.

27. Mirkes, P. E. 1987. Hyperthermia-induced heat shock response and thermotolerance in postimplantation rat embryos. *Dev. Biol.* 119:115–122.

28. Walsh, D. A., Klein, N. W., Hightower, L. E., and Edwards, M. J. 1987. Heat shock and thermotolerance during early rat embryo development. *Teratology* 36:181–191.

29. Kapron-Brás, C. M., and Hales, B. F. 1991. Heat-shock induced tolerance to the embryotoxic effects of hyperthermia and cadmium in mouse embryos *in vitro*. *Teratology* 43:83–97.

30. Anson, J. F., Laborde, J. B., Papkin, J. L., Hinson, W. G., Hansen, D. K., Sheehan, D. M., and Young, J. F. 1991. Target tissue specificity of retinoic acid-induced stress proteins and malformations in mice. *Teratology* 44:19–28.

31. Mirkes, P. E., Doggett, D., and Cornel, L. 1994. Induction of a heat shock response (HSP 72) in rat embryos exposed to selected chemical teratogens. *Teratology* 49:135–142.

32. Nover, L. 1991. Hear Shock Response. Boca Raton: CRC Press.

33. Seecof, R. L. 1980. Preparation of cell cultures from *Drosophila melanogaster* embryos. *Tissue Culture Assoc. Manual* 4:1019–1022.

34. Ashburner, M. 1989. Drosophila: *A laboratory manual*. Cold Spring Harbor, NY: Cold Spring Harbor Laboratory Press.

35. Duband, J. L., Lettre, F., Arrigo, A. P., and Tanguay, R. M. 1986. Expression and localization of hsp-23 in unstressed and heat-shocked *Drosophila* cultured cells. *Can. J. Genet. Cytol.* 28:1088–1092.

36. Ireland, R. C., Berger, E., Sirotkin, K., Yund, M. A., Ostebar, D., and Fristrom, J. 1982. Ecdysterone induces the transcription of four heat-shock genes in *Drosophila*. S3 cells and imaginal discs. *Dev. Biol.* 93:498–507.

37. Arrigo, A. P. 1987. Cellular localization of HSP23 during *Drosophila* development and following subsequent heat shock. *Dev. Biol.* 122:39–48.

38. Haass, C., Klein, U., and Kloetzel, P. M. 1990. Developmental expression of *Drosophila melanogaster* small heat-shock proteins. *J. Cell Sci.* 96:413–418.

39. Arrigo, A. P., Suhan, J. P., and Welch, W. J. 1988. Dynamic changes in the structure and intracellular locale of the mammalian low-molecular-weight heat shock protein. *Mol. Cell. Biol.* 8:5059–5071.

40. Mirkes, P. E., Grace, R. H., and Little, S. A. 1991. Developmental regulation of heat shock protein

synthesis and HSP 70 RNA accumulation during postimplantation rat embryogenesis. *Teratology* 44:77–89.

41. Mirkes, P. E., and Cornel, L. 1992. A comparison of sodium arsenite- and hyperthermia-induced stress responses and abnormal development in cultured postimplantation rat embryos. *Teratology* 46:251–259.

42. Hansen, D. K., Anson, J. F., Hinson, W. G., and Pipkil, J. L. 1988. Phenytoin-induced stress protein synthesis in mouse embryonic tissue. *Proc. Soc. Exp. Biol. Med.* 189:136–140.

43. Higo, H., Higo, K., Lee, J. Y., Hori, H., and Satow, Y. 1988. Effects of exposing rat embryos *in utero* to physical or chemical teratogens are expressed later as enhanced induction of heat-shock proteins when embryonic hearts are cultured *in vitro*. *Teratogen. Carcinogen. Mutagen.* 8:315–328.

44. Walsh, D. A., and Morris, V. R. 1989. Heat shock affects cell cycling in the neural plate of cultured rat embryos: A flow cytometric study. *Teratology* 40:583–592.

45. Walsh, D. A., Li, K., Speirs, J., Crowther, C. E., and Edwards, M. J. 1989. Regulation of the inducible heat shock 71 genes in early neural development of cultured rat embryos. *Teratology* 40:321–334.

46. Créte, P., and Landry, J. 1990. Induction of HSP 27 phosphorylation and thermoresistance in Chinese hamster cells by arsenite, cycloheximide, A23187 and EGTA. *Radia. Res.* 121:320–327.

47. Landry, J., Chrétien, P., Laszlo, A., and Lambert, H. 1991. Phosphorylation of HSP27 during development and decay of thermotolerance in Chinese hamster cells. *J. Cell. Physiol.* 147:93–101.

48. Amin, J., Mestril, R., and Voellmy, R. 1991. Genes for *Drosophila* small heat shock proteins are regulated differently by ecdysterone. *Mol. Cell. Biol.* 11:5937–5944.

49. Haass, C., Klein U., Kloetzel, P. 1990. Developmental Expression of *Drosophila melanogaster* small heat shock proteins. *J. Cell. Sci.* 96:413–418.

Chapter Thirteen

USING INVARIANTS OF SWIMMING MOTION IN BIOTOXICITY TESTING VIA COMPUTERIZED MICROSCOPY

David K. Cohoon, R. James Swanson, and Ronald J. Young

Conservation laws of physics described in Appleton[1] give rise naturally to the use of stochastic differential equations with partially deterministic and partially random driving forces (fueled by adenosinetriphosphate (ATP) to adenosinediphosphate (ADP) conversion) and parameters defined in Arnold.[2] The mathematical analysis of the observed motion of different types of spermatozoa described in Austin[3] led us to believe that there may be invariants among a small Barnsley type mathematical parameter set discussed in Berger and Soner[4] that can be used to represent or describe the motion of the individual swimmer over a given time period and that these apparently only slightly changing parameters may serve as a fingerprint that might permit us to keep track of the swimmer over an extended period of time. Keeping track of an individual swimmer while the chemical environment is changing may permit us to discover mechanisms by which chemical stressors or toxins might have affected the swimming motion. Prior work by Berrill and Karp[5] on the use of spermatozoa swimming parameters and Tetrahymena pyriformis swimming patterns in biotoxicity testing is discussed. Computer graphics showing the model fits to both human and rabbit spermatozoa are included and suggest that an improvement of the usual polygonal path and Box and Jenkins[6] analysis of swimming data may have been found. A survey of generalizations of the detailed flagella and cilia motion models of Brokaw[7,8] may give hope of being able to relate observed changes in structure in the filaments of flagella to observed changes in swimming parameters, with the analysis being aided by fluorescent probes emitting at different wavelengths being attached to different parts of the swimmer.

INDIVIDUALIZED SWIMMING PARAMETERS

As some single-celled microorganisms swim, they move back and forth across a curve, often a straight line, that describes their primary swimming direction. This curve could be a line joining

Thanks are given to Dr. R. M. Purcell[13] for assistance with the computer graphics. Thanks for the data go to Professor Katz[38,39] of Duke University and to Dr. R. Young[69-71] of the Life Sciences Department of the Edgewood Research Development and Engineering Center's Chemical and Biological Defense Command. Thanks go to Daniel Wagner and to Dr. Belkin,[51] President of Daniel Wagner Associates, for 2 days of support and access to their computers in 1990, when this work was done, and to Dr. J. Weaver, Chair of Computer Science, for allowing access to the computers at West Chester University at this time. For an understanding of equipment, thanks are given to Yves Laberge of Thomas Jefferson University and Dr. Vasquez[67] of Vanderbilt University for a demonstration of automated spermatozoa motion tracking equipment and the use of fluorescent probes in tracking motion of specific parts of the spermatozoa, respectively, and to Professor Swanson[64] of the Old Dominion University Biology Department for a tour of his spermatozoa motion analysis laboratory and electron microscope views of spermatozoa heads and flagellum cross sections.

the initial point to the endpoint of the portion of the swimming track being analyzed. The swimming of spermatozoa is observed by placing them in liquid in a low flat dish, called a Makler cell, that fits on the stage of a phase-contrast microscope. This chapter provides mathematical models that might describe this swimming motion of different types of spermatozoa observed by Katz,[38,39] Mahoney,[50] Olds-Clarke,[54] Robertson,[57] Swanson,[64] and the rabbit data of Young[69-71] and suggests that the primary cross-track frequency and the organism's swimming speed could serve as an identifier to keep track of an individual single-celled swimmer over a period of time while experiments concerning bioeffects of pharmaceuticals and other chemical stressors were being carried out. The term microorganism is used here to denote both an independent biosystem such as a protozoa and a single-celled swimmer such as a Makler-cell-confined spermatozoa. Computer analysis suggests that the theories of this chapter are valid for both human spermatozoa and rabbit spermatozoa; the analysis was carried out for human spermatozoa data provided by Katz[38,39] and rabbit spermatozoa data provided by Young.[69-71]

The concept of using swimming microorganisms to assess toxicity is not new, as Noever[53] and Silverman[62] have worked with *Tetrahymena* swimming pattern alteration by toxins with a view toward eliminating or reducing the need for rabbit eye testing for ocular irritation, and Young[69-71] has demonstrated that spermatozoa wobble motion changes are correlated with the presence of toxins. Prior work with phylum protozoa analyzed in the book of Hill[32] has included the work of Loefer and Mefferd[47,48] and others for the ciliate *Tetrahymena*, which was used in biotoxicity testing also by Noever[52,53] and Silverman.[60-62] Experimental work to a certain extent has focused on *Tetrahymena pyriformis*, regarded by many as the star performer of the phylum protozoa. The *Ohio Science Workbook* chapter by Silverman[62] pointed out that if one added a toxin to a dish of *Tetrahymena*, the normal zig-zag swimming pattern changes; Silverman[62] also pointed out that the most commonly observed changes are to a pattern of tight circles as though only the cilia on one side are functioning, or to marked decreases in swimming speed, or to conditions where two of the *Tetrahymena* stick together as though the toxin caused something to happen to their membrane. These observations are not mentioned in the other papers of Silverman,[60,61] where statistics for a variety of toxins are given. In their 1952 letter to the editor Loefer and Mefferd[47,48] describe pattern formation in swimming microorganisms by looking at a dense culture in a shallow medium. Loefer and Mefferd[47,48] noted that horizontal swimming streams form a polygonal network with four or five streams meeting at nodes of the network and observed that at these nodes where the organisms meet, they fall to the bottom of the shallow medium and then swim upward to rejoin the horizontal streams. Loefer and Mefferd[47,48] observed that under ideal circumstances, these patterns form in 10 s. Noever[52,53] and other NASA scientists using a side-looking microscope and examining *Tetrahymena thermophila* observed that large populations of these creatures, being sensitive to gravity, formed interesting geometrical patterns that were altered or were completely broken up when chemical stressors were added. Recently Young[69-71] published a paper that supports the thesis of this chapter, namely, that motion parameters of spermatozoa can indeed be used as a test of biotoxicity. Young[69-71] pointed out that a parameter called wobble, which is the curvilinear speed of the microorganism divided by the net speed along a best fitting straight line, seems to be related to toxicity. It appears from comparisons of model predictions to laboratory data that the wobble parameter used by Young[69-71] could be very accurately computed with the methods of Cohoon[14] for individual spermatozoa. Roberts and Berk[56] used changes in normal chemoattraction of protozoa to test the toxicity of water. The correlation of swimming speed with fertilization by Holt, Moore, and Hillier[34] and Olds-Clarke[54] would also seem to support the thesis that swimming parameters and statistics could measure the chemical environment of spermatozoa and that keeping track of affected individual swimmers could help us advance the understanding developed by Austin,[3] Berril,[5] Chang,[9] Dehehy,[17] Dresdner,[19] Goltz,[28] Gwatkin,[30] Kopf,[42] Mack,[49] Mahoney,[50] Olds-Clarke,[54] Robertson,[57] and others of changes in motion occurring when the chemical environment of the spermatozoa is similar to that occurring during fertilization. This understanding might be improved by application of the electron microscopy methods used by Swanson[64] after the motion has ceased, or by employment of the fluorescent probe methods used by Vasquez[67] while the motion is still being observed in a Makler cell. If water pollutant levels cause observable changes in motion parameters, this could be used as a warning that these levels could be dangerous to humans.

One considers low populations of uniflagelar microorganisms on a flat dish and looks down on them from above with the idea that one can keep track of individual swimmers over the course of time. A simple model, with a small number of parameters, gives a fair description of the motion of these organisms. A short data table is shown that seems to confirm this hypothesis. No attempt was made to weed out poor matches to the theory, except that in the case where the organism makes a sharp turn, it is necessary to look at a straight subsection of the track. Sample correlations of the speed were computed from randomly abbreviated and original tracks; the sample means and sample standard deviations of the differences of speeds and differences of cross-track oscillation frequencies for the randomly shortened and original tracks were computed. Data from longer swimming tracks would be needed to confirm the theory of this chapter. However, Noever,[52,53] Roberts and Berk,[56] Silverman,[60–62] and others are already using changes in other swimming motion patterns of *Tetrahymena pyriformis* as an in vitro test for chemical toxicity. Rigorous hydrodynamic models of Childress,[10] Cox,[16] Uldrick and Siekmann,[66] and others help us understand the interaction of the fluid with the swimmer. The work of Brokaw,[7,8] which modeled the flagellum of a swimmer, has been studied or extended with applications to swimmers with a flagellum such as a spermatozoa or else applied to ciliated swimmers such as bacteria or protozoa by Chwang,[12] Dresdner,[19] Fauci and Fogelson,[22] Higdom,[31] Holwill and Burge,[33] Keller and Rubinow,[40] and Lighthill.[44,45] Perhaps with a combination of birds-eye view and side-looking microscopes, one may discover other invariants of swimming microorganisms, perhaps enabling one to see, perhaps with fluorescent probes, the unique features of a swimmer's flagellum.

Straight-Line Swimmers

During observations of microorganisms under a microscope in Swanson's[64] laboratory, a large fraction of the swimmers seemed to travel in straight lines until they underwent a change in direction by bumping into one another, after which they seemed to go off along two different straight lines. The best fitting straight line seemed to be an encouraging aid in the analysis, and was used in the creation of our data; currently, care must be taken to choose a segment of a track that does not include a sharp bend, which, to the eye, appears to happen when two swimmers collide. With some effort, a best curve fitting model could probably be developed. Coordinates were transformed so that the line giving the best fit of the observed swimming coordinates became the abscissa of a laboratory coordinate system. A swimming speed along this line was calculated. The swimmer then seemed to bob above and below the new x-axis, giving us a function $y(t)$. A supremum norm fit of sinusoids was then carried out one frequency at a time. Fourier analysis did not work; when this was tried initially with fast Fourier transform packages or careful Gaussian quadrature, thousands of terms produced a poor fit to the data as apparently the frequencies that are needed are not integer multiples of some lowest frequency.

For many of the automated frame grabber recorded observations of Young[69–71] and Katz,[38,39] I could carry out a detrending by fitting their motions, their laboratory x abscissa and y ordinate coordinates on the microscope slide, to the best straight lines of the form given by

$$(x(t), y(t)) = (At + B, Ct + D) + (x^*(t), y^*(t))$$

in Cohoon[14] where (x, y) are affine functions of time in the form of the equation $(At + B, Ct + D)$ plus oscillatory zero mean functions $(x^*(t), y^*(t))$ also described in Cohoon.[14] I changed coordinates by a rotation so that the C of the equation just described is equal to zero in the new coordinate system and so that $y^*(t)$ is the motion perpendicular to the best fitting line that passes through the swimming coordinates, which means that the swimmer now seems to be traveling along the horizontal x axis of the new coordinate system. The oscillatory, zero-mean function $y^*(t)$, which simulates the cross-track motion, seems to contain biological information. The major thrust of the rest of the chapter is to find a small number of frequencies ω and a small number of linear combinations of the functions $\sin(\omega t)$ and $\cos(\omega t)$ such that after subtracting these linear combinations from the zero-mean functions, $x^*(t)$ and $y^*(t)$, what is left is a time series that is small with respect to some norm, or measure of the size of time series prescribed by a norm, such as the square root of the sum of the squares of the differences norm. The frequency appears to be a characteristic of the individual swimmer and may possibly be used as a highly sensitive measure of toxicity by looking at how much would have to be added to the microscope dish to change the creature's swimming frequency and other parameters.

Suppose there are N microscope slide swimming coordinates that are members of the set

$$C = \{(x_1, y_1), \ldots, (x_N, y_N)\}$$

and represent the observed laboratory coordinates of a microscopic swimmer moving on a dish-like microscope slide, where the time at which the swimmer has coordinates (x_{j+1}, y_{j+1}) is j times a known time between measurements. This effectively gives the (x, y) coordinates of the swimmer as a function of time. The first step is to find the slope b_1 and intercept b_0 of the best fitting straight line, so that the expression

$$S = (y_1 - b_1x_1 - b_0)^2 + (y_2 - b_1x_2 - b_0)^2 + \cdots$$
$$+ (y_{N-1} - b_1x_{N-1} - b_0)^2 + (y_N - b_1x_N - b_0)^2$$

is as small as possible. Regrouping terms in this equation so that the function $S(b_0, b_1)$ defined by this equation is more easily seen to be a polynomial in b_1 and b_0 gives the equation

$$S(b_0, b_1) = \left(\sum_{i=1}^{N} y_i^2\right) + \left(\sum_{i=1}^{N} x_i^2\right)b_1^2 + b_0^2 N$$
$$- \left(2\sum_{i=1}^{N} x_iy_i\right)b_1 - \left(2\sum_{i=1}^{N} y_i\right)b_0 + \left(2\sum_{i=1}^{N} x_i\right)b_0b_1$$

The average x coordinate of the swimmer is denoted by

$$\bar{x} = \frac{\sum_{i=1}^{N} x_i}{N}$$

and the swimmer's average or expected y coordinate is given by

$$\bar{y} = \frac{\sum_{i=1}^{N} y_i}{N}$$

Collecting terms and substituting these two expressions for the average values of x and y into the previous equation yields

$$S = N[b_0^2 - 2b_0(\bar{y} - b_1\bar{x})] + \left(\sum_{i=1}^{N} x_i^2\right)b_1^2 - 2\left(\sum_{i=1}^{N} x_iy_i\right)b_1 + \sum_{i=1}^{N} y_i^2$$

Adding the representation of zero as

$$N(\bar{y} - b_1\bar{x})^2 - N(\bar{y} - b_1\bar{x})^2 = 0$$

to the right side of this equation makes it easy to see the relationship

$$S = N[b_0^2 - 2b_0(\bar{y} - b_1\bar{x}) + (\bar{y} - b_1\bar{x})^2]$$
$$+ \left(\sum_{i=1}^{N} x_i^2\right)b_1^2 - N(\bar{y} - b_1\bar{x})^2 - 2\left(\sum_{i=1}^{N} x_iy_i\right)b_1 + \sum_{i=1}^{N} y_i^2$$

Simplifying this equation using the identity

$$[b_0 - (\bar{y} - b_1\bar{x})]^2 = b_0^2 - 2b_0(\bar{y} - b_1\bar{x}) + (\bar{y} - b_1\bar{x})^2$$

it can be seen that

$$S = N[b_0 - (\bar{y} - b_1\bar{x})]^2 + b_1^2\left[\sum_{i=1}^{N} x_i^2 - N(\bar{x})^2\right]$$

$$- 2b_1\left[\left(\sum_{i=1}^{N} x_iy_i\right) - N\bar{xy}\right] + \sum_{i=1}^{N} y_i^2 - N(\bar{y})^2$$

Collecting terms and completing the square, it follows that

$$S = N[b_0 - (\bar{y} - b_1\bar{x})]^2$$

$$+ \left(\sum_{i=1}^{N} x_i^2 - N(\bar{x})^2\right)\left(b_1 - \frac{\sum_{i=1}^{N} x_iy_i - N\bar{xy}}{\sum_{i=1}^{N} x_i^2 - N(\bar{x})^2}\right)^2$$

$$+ \frac{\left[\left(\sum_{i=1}^{N} y_i^2 - N(\bar{y})^2\right)\left(\sum_{i=1}^{N} x_i^2 - N(\bar{x})^2\right) - \left(\sum_{i=1}^{N} x_iy_i - N\bar{xy}\right)^2\right]}{\sum_{i=1}^{N} x_i^2 - N(\bar{x})^2}$$

This equation implies that S is minimized as a function of b_0 and b_1, provided that the first two positive terms, which are the only terms involving b_0 and b_1, vanish identically. The statistical interpretation of this is made transparent by setting

$$b_1 = \left(\frac{\sum_{i=1}^{N} x_iy_i - N\bar{xy}}{\sum_{i=1}^{N} x_i^2 - N(\bar{x})^2}\right) = \frac{\dfrac{\sum_{i=1}^{N} x_iy_i}{N} - \bar{xy}}{\dfrac{\sum_{i=1}^{N} x_i^2}{N} - (\bar{x})^2}$$

which is, according to Feller,[23] an estimate of the covariance of the x_i and the y_i divided by the estimate of the variance of the x_i, respectively; the intercept b_0 is defined by the rule

$$b_0 = \bar{y} - b_1\bar{x}$$

There need be no concern, here, over dividing by zero; just make use of the Cauchy Schwarz inequality, which is a special case of the Holder inequality described in Friedman[26] and Hormander[35] specialized to the square root of the sum of squares norm and which says that the square of the inner or dot product of two linearly independent vectors is strictly smaller than the product of the sums of the squares of their entries. Considering the vector of N consecutive swimmer's x coordinates given by

$$X = (x_1, x_2, \ldots, x_N)$$

and the N-tuple of ones denoted by

$$Y = (1, 1, \ldots, 1)$$

it is clear that if there are as many as two different coordinates of X, then X cannot possibly depend linearly on Y, which means that for all α and all β the dot product of $\alpha X - \beta Y$ with itself is strictly positive. In particular, letting α be the length of Y and β be the length of X, it follows that the length of X multiplied by the length of Y is strictly greater than the dot product of X and Y. For the particular case where Y is an N-tuple every entry of which is 1, this may be expressed by the relationship,

$$(x_1^2 + x_2^2 + \cdots + x_N^2)(1^2 + 1^2 + \cdots + 1^2) = (x_1^2 + x_2^2 + \cdots + x_N^2)N$$
$$> (x_1 + x_2 + \cdots + x_N)^2 = (X \cdot Y)^2$$

which may be rewritten in the form

$$(\bar{x})^2 = \left(\frac{x_1 + x_2 + \cdots + x_N}{N}\right)^2 < \left(\frac{x_1^2 + x_2^2 + \cdots + x_N^2}{N}\right)$$

whenever there are two distinct values of x_i, which means that as long as there are two different x coordinates, the estimate of the variance of the x_i described in Feller[23] is nonzero.

In the *Applied Sciences and Computation* paper of Cohoon[14] it is observed that the slope of the best fitting straight line through the swimmer coordinates is simply the estimate of the variance in Feller[23] of the microscopically observed x and y coordinates of the swimmer divided by the estimate of the variance in Feller[23] of the x coordinates of a swimmer described in Cohoon,[14] and the y intercept of the best fitting line is the mean value of the observed y coordinates of the swimmer minus the product of this slope and the mean value of the x coordinates of the swimmer, provided that there are at least two different x coordinates. The fact that the mean value of the y coordinates minus the slope times the mean value of the x coordinates is the y intercept means that if one obtains a new set of y coordinates, $y^*(t)$, via the relationship $y^*(t) = y - mx - b$, where m is the slope and b is the y intercept, then by derivation of the y intercept b of the best fitting line as the mean of y minus the product of the slope times the mean of the x coordinates, the coordinates $y^*(t)$ have to have zero mean. After a rotation so that the best fitting line describing the path of the swimmers is the x axis of a rotated coordinate system, consider the problem of analyzing the data $y^*(t)$ and extracting information from this data that is peculiar to and characteristic of the individual microscopic swimmer.

Autocorrelation matrices could probably be used effectively to understand low-degree polynomial fitting of non-straight-line motion. If the swimmers's coordinates are (x_i, y_i) then the numbers (b_0, b_1) can be determined through an analysis of the overdetermined system,

$$A\begin{pmatrix} b_0 \\ b_1 \end{pmatrix} = \begin{pmatrix} 1 & X_1 \\ 1 & X_2 \\ \vdots & \vdots \\ 1 & X_n \end{pmatrix}\begin{pmatrix} b_0 \\ b_1 \end{pmatrix} = \begin{pmatrix} Y_1 \\ Y_2 \\ \vdots \\ Y_n \end{pmatrix}$$

This equation, which admits an obvious generalization to higher order polynomials by adding columns of squares, cubes, and so on of the x coordinates of the swimmer to the matrix A, can be solved by multiplying both sides of the equation by A^t, which is the transpose of A, defined by

$$A^t = \begin{pmatrix} 1 & 1 & \cdots & 1 \\ x_1 & x_2 & \cdots & x_n \end{pmatrix}$$

obtaining the relationship

$$C \cdot \begin{pmatrix} b_0 \\ b_1 \end{pmatrix} = \begin{pmatrix} n & \sum_{i=1}^{n} x_i \\ \sum_{i=1}^{n} x_i & \sum_{i=1}^{n} x_i^2 \end{pmatrix}\begin{pmatrix} b_0 \\ b_1 \end{pmatrix} = \begin{pmatrix} \sum_{i=1}^{n} y_i \\ \sum_{i=1}^{n} x_i y_i \end{pmatrix}$$

which is exactly the same as the set of equations obtained with the previous analysis; in general, for higher order polynomial fits needed for curved swimming paths, the coefficient matrix C in this equation has the property that the entry in row i and column j is a function of $i + j$.

SINUSOIDAL SWIMMING PARAMETERS

A serious problem with microscope slide data is that there is a limited rate at which one can take snapshots of the swimmer that reveal the (x, y) coordinates of the swimmer at uniformly spaced time points, and if the swimming is fairly rapid, the digitized data may be quite sparse in the sense that for the purposes of analysis, one really would have liked to know where the swimmer was at several intermediate time points. Standard packages such as FFT, described in Elliott and Rao,[20] and standard Barnsley methods for processing images or time series, described in Berger and Soner[4] or Koopmans,[41] were totally ineffective in analyzing this type of data. The analysis that follows suggests that other numerical difficulties associated with finding a best frequency so that $y^*(t) - A \cos(\omega t) - B \sin(\omega t)$ is uniformly as small as possible would be alleviated if one did not use equally spaced sampling times, although equally spaced times certainly do aid in estimating swimming speeds.

An algebra of continuous functions of time is a collection of functions with the property that if $f(t)$ and $g(t)$ are in the collection and c and d are numbers, then $cf(t) + dg(t)$ and the product function $f(t)g(t)$ are also in the collection. An algebra of functions of time is said to separate points if whenever t_1 and t_2 are two different times, then there is a function $f(t)$ in the algebra being considered so that $f(t)$ is not equal to $f(t)$. The finite linear combinations of functions of the form $\sin(\omega t)$ and $\cos(\omega t)$ are an example of an algebra that separates points. The Stone Weirstrass theorem described in Friedman[26] tells us then that the swimmer's cross-track motion function $y^*(t)$ can be approximated uniformly arbitrarily closely by a finite linear combination of trigonometric functions. Our method of fitting trigonometric series to the detrended data is therefore based on the Stone Weirstrass theorem described lucidly by Friedman,[26] instead of being based on the theory of Fourier series found, for example, in the classic text by Whittaker and Watson.[68] One difference in the methods is that the frequencies may not be multiples of a primary frequency as they are with Fourier series.

Assume for the remainder of the chapter that swimmer coordinates have been rotated so that in the new coordinate system the best fitting straight line is the x axis of the new coordinate system. Let $y_i^*(t)$ denote the ith cross-track oscillation coordinate or, more simply, the y coordinate of the swimmer in this new coordinate system. Practically, therefore, begin by fitting a two-term trigonometric series.

$$F(A, B, \omega, t) = A \cos(\omega t) + B \sin(\omega t)$$

as closely as possible to a detrended time series,

$$T = \{(t_i, y_i^*): i \in \{1, 2, \ldots, N\}\}$$

Indeed, minimize the function $G(A, B, \omega)$ defined by

$$G(A, B, \omega) = \sum_{i=1}^{N} [A \cos(\omega t_i) + B \sin(\omega t_i) - y_i^*]^2$$

by setting its partial derivatives with respect to A, B and ω equal to zero. At a critical point of the function $G(A, B, \omega)$ observe that

$$\frac{\partial G}{\partial A} = 0 = \sum_{i=1}^{N} \{2[A \cos(\omega t_i) + B \sin(\omega t_i) - y_i^*] \cos(\omega t_i)\}$$

and

$$\frac{\partial G}{\partial B} = 0 = \sum_{i=1}^{N} \{2[A \cos(\omega t_i) + B \sin(\omega t_i) - y_i^*] \sin(\omega t_i)\}$$

These last two equations are linear in A and B, and these variables can be eliminated from the equations giving a single nonlinear equation,

$$\frac{\partial G}{\partial \omega} = 0 = \sum_{i=1}^{N} \{2[A \cos(\omega t_i) + B \sin(\omega t_i) - y_i^*][-A \sin(\omega t_i)t_i + B \cos(\omega t_i)t_i]\}$$

Although this equation has an infinite number of complex frequency solutions, go through all of them on a practical bounded real frequency interval and select that value of ω that minimizes the function $G(A, B, \omega)$. It is Picard's theorem that says that an entire function having only a finite number of complex zeros must be the product of a polynomial and an exponential, and that since the previous expression is not of this form, it must necessarily have an infinite number of solutions in the complex frequency domain. The dependence of A and B on ω is completely determined here if the function values $\tan^2(\omega t_i)$ are not the same constant for every i. This would mean that the two vectors whose ith components are respectively $\cos(\omega t_i)$ and $\sin(\omega t_i)$ are linearly independent and that the Cauchy Schwarz inequality, which states that

$$\left(\sum_{i=1}^{n} a_i \cdot b_i \right)^2 \leq \left(\sum_{i=1}^{n} a_i^2 \right) \cdot \left(\sum_{j=1}^{n} b_j^2 \right)$$

for all real numbers a_i and b_i is a strict inequality when each a_i is set equal to $\cos(\omega t_i)$ and each b_i is set equal to $\sin(\omega t_i)$, which means that the determinant of the linear system involving A and B, which is given by

$$\Delta = \left[\sum_{i=1}^{N} \cos^2(\omega t_i) \right]\left[\sum_{i=1}^{N} \sin^2(\omega t_i) \right] - \left\{ \sum_{i=1}^{N} [\cos(\omega t_i) \sin(\omega t_i)] \right\}^2$$

is strictly positive, and that under these circumstances one can always solve for A and B, and that furthermore A and B would be single-valued functions of ω. In other words, the only troublesome values of ω would be those satisfying for each i

$$\omega = \frac{n\pi}{t_i} \text{ or } \omega = \frac{(2n - 1)\pi}{2t_i}$$

for some integer n, and these would be found only with probability zero. In anticipation of eliminating the coefficients $A(\omega)$ and $B(\omega)$ from the nonlinear system of three equations whose solution represents the critical points of G, make the definitions of the entries of the 2 by 2 coefficient matrix of the system that is obtained by setting the partial derivatives of G with respect to A and B equal to zero by defining the entry in row one and column one by the rule

$$a_{(1,1)} = \sum_{i=1}^{N} \cos^2(\omega t_i)$$

defining the entries in row 1 and column 2 and row 2 and column 1 by

$$a_{(1,2)} = \sum_{i=1}^{N} [\sin(\omega t_i) \cos(\omega t_i)] = a_{(2,1)}$$

and defining the entry in row 2 and column 2 by

$$a_{(2,2)} = \sum_{i=1}^{N} \sin^2(\omega t_i)$$

Then since the right sides of the two linear equations involving A and B may be expressed as

$$c_1 = \sum_{i=1}^{N} y_i^* \cos(\omega t_i)$$

and

$$c_2 = \sum_{i=1}^{N} y_i^* \sin(\omega t_i)$$

Cramer's rule would then tell us, under the assumption that the terms $\tan^2(\omega t_i)$ do not all have the same value, that the determinant Δ defined earlier has to be nonzero and that the functions $A(\omega)$ and $B(\omega)$ are given by

$$A(\omega) = \frac{c_1 a_{(2,2)} - c_2 a_{(1,2)}}{\Delta}$$

and

$$B(\omega) = \frac{c_2 a_{(1,1)} - c_1 a_{(2,1)}}{\Delta}$$

Next simply expand the expression for the partial derivative of G with respect to ω and make use of these expressions for $A(\omega)$ and $B(\omega)$ to obtain the single nonlinear equation

$$\left(\tfrac{1}{2}\right) \frac{\partial G}{\partial \omega} = 0$$

$$= \sum_{i=1}^{N} [B(\omega)^2 - A(\omega)^2] \sin(\omega t_i) \cos(\omega t_i) t_i$$

$$+ \sum_{i=1}^{N} A(\omega)B(\omega)[\cos^2(\omega t_i) - \sin^2(\omega t_i)]t_i$$

$$+ \sum_{i=1}^{N} (-y_i^*)[B(\omega) \cos(\omega t_i) - A(\omega) \sin(\omega t_i)]t_i$$

The derivation of the formulas for fitting the data is described in detail in Cohoon.[14] In summary, the steps are to find the values of A and B that would make (A, B) a critical point of G for a given frequency ω and then to solve a single nonlinear equation in the one unknown ω for the frequencies that minimize the maximum difference over the time interval that the creature is observed of the detrended $y^*(t)$ and the $A \cos(\omega t) + B \sin(\omega t)$. After obtaining the best approximation involving a single frequency, the old y_i is replaced by

$$y_{(i,\text{new})}^* = y_i^* - A \cos(\omega t_i) - B \sin(\omega t_i)$$

and one simply repeats the process of subtracting best linear combinations of $\cos(\omega t)$ and $\sin(\omega t)$ until the residual function cannot be made significantly smaller. It turns out that by selecting a very small number of frequencies ω, which turn out not to be harmonically related as in music but which give a good match to the laboratory data at each stage, a good fit to the cross-track motion is obtained. The best frequency ω and the associated amplitude $A^2 + B^2$ of this mode seem to be peculiar to the individual swimmer in all swimming data that was analyzed.

Wobble is defined by the statement that wobble plus one is the ratio of the total length of the swimming path from the starting point to the ending point of the swimming track being examined divided by the straight line distance between these points. Neglecting the contribution of on track oscillation, this is given by

$$\text{wobble} + 1 = \frac{\int_0^T \left(\sqrt{V_0^2 + \left\{ \sum_{i=1}^{n} [(-A_i\omega_i) \sin(\omega_i t) + B_i\omega_i \cos(\omega_i t)] \right\}^2} \right) dt}{V_0 T}$$

Note that if wobble is equal to zero, then the motion is along a direct straight line from the beginning portion of the track being considered to the endpoint of this track.

TABLES, GRAPHS, AND LABORATORY OBSERVATIONS

As Katz,[38,39] Swanson,[64] and Young[69-71] observed with a microscope only a planar view of the motion, the natural dependent variables are the x and y coordinates specifying the position of the center of mass of the swimming microorganism. One can propose development of a stochastic differential equation model of the motion of the uniflagellar microorganism and the use of identified model parameters described in Sage,[58] such as the parameters defining the best fitting line or curve, the swimming oscillation frequencies, and their associated vibration amplitudes as a means of classifying the motions such as the artificial intelligence schemes described in Grenander[29] or in Patrick and Fattu.[55] The independent variables in the differential equation would be the coordinates of the center of mass of the moving microorganism. The studies suggest that this type of model could be used to rather precisely fit the data; for example, a fitting of the cross-track motion of one of these microorganisms is shown in the figures of the next section, along with the raw laboratory motion data provided by Katz,[37,38] Swanson,[64] or Young[69-71] or as seen by a phase-contrast microscope.

This chapter models the swimming as a coupled system of ordinary differential equations with sinusoidal driving terms plus a constant force and damping terms to give a bounded velocity motion. The fitting of this data to the model is shown further along in this section. The trajectories shown in Figures 1A, 2A, 3A, 4A, and 5A are among 93 laboratory observations recorded at 200 frames per second using high-speed videomicrographic methods by Katz.[37,38] Figures 6A and 7A are rabbit spermatozoa tracks recorded at 30 frames per second by Young.[69-71]

A stochastic differential equation model of the type described by Arnold,[2] Cohoon,[15] Friedman,[25] Huber,[36] Liu,[46] McCabe, Belkin, Wagner, and Sommer,[51] and Srinivasan and Rasudevan[63] that would be used to model the motion of a cell driven by a flagellum could be analyzed on a personal computer, and the software would generalize the standard packages, described by Donoho and Gasko,[18] Fisherkeller,[24] Holt,[34] Katz,[38] and Mack,[49] and be portable to motion analysis centers and clinics. The predictions of the model have been compared with actual data to demonstrate our capability of fitting the data. A physical basis is presented for a deterministic model that could be used in carrying out a detailed simulation of the motion, and that could serve as a possible solution of the inverse problem, finding parameters defining a mathematical model of uniflagellar microorganism motion from the observed motion.

The cluster analysis described by Everitt[21] can be used to classify into groups a sample of microorganisms, from an examination of their motions and the derived system parameters. Other potential applications may be to identify motion parameters using Brownian motion ideas of Uhlenbeck and Ornstein[65] in the stochastic differential equations described in Arnold,[2] Friedman,[25] or Srinivasan[63] to create the simplified models of Cohoon,[14] or to use the homotopy methods of Chow,[11] Cohoon,[13] or Garcia,[27] or to use Newtonian methods to solve large nonlinear systems such as those in Fauci[22] that attempt to model the details of the motion of the flagellum that may change under chemical stress. Statistical analysis would then discriminate between parameters that are in normal ranges and those that are characteristically abnormal and linked to environmental stressors. The combinations of swimming speeds and primary frequencies and oscillation amplitudes seem to be characteristic of the individual single-celled swimmer, like a human fingerprint. This could prove to be an extremely sensitive test of the influence of environmental stressors on the function of cells. The level of a toxin in parts per million is significant when one can see a change in the combination of swimming speed, primary frequency, and oscillation amplitude of a single celled swimmer after its addition. This could, as in the work of Noever,[52,53] Roberts,[56] Silverman,[60-62] and Young,[69-71] provide a sensitive measure of the influence of industrial effluent on the environment.

Table 1 contains the randomly shortened track data analysis results for tracks selected because they were observed for a long enough time to make calculations using the program with these randomly clipped data sets. These summary tables for the original data sets are given in Table 2.

The theory also appears to work for rabbit data of R. Young,[69-71] and tracks and comparisons are shown in figures 6A and 6B, and 7A and 7B. An abbreviated tale showing the A and B coefficients, the frequency omega, and the amplitude are shown in Tables 3, 4, and 5. Note that in Tables 3–5 the calculated speeds and the oscillation frequencies ω for the largest amplitude oscillatory component appear to be close for the original data track and the randomly shortened data track for two different rabbit spermatozoa tracks. The 30 frame per second data was harder to analyze as many of the swimmers were resting or had very short tracks, so swimming tracks were selected that seemed to have been so regular that they were well recorded by the 30 frame per second camera.

Calculation of wobble involves the calculation of the arc length of the swimming path, which cannot easily be determined in closed form. Because of the highly oscillatory nature of higher order sinusoids contributing to the approximation of the cross-track oscillations of the swimmer, traditional trapezoidal rules might require a million points to obtain a reasonable approximation to the integral. Gaussian quadrature can accurately calculate the area under a lobe of a sinusoid with seven points. The Gaussian quadrature formula can be easily understood by looking at the integration of the Lagrange interpolation formula approximating the integral of $f(t)$, the swimmer path length up to time t, which is given by

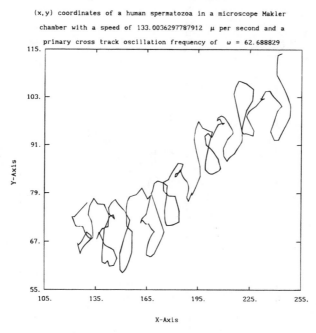

Figure 1A. The (x, y) coordinates of a swimming human spermatozoa.

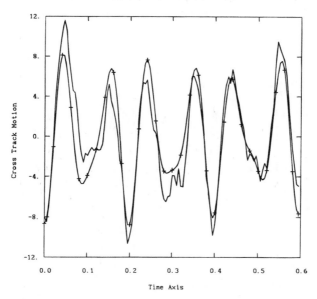

Figure 1B. The comparison of laboratory observations and model predictions of swimming oscillations across the best curve joining the starting and ending point of the swimming path for a human spermatozoa with a swimming speed of about 133 microns per second.

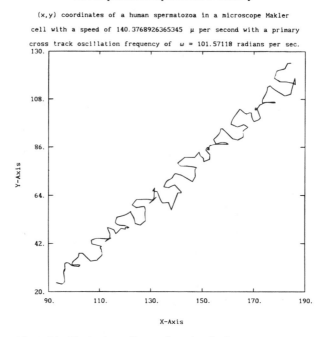

Figure 2A. The (*x*, *y*) coordinates of a swimming human spermatozoa.

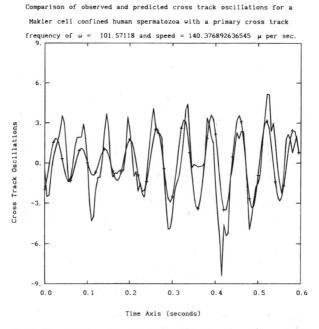

Figure 2B. The comparison of laboratory observations and model predictions of swimming oscillations across the best curve joining the starting and ending point of the swimming path for a human spermatozoa with a swimming speed of about 140 microns per second.

Observed (x,y) coordinates of swimming microorganism

ω = 54.827764; speed = 70.750041470749

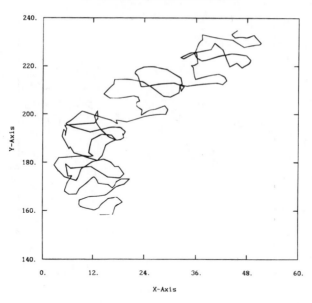

Figure 3A. The (x, y) coordinates of a swimming human spermatozoa.

Observed and predicted cross track oscillations

ω = 54.827764; v = 70.750041470749

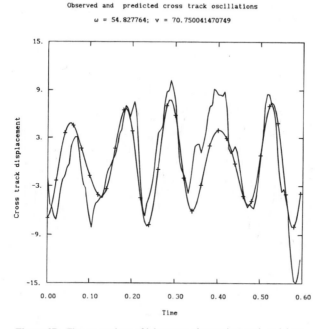

Figure 3B. The comparison of laboratory observations and model predictions of swimming oscillations across the best curve joining the starting and ending point of the swimming path for a human spermatozoa with a swimming speed of about 70.75 microns per second.

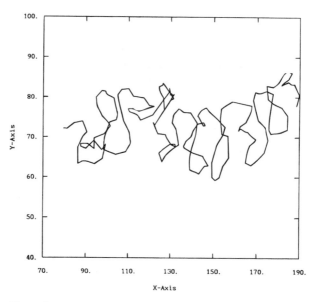

Figure 4A. The (x, y) coordinates of a swimming human spermatozoa.

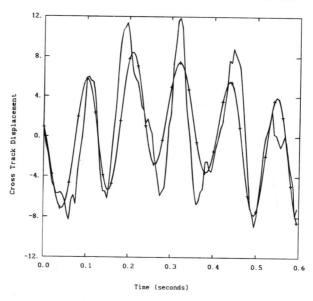

Figure 4B. The comparison of laboratory observations and model predictions of swimming oscillations across the best curve joining the starting and ending point of the swimming path for a human spermatozoa with a swimming speed of about 112.8 microns per second.

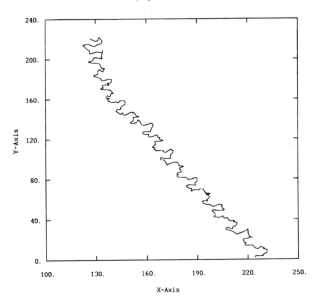

Figure 5A. The (x, y) coordinates of a swimming human spermatozoa.

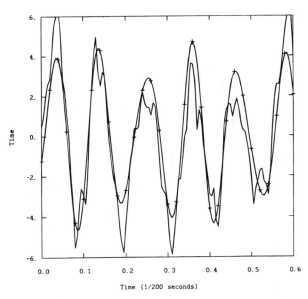

Figure 5B. The comparison of laboratory observations and model predictions of swimming oscillations across the best curve joining the starting and ending point of the swimming path for a human spermatozoa with a swimming speed of about 116 microns per second.

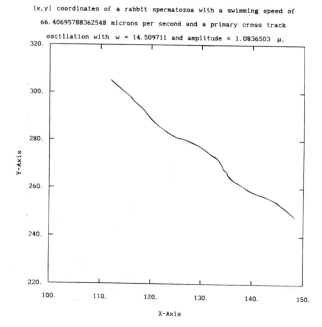

(x, y) coordinates of a rabbit spermatozoa with a swimming speed of
66.40695788362548 microns per second and a primary cross track
oscillation with ω = 14.509711 and amplitude = 1.0836503 μ.

Figure 6A. The (x, y) coordinates of a rabbit spermatozoa with a low value of wobble.

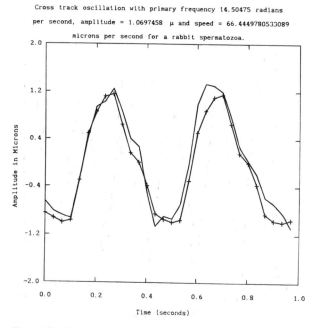

Cross track oscillation with primary frequency 14.50475 radians
per second, amplitude = 1.0697458 μ and speed = 66.4449780533089
microns per second for a rabbit spermatozoa.

Figure 6B. The comparison of laboratory observations and model predictions of swimming oscillations across the best curve joining the starting and ending point of the swimming path for a rabbit spermatozoa with a swimming speed of about 66.4 μ per second.

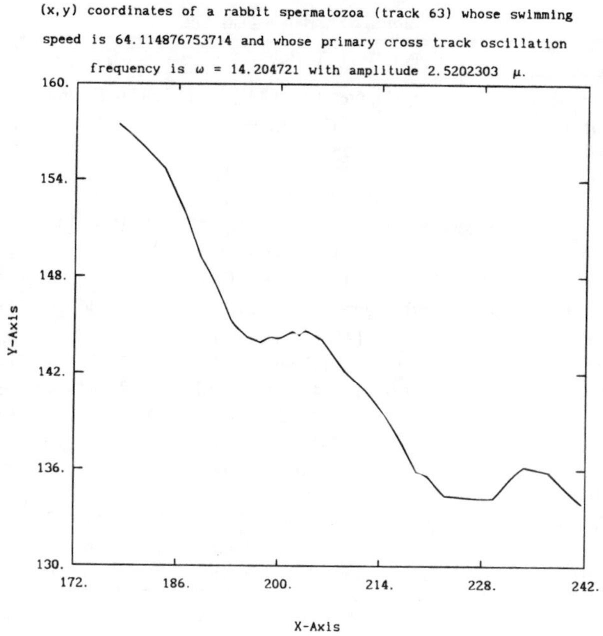

(x,y) coordinates of a rabbit spermatozoa (track 63) whose swimming
speed is 64.114876753714 and whose primary cross track oscillation
frequency is ω = 14.204721 with amplitude 2.5202303 μ.

Figure 7A. The (x, y) coordinates of a rabbit spermatozoa with a high value of wobble.

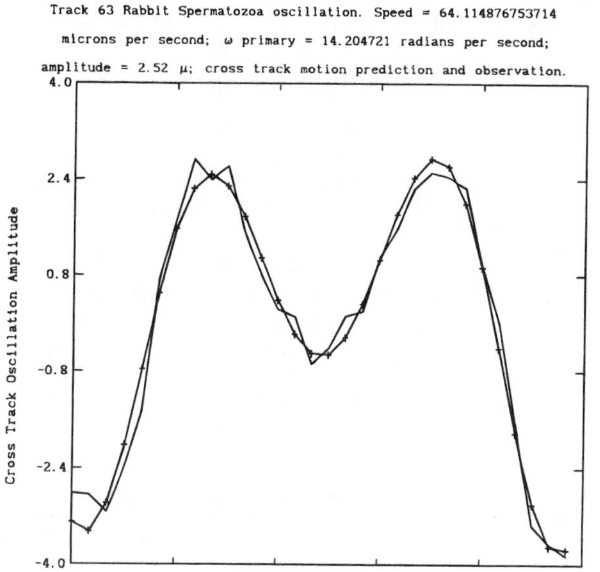

Track 63 Rabbit Spermatozoa oscillation. Speed = 64.114876753714
microns per second; ω primary = 14.204721 radians per second;
amplitude = 2.52 μ; cross track motion prediction and observation.

Figure 7B. The comparison of laboratory observations and model predictions of swimming oscillations across the best curve joining the starting and ending point of the swimming path for a rabbit spermatozoa with a swimming speed of about 64.1 microns per second.

Table 1. Shortened Data Set

A	B	ω
Track 1 (shortened data set) (Figures 1A and 1B) 133.1328278225963 = Speed		
−6.4704746D − 01	5.5674833D + 00	6.2923738D + 01
−4.2458780D − 01	2.5823514D + 00	9.7277125D + 01
2.0317620D + 00	−1.4516244D + 00	1.1319602D + 04
−7.3850331D − 01	1.8845679D − 01	1.3057649D + 03
Track 2 (shortened data set) (Figures 2A and 2B) 140.3632725503298 = Speed		
1.8004545D + 00	−1.5102951D + 00	1.0106251D + 02
7.7059398D − 01	5.1165881D − 01	3.8092375D + 03
Track 3 (shortened data set) (Figures 3A and 3B) 71.23877341346318 = Speed		
2.6584066D + 00	4.6009192D + 00	5.3147741D + 01
−2.1204264D + 00	6.7076895D − 02	1.2114599D + 03
Track 7 (shortened data set) (Figures 4A and 4B) 107.3705084841984 = Speed		
−6.0600213D + 00	−1.8789294D + 0	5.5299751D + 01
−2.2312068D + 00	2.3741636D + 00	1.2331658D + 03
2.3536239D + 00	2.3467561D + 00	9.1747164D + 01
−8.4950925D − 01	−1.1607427D + 00	2.5467910D + 03
Track 8 (shortened data set) (Figures 5A and 5B) 116.4707648859612 = Speed		
3.4916445D + 00	1.0523825D + 00	5.7021996D + 01
5.3786183D − 01	6.6969828D − 01	6.5483006D + 01

Table 2. Original Data Sets

A	B	ω
Track 1 (Figures 1A and 1B) 133.0036297787912 = Speed		
−5.8283928D + 00	1.2661289D + 00	6.2688829D + 01
−2.4017509D + 00	−8.4781384D − 01	9.6436953D + 01
−4.2443896D − 01	4.2246295D − 01	4.9553689D + 03
Track 2 (Figures 2A and 2B) 140.3768926365345 = Speed		
−1.0961883D + 00	2.0035001D + 00	1.0157118D + 02
−8.7836711D − 01	−9.9916870D − 01	9.1131715D + 01
Track 3 (Figures 3A and 3B) 70.75004147071490 = Speed		
−5.7746991D + 00	−1.5530989D + 00	5.4827764D + 01
−1.2001571D + 00	1.7599520D + 00	7.4573879D + 01
Track 7 (Figures 4A and 4B) 112.8201738398282 = Speed		
3.5779813D + 00	−4.3608130D + 00	5.5799884D + 01
−2.4933183D + 00	1.2416872D + 00	2.5230892D + 03
−1.6222680D − 01	7.8831595D − 01	2.5857511D + 03
Track 8 (Figures 5A and 5B) 116.5574909155900 = Speed		
−7.4504187D − 01	3.6563991D + 00	5.7499979D + 01
1.0479441D + 00	6.5367556D − 01	1.2480990D + 03
−5.6414503D − 01	−8.0276757D − 01	8.0815102D + 01
−5.9328640D − 02	6.6970228D − 01	2.1776566D + 02

Table 3. Rabbit Track Data of R. Young (Figures 6A and 6B), Low Wobble Swimmer, Speed = 66.44497805330089 μm/s

A	B	ω	Amplitude
−9.1626324D − 01	−5.5210297D − 01	1.4504750D + 01	1.0697458D + 00
1.8710259D − 01	−3.5687835D − 02	2.9082965D + 01	1.9047572D − 01
−1.1940143D − 01	−2.6396155D − 02	2.3927246D + 03	1.2228434D − 01

Table 4. Analysis of Shortened of Data Track (Figures 6A and 6B)

A	B	ω	Amplitude
-1.0814250D + 00	-6.9411365D - 02	1.4509711D + 01	1.0836503D + 00
1.4582872D - 01	-1.2287206D - 01	2.1312615D + 01	1.9069231D - 01
-5.3652283D - 02	-1.7867503D - 01	4.0490680D + 02	1.8655652D - 02
5.5043065D - 03	6.9092973D - 02	4.5452917D + 01	6.9311877D - 02

Table 5. Comparison of Summary Data Sets for Original and Shortened Data Sets for Track 63

A	B	ω	Amplitude
Original Data Set (Figures 7A and 7B), High Wobble Swimmer, 64.11487675371400 = Speed			
-1.9848009D + 00	-1.5531022D + 00	1.4204721D + 01	2.5202303D + 00
-1.0741154D + 00	7.2141000D - 01	4.1521171D + 03	1.2938919D + 00
-4.1825090D - 01	2.9748120D - 01	1.8116771D + 01	5.1325323D - 01
1.8007983D - 01	1.1760887D - 01	1.7836861D + 02	2.1508275D - 01
Randomly Shortened Data Set (Figures 7A and 7B), High Wobble Swimmer, 63.19020304141807 = Speed			
-2.3742481D + 00	7.8067326D - 02	1.4553227D + 01	2.3755312D + 00
-7.4273727D - 01	-8.2494682D - 02	2.1538045D + 01	7.4730451D - 01
-2.2176480D - 01	-8.6975349D - 02	2.8537341D + 01	2.3821070D - 01

$$\text{wobble} + 1 \equiv \int_0^{T_0} f(t)\, dt$$

$$\approx \sum_{i=1}^{n}\left[\int_0^{T_0}\left(\frac{\prod_{\substack{j=1\\j\neq i}}^{n}(s - Y_j)}{\prod_{\substack{j=1\\j\neq i}}^{n}(Y_i - Y_j)}\right)ds\right]f(Y_i) = \sum_{i=1}^{n} W_i f(Y_i)$$

where the W_i in this formula are computed once and for all and stored and then are reused to integrate different functions $f(t)$ over the interval $[0, T_0]$, which is the stretch of time over which the swimmer is being observed. One can do even better than this by considering the interval $[-1, 1]$ and setting the quadrature points y_i to be zeros of Legendre polynomials, calculating the weights w_i, and simply changing variables when one goes to a new interval so that an integration over each subdivision of the time interval from 0 to T_0 is transformed to an integral over $[-1, 1]$. This is the approach used in calculating wobble of the swimmer.

Wobble was calculated for the two rabbit data tracks using the trigonometric fit formula at the end of the last section. The time interval from 0 to T_0 was calculated by dividing this time interval into smaller subintervals and using 14-point Gaussian quadrature on each of the intervals. The reader can check the following calculations using the Gaussian quadrature algorithm,

$$\text{wobble} + 1 = \int_0^{T_0} f(t)\, dt \approx \sum_{j=1}^{N}\sum_{i=1}^{n}\left(\frac{b_j - a_j}{2}\right)w_i f\left[\frac{a_j + b_j}{2} + y_i\left(\frac{b_j - a_j}{2}\right)\right]$$

where N is the number of subdivisions of the time interval $[0, T_0]$ over which the swimmer is being observed, n is the number of Gaussian quadrature points, y_i is the Gaussian quadrature evaluation point in the subinterval $[-1, 1]$ of all real numbers between -1 and $+1$, w_i is the Gaussian quadrature weight for the integration over this interval, a_j is equal to $(j - 1)T_0/N$, b_j is equal to jT_0/N, and where $f(t)$ is defined by

$$f(t) = \frac{\sqrt{\left(\frac{dx}{dt}\right)^2 + \left(\frac{dy}{dt}\right)^2}}{V_0 T_0}$$

Table 6. Convergence of Wobble Calculations

Number of subdivisions	Figure 6A, track 35, wobble calculation of wobble + 1	Figure 7A, track 63, wobble calculation of wobble + 1
1	3.046549099618712	64.13802849818042
100	3.052186949921818	53.54809930506296
200	3.051888121975223	53.38552447699203
300	3.052032429782489	53.38151022715049
3000	3.051906485403135	53.38370757000511
30000	3.051906485403111	53.38371710379018

where $(x(t), y(t))$ signifies the coordinates of the swimmer at time t. The wobble values computed versus the number of subintervals into which the time interval was divided for the two sets of data are given in Table 6.

Part of the difficulty in convergence is that there are high-frequency terms with low-amplitude contributions that continue to influence the value of the integral. It would take many subdivisions to obtain an accurate answer, even with Gaussian quadrature, which is a nearly optimal integration algorithm for trigonometric functions. The reader will see in Figures 6A and 7A that the spermatozoa associated with track 7A would be expected intuitively to have a much higher wobble than the rabbit spermatozoa whose swimming track is shown in Figure 6A.

This data are presented as they were developed. No attempt was made to present only data that agreed with the our hypothesis that the combination of swimming speed and primary frequency served to identify the microorganism. The greatest discrepancy occurs in track 7, which is shown in Figure 4A, in the swimming speed, but you should note from the microscope data that the swimming path of organism 7 has quite a kink in it. It is conjectured that other observations of swimming tracks would fall in line with this theory; other investigators are encouraged to confirm or disprove the theory that locally these swimming speeds and primary cross-track oscillation frequencies might be used to keep track of swimming microorganisms for an extended period of time as they collide with one another and move about in a microscope observation dish. This would permit sensitive bioeffects tests and could cut the costs of drug development and provide sensitive measures of toxicity. It could also possibly be used to classify spermatozoa of farm animals and humans as fertile or nonfertile.

SAMPLE CORRELATIONS AND STANDARD DEVIATIONS

Are there really invariants in the swimming motion of spermatozoa? Are swimming speed, cross-track amplitude, and the primary frequency associated with cross-track motion really relatively independent of the portion of the swimming track that is used to calculate them? While a proof of this is not claimed, some correlation calculations giving correlations of estimations of swimming speed of long tracks and randomly shortened tracks and the correlations of primary frequency of cross-track oscillations or the frequency of the swimmer's wiggling above and below the line joining the swimmer's initial point and terminal point in the portion of the swimming track being analyzed are given in Table 7. Also given are the standard deviations of the differences between these estimations for the long track and the randomly shortened track. Here, a small standard deviation would suggest small differences in these quantities that the theory suggests are the same, while a correlation close to one would suggest a definite connection between the quantities. Table 7 gives a sample of 12 primary cross-track frequencies for a full data set and for the same data set randomly shortened in length.

Table 8 gives a sample of the same 12 data sets with the swimming speeds estimated from the original swimming tracks and the swimming speeds estimated when these 12 swimming tracks were randomly shortened in length.

In Table 7 observe similarities in the primary cross-track oscillation frequencies ω derived from the original swimming tracks and in the primary oscillation frequencies ω derived from the randomly shortened tracks, and in Table 8 notice the similarities in the swimming speeds estimated from the original tracks and those estimated from the randomly shortened data tracks.

Table 7. Primary Frequency Comparison Across Data Sets for Full Track and Track Subsets

I	OM(I)	OMSH(I)	DIFFOM	SMDFOM
1	6.2695190D + 01	6.2721959D + 01	−2.6769000D − 02	−2.6769000D − 02
2	1.0154358D + 02	1.0101565D + 02	5.2793000D − 01	5.0116100D − 01
3	5.4674718D + 01	5.4064519D + 01	6.1019900D − 01	1.1113600D + 00
4	7.0041734D + 01	6.8741068D + 01	1.3006660D + 00	2.4120260D + 00
5	5.4960178D + 01	5.5638503D + 01	−6.7832500D − 01	1.7337010D + 00
6	1.0259502D + 02	1.0291148D + 02	−3.1646000D − 01	1.4172410D + 00
7	5.5780267D + 01	5.5066741D + 01	7.1352600D − 01	2.1307670D + 00
8	6.6673173D + 01	6.8292726D + 01	−1.6195530D + 00	5.1121400D − 01
9	6.8833605D + 01	6.8650620D + 01	1.8298500D − 01	6.9419900D − 01
10	1.0292179D + 02	1.0196217D + 02	9.5962000D − 01	1.6538190D + 00
11	5.7369522D + 01	5.6998616D + 01	3.7090600D − 01	2.0247250D + 00
12	5.6404175D + 01	5.7433912D + 01	−1.0297370D + 00	9.9498800D − 01

Note. OM(I) and OMSH(I) denote the primary ω of the full and shortened tracks and DIFFOM and SMDFOM represent the difference of these oscillation frequencies and a running of these differences, respectively.

To quantify these observations, Table 9 will provide the reader with statistical calculations giving correlations between observations and variations in the differences. Also given in Table 8 are the mean difference in swimming speeds from the full and shortened data sets and the sample standard deviation. Back in Table 7 the third column gives the average difference of the angular frequencies of the cross track oscillations and the sample standard deviation. If v_i is the estimated swimming speed for the ith track, and if w_i is the estimated swimming speed for the random shortening of the ith data track, then the sample correlation of the v_i and the w_i is given by the ratio of the covariance of the v_i and the w_i and the products of the standard deviations of the v_i and the w_i, respectively. The formula is given specifically in Cohoon[14] and generally in Larsen and Marx.[43] The same statistical calculations are made for the primary cross-track oscillation frequencies ω_i for the full swimming tracks and the primary cross-track oscillation frequencies ω_i of the randomly shortened swimming tracks.

Table 8. Swimming Speed Comparison Across Data Sets for Full and Shortened Tracks

I	SP(I)	SPSH(I)	DIFFSP	SMDFSP
1	1.3312704D + 02	1.3315871D + 02	−3.1676989D − 02	−3.1676989D − 02
2	1.4065757D + 02	1.4045549D + 02	2.0208259D − 01	1.7040560D − 01
3	7.0698042D + 01	7.0142647D + 01	5.5539510D − 01	7.2580070D − 01
4	1.6721481D + 02	1.6275447D + 02	4.4603352D + 00	5.1861359D + 00
5	1.2482227D + 02	1.2574256D + 02	−9.2029432D − 01	4.2658416D + 00
6	1.5347475D + 02	1.5281828D + 02	6.5647106D − 01	4.9223127D + 00
7	1.1209639D + 02	1.0691714D + 02	5.1792541D + 00	1.0101567D + 01
8	8.5655219D + 01	8.1536269D + 01	4.1189501D + 00	1.4220517D + 01
9	1.6573157D + 02	1.6586454D + 02	−1.3296473D − 01	1.4087552D + 01
10	1.5571654D + 02	1.5642333D + 02	−7.0678902D − 01	1.3380763D + 01
11	1.1648461D + 02	1.1607946D + 02	4.0515394D − 01	1.3785917D + 01
12	1.2031227D + 02	1.2285925D + 02	−2.5469778D + 00	1.1238939D + 01

Note. SP(I) and SPSH(I) denote the estimated swimming speed for the full and randomly shortened tracks and DIFFSP and SMDFSP denote the differences and running sum of these differences in speeds, respectively.

Table 9. Summary Table of Correlations and Standard Deviations

0.9970674529864353	=	correlation coefficient for speeds
0.9990675146467306	=	sample correlation for omegas
0.9365782668885458	=	average difference of speeds
5.632322114394798	=	sample standard deviation speeds differences
8.2915666666664833E − 02	=	average difference of omegas
0.7368752771284255	=	sample standard deviation omegas differences

The sample correlation is given by

$$R(v, w) = \left(\frac{cov(v, w)}{\sigma_v \sigma_w}\right) = \frac{n \sum_{i=1}^{n} v_i w_i - \left(\sum_{i=1}^{n} v_i\right)\left(\sum_{i=1}^{n} w_i\right)}{\sqrt{\left[n\left(\sum_{i=1}^{n} v_i^2\right) - \left(\sum_{i=1}^{n} v_i\right)^2\right]\left[n\left(\sum_{i=1}^{n} w_i^2\right) - \left(\sum_{i=1}^{n} w_i\right)^2\right]}}$$

where v_i is the net speed of the ith swimmer for the normal track and where w_i is the net speed of the ith swimmer for the randomly shortened data track, and σ_v and σ_w are the standard deviations of the speeds of the original and shortened tracks.

To quantify how closely the swimming speeds of the shortened tracks agree with the estimated swimming speeds for the original data tracks, an estimation of the deviation from zero of the $(v_i - w_i)$ is measured using the sample variance cited in Larsen and Marx[43] for the differences for each data track index i between the swimming speed v_i of the original ith data track and the estimated swimming speed w_i of the randomly shortened ith data track; this sample variance is denoted by $s^2(v - w)$ and is defined in Cohoon[14] and in Larsen and Marx[43] by the ratio of the sum of the squares of the differences $(v_i - \bar{v})$ minus one over the number n of tracks being analyzed times the square of the sum of the differences $(v_i - \bar{v})$ all divided by $n - 1$. For the velocities this is given by

$$s^2(v - w) = \left(\frac{n\left[\sum_{i=1}^{n} (v_i - w_i)^2\right] - \left[\sum_{i=1}^{n} (v_i - w_i)\right]^2}{n(n - 1)}\right)$$

To quantify the differences in the primary cross-track oscillation frequencies the sample variance, $s^2(\omega - \bar{\omega})$, defined in Feller[23] of the differences in the primary frequencies associated with the full tracks and the randomly shortened tracks. The results of carrying out these computations for the data sets associated with 12 different swimming tracks with the speeds and frequencies listed are given in Table 9.

Note that the standard deviation is for both speed and omega down about two orders of magnitude from the actual values in Table 9.

A SAMPLE MODEL FROM BIOHYDRODYNAMICS

Sparse microscope slide data of Katz[37,38] and Young[69–71] were used to model the swimmer's driving force and the water's drag on the swimmer; the conservation laws of physics on which the modeling is based are described in this section.

Although theoretical models, such as those of Brokaw,[7,8] Chwang and Wu,[12] Dresdner,[19] Fauci,[22] Higdon,[31] Lighthill,[44,45] and Uldrick,[66] of the hydrodynamics of propulsion of a microorganism by a beating flagellum have been created, with details of the flagellum motion studied by Brokaw,[7,8] they do not lend themselves easily to computation. The characteristics of the motion have been studied by Goltz,[28] Gwatkin,[30] and Katz[38] using microscopic video observation. Researchers and practitioners advise that improvement in the various motility characterizations now in use is an important problem worthy of analytical investigation.

Current visualization programs like those of Donoho and Gasko,[18] Fisherkeller,[24] Katz,[38] and Mack[49] and newer methods permit observation and automated recording of forward velocity. Low concentrations of fluorescent probes have been used by Vasquez[67] for many types of motion analysis. Higher concentrations have been used to identify whether or not the addition of certain glycoproteins found in the cell membrane of the oocyte stimulated the acrosomal reaction in nonmoving spermatozoa cells. Standard statistics packages produced commercially for motion analysis give only crude estimates of velocity distributions. There is a need to develop system identification methods in the spirit of Grenander[29] and Patrick and Fattu[55] and statistical methods including ideas of Huber,[36] Jenkins,[37] Koopmens[41] and Liu[46] that are sufficient to classify and characterize these motions with a small number of variables.

While it would not be difficult to record the ratio of speed made good or net velocity to the speed along the swimming microorganism's path as a measure of efficiency, what seems to be missing is a fully developed mathematical model that could, with the utilization of proper parameters, simulate the observed motion, thereby permitting the utilization of model parameters as a quantitative characterization of the motion. The analysis of swimmer motion tracks suggests that additional parameters, other than the ones considered, may be useful; an elementary model based on a small number of characteristic frequencies and amplitudes of the driving forces for the swimming motion seems to be particularly promising.

BIOHYDRODYNAMICS

A description of the properties of spermatozoa, which are uniflagellar swimmers, and their transitions to other swimming states such as hyperactivation, acrosomal reaction, and capacitation is presented in Chang,[9] and descriptions of the fertilization process are found in Austin[3] and Gwatkin.[30] Motion of uniflagellar microorganism driven by flagellar propulsion has been observed by Dresdner[19] and Mahoney[50] using video micrography and is used to assess fertility of a sample.

Brokaw,[7,8] Keller,[40] and others worked on detailed physical modeling the motion of microscopic swimmers, including the uniflagellar microorganisms whose motion was described in the data presented in previous sections, or on finding parameters that represent the motion. The equations are based on conservation laws of physics described in Appleton[1] applied to a continuum. One could use concepts of fluxes of mass, of momentum, of kinetic energy, of internal energy, and of entropy. Using the concepts of fluxes, one can derive mass conservation equations, Navier Stokes equations, energy transfer equations, and entropy transfer equations from first principles. It has been pointed out by Lighthill,[44,45] however, that the overwhelming dominance of surface forces such as pressure and viscous stresses over volume forces, such as inertial effects, means that fluid accelerations can be neglected and the forces on each fluid element are therefore essentially in balance. This balance was used in the model of Cox.[16] This would mean that the motion may be adequately described using the linear differential equation model of Cohoon.[14] The idea is then, taking into account the conservation laws, to precisely compute the propulsive forces and velocities and dissipated power from a knowledge of the motion of the flagellum using a Brokaw[7,8] type of model.

The forces generated by the flagellum on the fluid are modeled as a distribution of fundamental solutions called Stokeslets and have been studied by Chwang,[12] Higdon,[31] Lighthill,[45] and others. The weights associated with this distribution could be determined by solving an inverse problem in the form of an integral equation with a time-dependent kernel.

Biologically, the transfer of ATP to ADP supplies power to the cell. Dresdner and Katz[19] (p. 927) calculated that the power needed to produce the swimming orbit in the fluid bearing the microorganism represented 30% of the total free energy potential available from ATP dephosphorylation described in Brokaw and Gibbons.[7] Computer models of flagellar waveforms have been generated, and these models can be used to predict the energy expended by the microorganisms. The swimming speed, a parameter that can be observed, was found to depend jointly on the flagellar length L and the beat frequency f, and the power output has been found to depend jointly on the viscosity, the square of the frequency and the cube of the flagellar length L. Keller and Rubinow[40] considered a linear velocity and an angular velocity. They noted that others have observed an asymmetry in the movement of the tip of the flagella; it could be suggested that this asymmetry might present us with a complex source term that depends nonlinearly on the system parameters whose analysis might require the methods of Cohoon[13] or Sage.[58] In this regard Swanson[64] pointed out that an electron microscope with 100,000 power magnification shows upon looking at the cross section of a sperm tail that there is along its core a doublet microtubule with radiating protein material spokes coming from this central structure out to the boundary, where one sees nine sets of microtubles whose structure is also described in Berrill,[5] and that there is a different structure near the end of the tail. No one, however, has linked this structure with the details of the movements of the flagellum, although this might be extremely useful in developing and refining predictive mathematical models. Moving cylindrical coordinates can be used to model helical motion; a point on the flagellum is selected and one supposes that the tail is wound in a helical manner around a cylinder whose axis is parallel to the direction of motion of the sperm or protozoan microorganism, and then the swimmer's velocity is decomposed into a velocity tangential to the cylinder axis and an angular velocity in the surface of the cylinder that just contains all points on the beating flagellum of the swimmer. Diagrams describing this motion are found in Chwang and Wu.[12] Keller and Rubinow[40] point out that the force and torque exerted on the fluid by the microorganism at each point on its surface can be separated into propulsive and drag components and may be described by the differential equation given by Cohoon,[14] where the column vector consisting of the force and the torque, the time derivative of the total angular momentum vector of the swimmer, is a combination of the sum of a column vector whose components are the propulsive ATP-to-ADP generated force described in Dresdner and Katz,[19] and propulsive torque minus a 6 by 6 drag coefficient tensor acting on the column vector whose components are the velocity that is tangential to the motion and the velocity tangential to a cylinder that circumscribes the beating flagellum of the swimmer. This coupled force and torque relationship is summarized by the equation

$$\begin{pmatrix} \vec{F} \\ \vec{T} \end{pmatrix} = \begin{pmatrix} \vec{F}_p \\ \vec{T}_p \end{pmatrix} = \bar{\bar{G}} \begin{pmatrix} \vec{w} \\ \vec{\Omega} \end{pmatrix}$$

In Cohoon[14] it was pointed out that this suggests that (x, y) coordinates of the center of mass of the swimmer might be represented by an equation where the column vector has two components, which are the acceleration in the x direction and the acceleration in the y direction, plus a 2 by 2 viscous drag matrix operating on the vector whose components are the velocity in the x direction and the velocity in the y direction, equal to a column vector whose components are functions of time that represent the propulsive forces of the individual swimmer.[14] Thus, momentum conservation suggests modeling using the equation

$$\frac{d^2}{dt^2} \begin{pmatrix} x(t) \\ y(t) \end{pmatrix} + \bar{\bar{\beta}} \cdot \frac{d}{dt} \begin{pmatrix} x(t) \\ y(t) \end{pmatrix} = \begin{pmatrix} F(t) \\ G(t) \end{pmatrix}$$

A momentum balance analysis with knowledge of the viscous and propulsive forces acting at each point of the microorganism and a work calculation would theoretically yield formulas for the power expended by the swimming process. The assumption of Keller and Robinow[40] is a helical motion, but Shack, Fray, and Lardner[59] give a general development using the velocity of an element of the flagellum in terms of the translational velocity of a moving frame, the angular velocity with respect to rotation about an axis parallel to this frame, and the motion of a point on the flagellum relative to this frame. A force balance, requiring that the net force acting on a microorganism moving with constant velocity is zero, gives relationships between these variables. Using the notion that the dot product of force and velocity is power, and using knowledge of the forces and torques and both transnational and angular velocities of all points on the uniflagellar microorganism, would enable us, from basic physics, to compute the power, or rate at which work is being done by the organism. Using the values of Shack, Fray, and Lardner[59] for the viscous force acting on the head of the spermatozoa, and the torque about the axis on which the spermatozoa is moving, the progressive velocity, and the angular velocity on the surface of a circumscribing cylinder and the velocity at each point on the flagellum, one can develop a formula for the total amount of work performed during the swimming process and it can be compared with the energy potentially available through ATP to ADP conversion. The drag coefficients and the propulsive velocity have been calculated by Chwang,[12] Dresdner,[19] Higdon,[31] Shack,[59] and others. Holwill and Burge[33] pointed out that the hydrodynamic efficiency is greater for propulsion by helical waves in a flagellum than by sinusoidal waves in a flagellum. The vigorous beating motion of the tail during the nonprogressive, hyperactivation state described by Goltz,[28] Robertson,[57] and others is not well understood, however.

An important step would be to make a careful derivation of the formulas describing the detailed motion of the organism with a view toward creating a computer graphics simulation of the motion that includes details of tail motion given the shape of the head. This is important in this analysis since, as Swanson[64] pointed out, the shapes of the uniflagellar microorganism head and the microfilament structure appear to vary from one microscopic swimmer to another.

CLUSTER THEORY ANALYSIS

Improved statistical masks such as those in Everitt[21] could be developed that will provide a better estimate of the actual probability distributions from the sample distributions. This will be accomplished through the use of larger samples, more accurate measurements, and the examination of the population of uniflagellar microorganism having the standard observables such as: (1) the speed made good or the distance between the terminal and initial point divided by the elapsed time described in Holt, Moore, and Hillier,[34] (2) the maximum speed along the curved path used in Young,[69–71] (3) velocity of the lateral head movement, (4) amplitude of the lateral head movement in a smaller interval than is usually provided by commercially available cell motility software, and (5) the characteristic frequencies used to model motion along with the weights attached to these frequencies described in Cohoon.[14]

Consider a mathematical model for the motion of uniflagellar microorganism based on a system of six coupled differential equations relating the 6 by 1 column vector whose first three entries are the force and whose last three entries are the total torque exerted by the microorganism on the fluid is balanced by the active propulsive force and torque components and the fluid drag components. Three factors will govern the choice of a model: (1) the physics of motion for a harmonically driven body in a viscous medium; (2) the identifiability of the model parameters with the characteristics of sperm motility believed to be related to male fertility (e.g., progressivity and lateral head movement); and (3) the availability of computationally efficient methods to estimate the model parameters from sperm data.

The model parameter estimation will be performed using methods of nonlinear parameter estimation for a cost function based on the minimization of the sum

$$S = \sum_{i=1}^{N} [(x_{(i,\text{predicted})} - x_{(i,\text{observed})})^2 + (y_{(i,\text{predicted})} - y_{(i,\text{observed})})^2]$$

of the squares of the differences between the (x, y) coordinates of model predictions and those for the observed motion based on a time-series analysis using Box and Jenkins[6] methods to understand the information content of the residual difference between model predictions and the actual observations.

Methods will be developed to characterize statistically a population of microorganisms based on their parameter values. The cluster analysis methods of Everitt[21] can be used to the extent that the aggregation of data is observed in motility parameter space. In addition, one or more metrics will be defined for comparing the motility parameter distribution of a test population of unknown fertility against a reference population of known fertility.

SOFTWARE PROBLEMS

The software described in Cohoon[14] appears to differ from commercial packages described by A. Donoho, D. Donoho, and Gasko[18] or Fisherkeller, Friedman, and Tukey.[24] It could be added to the motion analysis software that has been created for existing laboratory systems.

Several new approaches to the simulation problem have been developed, but the analysis objective includes, in addition, the consideration of the mathematical entropy of the information content versus stochastic or random content analyzed in Box and Jenkins,[6] McCabe,[51] Uhlenbeck,[65] and others of the difference between the raw data and predictions of a simple deterministic model where the apparent microscopically observed accelerations in the x and y directions plus a 2 by 2 drag matrix multiplied by the column vector whose entries are the x and y velocities is set equal to a column vector whose components are the propulsive forces driving the organism used in Cohoon.[14] Several new approaches to the simulation problem have been proposed, but the creation of these stochastic residuals has now reached some maturity, and the considerable software development described in Cohoon[14] remains nearly the same; the results of these calculations could be dovetailed with a Box and Jenkins[6] method to quantify the information content of the residuals, which represent the difference between observations and the simulations produced by the computations in Cohoon.[14]

Consider the problem of determining parameters in a model that will produce a computer simulation of an observed swimming motion. One of the more elementary inverse problems is to take this observed motion and recover the propulsive forces and drag matrices in systems such as the equation in Cohoon[14] that sets the acceleration in the (x, y) microscope coordinate directions plus a 2 by 2 drag matrix acting on the column vector consisting of the velocities in the x and y directions to the column vector whose entries are the apparent organisms driving forces F and G in the x and y directions respectively. One could use existing data files and the homotopy optimization methods of Chow,[11] Garcia,[27] and others or direct Newton methods used by Fauci and Fogelson[22] to attempt to recover representations of the functions F and G and the entries of the 2 by 2 drag matrices. One objective is to demonstrate by fitting data to a mathematical model simulating the observed motion and by using cluster analysis to group the parameters in the system that has been identified by Sage and Melsa[58] that a better discrimination between the different classes, such as for spermatozoa that of possessing a swimming state like purposeful one-direction swimming or the chaotic swimming that occurs at the time of fertilization, within the samples can be achieved.

Some possible applications include: (1) developing an improved predictive model for sperm motion, focusing on those aspects of that motion such as lateral head movement and forward progressivity believed to be related to fertility; (2) estimating the propulsive forces and viscous damping forces in the differential equation presented by the Cohoon[14] model whose solution will give the observed motion; (3) assessing the information content of the residual difference between the laboratory data and the solution of the deterministic differential equation model that has been hypothesized by the automated solution of Cohoon[14] for the system identification problem; (4) developing a computer graphics simulation of the motion based on a differential equation model and comparing model predictions with experimental data; and (5) developing a classification scheme for partitioning the observed motions into groups based on model parameters.

DIFFERENTIAL EQUATION MODEL

After taking out the best fitting progressive motion, roughly the straight-line motion of the organism from the initial point to the end point of the portion of the swimming track being examined, of the swimming microorganism (detrending), an examination of the residual motion reveals the center of mass of the body oscillating both along this line or curve and in a direction perpendicular to it. In general one could describe the motion by considering a moving system of coordinates with an axis tangent to the best fitting curve and another perpendicular to this curve. The motion perpendicular to this curve is called cross-track oscillation, and the motion along the path is called on-track motion (see Figure 1A). Methods created by Cohoon[14] permit one to accurately describe the oscillatory cross-track motion (see Figure 1B) with a very small number of characteristic frequencies and amplitudes; it turns out that these frequencies need to be determined with some precision. These characteristic frequencies and amplitudes of the motion are then used to model the driving force in an ordinary differential equation model of Cohoon.[14]

In what follows, x measures the movement along our best fitting curve or line, and y measures the perturbation perpendicular to this curve.

Here, the problem of creating a system of stochastic differential equations whose solution $x(t)$ and $y(t)$ gives the trajectory of the uniflagellar microorganism is considered. For a possible uncoupled differential equation model, the functions $x(t)$ and $y(t)$ that give the x and y coordinates of the center of mass of the swimmer according to someone looking at the swimmer through a microscope as the spermatozoa is swimming confined to a Makler cell could be assumed to satisfy an ordinary differential equation of the form given by Cohoon[14] where the acceleration in the x or y coordinate direction plus a drag constant times the x or y velocity plus a constant times the x or y coordinate is equal to a constant driving force plus a sum of sinusoidal terms plus a purely stochastic or random or other term $W_{(1,t)}$ for the differential equation in x and $W_{(2,t)}$ for the differential equation in the y coordinate. The functions $W_{(1,t)}$ and $W_{(2,t)}$ are the parts of the deterministic forces not representable explicitly by the forms indicated, a constant force plus a finite sum of sinusoids, or else are stochastic in form (Figure 1A suggests that these functions should provide a relatively small contribution to the motion). The drag coefficients multiplying the velocity or derivative with respect to time t of x or y, respectively, depend on the level of viscous damping of the motion. The coefficients appearing in Cohoon[14] that multiply the coordinate x

or y itself, respectively, represent the restorative force of the water that has been pushed aside by the flagella of the microorganism. In the x differential equation the sum of these three terms is set equal to a constant F_0 term, which is the net driving force that gives the organism its observed velocity, plus the sum of sinusoidal terms and the corrective term $W_{(1,t)}$. If the best fitting curve is a straight line, rotate coordinates so that the x axis of a new coordinate system coincides with this line. After this rotation Cohoon[14] assumed that there was no net velocity in the y direction so the sum of the y acceleration plus a drag constant times the y velocity plus a restorative term of the form of a constant times y is simply set equal to a sum of sinusoidal terms with phase shift plus the term $W_{(2,t)}$. Thus, the acceleration in the x direction satisfies the equation

$$\frac{d^2x}{dt^2} + \beta_1 \frac{dx}{dt} + \alpha_1^2 x = F_0 + \sum_{j=1}^{M} A_j \sin(\omega_{(1,j)}t + \phi_{(1,j)}) + W_{(1,t)}$$

where F_0 is the driving force along the swimming track, and the acceleration of the swimmer in the cross-track direction is satisfies the differential equation

$$\frac{d^2y}{dt^2} + \beta_2 \frac{dy}{dt} + \alpha_2^2 y = \sum_{j=1}^{N} B_j \sin(\omega_{(2,j)}t + \phi_{(1,j)}) + W_{(2,t)}$$

which has only oscillatory or stochastic driving terms. These differential equations can be solved in closed form by the methods of Cohoon[15] if there is no stochasticity in the parameters. However, as the coupling between on-track and cross-track motion is possibly quite significant, an effort in developing a coupled differential equation model could produce useful biological information. The model in Cohoon[14] should probably be only partially deterministic, as there are always some fluctuations in the response that do not seem to be able to be matched even though, mathematically, the Stone Weirstrass theorem described in Friedman[26] guarantees a perfect pointwise fit with a supremum norm matching of any continuous function with a finite linear combination of phase shifted sinusoids.

The differential equation models in Cohoon[14] are special cases of the Langevin equation described in Arnold.[2] For the uncoupled model of Cohoon,[14] a new differential equation is derived by subtracting the deterministic portions from the general solution x of the differential equation of Cohoon,[14] thereby defining an new dependent variable, U, which is set equal to x minus the portion of the solution x_p that is propulsive or equal to a net velocity times time and a deterministic on track oscillation term x_u, which is given by

$$U = x - x_p - x_\omega$$

and which satisfies a new second-order differential equation of Cohoon[14] in which the acceleration of U plus the drag times the velocity of U plus a restorative constant times U is set equal to $W_{(x,t)}$, which may be rewritten in the form

$$\frac{d^2U}{dt^2} + \beta_1 \frac{dU}{dt} + \alpha_1^2 U = W_{(1,t)}$$

Using this new differential equation it may be possible to develop a Fokker Planck equation like those analyzed in Liu and Cohoon[46] and Srinivasan[63] for the joint probability distribution of $U(t)$.

Spermatozoa swim in a low flat disk-shaped dish called a Makler cell, which fits on the observation stage of a phase-contrast microscope, and a camera, frame grabber, and computer can record (x, y) coordinates as a function of time. Given laboratory observations of swimming coordinates, one should find parameters for systems of differential equations so that the (x, y) coordinates of the orbit or solution of the differential equations matches as closely as possible the observed (x, y) swimming coordinates. This should be attempted first for uncoupled systems; then see if improvement in fitting results when this type of fitting is attempted for linear coupled systems of differential equations, and then for nonlinear models.

SYSTEM IDENTIFICATION

The simple differential equation proposed here can be solved exactly. Finding parameters in the differential equation model from observations might require special homotopy inversion methods of Chow, Mallet-Paret, and Yorke,[11] Cohoon and Purcell,[13] and Garcia and Zangwill.[27] However, if the driving force amplitude F_0 were known for the on-track equation, oscillatory plus propulsive, then β_1, the damping force constant, can be estimated by simply looking at the observed average speed, which would be approximately equal to F_0/β_1, or this force constant divided by the damping constant along the track under the assumption that the restorative force constant α_1 along the track associated with the water being moved aside by the swimmer is zero. Then one uses the same damping term initially for the cross-track motion, and initially sets the restorative force constant α_2 multiplying the displacement y from the main swimming path equal to zero. Computerized microscopes record $x(t)$ and $y(t)$ at a sequence of times t_j and then these observations are compared with the solution depending on general model parameters. The model still will not fit the raw data perfectly. Keeping the driving forces fixed, however, one would then use nonlinear analysis to see whether or not an adjustment of the coefficients would lead to a model and solution that more accurately matched the laboratory observations. Thus, by allowing the damping forces and restorative forces of the water to vary, and keeping everything else fixed, one can create a function that gives model predictions of on-track coordinates x and cross-track coordinates y in terms of damping and restorative forces or even coupling terms in a matrix model; then one can transform these model values back to the laboratory coordinate system giving model predictions of laboratory coordinates $\underline{x}$ and $\underline{y}$ that would give a solution that would better match the laboratory observations x_i and y_i.

BIOLOGICAL OBSERVATIONS

In this section, we provide electron microscope images (provided by Swanson[64]) of normally shaped and abnormally shaped spermatozoa heads and flagella that may provide a reason to believe that each microscopic swimmer might exhibit a unique and identifiable swimming pattern. The data in the paper suggest that the computer can find a small set of numbers or parameters that serve to describe a microscopic swimmer and that are significantly independent of the portion of the swimming track that is used to create the mathematical model in the sense that if a different portion of the swimming track is used, the identifying parameters from the two track segments are close to one another. Also, using this method of fitting the model, it appears that we may have a more accurate method of calculating wobble that has been shown by Young[69-71] to be influenced by the presence of small concentrations of chemical stressors. The parameter set describing the microscopic swimmers appears to be peculiar to each individual swimming spermatozoa. The following electron microscope images by Swanson[64] showing the 9-2 micro filament structure in a spermatozoa flagellum and the variability in head shape provide biological evidence that is in harmony with these observations.

The first figure shows the location of several parts of the spermatozoa that include the acrosome (Ac) or modified enzyme-filled Golgi apparatus vesicle, the centriolar adjunct (Ce) (lateral extension of the proximal centriole) in the midpiece, the cross striated (Cr) (segmented) columns of the connecting piece, the equatorial region (Eq), the mitochondrion (Mi), the nucleus, (Nu), the ribs (Ri) of the fibrous sheath, and several vacuoles (Va). There can be differences in swimming patterns due to differences in the shapes of the heads of the swimmers and to differences in the flagella that drive the swimmers. The $=>$ shows the central doublet microtubules of the principal piece axoneme, a * indicates a transverse cross section of the flagellum showing the typical 9 + 2 axoneme with surrounding fibrous sheath, and a ** shows a transverse cross section through the tail principal piece showing the defective 9 + 2 axoneme with surrounding fibrous sheath.

The following 4 figures are transmission electron micrographs (TEM), which show all or a major portion of eleven human spermatozoa heads with connecting piece (neck) and all or a portion of the midpiece. The 11 individuals labeled A, B, . . . , K, respectively, show all these features. The twelfth micrograph labeled G shows only the acrosomal portion of the spermatozoa. In the andrology laboratory sperm morphology is always evaluated with the compound light microscope at 1000 power magnification using oil immersion; thus, much more detail is evident in these TEM micrographs than is apparent in more common images obtained with a light microscope. Figure 8 was magnified 14,000 times, Figure 9 10,000 times, and Figures 10 and 11 were magnified 7,200 times.

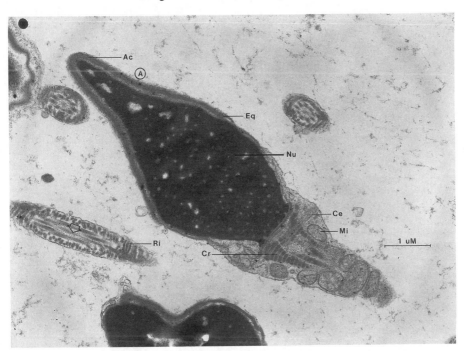

Figure 8. An illustration of a few important spermatozoal structures. The head and midpiece of cell A and the labeled tail of the second cell appear entirely normal in this micrograph. The numerous nonmembrane-bound vacuoles in the nucleus are typical in many heads and are not classified as abnormal. The morphology (shape) of the head does not preclude this swimmer from yielding a normal swimming pattern if the tail physiology is normal.

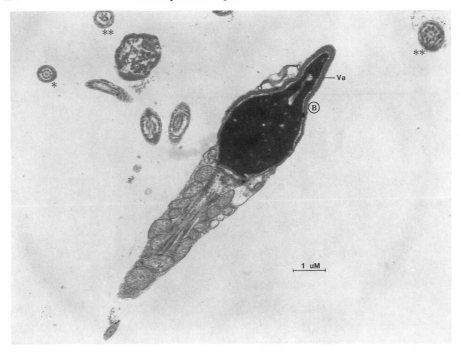

Figure 9. This shows sperm B with an aberration in the membranes of the head area opposite the identifying letter. This membrane defect is minor and by itself might result in a classification of slightly amorphous head (thus a slightly abnormal shape) if detected by light microscopy (LM) examination. Since the longitudinal axis (longest diameter) of the vacuole is greater than 1 micron, this cell is classified as severely abnormal when this defect is seen at the LM level. Because many defects observed with TEM, however, are not apparent with LM examination, this spermatozoan would be reasonably judged to be normal in most certified andrology laboratories using LM evaluation. The membrane defect in the shape of B would be expected to cause a deviation from straight line swimming. One normal and two abnormal tail cross sections are labeled in this transmission electron micrograph.

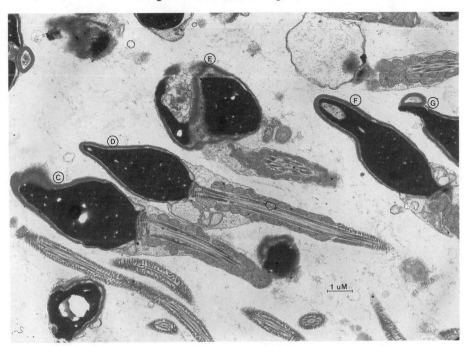

Figure 10. Five spermatozoa heads are labeled C, D, E, F, and G. Although C is slightly abnormally shaped at the tip of the head, the acrosome reaction (the change that occurs near the egg) is in progress and should be considered normal. The individual D is normal; the slight increase in cytoplasm (cytoplasmic droplet) around the neck and proximal midpiece is within normal limits. Although C and D are both normal, the shapes are clearly different, and one might expect quite different swimming patterns. Individual E is severely abnormal. Individual F is abnormal only in respect to the vacuole. Individual G cannot be fully evaluated because only a portion of the head is included on the electron microscope image. Individual G represents an interesting defect of the acrosome that might not be detected with light microscopy; this shape abnormality typically produces a dramatic effect on the swimming dynamics of the swimmer.

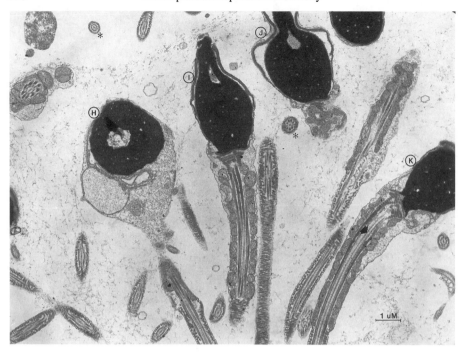

Figure 11. Four sperm heads are labeled H, I, J, and K. The sperm heads labeled H, J, and K have a severely abnormal shape. We regard individual I to have a normal morphology even though there is a slight perturbation at the tip of the nucleus and the acrosome. A typical tail cross section through the principal piece has been marked.

REFERENCES

1. Appleton, J. P., and Bray, K. N. C. 1964. The conservation equations for a nonequilibrium plasma. *J. Fluid Mechanics* 20:659–672.
2. Arnold, L. 1973. *Stochastic differential equations: Theory and applications.* New York: John Wiley and Sons.
3. Austin, C. R. 1972. Fertilization. In *Reproduction in mammals*, eds. C. R. Austin and R. V. Short, Chap. V. London: Cambridge University Press.
4. Barnsley, M. F., Berger, M. A., and Mete Soner, H. 1988. Mixing Markov chains and their images. In *Probability for the engineering and information sciences*, vol. 2, pp. 387–414.
5. Berrill, N. J., and Karp G. 1976. *Development.* New York: McGraw-Hill.
6. Box, G. E. P., and Jenkins, G. M. 1976. *Time series analysis. Forecasting and control.* San Francisco: Holden Day.
7. Brokaw, C. J., and Gibbons, I. R. 1975. Mechanisms of movement in flagella and cilia. In *Swimming and flying in nature*, eds. T. Y. C. Wu, J. Brokaw, and C. Brennon, pp. 89–125. New York: Plenum Press.
8. Brokaw, C. J. 1972. Computer simulation of flagellar movement. I. Demonstration of stable bend propagation and bend initiation by the sliding filament model. *Biophys. J.* 12:564–586.
9. Chang, M. C. 1958. The fertilization capacity of Spermatozoa deposited into Fallopian tubes. *Nature (Lond.)* 168:697–698.
10. Childress, S. 1964. The slow motion of a sphere in a rotating viscous fluid. *J. Fluid Mechanics* 20(Part 2):305–314.
11. Chow, S. N., Mallet-Paret, J., and Yorke. J. A. 1978. Finding zeros of maps: Homotopy methods that are constructive with probability one. *Math. Comp.* 32:887–889.
12. Chwang, A. T., and Wu, T. W. 1871. A note on the helical movement of microorganisms. *Proc. R. Soc. Lond.* 178:327–346.
13. Cohoon, D. K., and Purcell, R. M. 1989. Homotopy as an electromagnetic design method . . . . *J. Wave Material Interact.* 14:123–147.

14. Cohoon, D. K. 1995. Rugged individualism of swimming microorganisms. *J. Appl. Sci. Comp.* 1(3):408–436.
15. Cohoon, D. K. 1970. Free commutative semigroups of right invertible operators with decomposable kernels. *J. Math. Anal. Applications* 19(2):274–281.
16. Cox, R. G. 1970. The motion of long slender bodies in a viscous fluid . . . . *J. Fluid Mech.* 44:791–810.
17. Dehehy, M. A. 1975. The propulsion of nonrotating ram and oyster spermatoza. *Biol. Reprod.* 13:17–29.
18. Donoho, A. W., Donoho, D., and Gisko, M. 1985. MACSPIN Graphical Data Analysis Software User Manual, D^2. Austin, TX: Donoho and Donoho Software, Inc.
19. Dresdner, R. D., Katz, D. F., and Berger, S. A. 1980. The propulsion by large amplitude waves of uniflaggelar micro-organisms of finite length. *J. Fluid Mech.* 97:591–621.
20. Elliott, D. F., and Rao, K. R. 1982. *Fast transforms algorithms: Analysis, and applications*. New York: Academic Press.
21. Everitt, B. 1980. *Cluster analysis*. New York: Halsted Press.
22. Fauci, L. J., and Fogelson, A. L. 1993. Truncated Newton's methods and the modeling of complex immersed elastic structures. *Commun. Pure Appl. Math.* XLVI:787–818.
23. Feller, W. 1950. *An introduction to probability theory and its applications*. New York: Wiley.
24. Fisherkeller, M. A., Friedman, J. A., and Tukey, J. W. 1974. PRIM-9 An interactive multidimensional data display system. Stanford, CA: Stanford Linear Accelerator Publication 1408.
25. Friedman, A. 1975. *Stochastic differential equations and applications*. New York: Academic Press.
26. Friedman, A. 1970. *Foundations of modern analysis*. New York: Holt, Reinhart, and Winston.
27. Garcia, C. B., and Zangwill, W. I. 1981. *Pathways to solutions, fixed points, and equilibria*. Englewood Cliffs, NJ: Prentice Hall.
28. Goltz, J. S., Gardner, T. K., Kanous, K. S., and Lindemann, C. G. 1988. The interaction of pH and cyclic adenosine 3′, 5′-monophosphate on activation of motility in Triton X-100 extracted bull sperm. *Biol. Reprod.* 39:1129–1136.
29. Grenander, U. 1980. *Regular structures. Lectures in pattern theory*, vol. III. New York: Springer.
30. Gwatkin, R. B. L. 1977. *Fertilization mechanisms in men and animals*. New York: Plenum Press.
31. Higdon, J. J. L. 1979. A hydrodynamic analysis of flagellar propulsion. *J. Fluid Mech.* 90:685–711.
32. Hill, D. L. *The biochemistry and physiology of Tetrahymena*. New York: Academic Press.
33. Holwill, M. E. J., and Burge, R. E. 1963. A hydrodynamic study of the mobility of flagellated bacteria. *Arch. Bioch. Biophys.* 101:249–260.
34. Holt, W. V., Moore, H. D. M., and Hillier, S. G. 1985. Computer assisted swimming speed in human semen; Correlation of results with in vitro fertilization assays. London: Medical Research Institute, Gamete Biology Unit MRC/AFRC Comparative Psychology Research Group, Institute of Zoology, Zoological Society of London.
35. Hormander, L. 1963. *Linear partial differential operators*. New York: Academic Press.
36. Huber, P. J. 1985. Projection pursuit. *Ann. Stat.* 13:435–525.
37. Jenkins, G. M., and Watts, D. G. 1969. *Spectral analysis and its applications*. San Francisco: Holden Day.
38. Katz, D. F., Davis, R. O., Delandmeter, B. A., and Overstreet, J. W. 1985. Real time analysis of sperm motion using automatic video image digitization. *Comput. Methods Programs Biomed.* 21:173–182.
39. Katz, D. F., and Pedrotti, L. 1977. Geotaxis by motile spermatozoa: Hydrodynamic reorientation. *J. Theoret. Biol.* 67:723–732.
40. Keller, J. B., and Rubinow, S. I. 1976. Swimming of flagellated microorganisms. *Biophys. J.* 16:151–170.
41. Koopmans, L. H. 1974. *The spectral analysis of time series*. New York: Wiley.
42. Kopf, G. 1989. Mechanisms of signal transduction in mouse spermatozoa. In *Regulation of testicular function*, eds. L. C. Ewing and B. Robaire. *Ann. NY Acad. Sci.* 564: 289–302.
43. Larsen, R. J., and Marx, M. 1981. *An introduction to mathematical statistics and its application*. Englewood Cliffs, NJ: Prentice Hall.
44. Lighthill, J. 1975. *Mathematical biofluid dynamics*. Philadelphia: Society for Industrial and Applied Mathematics.
45. Lighthill, J. 1976. Flagellar hydrodynamics. *Soc. Ind. Appl. Math. Rev.* 18(2):161–230.
46. Liu, S. C., and Cohoon, D. K. 1970. Limiting behaviors of randomly excited hyperbolic tangent systems. *Bell Syst. Tech. J.* 49(4):543–560.
47. Loefer, J. B., and Mefferd, R. B. 1952. Concerning pattern formation by free swimming microorganisms' patterns. *Am. Nat.* 86:325–329.
48. Loefer, J. B., and Mefferd, R. B. 1952. Applications of the most probable number method to determine heat sensitivity of protozoa. *Proc. Ame. Soc. Protozoologists* 3:17.
49. Mack, S. O., Tash, J. S., and Wolf, D. P. 1989. Effect of measurement conditions on quantification of hyperactivated human sperm subpopulations by digital image analysis. *Biol. Reprod.* 40:1162–1169.
50. Mahoney, M. C., Alexander, N. J., and Swanson, R. J. 1988. Evaluation of semen parameters by means of automated sperm motion analyzers. *Fertil. Steril.* 49(5):876–880.

51. McCabe, B. J., Belkin, B., Wagner, D. H., and Sommer, K. M. 1987. Stochastic Models of Sperm Motion. Report to the National Science Foundation. Paoli, PA: Daniel Wagner Associates. September 30.

52. Noever, D. A., Matsos, H. C., Cronise, R. J., Looger, L. L., and Relwani, R. A. 1994. Computerized in vitro test for chemical toxicity based on *Tetrahymena* swimming patterns. In *Proc. 1994 Scientific Conf. Alternatives in Tests of Biotoxicity*, ed. J. Rhodes, pp. 627–638. Edgewood, MD: Batelle Edgewood Operations and the Chemical Research Development and Engineering Center.

53. Noever, D. A., Matsos, H. C., Cronise, R. J., Looger, L., Relwani, R. A., and Johnson, J. 1994. Computerized in vitro test for chemical toxicity based on *Tetrahymena* swimming patterns. *Chemosphere* 29:1373–1384.

54. Olds-Clarke, P. 1986. Motility characteristics of sperm from the uterus and oviducts of female mice after mating to congenic males differing in sperm transport and fertility. *Biol. Reprod.* 34:453–467.

55. Patrick, E. A., and Fattu, J. M. 1986. *Artificial intelligence with statistical pattern recognition*. Englewood Cliffs, NJ: Prentice Hall.

56. Roberts, R. O., and Berk, S. G. 1990. Development of a protozoan chemoattraction bioassay for evaluating toxicity of aquatic pollutants. *Toxicity Assess.* 5:279–287.

57. Robertson, L., Wolf, D. P., and Tash, J. S. 1988. Temporal changes in motility parameters related to acrosomal status: Identification and characterization of populations of hyperactivated sperm. *Biol. Reprod.* 39:797–805.

58. Sage, A. P., and Melsa, J. L. 1971. *System identification*. New York: Academic Press.

59. Shack, W. J., Fray, C. S., and Lardner, T. J. 1974. Observations on the hydrodynamics and swimming motions of mammalian spermatozoa. *Bull. Math. Biol.* 36:555–565.

60. Silverman, J. 1983. Preliminary findings on the use of protozoa (*Tetrahymena thermophila*) as models of ocular irritation testing in rabbits. *Lab. Anim. Sci.* 33:56–59.

61. Silverman, J., and Penisi, S. 1987. Evaluation of *Tetrahymena thermophila* as an in vitro alternative to ocular irritation studies in rabbits. *J. Toxicol. Cutaneous Ocul. Toxicol.* 6:33–42.

62. Silverman, J. 1993. Use of a protozoan to help determine if certain chemicals may be irritating to an animal's eye. In *Ohio Science Workbook: Biotechnology*, ed. S.E. Reames, pp. 165–167. Columbus, OH: Ohio Academy of Science.

63. Srinivasan, S. K., and Rasudevan, R. 1971. *Introduction to random differential equations and their applications*. New York: American Elsevier.

64. Swanson, R. J. 1990. Personal communication, Department of Biological Sciences. Old Dominion University, Norfolk, VA, May 31.

65. Uhlenbeck, G. E., and Ornstein, L. S. 1930. On the theory of Brownian motion. *Phys. Rev.* 36:823–841.

66. Uldrick, J. P., and Siekmann, J. 1964. On the swimming of a flexible plate of arbitrary finite thickness. *J. Fluid Mech.* 20:1–33.

67. Vasquez, J. M., 1990. Personal communication, Department of Obstetrics and Gynecology, Thomas Jefferson Medical School, Philadelphia.

68. Whittaker, E. T., and Watson, G. N. 1962. *A course of modern analysis*, 4th ed. Cambridge: Cambridge University Press.

69. Young, R. J., Bodt, B. A., Iturralde, T. G., and Starke, W. C. 1992. Automated analysis of rabbit sperm motility and the effect of chemicals on sperm motion parameters. *Mol. Reprod. Dev.* 33:347–356.

70. Young, R. J., and Bodt, B. A. 1994. Development of computer directed methods for the identification of hyperactivated motion using motion patterns developed by rabbit sperm during incubation under capacitation conditions. *J. Androl.* 15(4):362–377.

71. Young, R. J., Body, B. A., and Heitkamp, D. H. 1995. Action of metallic ions on the precocious development of rabbit sperm on motion patterns that are characteristic of hyperactivated motility. *Mol. Reprod. Dev.* 41:239–248.

Chapter Fourteen

COMPUTATION OF DEVELOPMENTAL TOXICITY POTENTIAL BY QSTR MODELS IN THE TOPKAT PROGRAM

Kurt Enslein, Vijay K. Gombar, Benjamin W. Blake, and James R. Carter

Quantitative structure–toxicity relationships (QSTR) were used to model developmental toxicity potential (DTP) for a set of 261 chemicals for which development toxicity assays have been performed in rats by the oral route. A scale based on malformations, maternal toxicity, fetal resorptions, fetal deaths, and fetal weight was used to summarize the DTP for each chemical. The 261 chemicals were grouped into 3 classes to enhance homogeneity of each group. The accuracy of the resulting equations, using E-state values on one- and two-atom fragments, symmetry indexes, and topological shape as descriptors for the chemicals, ranged between 90 and 93%. These equations have been incorporated into the TOPKAT program, and can be used for assessing DTP for untested compounds.

INTRODUCTION

The purpose of the research reported herein was to provide a method for the assessment of developmental toxicity potential (DTP) for chemicals that have not been assayed for that toxicity endpoint. Such computational assessments are useful in the development of new chemicals and the evaluation of existing compounds that do not merit the resources necessary for an animal bioassay. Quantitative structure–toxicity relationship (QSTR) techniques can be used to design such computational tools. This chapter describes the development and performance of a QSTR model and its application to the assessment of DTP.

METHODS

Database

In prior research, we identified 5559 open literature citations believed to contain data related to developmental toxicity in nonhuman mammals. From the subset of these citations for which publications were obtained and read, studies on 952 unique chemicals were identified. This subset contained 374 rat oral studies of single organic compounds of defined structure, and thus did not include mixtures and organometallics.

For these 374 studies, their authors reported the doses at which developmental toxicity (DT) and maternotoxicity (MT) occurred (Table 1). Two types of studies were removed from the 374 for the modeling data set: (a) those that were performed at only one dose and both DT and MT were observed at that dose, and (b) those in which neither DT nor MT were observed at even the highest exposure. These types of studies were inadequate for the purposes of the QSTR model, as a lower dose in the first type could well have produced a different result, and a higher dose in the second type could have altered the results as well. The remaining 273 chemicals formed the basis of the QSTR development.

Definition and Derivation of DTP Scores

Different degrees of DTP were derived based on the relation between the doses at which DT and MT occurred, as follows: Score 1 was assigned if no DT occurred even at maternotoxic doses; score 2 resulted if there was strict concordance between DT and MT, that is, DT nor MT at one dose, and both DT and MT at a higher dose; score 3 was assigned to chemicals that induced DT before the dose resulting in MT; and, finally, score 4 was assigned if DT was observed at least two doses below that which produced MT. This scoring scheme is summarized in Table 2.

One of the desirata for QSTR models is that the chemicals in the training set all produce their effects by the same mechanism or mode of action. Unfortunately, this information is usually unavailable. Since the training set consisted of heterogenous chemicals, we decided to divide them into broadly similar structures, each group containing preferably about the same number of chemicals.

Because of the relatively low frequency of occurrence of chemicals with DTP scores 2–4 and to permit the development of statistically valid models, we grouped these classes together. Thus we have a set of chemicals without DTP, and another set with DTP, without specification of strength of evidence. The numbers in each chemical class are shown in Table 3.

Table 1. Some Signs of Developmental and Maternal Toxicity

Developmental toxicity	Maternal toxicity
Reduced fetal growth	Reduced weight gain
Fetal death	Increased mortality
Resorptions	Alopecia
Skeletal anomalies	Rough fur
External malformations	Respiratory distress
Visceral defects	Behavioral
Runting	Vaginal bleeding

Table 2. Developmental Toxicity Potential Scores

Score	Definition
1	No DTP even at maternotoxic doses
2	Strict concordance between DTP and maternotoxicity
3	DTP at a dose approaching maternotoxicity
4	DTP at a non-maternotoxic dose

Table 3. Number[a] of Compounds by Chemical Class

Class	No DTP	DTP	Total
Aliphatics	35	44	79
Carboaromatics	39	53	92
Heteroaromatics	49	41	90
Total	123	138	261

[a] After removal of 12 chemicals during the modeling process.

QSTR Model Development

An outline of the steps involved in the development of QSTR equations is shown in Figure 1. Inasmuch as the toxicity endpoint consists of DTP and non-DTP chemicals, two-group linear discriminant analysis (LDA)[1] was used.

Given the screened database, the process starts with the generation of candidate structural descriptors (discussed later). After a correlation analysis to remove redundant descriptors, those descriptors that best explain the variation in DTP are selected by a stepwise procedure. At the end of this operation, a tentative model is obtained. The diagnostic procedures now begin. These are intended to assure that the QSTR model is robust. The procedures identify leverage chemicals, that is, those that have an undue influence on the equation, as well as poorly-behaved descriptors.[2] After each adjustment of the data and/or descriptor set the equation is recalculated, and the diagnostic procedures repeated, until a robust equation is obtained.

At this point it is necessary to validate the equation. We use two methods: the leave-one-out technique, and randomization tests. In leave-one-out, each compound is removed from the training set in turn, the equation recalculated, and the DTP of the left-out chemical calculated with the equation and compared with the experimental DTP score. For the randomization test, the equation

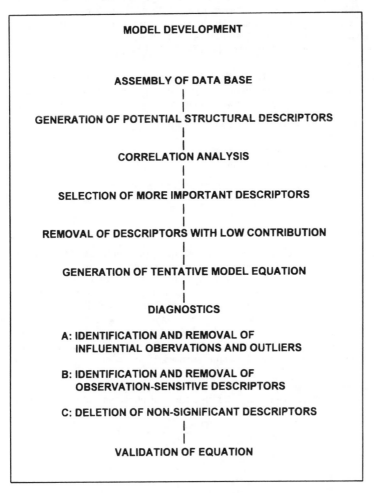

MODEL DEVELOPMENT

ASSEMBLY OF DATA BASE
|
|
GENERATION OF POTENTIAL STRUCTURAL DESCRIPTORS
|
|
CORRELATION ANALYSIS
|
|
SELECTION OF MORE IMPORTANT DESCRIPTORS
|
|
REMOVAL OF DESCRIPTORS WITH LOW CONTRIBUTION
|
|
GENERATION OF TENTATIVE MODEL EQUATION
|
|
DIAGNOSTICS

A: IDENTIFICATION AND REMOVAL OF
INFLUENTIAL OBERVATIONS AND OUTLIERS

B: IDENTIFICATION AND REMOVAL OF
OBSERVATION-SENSITIVE DESCRIPTORS

C: DELETION OF NON-SIGNIFICANT DESCRIPTORS
|
|
VALIDATION OF EQUATION

Figure 1. Steps in developing QSTR equations.

is recalculated with the DTP classes scrambled, and the classification accuracy is determined by comparison with the correct assignment.

Structural Descriptors

Effective structure quantification is the spirit of all structure–property relationship studies. It has been shown[3] that the structure descriptors should be able to quantify transport, bulk, and electronic attributes of a molecular structure.

Three classes of descriptors are used in this model: electrotopological state (E-state) values on a set of one-atom and two-atom fragments, topological shape, and symmetry indices.

Electronic Attributes

Theoretically it is possible to quantify electronic attributes at any desired level of complexity ranging from quantum mechanical to a mere count of lone pairs. In recent years a number of methods have been published that do not require knowledge of molecular geometry and are extremely fast in computing electronic properties[4,5] such as partial atomic charges, residual electronegativity, effective polarizability, etc. These algorithms have a practical advantage, especially for QSTR studies, because they can be calculated at modest cost for large sets of big molecules. We have shown,[6] through an example of mutagenicity of some triazenes, that the QSTRs obtained by using electronic descriptors computed from these non-geometry-based methods are of better or equal quality than that of QSTRs developed using sophisticated molecular orbital methods.

For the developmental toxicity models we have applied a rather new approach, which quantifies electronic attributes of molecules in terms of E-values.[7] Some of the advantages of this approach over the one used for the study of triazenes are:

1. Complete electrotopological information encoding
2. Greater statistical reliability
3. Easy comprehension and implementation
4. Suitable for validation of predictions

A brief description of the two-stage method for the calculation of E-values is given in the following sections.

Identification of Fragments

The first step in quantification of electronic attributes of a molecule is to parse the molecular structure for identification of one-atom and two-atom fragments that are present in our proprietary fragment library. If there are any atoms or hybridization states of atoms in a molecule that are not represented in the library, such molecules need to be excluded from the analysis. At present this library contains about 2500 fragments consisting of atoms H, B, C, N, O, F, Si, P, S, Cl, Br, and I in a variety of hybridization states and thus covers a wide range of organic molecules. If needed, the library can be expanded to include additional atoms of particular interest.

There are two sets of fragments in the library: general and specific fragments. Unlike general fragments, the specific fragments include attached H atoms and impose restrictions on the topological environment of atom(s). In our experience, the type, count, and E-values of one-atom and two-atom fragments collectively define a chemical structure uniquely, for all practical purposes. For 3-methoxy-1-propanol, for instance, four one-atom and four two-atom fragments are generated. They are:

One Atom	
Type	Count
$-CH_2$	3
$-O-$	1
$-OH$	1
$-CH_3$	1

Two Atom	
Type	Count
$-CH_2-CH_2-$	2
$-CH_2-OH$	1
$-CH_2-O-$	1
$-O-CH_3$	1

These fragments collectively will define 3-methoxy-1-propanol and *only* 3-methoxy-1-propanol.

Computation of Electrotopological State Values

After having identified the unique set of fragments in a molecule, the E-values of these fragments are computed. The E-value of a fragment encodes information about its electron content (valence, sigma, pi and lone-pair), topology, and environment. Since an E-value is computed by taking into account the effects of both intrinsic and environmental features, it changes even with remote variations in structure; of course, the magnitude of variation depends on the severity of the changes.

The computation of the E-value of any atom begins with assignment of intrinsic state value, I, to every nonhydrogen atom i in the molecule according to:

$$I_i = \frac{\delta^v + 1}{\delta}$$

where δ is the number of s-electrons and δ^v is the sum of sigma, pi, and lone-pair electrons. The I value is then corrected for the field influence ΔI_i on atom i. ΔI_i may be calculated as:

$$\Delta I_i = \frac{\Sigma(I_i - I_j)}{r_{ij}^2}$$

where r_{ij} is the number of atoms in the shortest path between atoms i and j, both inclusive. The sum of I_i and ΔI_i then gives the E-value for atom i. The E-value for a fragment is calculated by summing up the E-values of the atoms involved in the fragment. It is these E-values on all one-atom and two-atom fragments that are used here to quantify the electronic attributes of molecules.

Transport Attributes

Transport attributes are often expressed in terms of the logarithm of partition coefficient between n-octanol and water, log P.[8] Since log P is an additive–constitutive property, it can be calculated from the constant contributions of structural features of a molecule.[9-11] Considering these contributions as different weights associated with various structural fragments, we decided to use the counts of one-atom and two-atom fragments instead of log P and left the selection of fragments and the assignment of weights of the selected fragments to be determined by the statistical method used for developing the structure–toxicity relationship.

Since molecular shape and molecular symmetry also influence molecular transport, we included topological shape descriptors, k, of orders 1 through 7[12,13] and seven indices of molecular symmetry[14] for quantifying the transport attributes of molecules.

Bulk Attributes

Besides molecular weight, we used size-corrected E-values on one-atom and two-atom fragments for quantification of molecular bulk. The size-corrected E-values are computed from a rescaled count of valence electrons: $4\delta^v/n^2$ instead of δ^v.

Assessment of DTP

In order to produce a DTP assessment for a query compound, the procedure shown in Figure 2 is used. Note that the only action that need be taken by a user is to input the structure of the query chemical. All remaining operations, including generation of structural descriptors, are performed by the TOPKAT program.

The TOPKAT program is an integrated software system that incorporates QSTR models and permits the assessment of toxicity endpoints for new chemicals. Referring again to Figure 2, the assessment procedure starts with the identification of the structural descriptors in the query compound forming part of the QSTR model. The descriptor values are then calculated. TOPKAT checks whether the query structure is adequately covered by the data base chemicals. If there is one (or more) fragment in the query structure not present with sufficient frequency in the training set chemicals, TOPKAT will so indicate, and give the user the choice to terminate the assessment procedure. Otherwise, TOPKAT checks whether the structure is within the optimum prediction space for the DTP model, that is, whether the query structures falls within the multivariate space of the model. Thereafter, the discriminant score based on the descriptor values and their respective coefficients is calculated, followed by transformation of the score to a probability statement by means of a simple exponential equation.[1]

Evaluation of TOPKAT Assessment of DTP

TOPKAT version 3.0 incorporates features that permit objective decisions regarding the quality of DTP assessments. Several operations are automatically performed:

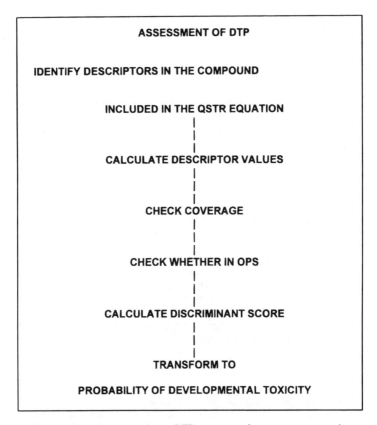

Figure 2. Procedure to produce a DTP assessment for a query compound.

Table 4. Statistical Parameters for DTP Models

Statistical parameter	Submodel		
	Aliphatics	Carboaromatics	Heteroaromatics
Number of compounds	79	92	90
Number of descriptors	22	29	29
Electronic	15	19	21
Shape	2	0	0
Symmetry	1	1	0
Fragment count	4	9	8
F-ratio	7.70	7.59	7.96
Wilk's	0.25	0.22	0.21

TOPKAT checks whether the query chemical contains one or more fragments that are not present in the training set. If all fragments are present, the query compound is considered "covered" by the training set.

TOPKAT next determines whether the query chemical falls within the optimum prediction space (OPS) associated with the developed QSTR model. OPS is determined from the range of the descriptors in the equation, and their interrelationships. In other words, TOPKAT checks whether the DTP equation is applicable to the query compound. If it is, the probability that the estimate will be correct is the same as the accuracy of the DTP equation. If, on the other hand, the query compound falls outside OPS, the confidence in the estimate will be reduced; in fact it may be wise to reject the estimate altogether.

If the estimate is acceptable TOPKAT can be used to check for database structures that are similar to the query compound. Note that similarity is computed in terms of E-values; that is, the most similar compounds will have the most similar pattern of E-values. The most similar compounds may well be quite different from those with conventional visual or substructural similarity.

RESULTS AND DISCUSSION

Equation and Statistics

In Table 4 we show the statistical parameters for the three submodels. Note that most of the structural descriptors are E-state variables. All equations are statistically highly significant, as indicated by the tabled F-ratios. The differences between the number of compounds in the database and the number of compounds in the training sets represents chemicals that were removed during the model development process. Thus, eight compounds were removed from the aliphatics subset, three from the carboaromatics, and one from the heteroaromatics.

Model Accuracy

In Table 5 are shown the classification accuracies for the 3 submodels. The overall accuracy ranges between 86% and 97.4%, depending on the submodel. These numbers take into account the indeterminates, that is, those chemicals for which, in the leave-one-out test, the model-computed posterior probability is between 0.30 to 0.69. One notes that sensitivity and specificity are remarkably well balanced, that is, that neither false negatives nor false positives predominate.

Table 5. Model Accuracy

Submodel	Indeterminates	Misclassified	Sensitivity	Specificity
Aliphatics	2.5%	8.9%	88.6%	88.6%
Carboaromatics	2.2%	6.5%	87.0%	97.4%
Heteroaromatics	6.5%	10.3%	86.1%	86.0%

In order to confirm that the accuracies in Table 5 were not due to chance, chemicals were randomly tagged DTP and non-DTP in each submodel while maintaining the original group populations, keeping the ratio of positives to negatives the same as in the original distributions. Using the descriptors of the submodels, discriminant functions were redeveloped. Again using the leave-one-out test, the maximum accuracy that was achieved for any submodel was 53%, that is, essentially chance, indicating that the original submodels do portray a real association between the descriptors and the DTP endpoint.

Some DTP Assessments

The QSTR models developed here were applied to several chemicals not included in the training set. The computed DTPs were compared with the experimental results, and these are indicated as Pos (for Positive) or Neg (for Negative) in Table 6.

Some Observations on Table 6

Diethyl phthalate: This compound is assessed as a non-DTP chemical. Its literature value is Positive. The assessment is clearly at variance with the literature data.

Thalidomide: The compound is in OPS, but, on the basis of this model developed from oral rat assays, its DTP is in the indeterminate zone. At this time we have not been able to identify an acceptable rat study for this chemical, thus the apparently paradoxical result.

Other compounds: All the other compounds for which literature data were available were correctly predicted.

SOME FURTHER COMMENTS

Data Limitations

As previously stated, any QSTR model is dependent on a database of measured endpoints. As such, a model's applicability is necessarily limited by the restricted set of chemicals in the training set. Thus it is important to abide by the diagnostics that TOPKAT provides, as these may reflect the inability of the training set to support the query compound estimate. As the training set grows and the model is redeveloped with an enlarged database, the model will become applicable to an ever larger subset of the chemical universe.

Table 6. Some Compounds Assessed with the DTP Model

Compound	DTP class	Probability from model
Acetaminophen		0.000 Not in OPS
Acyclovir	Pos	0.955
Amiloride		0.915 Not in OPS
Clonazepam		0.000
Chloramphenicol		1.000 Not in OPS
Chlordiazepoxide		0.999
Chlorpheniramine		0.025
Chlorpromazine		0.997 Not in OPS
Diazepam		0.000 Not in OPS
Diethyl phthalate	Pos	0.007
Meclizine	Pos	0.987
Metronidazole	Neg	0.003 Not in OPS
Nitroimidazole		0.011
Oxazepam		0.050 Not in OPS
Phenacetin		0.000 Not in OPS
Phenobarbital	Pos	0.369 Not in OPS
Thalidomide		0.449
Urethane	Pos	1.000
Valpromide		1.000

Note. For compounds for which DTP class is not indicated, data are not available from rat oral assays.

Distinction from Teratogenicity

We would like to emphasize that in this chapter we have described a computational model for developmental toxicity potential, not teratogenicity. While fetal malformations played a part in the scoring of DTP, these were only one component in the calculation of the score. Our teratogenicity model[15] only took presence or absence of fetal malformations into account. For further details we refer the interested reader to our published work on teratogenicity.

REFERENCES

1. Gombar, V. J., and Enslein, K. 1991. Structure-biodegradability relationship model by discriminant analysis. In *Applied multivariate analysis in SAR and environmental studies*, eds. J. Devillers, and W. Karcher, pp. 377–414. Dordrecht: Kluwer Academic.
2. Belsley, D. A., Kuh, E., and Welsch, R. E. 1980. *Regression diagnostics: Identifying influential data and sources of collinearity.* New York: Wiley.
3. Purcell, W. P., Bass, G. E., and Clayton, J. M. 1973. *Strategy of drug design: A guide to biological activity.* New York: Wiley.
4. Gasteiger, J., and Marsili, M. 1980. Quantification of effective polarizability. Applications in studies of x-ray photoelectron spectroscopy and alkylamine protonation. *Tetrahedron* 36:3219–3288.
5. Mullay, J. J. 1984. Atomic and group electronegativities *J. Am. Chem. Soc.* 106:5842–5847.
6. Gombar, V. K. and Enslein, K. 1990. Quantitative structure-activity relationship (QSAR) studies using electronic descriptors calculated from topological and molecular orbital (MO) methods. *Quant. Struct.-Act. Relat.* 9:321–325.
7. Hall, H. L., Mohney, B., and Kier, L. B. 1991. The electrotopological state: Structure information at the atomic level for molecular graphs. *J. Chem. Inf. Comput. Sci.* 31:76–82.
8. Fujita, T., Iwasa, J., and Hansch, C. 1964. A new substituent constant, pi, derived from partition coefficients. *J. Am. Chem. Soc.* 86:5175–5180.
9. Rekker, R. F., and de Kort, H. M. 1979. The hydrophobic fragmental constant. An extension to a 1000 data point set. *Eur. J. Med. Chem.* 14:479–488.
10. Hansch, C., and Leo, A. 1979. *Substituent constants for correlation analysis in chemistry and biology.* New York: Wiley.
11. Ghose, A. K., and Crippen, G. M. 1986. Atomic physicochemical parameters for three-dimensional structure-directed quantitative structure-activity relationships. I. Partition coefficients as a measure of hydrophobicity. *J. Comput. Chem.* 7:565–577.
12. Gombar, V. K., and Jain, D. V. S. 1988. Quantification of molecular shape and its correlation with physicochemical properties. *Indian J. Chem.* 26A:554–555.
13. Kier, L. B. 1986. Shape indexes of order one and three from molecular graphs. *Quant. Struct.-Act. Relat.* 5:1–7.
14. Mumtaz, M. M., Knauf, L. A., Reisman, D. J., Peirano, W. B., Derosa, C. T., Gombar, V. K., Enslein, K., Carter, J. C., Blake, B. W., Huque, K. I., and Ramanujam, V. M. S. 1995. Estimation of effect levels of chemicals from quantitative structure-activity relationship (QSAR) models. I. Chronic Lowest-Observed-Adverse-Effect-Level (LOAEL). *Toxicol. Lett.* 79:131–143.
15. Gombar, V. K., Borgstedt, H. H., Enslein, K., Hart, J. B., and Blake, B. W. 1991. A QSAR model of teratogenesis. *Quant. Struct.-Act. Relat.* 10:306–322.

Chapter Fifteen

ACTIVITY PROFILES OF DEVELOPMENTAL TOXICITY

Robert J. Kavlock

The available literature was searched for quantitative test results from both in vitro and in vivo assays for developmental toxicity for five model compounds: cyclophosphamide, methotrexate, hydroxyurea, caffeine, and ethylenethiourea. These compounds were chosen on the basis of their extensive utilization in a variety of assay systems for developmental toxicity as evidenced by their representation in the ETIC database (each generally has 100–500 citations encompassing multiple test systems). Nine cellular-based assays and six assays using whole embryos in culture, as well as Segment II and abbreviated exposure test for mammalian test species, are included in the database. For each assay, the critical endpoints were identified, each of which was then provided a three-letter code, and the criteria for extraction of quantitative information were established. The extracted information was placed into a computerized reference file and subsequently plotted such that the qualitative (positive/negative) and quantitative [e.g., IC50, highest ineffective dose (HID), lowest effective dose (LED)] results across all test systems could be displayed. The information contained in these profiles can be used to compare qualitative and quantitative results across multiple assay systems, to identify data gaps in the literature, to evaluate the concordance of the assays, to calculate relative potencies, and to examine structure–activity relationships. Examples are provided from the field of mutagenesis, where this approach is now allowing sophisticated polling of the available database. Efforts to produce a uniform, agreed-upon standard by which alternative tests for developmental toxicity can be judged have recently stalled, however, thus dimming the prospect for much advance in this area.

Recent developments in the field of developmental toxicology have resulted in the proliferation of assays designed to detect agents which may be hazardous to the embryo or fetus. Increasing amounts of data from in vitro and other short-term assays have created the need for a peer-compiled and reviewed database of quantitative test results. Such a database would help identify data gaps in the literature, provide a coherent basis for reporting assay results, and potentially form a central repository of test results. If verified results from standard in vivo testing protocols (i.e., FDA Segment II, EPA Developmental Toxicity Test, or ICH 4.1.3) that are the "gold standards" by which any alternate test performance must be judged are included in this database, it would provide the framework to establish the sensitivity, specificity, and accuracy of assays used for hazard identification, and to select assays for monitoring mechanisms relevant to the developmental toxicity of particular classes of compounds. The agreed-upon standard assay

This chapter is based in part upon work published in *Teratology* 43:159–185 (1991).[4] The information in that document was funded by the U.S. Environmental Protection Agency. It was subject to the agency's peer and administrative review, and was approved for publication. Mention of trade names or commercial products does not constitute endorsement or recommendations for use.

results would enable all developers and users of alternative tests to judge performance against the same information base. At present, assay developers have to either depend upon a list, suggested in the early 1980s by an expert panel[1] that has since been criticized as being biased toward cytotoxic agents and for deemphasizing maternal toxicity as a potential confounder, or to assess the literature themselves. These approaches are neither efficient nor reflective of a contemporary consensus of experts.

To accomplish this task, an approach developed by Garrett et al.[2] for mutagenesis assays was used to create a database for developmental toxicity test results. In this approach, a bar graph for each chemical is used to present the data from various short term genetic toxicity tests. On the x-axis, individual assays are grouped by some criteria, and each assay (or endpoint within an assay) is given a three-letter code. The y-axis is a bidirectional logarithmic dose/concentration scale, with zero dose units placed midway on the axis. Assay results are plotted on the y-axis and indicate whether the results were positive (a bar rising above the midline) or negative (a bar pointing down from the midline). Due to the logarithmic scale, the length of the line is directly proportional to the agent's potency or lack thereof. A caret at the end of a particular assay result indicates that the result was from a situation in which an exogenous metabolic assay system was included. Should multiple results be available for any test, the arithmetic mean of the results is plotted (individual hatched lines on bar graph). In cases where both negative and positive results are available for an endpoint, a solid line is drawn to the mean of the majority results, and a dotted line to the mean of the minority results. The condensed format of the data presentation facilitates the rapid visualization of the biological effects induced by a chemical and provides a mechanism for quick comparison of effects among different chemicals. The profile system for mutagenic assays has been adapted for standard use by the International Agency for Research on Cancer Monograph series since Supplement 2.[3]

With the exception of the present effort, there has been no centralized summary of quantitative results for developmental toxicants, although a number of qualitative summary efforts are available. After a review of assays for developmental toxicity, the following groupings were identified: cellular-based assays; embryos grown in vitro; full organogenesis-stage exposures for mice, rats, rabbits; miscellaneous species (e.g., cats, dogs, guinea pigs); nonhuman primates; and human studies. Studies that used exposures that encompassed all of organogenesis were separated from those using abbreviated exposure durations. For the cellular-based systems, eight types of assays were identified: pox virus expression, mouse ovarian tumor assay, palatal mesenchyme proliferation, *Drosophila* cell culture, neuroblastoma differentiation, rodent and chick limb bud and neuroblast micromass culture, chick embryo retinal cell assay, and mammalian organ culture (primarily limbs and palate). Six assays were identified that utilized embryos grown in vitro: *Hydra attenuata*, *Drosophila* larva culture, frog embryo culture, fish embryo culture, chick embryo culture, and mammalian whole embryo culture. The in vivo test assays generally followed the approach requested by federal regulatory agencies.

To evaluate the feasibility of presenting information in this manner, the ETIC (Environmental Teratogen Information Center) database was searched to identify chemicals that were tested in a variety of assays and that had a large literature base (between 100 and 500 peer-reviewed publications). From these criteria, five chemicals were selected for full data extraction: cyclophosphamide, methotrexate, hydroxyurea, caffeine, and ethylenethiourea. For each assay/endpoint in the literature, a panel of experts identified the lowest effected dose (LED) level for a positive compound, and the highest ineffective dose (HID) level for a negative. An example of a profile for cyclophosphamide is displayed in Figure 1. The reader is referred to the original publication of this effort[4] for details of the profile methodologies, assay coding nomenclature, and summary evaluation of the data.

Analysis of the five profiles generated in the evaluation process suggested that few interlaboratory comparisons are available (most results were from individual laboratories with particular interest in that assay), and that relatively few high quality standard in vivo test results are available for these agents, which are probably among the most tested chemicals (their developmental toxicity was largely detected years ago, and most studies in the literature are pursuing hypothesis testing rather than attempting hazard identification for a new chemical). A major limitation of the profile methodology is a general inability to graphically convey certain important aspects of experimental design, including strain, route of exposure, duration of exposure, vehicle,

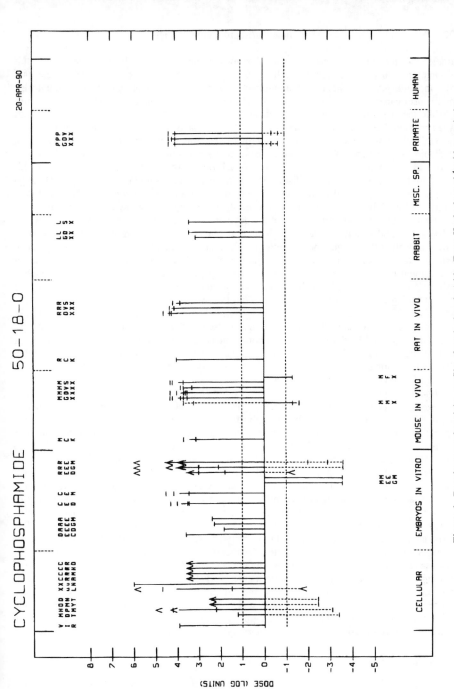

Figure 1. Developmental toxicity profile of cyclophsophamide. From Kavlock et al.[4] with permission.

sample size, and statistical analysis. One must look to the underlying database for some of this information, and to the complete publication for other parts. Nevertheless, much of the hard work in identifying the important literature and relevant effects is readily displayed graphically, and the user can easily obtained the primary report for more detailed presentation of the results.

While the original paper describing this system is almost 4 years old, no new assay systems have appeared that would suggest a revision of the approach is necessary to meet contemporary standards. What is lacking, however, is a strong consensus on whether the overall approach of developing screens for chemicals with unknown mechanisms of action is at all feasible. An effort was underway at the National Toxicology Program (NTP) during the early part of this decade to develop a gold standard list of developmental toxicants upon which to base validation studies. This effort, chaired by Bernard Schwetz, eventually came to a consensus that an in vitro test must ultimately predict the outcome of a full-scale in vivo bioassay in terms of effects on the viability, growth, and morphology of the developing conceptus. A list of agents upon which to develop a validation effort was to be the next product of this effort. However, while a scoring system reflecting the weight and strength of the evidence that a chemical causes developmental toxicity was developed, it has yet to be implemented. Thus, we are left with little further development of test methodologies over the last 5 years, no consensus list of developmental toxicants/nondevelopmental toxicants that would form the basis for a validation effort, and little hope of seeing progress in the near future. With the exception of the chick embryo retinal cell assay, FETAX (the frog embryo assay), and whole embryo culture, little effort is being placed in using or developing and validating new in vitro systems. Some efforts to integrate the concepts behind the Chernoff/Kavlock assay into a comprehensive preliminary assessment of toxicity for existing chemicals in widespread commerce has been recently initiated by the OECD in its SIDS (Screening Information Data Set). Comprehensive assay results are not yet available to support any significant conclusions on the merits of that approach.

While much progress has not occurred in development of either alternate testing approaches for developmental toxicity or for a centralized database, results from the effort with mutagenesis assays have advanced considerably, partially the result of adoption by the IARC Monograph process for organizing such data. The size of the database now allows sophisticated inquiries on various aspects of biological activity to be made. For example, one approach has been to compare profiles of different chemicals against one another and generate similarity values for the extent of concordance and nonconcordance.[5] It is also possible to extract profiles of two chemicals and directly and quantitatively compare them.[6] Thus, it is quite easy to examine structure–activity relationships for chemicals and begin to develop confidence in the ability of one test to do well with agents of type A mechanisms, and of other tests to be more reliable for type B mechanisms, etc.

The next steps in this process are (1) to identify and rank order by level of concern a number of agents for use in validation assays, and to extract the relevant information into a computerized database (i.e., continue the effort initiated by the NTP), and (2) to establish a system or process by which the qualitative and quantitative nature of all test results are either retrospectively or prospectively added to a database such as the one proposed here. Without these steps, we are doomed to repeat the failures of the past, and probably to abandon the development of new assays as a impossible task. Clearly, for progress to made, we need a readily available consensus database on what constitutes accuracy, specificity, and overall predictiveness of a test system.

REFERENCES

1. Smith, M. K., Kimmel, G. L., Kochhar, D. M., Shepard, T. H., Spielberg, S. P., and Wilson, J. G. 1983. A selection of candidate compounds for in vitro teratogenesis test validation. *Teratogen. Carcinogen. Mutagen.* 3:461–480.
2. Garrett, N. E., Stack, H. F., Gross, M. R., and Waters, M. D. 1984. An analysis of the spectra of genetic activity produced by known or suspected human carcinogens. *Mutat. Res.* 168:301–325.
3. IARC. 1987. *IARC Monogr. Eval. Carcinogen. Risks Hum.: Genetic and Related Effects: An Update of Selected IARC Monographs from Vol. 1 to 42*, Suppl. 7. Lyon: International Agency for Research on Cancer.
4. Kavlock, R. J., Greene, J. A., Kimmel, G. L., Morrissey, R. E., Owens, E., Rogers, J. M., Sadler, T. W., Stack, H. F., Waters, M. D., and Welsch, F. 1991. Activity profiles of developmental toxicity: Design considerations and pilot implementation. *Teratology* 43:159–185.

5. Garrett, N. E., Stack, H. F., Jackson, M. A., and Waters, M. D. 1992. Genotoxic and carcinogenic potential of anticholinesterases. In *Clinical and experimental toxicology of organophosphates and carbamates*, eds. B. Ballantyne and T. C. Marrs, pp. 223–240. Oxford: Butterworth-Heinemann.
6. Lohman, P. H. M., Mendelsohn, M. L., Moore, D. H. II, Waters, M. D. Brusick, D. J., Ashby, J., and Lohman, W. J. A. 1992. A method for comparing and combining short-term genotoxicity test data: The basic system. *Mutat. Res.* 266:7–25.

Chapter Sixteen

SCREENING OF POPULATIONS OF WOMEN AT RISK FOR REPRODUCTIVE FAILURE USING CULTURED RODENT EMBRYOS

Norman W. Klein

The single most important issue in reproductive toxicology has been the need to identify human reproductive toxins and teratogens. We have attempted to use cultures of whole rat embryos to detect and to identify embryotoxins as well as nutrient deficiencies in sera from individuals who have experienced reproductive failures. Additionally, these embryo cultures have been used to understand the mechanisms of toxicity, which have provided the basis for treatment. Examples of an embryotoxic substance, autoantibodies to laminin, and the requirement for a specific nutrient for neural tube closure, methionine, have provided the basis for a comprehensive approach to the identification of human reproductive toxins and teratogens.

OBJECTIVES AND APPROACH

The objectives of this work have been to identify human reproductive toxins and through an understanding of their mechanism of toxicity to develop appropriate treatments. These objectives have been based on the fact that most causes of human reproductive failure have not been identified. For example, although birth defects occur at incidences of between 3% and 7% of all births, the Teratology Society usually estimates unknown etiologies as high as 80%. Similarly, although fetal losses (such as spontaneous abortions) during pregnancies have been found to be as high as 62% of all initiated pregnancies, again, causes have rarely been identified. Epidemiological approaches, although essential to confirm the identity of such toxins, have been too insensitive for the initial identifications of reproductive toxins. Animal studies, although essential to investigate mechanisms of toxicity, have not been useful to identify human reproductive toxins because of differences in sensitivities between humans and animals as well as between individuals.

Our approach has involved the use of whole rat embryo cultures starting with the head fold stage or after approximately 9.5 d of gestation. The procedure used follows that of D.A.T. New of Cambridge, U.K., including the isolation of embryos with intact yolk sac but Reichert's membrane removed.[1] Cultures last for 48 h, and a medium has been used consisting of blood sera obtained from immediately centrifuged whole blood, heat inactivated and filtered for sterility. Embryos have been then cultured in a hot room maintained at 37.5°C, in culture bottles rotated at 30 rpm and gassed with increasing amounts of oxygen during the course of the culture.

Several factors have contributed to the successful use of this whole embryo culture system.

This work has been supported over the years by the Storrs Agricultural Experiment Station and Research Foundation of the University of Connecticut. Additional funding have been provided by grants from the Department of Energy and more recently by NIEHS grant ESO4312. This is Scientific Contribution 3001 of the Storrs Agricultural Experiment Station.

For example, the stages of development used during the 48-h culture period corresponds to the most rapid phase of organogenesis (equivalent to wk 3–6 in women). Embryos have been cultured on 90% serum, making it possible to detect in embryo responses toxins present in relatively low concentrations. One additional critical factor has been the selection of a narrow range of developmental stages for experiments, as embryo sensitivities to all agents have been found to change dramatically with stage of development at initial exposure.

BACKGROUND AND VALIDATIONS

To demonstrate the feasibility of using whole rat embryo cultures to detect embryotoxic (embryo-lethal plus teratogenic) substances in blood sera, rats were injected with either cadmium chloride or cyclophosphamide and their blood sera were used as culture media for rat embryos taken from uninjected pregnant rats. Depending on dosage and time following the injections, reproducible embryo responses were obtained.[2] It should be noted that one of the originally selected substances, cadmium chloride, probably acted directly as a reproductive toxin while the other, cyclophosphamide, probably required metabolic activation to become the proximal reproductive toxin.

We then found that rat embryos could be cultured on human sera if given additional glucose (300 mg%) and that embryotoxins could be detected in the sera if taken from patients receiving either drugs for cancer chemotherapy or medication for epilepsy (anticonvulsant).[3] Both groups of substances have been recognized as human teratogens.

Next, we tried to compare the embryotoxicities of several of the most frequently used anticonvulsants by culturing embryos in serum samples from a rather large number of individuals (128) receiving monotherapy (single drug) for epilepsy.[4] (It should be noted that epilepsy has placed women in a high-risk group for reproductive problems including birth defects.) The results from the study, in general, agreed with the present practices of medicating women during pregnancy, but drug levels were not predictive of toxicities to cultured rat embryos, suggesting that drug metabolites were the proximal teratogens.

As various drugs, including the anticonvulsant phenytoin and the infamous morning sickness drug thalidomide, were found not to be toxic or teratogenic to rodents, we thought a useful approach for dealing with this species specificity could involve the dosing of monkeys with drugs of interest followed by the use of their sera as culture media for whole rat embryos. For this purpose we attempted to culture rat embryos on blood serum samples drawn from untreated monkeys in collaboration with the Primate Center of the University of California at Davis. Of 18 monkeys tested, sera from only two failed to support normal rat embryo development.[5] In checking the records it was found that the rat embryo cultures had detected the only monkeys in the group that had failed to reproduce successfully. A second group of monkeys with poor reproductive histories was found at the Primate Center of the University of Washington, Seattle under the direction of Dr. G. P. Sackett. In blind trials, sera from 86% of the poor reproducers ($n = 14$) failed to support normal rat embryo development, while this figure was only 33% ($n = 12$) for sera from good reproducers. These observations immediately changed the direction of our research as we felt that determining the basis for the embryo toxicity of these sera could be of potentially greater value to humanity than simply testing drugs.

THE IDENTIFICATION OF EMBRYOTOXIC FACTORS

For our first attempt to use whole embryo cultures to identify reproductive toxins in sera, we selected a group of monkeys whose sera remained embryotoxic after dialysis.[6] This suggested that a molecule(s) of over 5000 kD was the culprit. Using classical ammonium sulfate fractionation along with polyacrylamide gel electrophoresis, we detected a fraction that was highly embryotoxic when added to control rat serum. This fraction contained primarily immunoglobulin (IgG). To determine which of the numerous antigens were involved with the toxicity, we turned to indirect immunofluorescence and found that the antibody bound strongly to Reichert's membrane and other basement membranes in the embryo proper. We then collected Reichert's membranes, solubilized these acellular membranes, and used this material for Western blots. Reichert's membrane has been known to consist primarily of the extracellular matrix proteins: laminin, fibronectin, and type IV collagen, and in this case most of the antibody reactivity was directed at laminin.

To confirm the importance of this antibody, monkeys with excellent reproductive histories were immunized with pure laminin.[7] Subsequently, the sera from these monkeys became toxic to cultured rat embryos, and these monkeys became aborters and failed to reproduce successfully.

Recently, we have conducted studies on laminin epitope mapping, as it became apparent that having antibodies to laminin alone was insufficient to predict either sera toxicity to cultured rat embryos or reproductive outcomes. First, testing a series of laminin monoclonal antibodies in whole embryo cultures, some were found to be highly lethal, some caused embryo abnormalities, and still others were found to be nontoxic.[8] In a second approach, monkeys with excellent reproductive histories were immunized with four different synthetic laminin sequences: YIGSR, RGD, IKVAV, and a nonactive control sequence referred to as YD.[9] Of the four peptides, serum samples from the YIGSR-immunized monkey were the most consistently teratogenic to cultured rat embryos over the longest period of time, and the YIGSR-immunized monkey became an aborter. This sequence, YIGSR, has now been detected in the serum of some women at high reproductive risk such as women suffering from systemic lupus erythematosus.

In regard to mechanisms of toxicity we have observed that these autoantibodies to laminin bind exclusively on the surfaces of the endodermal cells of the rat visceral yolk sac. At this site, they caused disruption and breakdown of microvilli, which in turn reduced the uptake of nutrients by the yolk sac, limiting the availability of nutrients to the developing embryo. Clearly, these observations suggested that if such interference by antibodies could occur also at the levels of the human trophoblast cells, yolk sac, or placenta, the treatment of autoimmune diseases with regard to reproduction should involve dietary supplements with critical nutrients.

THE IDENTIFICATION OF NUTRIENT DEFICIENCIES

Although women suffering from epilepsy have been known to be at risk for reproductive problems including birth defects, the causes have not been identified. However, in general, the possible causes recognized have included the anticonvulsant drugs as well as their metabolites, the epilepsy itself, or nutritional problems, as many anticonvulsant drugs have been considered to be antimetabolites of such nutrients as folic acid. For this reason, in the large epilepsy study previously noted,[4] a mixture of water-soluble vitamins and essential amino acids was added to embryotoxic human sera and retested in whole embryo culture. Most striking and unpredicted was the observation that this supplement completely overcame the embryotoxicity of 60% of the 53 samples tested in this manner. In attempting to identify the nutrient or nutrients involved, groups of nutrients or individual nutrients were systematically omitted from the supplements. Some sera appeared to require vitamins, others amino acids, and still others required contributions from both groups of nutrients. Of particular interest, several serum samples required methionine alone, and this corresponded to reduced levels of free methionine in their serum.

Subsequently, we attempted to culture rat embryos on bovine sera for several reasons. For example, we were interested in finding a source of sera that was available at low cost and we had received several requests to study sera from herds of cows experiencing high rates of fetal loss (spontaneous abortions). When embryos were cultured on cow sera they developed abnormalities and, particularly, the developing neural tubes failed to close.[10] We tested several herds in Connecticut as well as herds in the states of New York, Pennsylvania, and California and the results were consistent: All caused neural tube defects. Next, we added the mixture of vitamins and amino acids previously used in the epilepsy study to the cow sera, and much to our surprise this nutrient supplement completely overcame the embryotoxicity of these cow sera. By systematically eliminating individual nutrients from the nutrient supplements, we determined that the only essential nutrient was the amino acid methionine. Cow sera were found to have extremely low levels of this amino acid, and the cultured rat embryos required this supplement only during the short period immediately preceding neural tube closure.

Subsequently, we observed that methylation of amino acids in the proteins of the neural tube was reduced providing one possible explanation for this requirement.[11] Further studies with methionine have shown that in addition to overcoming outright deficiencies as in cow sera, methionine could also reduce the toxicities of substances present in sera,[12,13] as well as a genetic defect in the mice responsible for neural tube defects.[14,15] Even more striking, preliminary trials have suggested that methionine as a dietary supplement could improve reproductive outcomes in women suffering from recurrent spontaneous abortions.[16]

The requirement for methionine appears to be involved at the level of the developing neural tube with specific protein methylation steps for closure. But, why does it appear that additional methionine is essential under a variety of conditions? This, we feel, could be caused by any factor restricting the general (nonspecific) flow of nutrients to the embryo. This has been particularly evident at the level of the rat embryo yolk sac in the studies with autoantibodies to laminin.[12] In this case, we feel that microvilli disruption caused the reduction in nutrient uptake and in turn reduction of nutrients reaching the embryo. Similarly, we believe that such autoantibodies could restrict nutrient passage across the trophoblast cells, the transient primate yolk sac, or the placenta. Thus, any substance that reduced nutrient passage to the embryo could respond favorably to methionine during the preneural tube closure stage.

AN OVERALL APPROACH TO IDENTIFY HUMAN REPRODUCTIVE TOXINS

Based on the observations described here we have been attempting to develop a logical sequence of steps using whole rat embryo cultures to identify reproductive toxins. However, it should be appreciated that simple techniques could be used to determine the presence of a reproductive toxin once the embryo cultures provide the initial identification. For example, we no longer need embryo cultures to identify antilaminin antibodies or anti-YIGSR antibodies in sera, as we now can use such simple inexpensive analytical techniques as enzyme-linked immunosorbent assay (ELISA).

The first step is to culture embryos directly on sera with only glucose as a supplement (Figure 1). If the serum is taken from an individual who had experienced reproductive failures and the serum supports normal rat embryo development, the analysis ends and one might only conclude that whatever the problem it is probably not a factor expressed in the blood serum. Next, if the serum is embryotoxic or teratogenic the mixture of vitamins and amino acids are added and the serum is retested in embryo cultures. If the serum is still teratogenic in the presence of these supplements, we assume that the serum contains a toxic agent and dialyze the serum for a short period (30 min) against Tyrode's solution. As dialysis might remove essential small nutrients as well as small toxic substances, retesting after dialysis in embryo cultures requires the addition

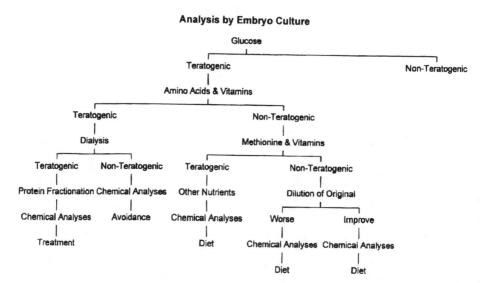

Figure 1. A comprehensive procedure for the identification of reproductive toxins and nutrient deficiencies in sera by whole rat embryo culture.

of the nutrient mix as well as glucose. If the embryotoxicity is reduced or eliminated by dialysis, we turn the serum over to an analytical laboratory for heavy metal analyses including lead, mercury, and cadmium. Returning back to the dialysis step, if dialysis does not reduce the embryotoxicity of the serum, we assume the toxicity is associated with a protein and based on past experience we usually proceed directly to the testing of the IgG serum fraction for embryotoxicity, and this may then lead to the identification of an autoimmune problem.

Returning back to a serum sample that responds favorably to nutrient supplements, one cannot conclude simply that this response indicates a nutrient deficiency. This is a special problem as nutrients such as methionine can overcome not only the embryotoxicity of a nutrient deficiency but also toxic substances (recall, autoantibodies and valproic acid). For this problem we developed a special approach based on the following rationale. If serum is embryotoxic and responds favorably to nutrients, for the next step we simply dilute the serum, from 90% (the usual level) to 70% or 80%, with Tyrode's salts and retest in embryo culture (without added nutrients). If following dilution of the serum the embryo responses are favorable (the embryos are closer to normal) we conclude that we have diluted out a "toxic substance." However, on the other hand, if this dilution leads to even greater embryotoxicity, we now conclude that we have diluted an essential nutrient that was present in only marginal amounts in the first place and conclude that we are dealing with a nutritional deficiency. Nevertheless, regarding potential treatment for the individual, it might not be relevant if the favorable nutrient response of the cultured embryo is related to a toxic substance or a metabolic disorder leading to a deficiency.

It should be noted that throughout the flow diagram (Figure 1), embryo findings are confirmed by chemical analyses of the sera. To date we have applied this approach to several situations. In brief, we have observed more embryotoxic IgG fractions than one might expect suggestive of rather extensive subclinical autoimmune diseases. Also, we have observed large numbers of individuals whose sera respond favorably to methionine supplements. This, we feel, is probably caused either by dietary deficiencies or alternatively by metabolic disorders. The dietary deficiency is of interest as we attempt to avoid studies of poverty (an economic problem of poor nutrition). This has suggested that middle-class American women may be avoiding favorable sources of methionine such as beef, fish, and poultry for a diet consisting mainly of vegetables. Finally, in addition to toxic IgGs and methionine, serum samples that improved by dialysis have shown on analyses, to contain elevated levels of lead.

REFERENCES

1. New, D. A. T., Coppola, P. T., and Cockroft, D. L. 1976. Comparison of growth *in vitro* and *in vivo* of postimplantation rat embryos. *J. Embryol. Exp. Morphol.* 36:133–144.
2. Klein, N. W., Vogler, M. A., Chatot, C. L., and Pierro, L. J. 1980. The use of cultured rat embryos to evaluate the teratogenic activity of serum: Cadmium and cyclophosphamide. *Teratology* 21:199–208.
3. Chatot, C. L., Klein, N. W. Piatek, J., and Pierro, L. J. 1980. Successful culture of rat embryos on human serum: Use in the detection of teratogens. *Science* 207:1471–1473.
4. Chatot, C. L., Klein, N. W., Clapper, M. L., Resor, S. R., Singer, W. D., Russman, B. S., Holmes, G. L., Mattson, R. H., and Cramer, J. A. 1984. Human serum teratogenicity studied by rat embryo culture: Epilepsy, anticonvulsant drugs and nutrition. *Epilepsia* 25:205–216.
5. Klein, N. W., Plenefisch, J. D., and Carey, S. W. 1982. Serum from monkeys with histories of fetal wastage causes abnormalities in cultured rat embryos. *Science* 215:66–69.
6. Carey, S. W., and Klein, N. W. 1989. Autoantibodies to laminin and other basement membrane proteins in sera from monkeys with histories of reproductive failure identified by cultures of whole rat embryos. *Fertil. Steril.* 51:711–718.
7. Weeks, B. S., Klein, N. W., Kleinman H., Fredrickson, T., and Sackett, G. P. 1989. Laminin immunized monkeys develop sera toxic to cultured rat embryos and fail to reproduce. *Teratology* 40:47–57.
8. Rasmussen, M. V., Klein, N. W., Abrahamson, D. R., and Chung, A. E. 1994. Effects of laminin monoclonal antibodies on the development of cultured rat embryos. *Teratology* 49:20–28.
9. Chambers. B. J., Klein, N. W., Conrad, S. H., Ruppenthal, G. C., Sackett, G. P., Weeks, B. S., and Kleinman, H. K. 1995. Reproduction and sera embryotoxicity following the immunization of monkeys with the laminin peptides YIGSR, RGD and IKVAV. *Proc. Nat. Acad. Sci. USA* 92:6818–6822.
10. Coelho, C. N. D., Weber, J. A., Klein, N. W., Daniels, W. G., and Hoagland, T. A. 1989. Whole rat embryos require methionine for neural tube closure when cultured on cow serum. *J. Nutr.* 119:1716–1725.
11. Coelho, C. N. D., and Klein, N. W. 1990. Methionine and neural tube closure in cultured rat embryos: Morphological and biochemical analyses. *Teratology* 42:437–451.

12. Chambers, B. J., Klein, N. W., Nosel, P. G., Khairallah, L., and Romanow, J. 1995. Methionine overcomes neural tube defects caused by antilaminin antibodies. *J. Nutr.* 125:1587–1599.

13. Nosel, P. G., and Klein, N. W. 1992. Methionine decreases the embryotoxicity of sodium valproate in the rat: *In vivo* and *in vitro* observations. *Teratology* 46:499–507.

14. Essien, F. B. 1992. Maternal methionine supplementation promotes the remediation of axial defects in Axd mouse neural tube mutants. *Teratology* 45:205–212.

15. Essien, F. B., and Wannberg, S. L. 1993. Methionine but not folinic acid or vitamin B-12 alters the frequency of neural tube defects in Axd mutant mice. *J. Nutr.* 123:27–34.

16. Ferrari, D. A., Gilles, P. A., Klein, N. W., Nadler, D., Weeks, B. S., Lammi-Keefe, C. J., Hillman, R. E., Carey, S. W., Ying, Y.-K., Maier, D., Olsen, P., Wemple, D. W., Greenstein, R., Meuchler, E. K., Miller, R. K., and Mariona, F. G. 1994. Rat embryo development on human sera in related to numbers of previous spontaneous abortions and nutritional factors. *Am. J. Obstet. Gynecol.* 170:228–236.

Chapter Seventeen

CONTINUED EVALUATION AND APPLICATION OF A BIOLUMINESCENT BACTERIAL GENOTOXICITY TEST

W.-D. Wang, T. S. C. Sun, and H. M. Stahr

The objective of genetic toxicology is to detect and understand the properties of agents that produce deleterious effects in genetic elements at subtoxic concentrations. Due to the high cost of animal testing and its long duration to see the effect of sublethal exposure, many short-term genetic toxicology assay systems have evolved, and some are proven with value and relevance for real genotoxic assessment such as the Ames test. Results of the Ames test on mutagenicity have shown 85–95% correlation with results of the animal carcinogenicity testing.

We investigated a new genotoxicity test, Mutatox, which has shown promise as a simple, sensitive, fast, and low-cost alternative test for chemical screening and risk assessment. This test utilizes a dark mutant of Vibrio fischeri *that exhibits light production when grown in the presence of sublethal concentrations of genotoxic agents. Our data and other published results have indeed shown that many known direct mutagen agents (either base substitution or frameshift), DNA-damaging agents, DNA intercalatory agents, and DNA synthesis inhibitors can restore the light production of the bacterial dark mutant. Mutagenicity testing results correlate well with that of the Ames test. Comparing to the Ames test, the Mutatox genotoxicity test is not affected by the presence of amino acid or other nutrients. Therefore, it is possible to assay complex organic matter such as food/feed and biological fluids. This chapter shows results of genotoxicity test on some known chemicals, and discusses results of some complex sample matrices such as cooking oil, poultry, sausage, and vegetable processing water, and feed additives (antioxidant) for their potential genotoxicity. We show not only that the total genotoxicity of sample matrices can be evaluated; it is also possible to isolate genotoxic substances into aqueous, alcohol, methylene chloride fractions to further test and identify the chemicals.*

INTRODUCTION AND OVERVIEW

There is an urgent need for techniques to be used in monitoring chemical genotoxicity. Our environment contains a vast variety of agents that are detrimental to human health. Agents that are acutely toxic are readily detected because the immediate effects allow rapid identification of the source of toxicity. Mutation or tumors are not the immediate result of an exposure to mutagenic or carcinogenic agent. The latent period for tumor induction in humans may be as long as 20 years. A source of mutagenic or carcinogenic activity may only be detected after many persons have been exposed for many years.

Correlation between mutagenicity and carcinogenicity has become apparent since the first

Support from a USDA/CSRS special grant made to the Food Safety Consortium is recognized.

published list of carcinogenic mutagens by Ames and colleagues.[1] Mutation assays are shorter and much less costly than classical carcinogenicity tests. Comparing with analytical chemistry tests, a biological test can be used on samples of complex mixture with minimal fractionation. Therefore biological mutation assays are indispensable tools in complex environmental and food monitoring.

There are two major requirements in mutagenicity testing. One is comparatively simple. Mutagenicity testing is necessary for any chemical that is newly introduced into our environment as a pesticide, preservative, drug, food additive, or for any other use that could lead to exposure of humans to it. The other is that changes detected be genetically defined and, above all, not mimicked by effects unrelated to genotypic change. Most mutation tests are based on the detection of phenotypic changes, such as the Ames test. Very few are designed to detect directly changes of chromosome structure or chemical-physical alterations in DNA.

MECHANISM AND THEORY OF MUTATOX* TEST

The Mutatox test applies a dark mutant (strain M/1/69) of *Vibrio fischeri* that exhibits light production when grown in the presence of genotoxic agents. It is understood that light production by luminous marine bacteria is catalyzed by the enzyme luciferase, whose gene expression is normally repressed until such conditions as starvation, heat shock, or the presence of toxic substances occur. A small sensory molecule, called an autoinducer, is synthesized by the bacteria. The autoinducer grows exponentially once luciferase is activated. The activation of luciferase synthesis is believed to occur at levels of DNA transcription.[2] The genetic mechanisms that regulate expression of genes for luminescence have been postulated by Engebrecht et al.[3] and Ulitzur et al.[4] as shown in Figure 1.

It is postulated that the autoinduction process is a multi-endpoint process. The accumulation of autoinducer in the bacteria, the enhanced affinity of Lex-A protein to its DNA binding site, and the induction of the htpR σ32 gene can all advance the onset of luminescence in the bacteria.

EXPERIMENT PROCEDURES AND RESULT DISCUSSION

The dark mutant bacteria is provided by Microbics (Carlsbad, CA) in lyophilized form. Rehydrate the bacteria medium (direct or S9 activated) with double deionized water and add serially diluted samples or positive controls to each 1 ml of rehydrated bacteria medium for testing. The photometer used for the bioluminescence determination in the Mutatox test is the Tri-Carb model 1600 liquid scintillation spectrometer (Packard Instrument Co., Downer's Grove, IL). Prepared samples are measured for light intensity immediately for a continuous 24-h period at every 1-h interval. If the maximal luminescence value reached at any time during a test is higher than three times that of a negative control, the test is designated as positive. Duplicate or triplicate samples are run in each Mutatox test to ensure reliability of results. Either proflavine (a known DNA intercalating agent) or N-methyl-N'-nitro-nitrosoguanidine (MNNG, a known carcinogen) is used as a positive control for direct assay, and benzo[a]pyrene (a known carcinogen) or aflatoxin B1 (a known carcinogen) for S9 assay. A typical positive response curve in shown in Figure 2.

The exponentially increasing mutation rate of the dark mutant can be observed clearly in Figure 3, where logarithmic transformation converts the light intensity curve (Figure 2) into a linear curve. The Mutatox test can also be used for quantitative dose-response relationship study. Figure 4 shows results of 2 positive control samples at 0.5 μg and 2.0 μg. The higher dose yields about twice as high light intensity. This dose response only holds within a certain concentration range for all chemicals or complex sample matrices we tested. Concentrations above the upper limit seem to completely inhibit the light production. Figure 5 shows Mutatox test results of several pure natural mycotoxins. Note that the luminescence starts at different time. Also, the maximal luminescence of different chemicals varies substantially. Precision and reliability of the test can be observed in Figure 6, where duplicate measurements are shown to yield a reasonably consistent readings. Other results presented here are an average of replicate readings

---

* Patented product of Microbics, Inc., Carlsbad, CA.

THE REGULATORY CONTROL OF
V. fischeri LUX SYSTEM

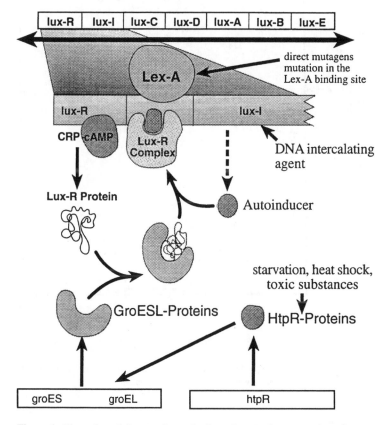

Figure 1. Illustration of the genetic mechanisms that regulate expression of genes for luminescence.

at any time. Table 1 shows the Mutatox test results of several heterocyclic amines such as MeIQ, Trp-p-1, and Trp-p-2. All three responded negatively for direct assay and positively for the S9 assay. It is known that heterocyclic amines are not themselves mutagenic to *Salmonella typhimurium* strains, but only exert mutagenic activity in the presence of S9 fraction.[5] Our study further confirmed the necessity of the S9 fraction activation system for heterocyclic amines to exhibit genotoxicity in the Mutatox test.

Results of Autoxidized Fatty Acids, Chlorinated Fatty Acids, and Heated Cooking Oil

It is known that fatty acid autoxidation products, fatty acid hydroperoxides, are very toxic to animals. Some studies have demonstrated that various hydroperoxides can initiate free radical oxidation of carcinogens to the ultimate active form. Highly oxidized fats that contain high concentrations of C_{20}–C_{22} polyunsaturated fatty acids are reported to cause injurious effects to animals. Cholesterol autoxidation products are also reported to be toxic. Therefore there are considerable concerns over the mutagenic potential of continually reused frying fats in the fast-food and ready-to-eat meal preparation. The experiment protocol used was bubbling of air

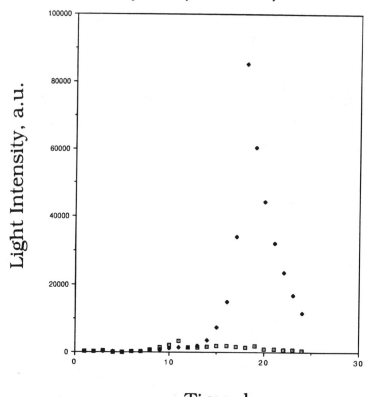

Figure 2. A typical light production curve. Shown here are responses of a blank control and 0.5 μg proflavin were added to the dark mutant.

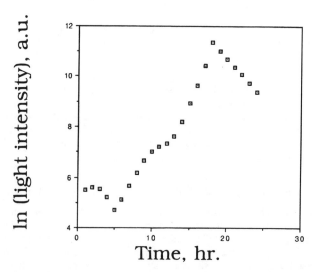

Figure 3. Logarithmic transformation of light intensity of Figure 2 results in a nearly linear curve.

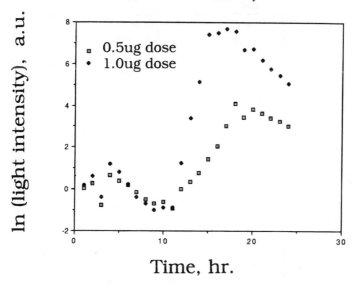

Figure 4. For 0.5-μg and 1.0-μg doses of 3,6-diaminoacridine, the latter shows about twice the intensity of the former. Original light intensity values are mathematically treated by taking logarithmics and subtracting that of the blank control.

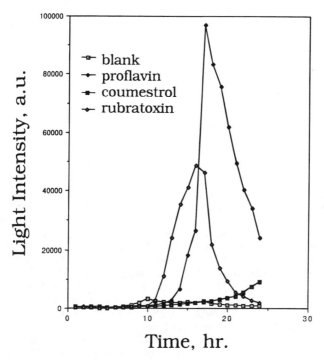

Figure 5. Measured light intensity of several pure mycotoxins. Note the variation in maximal luminescence and onset of luminescence.

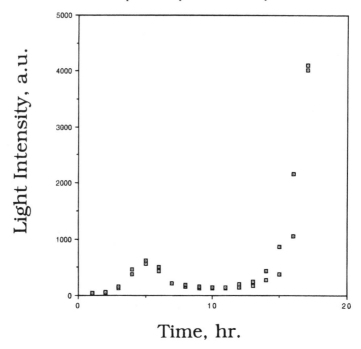

Figure 6. Shows reliability and reproducibility of the test, where replica readings are fairly consistent.

Table 1. Genotoxicity of Some Heterocyclic Amines

Chemical	Direct assay	S9 assay	Concentration range for positive response (μg/ml media)	Toxic concentration (μg/ml media)
MeIQ	−	+	0.5–10.0	30
Trp-p-1	−	+	0.5–7.5	40
Trp-p-2	−	+	0.5–7.5	40

through the fatty acids esters methyl linoleate and linolenate in a water bath at 37–40°C for 72 and 144 h. Then the autoxidized products are resolved into five fractions in increased polarity order: diethyl ether/hexane, 1:9, 2:8, 3:7, 5:5, and 7:3. Four different chlorinated fatty acids that were identified in food sources were tested. Heated cooking oil and cooking oil with 1% pure cholesterol addition were heated at 180–190°C for 8 h each day for 5 consecutive days. Aliquots of each sample were taken at the end of each day. Results are presented in Tables 2–6.

The fatty acids esters and fatty acids tested were nongenotoxic. Chlorinated fatty acids from spices were analyzed. The esters of capric, lauric, palmitic, and linoleic acids were identified at levels up to 1400 ppm. They are all negative in direct assay and positive in S9 assay. Cooking oil after repeated heating starts to show positive effect at d 4. The genotoxic response of cooking oil after repeated heating is attributed to possible heterocyclic amines or other pyrolysis breakdown products of fatty acids. It can be concluded that overused and abused oils undoubtedly contain oxidized materials that, if chronically consumed, could pose a human health risk. Cooking oil with 1% cholesterol addition provokes a higher genotoxicity effect with the same repeated heating process.

Table 2. Genotoxicity of Autoxidized Products of Methyl Linoleate

Chemical	Direct assay	S9 assay	Concentration range used (μg/ml media)	Toxic concentration (μg/ml media)
Whole autoxidized fatty acid	−	−	0.001–50	15
Pure fatty acid	−	−	0.001–50	N.D.[a]
Fraction 1	−	−	0.001–50	N.D.
Fraction 2	−	−	0.001–50	15
Fraction 3	−	−	0.001–50	10
Fraction 4	−	−	0.001–50	10
Fraction 5	−	−	0.001–50	10

[a] N.D., not determined within the concentration range used.

Table 3. Genotoxicity of Autoxidized Products of Methyl Linolenate

Chemical	Direct assay	S9 assay	Concentration range used (μg/ml media)	Toxic concentration (μg/ml media)
Whole autoxidized fatty acid	−	−	0.001–50	15
Pure fatty acid	−	−	0.001–50	N.D.[a]
Fraction 1	−	−	0.001–50	N.D.
Fraction 2	−	−	0.001–50	15
Fraction 3	−	−	0.001–50	10
Fraction 4	−	−	0.001–50	10
Fraction 5	−	−	0.001–50	10

[a] N.D., not determined within the concentration range used.

Table 4. Genotoxicity of Chlorinated Fatty Acids

Chemical	Direct assay	S9 assay	Concentration range for positive response (μg/ml media)	Toxic concentration (μg/ml media)
2-chloroethyl caprate	−	+	10–100	150
2-chloroethyl laurate	−	+	10–100	150
2-chloroethyl palmitate	−	+	10–100	150
2-chloroethyl linoleate	−	+	10–100	150

Table 5. Genotoxicity of Heated Cooking Oil

Days of heating	Direct assay	S9 assay	Concentration range used (μg/ml media)	Toxic concentration (μg/ml media)
0	−	−	0.01–150	N.D.[a]
1	−	−	0.01–150	N.D.
2	−	−	0.01–150	N.D.
3	−	−	0.01–150	120
4	+	+	0.01–150 (1–75)[b]	100
5	+	+	0.01–150 (1–75)[c]	100

[a] N.D., not determined within the concentration range used.
[b,c] The concentration range responded positive.

Table 6. Genotoxicity of Heated Cooking Oil with Addition of 1% Cholesterol

Days of heating	Direct assay	S9 assay	Concentration range used (μg/ml media)	Toxic concentration (μg/ml media)
0	−	−	0.01–150	N.D.[a]
1	−	−	0.01–150	N.D.
2	+	+	0.01–150 (0.5–40)[b]	100
3	+	+	0.01–150 (0.5–40)[c]	75
4	+	+	0.01–150 (0.5–40)[d]	75
5	+	+	0.01–150 (0.5–40)[e]	75

[a] N.D., not determined within the concentration range used.
[b=e] The concentration range responded positive.

Table 7. Genotoxicity of Methanol Extraction of Onion

Compound	Direct assay	S9 assay
Quercetin standard	−	+
Lower band	−	+

Results of Poultry and Sausage Processing Water and Ozonated Vegetable

Poultry processing water is recycled after ozonation. Water samples collected over several days from a poultry processing plant at every operation stage were tested for mutagens. Negative responses were obtained for all samples. Chlorinated (400 ppm) chiller water, on the other hand, was highly positive in the Mutatox test. Chloroform/methanol extraction and gas-liquid chromatography (GLC) analysis show that chlorinated fatty acids were present, which were previously tested in our laboratory as positive for genotoxicity.

Sausage processing waters were treated with ultraviolet (UV) light for sanitation purposes and tested for mutagens in comparison with control brine water. We incidentally discovered that NaCl can interfere with the Mutatox test result when we directly put the control brine and used processing water in a run. A higher light response is obtained from control brine, which contains 9% NaCl, while used processing water contains 24% NaCl. After water samples are extracted with methylene chloride, residues in the organic phase yield positive response from used processing water and negative from control brine as shown in Figure 7. Different concentrations of NaCl solution were run with the Mutatox test. Results are shown in Figure 8, where a concentration of 10–15% yields maximal luminescence. It is not clear why the electrolyte yields this false mutagenic response. The genotoxicity of sausage processing water could be attributed to aflatoxin, which is reported to be present in smoked meat products. The genotoxicity test of methanol extract of onion was conducted. Results indicated that quercetin and another substance (lower band), which was extracted from onion was positive for genotoxic (Table 7).

Vegetables (potato, carrot) were treated in ozonated water and ozonated atmosphere for sanitation and storage purposes, respectively. Vegetables were dipped in ozonated water momentarily, then extracted with water and methanol to test for possible mutagens generated by this ozonation process. The result was negative. Long-term storage of vegetables in a controlled ozonated atmosphere did not yield positive response.

Results of Feed Additives (Antioxidant)

Unknown compositions of some feed additives (as antioxidant) were tested for comparing relative levels of genotoxicity. The luminescence levels were all about the same except one was consistently higher than the rest, but it was less than twice of the blank, that is not positive, for mutagenicity. From work conducted in our laboratory on various subjects, we conclude that the Mutatox genotoxicity test combined with analytical chemistry can be a simple, rapid, and cost-effective tool in identifying toxicity sources in not only pure chemicals but also complex environmental and food sample matrices. Results from the Mutatox test on hundreds of chemicals correlate well with those of the Ames test.[6]

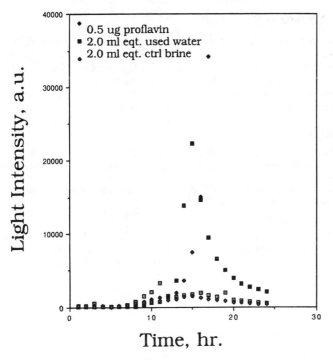

Figure 7. Results of sausage processing water. Shown here are responses of positive control, MeCl$_2$ extracts of used and control brine water.

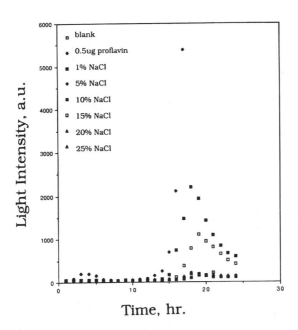

Figure 8. Results of NaCl solution. Tested at NaCl concentration 1%, 5%, 10%, 15%, 20%, and 25%.

FURTHER RESEARCH NEEDED

Continued genotoxicity test on more known carcinogenic mutagens is needed. A large database of Mutatox test results is needed for the validation of the test. Also, for every unknown sample tested positive, more analytical chemistry study needs to be done. That includes isolation of toxic substances and structure elucidation. The fact that the Mutatox positive samples indeed show the presence of some known or new genotoxic chemicals will be the best support for this validation process. Study of the ozone-treated onion is an example.

REFERENCES

1. Ames, B. N., Durston, W. E., Yamasaki, E., and Lee, F. D. 1973. Carcinogens are mutagens: A single test system combining liver homogenates for activation and bacteria for detection. *Proc. Natl. Acad. Sci. USA* 70:2281.
2. Nealson, K. H., Platt, T., and Hastings, J. W. 1970. Cellular control of the synthesis and activity of the bacteria luminescent system. *J. Bacteriol.* 104:313.
3. Engebrecht, J., Nealson, K., and Silverman, M. 1983. Bacterial bioluminescence: Isolation and genetic analysis of functions from Vibrio fischeri marine bacterium. *Cell* 32:773.
4. Adar, Y. Y., Simaan, M., and Ulitzur, S. 1992. Formation of the Lux R protein in the Vibrio fischeri Lux system is controlled by HtpR through the GroESL proteins. *J. Bacteriol.* 174:7138.
5. Sugimura, T., Sato, S., Ohgaki, H., Takayama, S., Nagao, M., and Wakabayashi, K. 1986. In *Genetic toxicology of the diet, 1,* ed. I. Knudsen, pp. 85–107. New York: A. R. Liss.
6. Document of Microbics, Inc. 1993. Mutatox test data for prechemicals. Carlsbad, CA: Author.

PART III

IMMUNOTOXICITY

Chapter Eighteen

CYTOKINE GENE EXPRESSION AND ALLERGIC CONTACT DERMATITIS

Craig A. Elmets

Current methods of screening for potential contact allergens in the premarketing evaluation of new products require testing procedures that employ significant numbers of animals. Efforts from this laboratory have been directed at obtaining a greater understanding of the role that cytokines play in allergic contact dermatitis and at using that information to devise a sensitive in vitro assay to predict the allergenicity of new products and chemicals that may come in contact with the skin. Using urushiol as a prototype, we found, using in situ hybridization techniques, contact allergens augmented steady-state levels of such epidermal cytokine genes as interleukin 1α (IL-1α), IL-1β, and tumor necrosis factor α (TNF-α) in vivo. These changes were present in the skin of allergic patients but did not occur in nonallergic individuals. Moreover, when the RNA of cultured keratinocytes from nonallergic and allergic donors treated with urushiol were compared using the technique of semiquantitative reverse transcriptase PCR, similar disparities in cytokine gene expression were observed. Differences in cytokine gene expression were present both for IL-1α and IL-1β and IL-6 and IL-8. These observations provide evidence of changes in cytokine gene expression in cultured epidermal cells following exposure to new compounds in vitro and may form the basis for a predictive assay that could supplant animal testing for the detection of contact allergens.

Allergic contact hypersensitivity is a common human experience that is responsible for considerable morbidity. In the United States, skin disorders account for 40% of all reported occupationally related diseases,[1] and allergic contact dermatitis is responsible for a significant percentage of those. It is also a major problem in industry since it represents a major impediment to the development of new cosmetics, personal hygiene products, and topical medications. Until recently, the toxicological evaluation of new products introduced into the marketplace has included extensive testing in animals. The use of animals for this purpose, however, is less than ideal for a number of reasons. First, there are marked species differences between humans and the various species of rodents used to test for potential contact sensitizing compounds. Second, animals are expensive. Finally, the use of animals in product testing raises ethical issues that could be avoided if an in vitro alternative could be developed.

The conceptual framework for any in vitro assay that might serve as an alternative to animal testing for screening potential contact allergens will inevitably depend on the new knowledge that has been generated about the pathophysiology of the skin disorder it causes. Allergic contact dermatitis is a cutaneous T-lymphocyte-mediated response to topically applied small molecules. The skin is an active participant in the response. Epicutaneous application of hapten results in

This work was supported by the Avon Program Project of the Johns Hopkins Center for the Alternatives to Animal Testing.

avid binding to protein and cell membrane carriers within the epidermis. The complete antigen that is formed by this conjugation reaction is taken up by epidermal Langerhans cells,[3,4] which process it and display it on the cell surface in association with class I and II major histocompatibility complex determinants.[3,5-7] Langerhans cells (LC) present haptens, within the regional lymph nodes, to clones of T cells that bear T cell receptors for antigen. Once this has transpired, T cells proliferate and differentiate and return to the site of hapten application, where they are responsible for creating an inflammatory response that is recognized clinically as allergic contact dermatitis.

Keratinocytes, the predominant epidermal cell type, are also believed to contribute to the immunopathogenesis of allergic contact dermatitis by synthesizing and secreting a variety of soluble polypeptide cytokines, some of which promote the inflammatory response, and others of which confine that same process.[8] In so doing, it is widely believed that keratinocytes play a key role in controlling the overall magnitude of such reactions. Keratinocytes produce many cytokines.[9-13] Included among these are the multifunctional cytokines interleukin-1α (IL-1α)[14] and IL-1β,[14] IL-6,[15-17] and tumor necrosis factor α (TNF-α)[18,19] the chemokine IL-8,[20] and the colony-stimulating factor GM-CSF.[21]

IL-1α and IL-1β are 17-kD polypeptides in their secreted forms and are the products of two distinct genes.[22] Normal and transformed cultured keratinocytes synthesize both IL-1α and IL-1β. Langerhans cells produce IL-1β when stimulated with PMA or LPS.[24] Biologically active IL-1 has been detected in normal human epidermis,[25,26] indicating production of this cytokine in situ as well. Functionally, IL-1 appears to be a mediator of the acute-phase response;[27,28] a necessary cofactor in the process of antigen presentation to T cells by LC[10,29] and macrophages;[30] a possible chemotactic factor for T cells;[31] and an inducer of the production of other cytokines such as IL-8[20] and GM-CSF[21] from keratinocytes and IL-6[32] and IL-8[20] from fibroblasts. Lastly, IL-1 has been shown to mediate LC differentiation in culture.[5,33]

IL-6 is a multifunctional cytokine produced by many cell types.[15-17,34] At least six different IL-6 polypeptides have been detected that range in size from 19 to 70 kD.[35] These proteins are all the product of a single polymorphic gene.[36] Size differences appear to be due to differential phosphorylation, glycosylation, or sulfation.[35] IL-6 is a mediator of the acute-phase response; can stimulate B- and T-cell growth; and is a thymocyte, T-cell, B-cell, and macrophage activator. Keratinocytes are among the cell types that produce IL-6.[15-17] IL-6 and its mRNA have been observed to be elevated in psoriatic skin sections, and IL-6 was shown to be a growth factor for cultured keratinocytes.[37] It has been shown that IL-1 and TNF-α are potent inducers of IL-6 mRNA in cultured fibroblasts.[32]

IL-8 is a member of the chemokine family of cytokines. It is an 8-kD heparin-binding basic polypeptide that acts as a chemotactic factor for T cells.[38] This cytokine also is a chemotactic and activating factor for neutrophils.[38-40] IL-8 mRNA can be induced in cultured keratinocytes in response to IL-1α, but in contrast to fibroblasts, no effect was seen upon administration of TNF-α.[20]

TNF-α is a multimeric polypeptide whose subunits have a relative M_w of 17 kD.[41-48] It was originally detected as a macrophage product that is biologically inactive until cleaved at several sites.[45-47] Aside from its cytostatic and cytolytic effects on tumor cell lines,[48] TNF-α stimulates prostaglandin E$_2$ (PGE$_2$) release;[49-51] production of IL-1 and IL-6,[49,51] expression of MHC class I and II antigens on fibroblasts;[52] and the activity of cytotoxic T lymphocytes.[53-55] Immunoreactive TNF-α and TNF-α mRNA have been detected in epidermal cells and epidermoid cell lines.[18,19] TNF-α maintains the viability of cultured epidermal LC[33] and stimulates IL-6[32] and IL-8[20] secretion by fibroblasts. Lastly, TNF-α can downregulate the induction of contact hypersensitivity responses in mice.[56]

Efforts in my laboratory to develop an assay that might serve as an in vitro alternative to animal testing have focused on individual differences in cutaneous cytokine mRNA expression following contact with allergenic compounds. For this purpose, urushiol, the active moiety in poison ivy/oak, has been employed as a prototypic contact allergen and the cytokines IL-1α, IL-1β, IL-6, IL-8, GM-CSF, and TNF-α have been examined as cytokines whose synthesis is likely to be altered following urushiol exposure.

IN SITU DETECTION OF CYTOKINE mRNA IN NORMAL HUMAN SKIN

Initial studies were conducted to identify the sites of IL-1α, IL-1β, and TNF-α mRNA synthesis in normal human skin. The method of in situ hybridization was used for this purpose. IL-1α, IL-1β, and TNF-α messenger RNAs were detected at multiple sites including the epidermis, hair follicles, sebaceous glands, the dermal microvasculature, and arrectores pilorum smooth muscle. Within the epidermis, transcripts for the cytokines were localized primarily within the granular and basal layers. IL-1α, IL-1β, and TNF-α mRNAs were also present in normal human eccrine sweat glands and in secretory coil epithelium.[57,58] The conclusion from these experiments was that there are multiple sites of cytokine mRNA expression within the skin in situ, including the epidermis.

UPREGULATION OF CYTOKINE mRNAS IN HUMAN SKIN TREATED WITH URUSHIOL

Based on the findings in normal skin, six subjects allergic to urushiol were biopsied prior to and at various times after patch testing with urushiol (poison ivy).[59] In all six subjects, significant elevations of IL-1β mRNA were detected as early as 6 h after urushiol application. This was at a time prior to clinical or histological evidence of a contact allergic reaction. IL-1β mRNA had returned to background levels by 72 h even though a vigorous inflammatory reaction was present at that time. Elevation of IL-1α and TNF-α mRNAs was not present until 24 h after urushiol application, coincident with clinical and histological evidence of contact dermatitis. Levels of IL-1α and TNF-α mRNAs continued to rise in epidermis for at least the next 48 h. In subjects in whom no clinical or histological evidence of reactivity to urushiol was present, no elevation in cytokine mRNAs was observed, indicating that the changes in cytokine mRNAs correlated well with the contact allergic reaction.

The results provide evidence for differential temporal regulation of epidermal cytokine mRNAs following exposure to contact allergens and implicate them in the pathogenesis of this disorder. They also indicate that in vivo there is a close correlation between the status of individuals to become sensitized to urushiol and the level of IL-1α, IL-1β, and TNF-α mRNAs the produce following in vivo exposure to that contact allergen.

CYTOKINE RNA PROFILES IN CULTURED KERATINOCYTES EXPOSED TO POISON IVY IN VITRO

In order to further examine the hypothesis that differences in cytokine levels could be used to distinguish between subjects who were allergic and were not allergic to a particular compound and to begin to develop an in vitro system with which to assess the potential of compounds to elicit a contact hypersensitivity response, further studies were conducted to address the following issues. First, does urushiol increase the transcription of other epidermal cytokine mRNAs besides IL-1α, IL-1β, and TNF-α? Second, can the upregulation of cytokine mRNAs by urushiol be detected in cultured keratinocytes?

This was accomplished by examining the kinetics and magnitude of the expression of IL-1α, IL-1β, IL-6, IL-8, and GM-CSF mRNAs in cultures of normal human keratinocytes was examined following exposure to 5 mM extracts of urushiol. At various intervals between 2 and 24 h, RNA was extracted and was analyzed for cytokine mRNA expression using semiquantitative reverse transcriptase PCR. Cytokine signal strength was normalized to that of hypoxanthine guanine phosphoribosyl transferase (HGPRT), which was not upregulated following urushiol exposure. All cytokines examined were constitutively expressed in cultured keratinocytes.[60] Following exposure to urushiol a modest increase in the expression of IL-1α and IL-1β mRNAs was observed; a much greater increase in IL-6 and IL-8 mRNAs was present and the maximum increase tended to occur at a later time point than that of IL-1α and IL-1β mRNAs. GM-CSF was not upregulated following urushiol exposure. The findings indicate that cytokine mRNAs are upregulated in urushiol-exposed keratinocytes that have been cultured in vitro.

Finally, cytokine mRNA expression in keratinocyte cultures from donors who were allergic to urushiol and from donors who were not allergic to urushiol was compared following exposure to that allergen. Cytokines were only upregulated in keratinocyte cultures derived from allergic donors and not from keratinocyte cultures from nonallergic subjects. This parallels what was observed in the in situ hybridization studies when skin was sensitized to urushiol in vivo.

This model may therefore be useful in further development of an in vitro correlate of the in vivo contact dermatitis response.

SUMMARY

As assessment of contact allergy is an essential component of the premarketing evaluation of new household products, soaps and cosmetics. Traditionally, in vivo assays using various species of animals have been employed for this purpose. The pain and distress that animals undergo during safety evaluation for cutaneous allergy represents a serious disadvantage to this type of testing procedure. In other biomedical disciplines, the use of animal models has largely been supplanted by in vitro assays that are at least as sensitive and as predictive as the in vivo assays. Experimentation from this laboratory using urushiol as a prototypic agent indicates that evaluation of cytokine mRNA profiles in cultured skin cells or their equivalents has the potential to supplant these in vivo assays that utilize animals.

REFERENCES

1. Tucker, S. B. 1988. Prevention of occupational skin disease. *Dermatol. Clin.* 6:87–96.
2. Shelley, W. B., and Juhlin, L. 1976. Langerhans cells form a reticuloepithelial trap for external contact antigens. *Nature* 261:46–47.
3. Cruickshank, C. N. D., and Cooper, J. R. 1975. Langerhans cells in tissue cultures of guinea-pig epidermal cells. *Br. J. Dermatol.* 92:121–130.
4. Silberberg-Sinakin, I., Thorbecke, G. J., Baer, R. L., Rosenthal, S. A., and Berezowsky, V. 1985. Antigen-bearing Langerhans cells in skin, dermal lymphatics and in lymph nodes. *Cell. Immunol.* 25:137–151.
5. Schuler, G., and Steinman, R. M. 1985. Murine epidermal Langerhans cells mature into potent immuno-stimulatory dendritic cells *in vitro*. *J. Exp. Med.* 161:526–546.
6. Sullivan, S., Bergstresser, P. R., Tigelaar, R. E., and Streilein, J. W. 1986. Induction and regulation of contact hypersensitivity by resident, bone marrow-derived, dendritic epidermal cells: Langerhans cells and Thy-1⁺ epidermal cells. *J. Immunol.* 137:2460–2467.
7. Volc-Platzer, B., Majdic, O., Knapp, W., Wolff, K., Hinterberger, W., Lechner, K., and Stingl, G. 1984. Evidence of HLA-DR antigen biosynthesis by human keratinocytes in disease. *J. Exp. Med.* 159:1784–1789.
8. Kupper, T. S. 1990. The activated keratinocyte: A model for inducible cytokine production by non-bone marrow-derived cells in cutaneous inflammatory and immune responses. *J. Invest. Dermatol.* 94:146S–150S.
9. Barker, J. N. 1992. Role of keratinocytes in allergic contact dermatitis. *Contact Dermatitis* 26:145–148.
10. Sauder, D. N., Carter, C., Katz, S. I., and Oppenheim, J. J. 1982. Epidermal cell production of thymocyte activating factor (ETAF). *J. Invest. Dermatol.* 79:34–38.
11. Luger, T. A., Stadler, B. M., Katz, S. I., and Oppenheim, J. J. 1981. Epidermal cell (keratinocyte)-derived thymocyte-activating factor (ETAF). *J. Immunol.* 127:1493–1498.
12. Enk, A. H., and Katz, S. I. 1992. Early molecular events in the induction phase of contact sensitivity. *Proc. Natl. Acad. Sci. USA* 89:1398–1402.
13. Enk, A. H., Angeloni, V. L., Udey, M. C., and Katz, S. I. 1993. Inhibition of Langerhans cell antigen-presenting function by IL-10. A role for IL-10 in induction of tolerance. *J. Immunol.* 151:2390–2398.
14. Kupper, T. S., Ballard, D. W., Chua, A. O., McGuire, J. S., Flood, P. M., Horowitz, M. C., Langdon, R., Lightfoot, L., and Gubler, U. 1986. Human keratinocytes contain mRNA indistinguishable from monocyte interleukin 1 alpha and beta mRNA. Keratinocyte epidermal cell-derived thymocyte-activating factor is identical to interleukin 1. *J. Exp. Med.* 164:2095–2100.
15. Kirnbauer, R., Kock, A., Schwarz, T., Urbanski, A., Krutmann, J., Borth, W., Damm, D., Shipley, G., Ansel, J. C., and Luger, T. A. 1989. IFN-beta 2, B cell differentiation factor 2, or hybridoma growth factor (IL-6) is expressed and released by human epidermal cells and epidermoid carcinoma cell lines. *J. Immunol.* 142:1922–1928.
16. Kupper, T. S., Min, K., Sehgal, P., Mizutani, H., Birchall, N., Ray, A. and May, L. 1989. Production of IL-6 by keratinocytes. Implications for epidermal inflammation and immunity. *Ann. NY Acad. Sci.* 557:454–465.
17. Luger, T. A., Schwarz, T., Krutmann, J., Kirnbauer, R., Neuner, P., Kock, A., Urbanski, A., Borth, W., and Schauer, E. 1989. Interleukin-6 is produced by epidermal cells and plays an important role in the activation of human T-lymphocytes and natural killer cells. *Ann. NY Acad. Sci.* 557:405–414.

18. Oxholm, A., Oxholm, P., Staberg, B., and Bendtzen, K. 1988. Immunohistological detection of interleukin I-like molecules and tumour necrosis factor in human epidermis before and after UVB-irradiation in vivo. *Br. J. Dermatol.* 118:369–376.

19. Kock, A., Schwarz, T., Kirnbauer, R., Urbanski, A., Perry, P., Ansel, J. C., and Luger, T. A. 1990. Human keratinocytes are a source for tumor necrosis factor alpha: Evidence for synthesis and release upon stimulation with enditoxin or ultraviolet light. *J. Exp. Med.* 172:1609–1614.

20. Larsen, C. G., Anderson, A. O., Oppenheim, J. J., and Matsushima, K. 1989. Production of interleukin-8 by human dermal fibroblasts and keratinocytes in response to interleukin-1 or tumour necrosis factor. *Immunology* 68:31–36.

21. Kupper, T. S., Lee, F., Coleman, D., Chodakewitz, J., Flood, P., and Horowitz, M. 1988. Keratinocyte derived T-cell growth factor (KTGF) is identical to granulocyte macrophage colony stimulating factor (GM-CSF). *J. Invest. Dermatol.* 91:185–188.

22. Nozaki, S., Feliciani, C., and Sauder, D. N. 1992. Keratinocyte cytokines. *Adv. Dermatol.* 7:83–101.

23. Mizutani, H., Black, R., and Kupper, T. S. 1991. Human keratinocytes produce but do not process pro-interleukin-1 (IL-1) beta. Different strategies of IL-1 production and processing in monocytes and keratinocytes. *J. Clin. Invest.* 87:1066–1071.

24. Morhenn, V. B., Lee, S. W., Ilnicka, M., and Eugui, E. M. Activated human Langerhans cells express mRNA for IL-1 alpha and IL-1 beta and produce these cytokines but do not secrete them. *Cytokine* 4:500–505.

25. Gahring, L. C., Buckley, A., and Daynes, R. A. 1985. Presence of epidermal-derived thymocyte activating factor/interleukin 1 in normal human stratum corneum. *J. Clin. Invest.* 76:1585–1591.

26. Hauser, C., Saurat, J. H., Schmitt, A., Jaunin, F., and Dayer, J. M. 1986. Interleukin 1 is present in normal human epidermis. *J. Immunol.* 136:3317–3323.

27. Gery, I., and Waksman, B. H. 1972. Potentiation of the T-lymphocyte response to mitogens. II. The cellular source of potentiating mediator(s). *J. Exp. Med.* 136:143–155.

28. Ristow, H. J. 1987. A major factor contributing to epidermal proliferation in inflammatory skin diseases appears to be interleukin 1 or a related protein. *Proc. Natl. Acad. Sci. USA* 84:1940–1944.

29. Laub, R., Schreiber, S., and Stingl, G. 1994. Functional significance of Langerhans cell derived IL-1β and IL-6 for the initiation of primary allogenic T-cell responses. *J. Invest. Dermatol.* 102:526.

30. Kurt-Jones, E. A., Beller, D. I., Mizel, S. B., and Unanue, E. R. 1985. Identification of a membrane-associated interleukin 1 in macrophages. *Proc. Natl. Acad. Sci. USA* 82:1204–1208.

31. Sauder, D. N., Monick, M. M., and Hunninghake, G. W. 1985. Epidermal cell-derived thymocyte activating factor (ETAF) is a potent T-cell chemoattractant. *J. Invest. Dermatol.* 85:431–433.

32. Zhang, Y. H., Lin, J. X., Yip, Y. K., and Vilcek, J. 1988. Enhancement of cAMP levels and of protein kinase activity by tumor necrosis factor and interleukin 1 in human fibroblasts: Role in the induction of interleukin 6. *Proc. Natl. Acad. Sci. USA* 85:6802–6805.

33. Heufler, C., Koch, F., and Schuler, G. 1988. Granulocyte-macrophage colony-stimulating factor and interleukin-1 mediate the maturation of murine epidermal Langerhans cells into potent immunostimulatory denditic cells. *J. Exp. Med.* 167:700–705.

34. Clark, S. C. 1989. Interleukin-6. Multiple activities in regulation of the hematopoietic and immune systems. *Ann. NY Acad. Sci.* 557:438–443.

35. May, L. T., Santhanam, U., Tatter, S. B., Ghrayeb, J., and Sehgal, P. B. 1989. Multiple forms of human interleukin-6. Phosphoglycoproteins secreted by many different tissues. *Ann. NY Acad. Sci.* 557:114–121.

36. Zilberstein, A., Ruggieri, R., Korn, J. H., and Revel, M. 1986. Structure and expression of cDNA and genes for human interferon-beta-2, a distinct species inducible by growth-stimulatory cytokines. *EMBO J.* 5:2529–2537.

37. Grossman, R. M., Krueger, J., Yourish, D., Granelli-Piperno, A., Murphy, D. P., May, L. T., Kupper, T. S., Sehgal, P. B., and Gottlieb, A. B., 1989. Interleukin 6 is expressed in high levels in psoriatic skin and stimulates proliferation of cultured human keratinocytes. *Proc. Natl. Acad. Sci. USA* 86:6367–6371.

38. Larsen, C. G., Anderson, A. O., Appella, E., Oppenheim, J. J., and Matsushima, K. 1989. The neutrophil-activating protein (NAP-1) is also chemotactic for T lymphocytes. *Science* 243:1464–1466.

39. Matsushima, K., Morishita, K., Yoshimura, T., Lavu, S., Kobayashi, Y., Lew, W., Appella, E., Kung, H. F., Leonard, E. J., and Oppenheim, J. J. 1988. Molecular cloning of a human monocyte-derived neutrophil chemotactic factor (MDNCF) and the induction of MDNCF mRNA by interleukin 1 and tumor necrosis factor. *J. Exp. Med.* 167:1883–1893.

40. Yoshimura, T., Matsushima, K., Tanaka, S., Robinson, E. A., Appella, E., Oppenheim, J. J., and Leonard, E. J. 1987. Purification of a human monocyte-derived neutrophil chemotactic factor that has peptide sequence similarity to other host defense cytokines. *Proc. Natl. Acad. Sci. USA* 84:9233–9237.

41. Mestan, J., Digel, W., Mittnacht, S., Hillen, H., Blohm, D., Moller, A., Jacobsen, H., and Kirchner, H. 1986. Antiviral effects of recombinant tumour necrosis factor in vitro. *Nature* 323:816–819.

42. Munker, R., Gasson, J., Ogawa, M., and Koeffler, H. P. 1986. Recombinant human TNF induces production of granulocyte-monocyte colony-stimulating factor. *Nature* 323:79–82.

43. Ranges, G. E., Zlotnik, A., Espevik, T., Dinarello, C. A., Cerami, A., and Palladino, M. A., Jr. 1988. Tumor necrosis factor alpha/cachectin is a growth factor for thymocytes. Synergistic interactions with other cytokines. *J. Exp. Med.* 167:1472–1478.

44. Tracey, K. J., Wei, H., Manogue, K. R., Fong, Y., Hesse, D. G., Nguyen, H. T., Kuo, G. C., Beutler, B., Cotran, R. S., Cerami, A., and Lowry, S. F. 1988. Cachectin/tumor necrosis factor induces cachexia, anemia, and inflammation. *J. Exp. Med.* 167:1211–1227.

45. Beutler, B., and Cerami, A. 1986. Cachectin and tumour necrosis factor as two sides of the same biological coin. *Nature* 320:584–588.

46. Beutler, B., and Cerami, A. 1987. Cachectin: More than a tumor necrosis factor. *N. Engl. J. Med.* 316:379–385.

47. Beutler, B., Greenwald, D., Hulmes, J. D., Chang, M., Pan, Y. C., Mathison, J., Ulevitch, R., and Cerami, A. 1985. Identity of tumour necrosis factor and the macrophage-secreted factor cachectin. *Nature* 316:552–554.

48. Carswell, E. A., Old, L. J., Kassel, R. L., Green, S., Fiore, N., and Williamson, B. 1975. An endotoxin-induced serum factor that causes necrosis of tumors. *Proc. Natl. Acad. Sci. USA* 72:3666–3670.

49. Dinarello, C. A., Cannon, J. G., Wolff, S. M., Bernheim, H. A., Beutler, B., Cerami, A., Figari, I. S., Palladino, M. A., Jr., and O'Connor, J. V. 1986. Tumor necrosis factor (cachectin) is an endogenous pyrogen and induces production of interleukin 1. *J. Exp. Med.* 163:1433–1450.

50. Dayer, J. M., Beutler, B., and Cerami, A. 1985. Cachectin/tumor necrosis factor stimulates collagenase and prostaglandin E2 production by human synovial cells and dermal fibroblasts. *J. Exp. Med.* 162(6):2163–2168.

51. Dinarello, C. A., Cannon, J. G., Wolff, S. M., Bernheim, H. A., Beutler, B., Cerami, A., Figari, I. S., Palladino, M. A., Jr., and O'Connor, J. V. 1986. Tumor necrosis factor (cachectin) is an endogenous pyrogen and induces production of interleukin 1. *J. Exp. Med.* 163:1433–1450.

52. Collins, T., Lapierre, L. A., Fiers, W., Strominger, J. L., and Pober, J. S. 1986. Recombinant human tumor necrosis factor increases mRNA levels and surface expression of HLA-A, B antigens in vascular endothelial cells and dermal fibroblasts in vitro. *Proc. Natl. Acad. Sci. USA* 83:446–450.

53. Kehrl, J. H., Miller, A., and Fauci, A. S. 1987. Effect of tumor necrosis factor alpha on mitogen-activated human B cells. *J. Exp. Med.* 166:786–791.

54. Kohase, M., Henriksen-DeStefano, D., May, L. T., Vilcek, J., and Sehgal, P. B. 1986. Induction of beta 2-interferon by tumor necrosis factor: A homeostatic mechanism in the control of cell proliferation. *Cell* 45:659–666.

55. Philip, R., and Epstein, L. B. 1986. Tumour necrosis factor as immunomodulator and mediator of monocyte cytotoxicity induced by itself, gamma-interferon and interleukin-1. *Nature* 323:86–89.

56. Yoshikawa, T., and Streilein, J. W. 1990. Genetic basis of the effects of ultraviolet light B on cutaneous immunity. Evidence that polymorphism at the Tnf and Lps loci governs susceptibility. *Immunogenetics* 32:398–405.

57. Boehm, K. D., Yun, J. K., Garner, C., Strohl, K. P., and Elmets, C. A. 1994. *In situ* detection of cytokine messenger RNAs in the eccrine sweat gland of normal human skin. *Lymphokine Cytokine Res.* 13:9–13.

58. Boehm, K. D., Yun, J. K., and Elmets, C. A. 1991. Demonstration of IL-1 and TNF-alpha mRNAs *in situ* in normal human skin. *Clin. Res.* 39:516A.

59. Boehm, K. D., Yun, J. K., Strohl, K. P., and Elmets, C. 1992. Human epidermal cytokine transcript level changes *in situ* following urushiol application. *Clin. Res.* 40:465A.

60. Soohoo, L., Tang, H., Haqqi, T., and Elmets, C. A. 1993. Cytokine RNA profiles in human keratinocytes exposed to the contact allergen urushiol. *J. Invest. Dermatol.* 100:507.

Chapter Nineteen

STRATEGIES FOR DEVELOPING ALTERNATIVE METHODS TO ASSESS CONTACT ALLERGENS

Anthony A. Gaspari

Because allergic contact dermatitis (ACD) is an example of a T-helper-cell-mediated delayed-type hypersensitivity (DTH), we hypothesized that the study of the regulation of the expression of the B7 antigen would be highly relevant to understanding the immune mechanisms of ACD. Immunohistochemical studies that compared normal human skin to that of a 48-h patch-test reaction indicated that there is a dramatic upregulation of the expression of B7 antigen by epidermal keratinocytes (KC). Current studies are focusing on developing an in vitro model for the unregulation of adhesion molecules by KC with special interest on the transcriptional regulation of KC-derived B7 by allergens.

ANIMAL MODELS FOR ALLERGIC CONTACT HYPERSENSITIVITY: A NEED FOR IN VITRO ALTERNATIVES

Animal models have been used for years to study contact hypersensitivity.[1-5] These studies have been important because they have defined the mechanisms of this type of allergic reaction. Furthermore, comparative studies of the skin immune system of rodents and humans confirmed that there is a remarkable similarity between these species. Because of these similarities, rodent models of contact hypersensitivity are widely used as attempts to predict contact allergens in humans.[6-9] In an attempt to eliminate animal testing or a reliance on tissues derived from animals or the direct study of human volunteers, there is a strong impetus to develop in vitro models of allergic contact hypersensitivity. Such an in vitro model would replace human and/or animal predictive testing. The characteristics of an idealized version of such an in vitro test would include sensitivity, specificity, reproducibility, simplicity, and economy. Advances in the understanding of contact hypersensitivity have made it apparent that the immunobiology of this type of allergy is complex, and that the development of such an idealized in vitro alternative test would be a challenging task. Intuitively, the ideal in vitro predictive test(s) should examine the multiple aspects of the immunobiology of contact hypersensitivity. Presumably, risk assessment of allergenicity in humans will be based on the evaluation of multiple endpoints of the critical pathway(s) of contact dermatitis. Fortunately, advances in the areas of biotechnology and cellular and molecular immunology will facilitate the development of in vitro screening tests for contact

I wish to acknowledge Dr. Alan Goldberg and the Center for Alternatives to Animal Testing for their grant support and scientific resources, which have been critical to completing a number of these studies. I also acknowledge Dr. Adnan Nasir for his scientific contributions; Barbara Ferbel for her technical assistance; and Margaret Piscitello for preparing the manuscript.

allergens. The application of such advances to the study of contact hypersensitivity will undoubt-edly lead to better understanding of this allergy and possibly to an in vitro alternative test that is based on multiple endpoints that are developed based on a deep understanding of the critical "control points" of contact hypersensitivity.

THE DUAL PHASE MODEL OF CONTACT HYPERSENSITIVITY

Experimental data and clinical observations support the dual phase model of contact hypersensitiv-ity. Briefly, the afferent phase of contact sensitivity involves the penetration of a low-molecular-weight hapten into the skin, which then couples to a host component. This hapten–self component is then presented to antigen-reactive T cells by Langerhans cells (LC), which migrate from the skin to draining lymph nodes, particularly T-dependent areas of lymph nodes. In the draining lymph nodes, Langerhans cells encounter antigen-reactive T cells, and present antigen (hapten–self complex) to such helper T cells. This antigen presentation results in a clonal expansion of T cells that may migrate to the skin, peripheral blood, or other sites and serve as a pool of memory T cells.[10–12] In the efferent phase of contact hypersensitivity, a reexposure to the hapten again results in antigen presentation by LC to memory T cells, probably in the skin as well as regional lymph nodes. This results in a vigorous T-cell-mediated immune response. This T-cell-mediated inflammatory response is mediated by a variety of lymphokines and cytokines and becomes maximal at 24–48 h.

LC are the principal antigen-presenting cells (APC) in the afferent phase of contact hypersensi-tivity, which is a prototype of delayed-type hypersensitivity reactions, predominantly mediated by CD4+ T cells. One of the earliest observations suggesting LC played a role in contact hypersensitivity was the morphologic observation that lymphocytes were found in close apposition to LC.[10,13] This finding was an initial stimulus to a number of subsequent morphologic, immuno-logic, cellular, and histochemical investigations into the role of LC in allergic contact derma-titis (ACD).

After epicutaneous application of an allergen to the skin, LC undergo a variety of phenotypic and morphologic changes.[14–16] These changes indicate that allergens induce LC to become metabolically active. However, it is not known whether these changes are direct or indirect effects of allergens on LC (discussed later). The application of allergens also induces a decrease in the number of epidermal LC, in which the number of epidermal LC may decrease by as much as 50% after the application of an allergen. This decrease in number is not the result of LC death, but the emigration of LC from the epidermis.[10,17] These emigrating LC travel through dermal lymphatics and migrate to the paracortical (T-dependent) areas of draining lymph nodes. It is in the draining lymph node that the primary immune response responsible for the induction of ACD occurs. LC are thought to process and present exogenous antigens such as haptens to virgin CD4+ type 1 T-helper cells (TH1). This results in a clonal expansion of antigen-specific, self–major histocompatibility complex (self-MHC) restricted TH1 that form the basis of "immu-nologic memory." It is in this regard that LC and possibly dendritic APC in general are unique in their ability to present antigen to resting, virgin T cells.[18–20] Many other classical APC such as monocytes and macrophages have the ability to activate memory T cells, but cannot activate resting, virgin T cells as do LC. One study indicated that LC presented haptens to resting, virgin CD4+ T cells in vitro. Such in vitro sentisized T cells when adoptively transferred to naive mice were able to mediate contact hypersensitivity, providing strong support for the hypothesis that LC subserve the same role in vivo.[21] The unique ability of LC to initiate a primary immune T-cell response may be related to their abilities to express a variety of adhesion molecules that allow them to effectively "cross-talk" to T cells during the critical cell–cell interactions necessary for productive antigen presentation.[22,23]

LC are also likely to play a critical role in recall phenomenon in the previously sensitized host (the efferent limb of contact hypersensitivity). In this setting, reexposure to the allergen (either an accidental exposure or in the controlled environment of an epicutaneous patch test) induces LC to undergo a similar migration from the epidermis to draining lymph nodes, where they encounter memory T lymphocytes (hapten-specific T cells). Since such memory T cells have clonally expanded, there is a high frequency of allergen-reactive T cells, which are activated, proliferate, and produce lymphokines and initiate a cascade of cellular events, resulting in a delayed-type hypersensitivity (DTH) reaction. Laboratory investigations have not determined the mechanism of the induced migration of T lymphocytes to the epidermis in both the afferent and the efferent limbs of contact hypersensitivity. However, it is likely that various factors are responsible for the migration of TH cells to the skin: chemotactic cytokines (which may act locally in the microenvironment of the skin as well as distantly at draining lymph nodes), adherence molecules that are unregulated in the microenvironment of the skin (in the vascular endothelium, stromal cells as well as the cells of the epidermis), and antigen-bearing LC in the epidermis as well as LC that are in transit from the epidermis to the lymph nodes, which may serve as "beacons" to guide TH cells to the site of the allergen in the skin. In efferent responses, it is known that memory T cells reside in the dermis around dermal capillaries.[24] Such TH cells would certainly provide a local reservoir to trigger DTH and further recruit other TH cells.

Based on these mechanisms of contact hypersensitivity, it is possible to design a number of "tests" based on the assumptions that are inherent in the molecules and cells that are critical control points of contact hypersensitivity. A hypothetical "list" of critical control points is given in Table 1. As evidenced by the diverse areas of immunobiology that are relevant "control points" for contact sensitivity, there are multiple potential endpoints that could potentially lead to in vitro alternatives to animal testing. Some of these areas, particularly the role of epidermal cytokines (by both Langerhans cells and keratinocytes) and its role in the mechanisms of inflammation of irritant versus allergic contact dermatitis, have been the subject of intensive investigation by a number of investigators. It is also noteworthy that although there are multiple, diverse control points for contact hypersensitivity, it is apparent that these different endpoints are closely interconnected. For instance, it is now recognized that the maturation of epidermal Langerhans cells into potent antigen-presenting cells occurs in response to keratinocyte-derived cytokines such as IL-1, GM-CSF, and TNF.[25-27]

RELEVANCE OF THE EXPRESSION OF COSTIMULATORY MOLECULES TO CONTACT HYPERSENSITIVITY

We have been studying the relationship between the regulation of the expression of adherence molecules by keratinocytes, their ability to signal TH lymphocytes, and the relationship to contact hypersensitivity. The rationale for our approach is based on observations that antigen recognition by allergen-specific helper T lymphocytes that interact with antigen-presenting cells of the epidermis can result in two potential outcomes: activation (resulting in delayed-type hypersensitivity) or clonal anergy (immune tolerance). The characteristics of the antigen-presenting cells determine whether activation or anergy is induced during such cell–cell interactions. These two different outcomes of antigen recognition by T lymphocytes may be explained by the two signal model of T-cell activation first proposed by Bretscher and Cohn[28] and recently validated by Jenkins and Schwartz.[29-31] In this model, T-cell antigen receptor occupancy by nominal antigen

Table 1. Contact Hypersensitivity Control Points

Cytokine regulation and production by epidermal cells
  Keratinocyte and Langerhans cell cytokine patterns in response to allergens and/or irritants in vitro and in vivo
Antigen-presenting cell/accessory cell functions
  Enhancement of Langerhans cell or keratinocyte antigen-presenting cell function(s) by allergens and/or irritants
Antigen processing of the hapten–self complex
  Studies of the self molecules that are modified by hapten, and degradative pathway used by antigen-presenting cells (Langerhans cells and keratinocytes) to generate nominal antigen to specific T lymphocytes
Regulation of the expression of adherence molecules
  Effects of allergens/irritants on Langerhans cell or keratinocyte expression on the cell surface adherence molecules
Cell migration studies
  Migration of Langerhan cells and T cells to and from the skin or draining lymph nodes

in the context of self class II MHC is the first signal for T-cell activation, which by itself is a tolerogenic signal. When the first signal for T-cell activation is accompanied by a second signal, this results in T-cell activation. Further studies of the characteristics of this second signal indicated that the B7/BB-1 antigen was the critical second signal that provided APC-derived costimulatory activity for both mouse and human TH cells, resulting in IL-2 production and TH activation.[32–36] In parallel, studies of CD28 (the physiologic ligand for B7/BB-1) are consistent with this molecule being the receptor for this costimulatory activity, since monoclonal antibodies that cross-link cell surface CD28 expressed by T-cells can mimic the functions of the APC-derived costimulatory activity provided by the B7/BB-1 antigen.[37–43] Table 2 lists factors of T-cell biology.

In vivo, small numbers of human keratinocytes (KC) also express B7/BB-1 antigen.[44–46] In vitro, we have demonstrated that the state of differentiation of KC modulates their expression of B7/BB-1 antigen.[47]

This implies that there may be subsets of KC that can present antigen. Using immunohistochemistry on formalin-fixed, paraffin-embedded tissue sections, we have studied epidermal expression of B7/BB-1 during human contact hypersensitivity reactions (our unpublished data). Skin biopsy specimens were obtained from 48-h positive patch-test reactions. This time point was selected because this is when there is a peak in the clinical (i.e., observable erythema and edema) as well as histologic (T-cell infiltrate, epidermal spongiosis, and dermal edema) inflammatory response.[48,49] In normal human skin, there were rare B7/BB-1+ dendritic epidermal cells.[47] However, in ACD (48-h positive patch-test reactions) there was a marked increase in the epidermal expression of B7/BB-1 by KC during ACD. The B7/BB-1 antigen was predominantly by epidermal KC, although LC expression was also detected, particularly in LC that had migrated from the epidermis into the dermis (not shown). This pattern of epidermal B7/BB-1 antigen expression by KC was highly reproducible in biopsy specimens from 48-h patch-test readings from a number of different human volunteers, as well as a number of different allergens (such as nickel sulfate, formaldehyde, formaldehyde resin, potassium dichromate, tuliposide A, and dipivalyl epinephrine HCl). We and others[46,50] have confirmed these immunohistochemical studies using the polymerase chain reaction, detecting the presence of B7/BB-1 transcripts in human epidermis (data not shown). These data indicate that B7/BB-1 antigen, an important APC-derived signaling molecule for TH1 activation, is expressed in human epidermis. More importantly, the expression of this molecule is reproducibly upregulated by both KC and LC during ACD reactions in the skin. These data suggest that the upregulation of second signal molecules by epidermal cells is tightly coupled to, and highly relevant to, contact hypersensitivity. We also have preliminary data that suggests that allergens directly induce the upregulation of B7/BB-1 by keratinocytes in vitro and possibly in vivo. If this finding is confirmed, it could imply that this event is a primary event in contact hypersensitivity, not a secondary event related to T-helper cell-derived lymphokines such as interferon-gamma, which is known to upregulate class II major histocompatibility antigens and ICAM-1 (intercellular adhesion molecule) expression by human keratinocytes. Another important demonstration of the relevance of B7/BB-1 expression by keratinocytes to the pathogenesis of contact hypersensitivity is our study of transgenic mice whose keratinocytes constitutively expressed high cell surface levels of B7-1. To accomplish this, we used a recombinant DNA construct to targeted the B7-1 antigen to basal keratinocytes of transgenic mice.[51] This construct is depicted in Figure 1. Transgenic mice were produced using standard technology. We identified transgenic mice using immunochemical methods and confirmed these data using southern blotting.[51]

To test our hypothesis that altered regulation of the expression of B7-1 by epidermal keratino-

Table 2. T-Cell Biology

Signaling requirements of allergen-specific T-lymphocytes.
Lymphokine patterns in response to allergens or irritants.
Effector functions of allergen-specific T lymphocytes.
Repertoire of T-cell receptor by allergen-specific T lymphocytes.
T-cell epitopes of hapten–self complex.

pKmB7C_ß

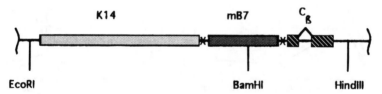

Figure 1. Expression vector construct. K14-mBY-C$_\beta$ construct was linearized by digestion of pKmB7C$_\beta$ with EcoRI and HindIII. The linearized DNA was further digested with ScaI and separated from pGEM3Z vector (flanking K14-mB7-C$_\beta$ not shown) by centrifugation over a 10–40% sucrose gradient. The resultant DNA was dialyzed and microinjected into the pronuclei of fertilized mouse eggs, which were transferred to pseudo-pregnant females as described in the text to create B7-1 transgenic mice.

cytes would have profound effects on contact hypersensitivity, we compared transgenic mice to their non-transgenic littermates for their ear swelling responses to the hapten fluorescein isothiocyanate.[52] At 24 h, the peak of the typical ear swelling response, there was no significant difference when comparing transgenic to non-transgenic littermates (see Figure 2, A and B). However, at later time points in the transgenic mice, but not the non-transgenic mice, there was a continued crescendo in the ear swelling that persisted for 144 h. This difference between transgenic and non-transgenic mice at the 84-h time point was statistically significant ($p < .05$). This same pattern of exaggerated and persistent ear swelling was noted in a second line of B7-1 transgenic mice (24-h ear swelling of sensitized mice: transgenic $\Delta T = 16 + 3$; non-transgenic $\Delta T = 11 + 2$; 144-h ear swelling of sensitized mice: transgenic $\Delta T = 14 + 4$; non-transgenic $= 2 + 1$).

Interestingly, there was also a difference in the kinetics of the ear swelling response of naive control animals, with the transgenic mice again demonstrating a crescendo in ear swelling up to 144 h. The progressive in vivo ear swelling response in transgenic mice was dependent on B7-1 expression, as a single subcutaneous injection of 20 μg of Cytotoxic T-lymphocyte antigen-4/Ig fusion protein (CTLA-4/Ig, immunoglobulin) prior to the epicutaneous application of hapten prevented this phenomenon in CTLA-4/Ig-treated, but not sham-treated, mice (see Figure 2C).

Thus, altered regulation of B7-1 by epidermal keratinocytes is highly relevant to the pathophysiology of contact hypersensitivity. In our transgenic mice, we observed profound alterations in the later phases of contact hypersensitivity, with our B7-1 transgenic mice demonstrating an exaggerated and persistent contact hypersensitivity reactions.

These data, along with our observations in the study of human contact hypersensitivity reactions, indicate that the study of the regulation of the expression of B7 by epidermal cells such as keratinocytes and Langerhans cells and its modulation by allergens has potential to lead to an in vitro alternative to screen for allergens. We are attempting to clone the 5' regulatory (promoter) region for epidermal B7-1. If we are successful, we will then develop a semiquantitative assay (B7/BB-1 promoter-driven chloramphenicol acetate transferase activity) to screen characterized as well as unknown allergens. We hypothesize that the chemical properties of allergens induce epidermal cells to assume the phenotype of activated antigen-presenting cells. If our hypothesis is correct, allergens may directly (or indirectly via cytokines) increase epidermal B7 promoter activity. It remains to be determined whether this test will be sensitive and specific for allergens. These studies nonetheless will reveal a great deal of information regarding the cellular and molecular mechanisms of contact hypersensitivity in humans.

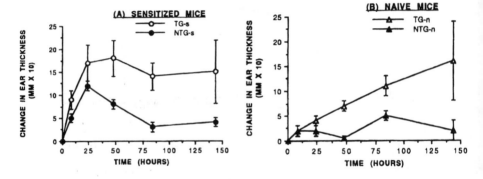

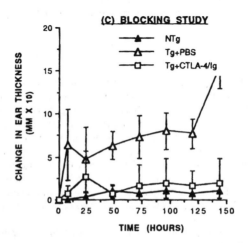

Figure 2. Time course of the ear swelling response to epicutaneous hapten application in sensitized and naive mice and blocking with anti-B7 reagents. Transgenic or nontransgenic animals were challenged on the pinna of the ear 6 after painting abdominal skin with 0.5% fluorescein isothiocyanate (FITC, sensitized) (A) or without previous painting (naive) (B). In both the sensitized and naive groups, the transgenic mice developed a persistent ear swelling response. To block the progressive ear swelling response, we treated a group of transgenic mice with a single subcutaneous injection of CTLA-4/Ig (200 μg in a 20 μl volume): another group of transgenic mice received 20 μl phosphate buffered saline (PHS) before being challenged with an epicutaneous application of 20 μl of 0.5% FITC: and a group of nontransgenic mice served as a negative control, and received only a 0.5 % FITC challenge (C).

REFERENCES

1. Bloch, B., and Steiner-Wourlisch, A. 1930. die Sensibilisierung des Meerschweinchens gegen Primeln. *Arch. Dermatol. Syph.* 162:349.
2. Landsteiner, K., and Chase, M. W. 1937. Studies on the sensitization of animals with simple chemical compounds. IV. Anaphylaxis induced by picryl chloride and 2,4-dinitrochlorobenzene. *J. Exp. Med.* 66:337.
3. Landsteiner, K., and Jacobs, J. 1935. Studies on the sensitization of animals with simple chemical compounds. *J. Exp. Med.* 61:643.
4. Landsteiner, K., and Jacobs, J. 1936. Studies on the sensitization of animals with simple chemical compounds. II. *J. Exp. Med.* 61:625.

5. Asherson, G. L., and Ptak, W. 1968. Contact and delayed hypersensitivity in the mouse. I. Active sensitization and passive transfer. *Immunology* 15:405.

6. Code of Federal Regulations. 1985. Office of the Federal Registrar, National Archives of Records in Service. General Services Administration, title 16, part 1500.50.

7. U.S. Environmental Protection Agency. 1982. Pesticides registrations: Proposed data requirements, sect 158.135: Toxicology data requirements. *Fed. Reg.* 47:53192.

8. National Academy of Sciences, Committee for the Revision of NAS Publication 1138. 1977. Principles and Procedures for Evaluating the Toxicity of Household Substances, pp. 23–59. Washington, DC: National Academy of Sciences.

9. Organization for Economic Cooperation and Development. 1981. OECD Guidelines for Testing Chemicals, 4. Paris: OECD.

10. Silberberg-Sinakin, I., Thorbecke, G. J., Bear, R. L., Rosenthal, S. A., and Berezowsky, V. 1976. Antigen-bearing Langerhans cells in skin, dermal lymphatics and in lymph nodes. *Cell. Immunol.* 25:137.

11. Knight, S. C., Krejci, J., Malkovsky, M., Colizzi, V., Gautam, A., and Asherson, G. L. 1985. The role of dendritic cells in the initiation of immune responses to contact sensitizers. I. *In vivo* exposure to antigen. *Cell Immunol.* 94:427.

12. Knight, S. C., Bedford, P., and Hunt, R. 1985. The role of dendritic cells in the initiation of immune response to contact sensitizers. II. Studies in nude mice. *Cell Immunol.* 94:435.

13. Silberberg, I. 1973. Apposition of mononuclear cells to Langerhans cells in contact allergic reactions. An ultrastructural study. *Acta Derm. Venereol. (Stockh.)* 53:1.

14. Picut, C. A., Lee, C. S., and Lewis, R. M. 1987. Ultrastructural and phenotypic changes in Langerhans cells induced in vitro by contact allergens. *Br. J. Dermatol.* 116:773.

15. Aiba, S., and Katz, S. I. 1990. Phenotypic and functional characteristics of in vivo activated Langerhans cells. *J. Immunol.* 145:2791.

16. Kolde, G., and Knop, J. 1987. Different cellular reaction patterns of epidermal Langerhans cells after application of contact sensitizing, toxic and tolerogenic compounds. A comparative ultrastructural and morphometric time-course analysis. *J. Invest. Dermatol.* 89:19.

17. Weinlich, G., Sepp, N., Koch, F., Schuler, G., and Romani, N. 1989. Evidence that Langerhans cells rapidly disappear from the epidermis in response to contact sensitizers but not to tolerogens/nonsensitizers. *Arch. Dermatol. Res.* 281:556A.

18. Knight, S. C., Krejci, J., Malkovsky, M., Colizzi, V., Gautam, A., and Asherson, G. L. 1985. The role of dendritic cells in the initiation of immune responses to contact sensitizers. I. In vivo exposure to antigen. *Cell Immunol.* 94:427.

19. Knight, S. C., Bedford, P., and Hunt, R. 1985. The role of dendritic cells in the initiation of immune response to contact sensitizers. II. Studies in nude mice. *Cell Immunol.* 94:435.

20. Hauser, C., and Katz, S. I. 1988. Activation and expansion of hapten- and protein-specific T helper cells from nonsensitized mice. *Proc. Natl. Acad. Sci. USA* 85:5625.

21. Hauser, C. 1990. Cultured epidermal Langerhans cells activate effector T cells for contact sensitivity. *J. Invest. Dermatol.* 95:436.

22. Springer, T. A. 1990. Adhesion receptors of the immune system. *Nature* 346:425.

23. Jenkins, M. K., Taylor, P. S., Norton, S. D., and Urdahl, K. B. 1991. CD28 delivers a co-stimulatory signal involved in antigen specific IL-2 production by human T-cells. *J. Immunol.* 147(8):2461.

24. Streilein, J. 1978. Lymphocyte traffic, T-cell malignancies and the skin. *J. Invest. Dermatol.* 71:167.

25. Witmer-Pack, M. D., Olivier, W., Valinsky, J., Schuler, G., and Steinman, R. M. 1987. Granulocyte/macrophage colony-stimulating factor is essential for the viability and function of cultured murine epidermal Langerhans cells. *J. Exp. Med.* 166:1484.

26. Heufler, C., Koch, F., and Schuler, G. 1988. GM-CSF and IL-1 mediate the maturation of murine epidermal Langerhans cells into potent immuno-stimulatory dendritic cells. *J. Exp. Med.* 167:700.

27. Koch, F., Heufler, C., Scheeweiss, D., Kaempgen, E., and Schuler, G. 1989. Tumor necrosis factor alpha maintains the viability of murine epidermal Langerhans cells in culture but in contrast to GM-CSF without inducing functional maturation. *J. Invest. Dermatol.* 92:461.

28. Bretscher, P. A., and Cohn, M. 1970. A theory of self-nonself discrimination. Paralysis and induction involve recognition of one and two determinants on an antigen, respectively. *Science* 169:1042.

29. Jenkins, M. K. and Schwartz, R. S. 1987. Antigen presentation by chemically modified splenocytes induces antigen-specific T cell unresponsiveness *in vitro* and *in vivo*. *J. Exp. Med.* 165:302.

30. Mueller, D. L., Jenkins, M. K., and Schwartz, R. H. 1989. Clonal expansion versus functional clonal inactivation: A co-stimulatory signaling pathway determines the outcome of T cell antigen receptor occupancy. *Annu. Rev. Immunol.* 7:445.

31. Jenkins, M. K. 1992. The role of cell division in the induction of clonal anergy. *Immunol. Today* 13(2):69.

32. Koulova L, Clark, E. A., Shu, G., and DuPont, B. 1991. The CD28 ligand B7/BB-1 provides co-stimulatory signal for alloactivation of CD4+ T cells. *J. Exp. Med.* 173:759.

33. Linsley, P. S., Brady, W., Grosmaire, L., Aruffo, A., Damle, N. K., and Ledbetter, J. A. 1991. Binding

of the B cell activation antigen B7 to CD28 costimulates T cell proliferation and interleukin 2 accumulation. *J. Exp. Med.* 179:721.

34. Norton, S. D., Zuckerman, L., Urdahl, K. B., Shefner, R., Miller, J., and Jenkins, M. K. 1992. The CD28 ligand, B7, enhances IL-2 production by providing a co-stimulatory signal to T-cells. *J. Immunol.* 149:1556.

35. Reiser, H., Freeman, G. J., Razi-Wolf, Z., Gimmi, C. D., Benacerraf, B., and Nadler, L. M. 1992. Murine B7 antigen provides an efficient co-stimulatory signal for activation of murine T lymphocytes via the T-cell receptor/CD3 complex. *Proc. Natl. Acad. Sci. USA* 89:271.

36. Freeman, G. J., Gray, G. S., Gimmi, C. D., Lombard, D. B., Zhou, L.-J., White, M., Fingeroth, J. D., Gribben, J. G., and Nadler, L. M., 1991. Structure, expression, and T cell co-stimulatory activity of the murine homologue of the human B lymphocyte activation antigen B7. *J. Exp. Med.* 174:625.

37. Hara, T., Fu., S. M., and Hansen, J. A. 1985. A new activation pathway use by a major T cell population via a disulfide-bonded dimer of a 44 kilodalton polypeptide (9.3 antigen). *J. Exp. Med.* 161:1513.

38. Moretta, A., Pantaleo, G., Lopez-Botet, M., and Moretta, L. 1985. Involvement of T44 Molecules in an antigen independent pathway of T cell activation. *J. Exp. Med.* 162:823.

39. Lesslauer, W., Koning, F., Ottenhoff, T., Giphart, M., Goulmy E., and van Rood, J. J. 1986. T90/44 (9.3 antigen). A cell surface molecule with a function in human T cell activation. *Eur. J. Immunol.* 16:1289.

40. Lindsten, T., June, C. H., Ledbetter, J. A., Stella, G., and Thompson, C. B. 1989. Regulation of lymphokine messenger RNA stability by a surface-mediated T cell activation pathway. *Science* 244:339.

41. Thompson, C. B., Lindsten, T., Ledbetter, J. A., Kunkel, S. L., Young, H. A., Emerson, S. G., Leiden J. M., and June, C. H. 1989. CD28 activation pathway regulates the production of multiple T-cell-derived lymphokines/cytokines. *Proc. Natl. Acad. Sci. USA* 86:1333.

42. June, C. H., Ledbetter, J. A., Linsley, P. S., and Thompson, C. 1990. Role of the CD28 receptor in T-cell activation. *Immunol. Today* 11(6):211–216.

43. Harding, F. A., McArthur, J. G., Gross, J. A., Raulet, D. H., and Allison, J. P. 1992. CD28-mediated signalling co-stimulates murine T cells and prevents induction of anergy in T-cell clones. *Nature* 356:607.

44. Fleming, T. E., Mirando, W. S., and Elmets, C. A. 1992. Expression of the activation antigen BB-1/B7 on cells of non-hematopoietic origin: Keratinocytes from human epidermis. *J. Invest. Dermatol.* 98(4):577A.

45. Ferbel, B., and Gaspari, A. A. 1992. Expression of the antigen presenting cell molecule, B7 in normal human skin. *Proc. 8th Int. Cong. Immunology*, Budapest, Hungary, p. 671A. Springer-Verlag.

46. Gaspari, A. A., Nasir, A., Ferbel, B., and Polakowska R. 1993. Cloning of a cDNA encoding an isoform of the B7/BB-1 antigen expressed by cultured human epidermal Langerhans cells. *J. Invest. Dermatol.* 100(94):520 (abstr.).

47. Nasir, A., Ferbel, B., and Gaspari, A. A. 1995. Keratinocytes regulate their expression of B7/BB-1 by a unique, calcium dependent mechanism. *J. Invest. Dermatol.* 104:763–767.

48. Brasch, J., Mielke, V., Kunne, N., Weber-Matthiesen, V., Bruhn, S., and Sterry, W. 1990. Immigration of cells and composition of cell infiltrates in patch test reactions. *Contact Dermatitis* 23:238.

49. Kanerva, L., Ranki, A., and Lauharanta, J. 1984. Lymphocytes and Langerhans cells in patch tests. An immunohistochemical and electron microscopic study. *Contact Dermatitis* 11:150.

50. Symington, F., Brady, W., and Linsley, P. S. 1993. Expression and function of B7 on human epidermal Langerhans cells. *J. Immunol.* 150(4):1286.

51. Nasir, A., Ferbel, B., Salminen, W., Barth, R. K., and Gaspari, A. A. 1994. Exaggerated and persistent cutaneous delayed type hypersensitivity in transgenic mice whose epidermal keratinocytes constitutively express B7-1 antigen. *J. Clin. Invest.* 94:892–898.

52. Gaspari, A. A., and Katz, S. I. 1991. Contact hypersensitivity. In *Current protocols in immunology*, eds. J. E. Coligan, A. M. Kruisbeek, D. H. Marguilies, E. M. Shevach, and W. Strober, Section 4.2:1–5. New York: John Wiley & Sons.

PART IV

NEUROTOXICITY

Chapter Twenty

ASTROCYTES AS TARGET SITE
FOR NEUROTOXICITY

Michael Aschner

This review starts with a brief review of recent research on the role of astrocytes in homeostatic central nervous system (CNS) mechanisms such as the maintenance of normal extracellular ion concentrations, the uptake of extracellular K^+, and the control of extracellular pH. Astrocytes in primary culture have been found to contain the whole plethora of receptors and also some of the uptake systems for CNS transmitters. The potential for astrocytic cultures to serve in assaying CNS toxicity is discussed, outlining both the advantages and disadvantages of in vitro methodologies. Current methodologies for the assessment of astrocytic homeostasis, namely, neurotransmitter efflux, measurements of astrocytic volume, and probing for protein and mRNA levels, are subsequently outlined. Finally, the information on how methylmercury (MeHg) interferes with astrocytic functions is briefly surveyed, and the potential role of astrocytes in facilitating and protecting against MeHg neurotoxicity is discussed.

INTRODUCTION

Advances in methodology have been critical to the rapid advances in the understanding of the functioning central nervous system (CNS). A tacit concept unique to the mammalian brain is that its functions are overwhelmingly due to the properties of its electrically excitable cells, the neurons. However, nonexcitable cells within the CNS outnumber the neurons; a class of these is collectively referred to as the neuroglia. The neuroglia are comprised of the astroglia or astrocytes, oligodendroglia or oligodendrocytes, and microglia. The term neuroglia was erroneously coined by the German pathologist Virchow in 1850, postulating that neurons were embedded in a connective tissue matrix to which he gave the name neuroglia, or nerve glue. Although erroneous, this term, has persisted for over a century as the preferred generic term for these cells.[1,2] Two forms of astrocytes have been recognized in mammalian CNS, commonly referred to as the fibrous astrocyte and protoplasmic astrocyte.[2] The fibrous astrocytes possess many thin processes, which are filled with bundles of filaments, consisting predominantly of the astrocyte-specific glial fibrillary acidic protein (GFAP). The protoplasmic astrocyte also possesses numerous processes, but they are shorter and in situ tend to insinuate in complex patterns between the neurons and their processes right down to the synaptic boutons where they contact the neuronal soma or dendritic processes. The protoplasmic astrocyte has a much lower density of intermediate filaments and often will not stain for GFAP in situ, but will stain for the nonspecific intermediate filament component vimentin,[3] glutamine synthetase (GS), or S100

Preparation of this review was written while the author's work was supported in part by NIEHS grant 05223 and U.S. EPA award 819210.

protein.[4] In situ the fibrous astrocytes are localized to the white matter whereas protoplasmic astrocytes are found exclusively in the gray matter.

The functions of astrocytes have begun to be delineated only over the last three decades with the pioneering work by Kuffler et al.[5] (discussed later). Indeed, the prevailing view that astrocytes exclusively function as passive physical support for neurons has rapidly faded, and it is now appreciated that if we are to understand the physiology and pathology of both the developing and the mature brain we must also understand the roles assumed by astrocytes, for they function prominently, not only in normal brain physiology and development, but also in the pathology of the nervous system. The modern experimental approach to glial cells, and specifically astrocytes with which this brief review is concerned, is considered to have started with the pioneering electrophysiologic studies of Kuffler and his colleagues on astrocyte-like glial cells in primitive animals such as the leech and in lower vertebrates.[5] Disposing of perhaps the last remnant of the old speculative approach that had led many to propose that astrocytes formed the extracellular space of the brain, Kuffler and his associates clearly showed that this, at least for the glia in the nervous system of leech and the optic nerve of amphibians, and only by implication for other glial cells, was totally wrong. The amphibian glial cells were found to have a normal high intracellular K^+ and, in fact, to be characterized by a membrane potential that was essentially the same as the Nernst potential for K^+, or -80 to -90 mV intracellular negative. Later work on "electrically silent" cells in the mammalian CNS identified glial cells that had the same characteristics as the leech. Kuffler's pioneering work led to one of the earliest functions proposed for glial cells, namely, the control of extracellular K^+ by astrocytes, in taking up K^+ released by active neutrons.[5] A localized released of K^+ from neurons during excitation would depolarize the astrocyte at this point with a 60-mV depolarization for a 10-fold increase in $[K^+]_o$. This would set up a current loop with other nondepolarized parts of the cell, and since the membrane was permeable only to K^+, there would be an inward current at the depolarized point carried by extracellular K^+ crossing the membrane. Since K^+ is the major electrolyte inside the cell it would also be the major current carrier inside the cell, and the current loop would be connected by efflux of K^+ at some distant point since only K^+ could cross the membrane. The return part of the loop would be carried by major extracellular ions, such as Na^+. This led to the concept of "K^+ spatial buffering" in which K^+ is transferred from a region of localized release to some distant point through the astrocyte or even though as an astrocytic syncytium. It also led to studies on other K^+ transport systems in glial cells with the emphasis that a major function of glial cells was to maintain $[K^+]_o$ homeostasis in the brain.

The next major advance in astrocytic research was that primary cultures prepared from neonatal or late-stage fetal rodent brains were found to lead to predominately, and with appropriate manipulations almost exclusively, to monolayer cultures consisting of astrocytes.[6] Confirmation of the astrocytic nature of these cultures came when it was discovered in the early 1970s[7] that the intermediate filaments of astrocytes were comprised of a unique protein, GFAP, and that almost all the cells in these primary cultures stained positively for GFAP. The development of methods for routinely preparing >95% GFAP positive cell cultures by methods such as that of McCarthy and De Vellis[8] enabled state-of-the-art experimental techniques in cell biology to be brought to bear on the study of these cultures. The cell culture approach also led to lineage studies, which were initiated by reports of type 1 and type 2 astrocytes.[9]

SURVEY OF ASTROCYTIC FUNCTIONS

Ion Channels

The control of extracellular K^+ was one of the earliest physiological functions attributed to astrocytes (discussed earlier), and studies associated with it led to considerable information about the K^+ transporting systems in these cells. These include different K^+ channels, carrier systems for K^+, and the the Na^+/K^+ pump. Astrocytic buffering plays a vital role in maintaining normal nerve function, but exactly how astrocytes buffer $[K^+]_o$ is unknown. Three models have been proposed: (1) spatial buffering of K^+, which involves diffusion of K^+ in an electrically coupled glial syncytium driven by differences in the electrical potential between different regions, (2) the related K^+ siphoning, and (3) K^+ accumulation associated with passive influx of K^+, Cl^-, and water (see refs. 10–12 for a review). Although it is beyond the scope of this review to discuss the details of all these models, common basic principles to all three models include reduction of locally increased $[K^+]_o$ by uptake of K^+ and subsequent spatial redistribution of K^+ ions. How sequestered K^+ is returned to the neuron is unknown.

K^+ channels are the most diverse ionic channel type in astrocytes. (This topic has been recently reviewed by Barres and Chun[10] and by Duffy and MacVicar.[13]) A wide variety of K^+ channels have been found in astrocytes, including inward rectifying K^+ channel (K_{in}), a Ca^{2+}-dependent K^+ channel (K_{Ca}^+), delayed rectifying channels (K_d) and an inactivating potassium channel (K_a). K^+ channels sensitive to ATP have also been found in astrocytes.

Similar in their properties to the those found in neurons where they are responsible for electrical excitability, voltage-dependent Na^+ channels are surprisingly also found in cultured primary astrocytes.[11,14] Their precise role remains elusive. Like their neuronal counterparts, some astrocytic Na^+ channels have been found to be sensitive to tetrodotoxin (TTX). However, astrocytes possess both TTX-sensitive and relatively TTX-insensitive Na^+ channels, which have different characteristics in terms of the depolarization required to activate them.[15] Work by Sontheimer et al.[16] has also identified that astrocytes from certain CNS regions, such as the spinal cord, have a very high density of Na^+ channels that have open probability at the resting membrane potential of these cells (approximately -70 mV). It was hypothesized that the Na^+ channels function in regulating Na^+ entry into the astrocytes to activate the Na^+/K^+ pump when active uptake of K^+ is required, such as when $[K^+]_o$ rises from its normal level of 3 mM to 5–10 mM during periods of sustained neuronal activity. It is postulated that these Na^+ channels represent an autoregulating mechanism for active K^+ clearance by astrocytes that does not require any special properties of the Na^+/K^+ pump.[15,16]

Astrocytes, at least those grown in primary cultures, also contain voltage-gated L-type Ca^{2+} channels.[17] This finding was surprising because such channels were thought to be exclusive to neurons, and were responsible for such properties as Ca^{2+} action potential and the depolarization-induced Ca^{2+} influx at nerve terminals required for transmitter exocytosis. The occurrence of large changes in $[Ca^{2+}]_i$, levels in astrocytes upon stimulation by receptor agonists or neurotransmitters (discussed later), such as glutamate, as well as mechanical stimulation and swelling suggests that such channels are needed for Ca^{2+} to enter the cells under such conditions to raise $[Ca^{2+}]_i$, or replenish intracellular Ca^{2+} (reviewed by Duffy and MacVicar[13]). In addition, as in many other cell types, an array of regulatory processes in astrocytes requires the release of Ca^{2+} from intracellular stores.

Anion Channels

A number of anion channels have been described in astrocytes, including low-conductance chloride channels (Cl_s) and a high-conductance chloride channel (Cl_H)[18,19]. These channels transport both Cl^- and HCO_3^-, and they are likely to be involved in the uptake of HCO_3^- or Cl^- when $[K^+]_o$ rises, or release of KCl and/or amino acids during volume regulation. They can be both chemically and voltage gated, so they will contribute to current flow across the membrane and change the membrane potential.

Ion Carriers

Ion carriers are distinct from ion channels in that a synchronous movement of more than one ion always occurs, rather than the independent diffusional movement of a single ion down its electrochemical gradient characteristics of channels. An important ion carrier is the $Na^+/K^+/2Cl^-$ uptake system, utilized by cells for active uptake of Cl^- driven by the inward Na^+ gradient and involved in volume regulation and active absorption of Cl^-. Like many other cell types, astrocytes are known to express this carrier in primary culture (reviewed by Kimelberg et al.[19]). Intracellular Cl^- concentrations in astrocyte cultures have been found to be severalfold higher than expected from the electrochemical equilibrium. This high Cl^- concentration may serve, when required, to maintain extracellular Cl^- levels, or for the efflux of KCl during volume regulatory processes.[20]

Na$^+$/K$^+$ Pump

Like all mammalian cells, astrocytes contain an active Na$^+$/K$^+$ pump. This pump functions to accumulate K$^+$ and extrude intracellular Na$^+$. A number of isoforms (α1, α2, and α3) comprise this pump. Although neurons exhibit all three isoforms, astrocytes express[21] α1 or α2 or both, but not α3. In terms of the kinetics of the different isoforms, there is evidence[21] both for and against a specialized role of astrocytic Na$^+$/K$^+$-ATPase in uptake of K$^+$. As with other Na$^+$ pumps, the astrocytic Na$^+$ seems likely to be driven mainly by intracellular Na$^+$. It has a high affinity for K$^+$ on the outside, and a midactivation level for Na$^+$ of about 10 mM on the inside.

pH Carrier

Other carrier systems for Cl$^-$ or Na$^+$ involve cotransport or exchange transport with pH equivalents, such as H$^+$, HCO$_3^-$ or OH$^-$. These carrier systems in astrocytes include the Na$^+$/H$^+$ and Cl$^-$/HCO$_3^-$, or OH$^-$ exchangers, as well as a variety of electrogenic or non-electrogenic contransport systems of Na$^+$ plus nHCO$_3^-$ (where n can be 1–3[22]). Since astrocytes in situ can undergo large pH changes (such as in ischemia), often in the direction opposite to the extracellular pH, it has been postulated that the existence of these carriers on astrocytes renders them critically important in pH homeostasis in the CNS.[23] The operation of such pH transporting systems may also be important in astrocytic volume changes. For example, the simultaneous operation of the Na$^+$/H$^+$ and Cl$^-$/HCO$_3^-$ exchangers, driven by intracellular hydration of CO$_2$ to H$^+$ and HCO$_3^-$ could lead to a net uptake of Na$^+$ and Cl$^-$ with concomitant astrocytic swelling.

Neurotransmitter Uptake Systems

Uptake systems for a number of amino acid neutrotransmitters, such as glutamate, glycine, taurine, and γ-aminobutyric acid (GABA), have been identified on the astrocytic membrane. These systems are Na$^+$-dependent and can also be electrogenic. There is considerable evidence for extremely active electrogenic uptake of glutamate in both cultured and acutely isolated astrocytes. Uptake in situ has been shown by means of autoradiography and immunocytochemistry. Three members of a family of glutamate transporters have been recently identified, two of which are exclusively located on astrocytes.[24]

Uptake of a number of monoamine transmitters has also been reported in cultured astrocytes (reviewed by Kimelberg et al.[19]) These uptake systems resemble their counterparts in nerve terminals, in being both Na$^+$-dependent and inhibitable by specific inhibitors such as antidepressants (fluoxetine). Uptake systems for adenosine,[25] taurine,[26–28] and histamine[29] have also been described. The relevance of these uptake systems to both astrocytic function and brain homeostasis has not yet been clearly determined.

Receptors for Neurotransmitters

β-Adrenergic and the ionotropic kainic acid/alpha-amino-3-hydroxy-5-methyl-isoxazole (AMPA) receptors have also been identified on astrocytes in vivo. Thus, it appears likely that astrocytes respond to the very same transmitters that at one time were thought to be exclusively located on post- or presynaptic neuronal membranes. The perisynaptic location of many astrocyte processes that form glial nets around neurons[4] puts both transmitter receptors and uptake systems in direct opposition to their sites of release (namely, presynaptic boutons on the neuronal soma or dendrites), and thus optimizes their potential for neurotransmission and neuromodulation. Indeed, electron microscopy studies combined with immunocytochemistry[30] show that β2 receptors are located on astrocytes processes close to the synaptic cleft, and Derouiche et al.[31] have described glutamine-positive astrocyne processes directly next to, or even penetrating to a limited extent into, glutamatergic synapses.

The functional implications of these receptors on the astrocytic membrane are still subject to speculation. These, of course, initially include the activation of second-messenger systems, in turn leading to a variety of functional effects. For example, the activation of the KA/AMPA glutamate receptors has been shown to lead to membrane potential depolarization and Na$^+$ and

K$^+$ inward currents.[32,33] New studies have implicated this receptor as a glial-specific type of AMPA receptor, which can also transport Ca^{2+}.[34] Like their neuronal counterparts, astrocytes are known to possess serotonin, histamine, GABA, angiotensin II, endothelin, bradykinins, substance P, vasoactive intestinal peptide (VIP), natriuretic, and opioid receptors.[35]

DEVELOPMENT AND NEUROTROPHIC FACTORS

Interactions between astrocytes and developing neurons are of the utmost importance in the development of the CNS. In the immature CNS, neuronal cell body migration and axonal outgrowth occur on radial glia, which later on lose their longitudinal orientation and are thought to form mature astrocytes.[36–38] Neuronal migration is the basis of CNS pattern formation and layering and is characterized by astrocyte-guided translocation of nerve cells from the site of cell division (subventricular zone) to their final destination. This process is perhaps best exemplified by the "outside-in" migration of cerebellar granule cells along radial fibers of the Bergmann glial cells.[36,39]

Astrocyte–neuron interactions are now recognized as being due to a number of adhesive and recognition molecules that are expressed by both cell types. Astrocyte–neuron cell-to-cell contact mediated by adhesion molecules is again perhaps best exemplified by the migration of cerebellar granule cells along Bergmann fibers. Translocation of neuronal cell bodies requires the coordinated temporal and spatial expression of different adhesive molecules, such as N-CAM, astrotactin, and L1.[36,40,41] Similarly, neurite outgrowth along astrocytic cell surfaces and the extracellular matrix (ECM) is characterized by a specific spatiotemporal elaboration of several adhesive molecules including L1, N-CAM, N-cadherin, and integrin-class extracellular matrix receptors.[42] Moreover, adhesion molecule binding mediates a number of additional processes that are also critical for development and regeneration: nerve fiber fasciculation (e.g., fasciclins, cadherins), pathway cues for guidance and target connectivity (e.g., L2/HNK-1 carbohydrate epitope), demarcation of topographic boundaries between laminar neuronal assemblies (e.g., J1 anti-adhesion molecules), astroglial differentiation (e.g., L1), regulation of intra- and extracellular ion composition (i.e., adhesion molecule on glia, AMOG; see section on Na$^+$/K$^+$ pump), and nerve-target adhesion (e.g., N-CAM).[43–45] Adhesion molecule interactions promote growth cone motility along astrocytic surfaces, and also provide the neurite with directional cues and other pertinent information regarding the surrounding microenvironment. Processing of this information clearly requires complex signal transduction and intracellular integration. How this occurs is not currently known, although it has been shown that the cytoplasmic domains of certain adhesion molecules (e.g., integrins, N-CAM 180, L1) are linked to various cytoskeletal elements.[46,47] In addition, specific binding-induced changes in these membrane-cytoskeleton linkage complexes might be responsible for alterations in cytoskeletal components that are the basis of cell–cell stabilization and growth cone extension.[40] In vitro evidence suggests that adhesion molecule binding influences second-messenger turnover (i.e., inositol phosphates, Ca^{2+}), which might mediate appropriate and necessary changes in neurite metabolism and membrane ion channel function.[48–50]

Astrocytes are also implicated in the lineage development of oligodendrocytes, the myelin-producing glial cells of the CNS. Comparing the differentiation of enriched oligodendroglia in subculture with their counterparts remaining on an astrocyte underlayer, the oligodendrocyte lineage exhibits signs of impaired cytoskeletal progression and plasticity in the absence of the astrocyte bed layer, exemplified by the prolonged retention of vimentin (indicating immaturity) and induced expression of glial-fibrillary acidic protein (GFAP).[51] With respect to myelinogenic products, newly separated cells within the oligodendrocyte lineage fail to initiate or sustain production of the oligodendrocyte-specific differentiation marker galactocerebroside (GalC).[51,52] Coculture experiments suggest that GalC expression and the loss of vimentin, two events that normally coincide with terminal oligodendrocyte differentiation in vivo,[53] require direct cell–cell contact with the astrocytes.[54,55]

SYSTEMS FOR STUDYING ASTROCYTES

In Situ Studies

As noted at the beginning of this review, methodology is critical to advances in our understanding the empirical sciences. Thus, the question of "how does one study astrocytes?" remains an important one. As noted in the introduction, a large stimulus was provided to studies of glial cells by the demonstration by Kuffler and his colleagues[5] that glia in vertebrates and lower vertebrates could be studied by the electrophysiological techniques current in the mid-1960s. These techniques have advanced considerably, and people are now studying the electrophysiological properties of mammalian astrocytes in situ by whole cell patch-camp techniques and in addition by imaging with intracellular pH or ion-sensitive fluorescent dyes, sometimes simultaneously with electrophysiological recordings. The traditional methods of light microscopy using specific labeling with astrocyte markers and electron microscopy still allow one to look at astrocyte morphology and their interactions with neurons in situ. When coupled with immunocytochemistry or in situ hybridization, these techniques allow one to localize specific proteins or their mRNAs to astrocytes and look for evidence of increased synthesis by measuring changes in mRNA levels.

In Vitro Studies

The evaluation of chemically induced cytotoxicity, particularly in heterogeneous system such as the brain, is often difficult in the intact animal because numerous factors (neural, hormonal, and hemodynamic) are not under experimental control. Hence, a simplified model, such as tissue culture, is indispensable as a tool for understanding basic physiology and pathology.

Once the cellular purity, content, and degree of maturation have been established, astrocytic and oligodendrytic cultures afford a host of advantages over in vivo techniques. Cell morphology, protein synthesis and release (myelin), energy metabolism, receptor interaction, neurotransmitter uptake and release, and electrolyte and nonelectrolyte uptake and release can be easily studied. Dispersion of cells in culture permits access to clean membrane surfaces for electrophysiological studies utilizing patch clamping and allows for rapid and reliable exchange of solutions. These are but a few of the parameters that can be probed over time. Direct effects of chemicals on a relatively homogeneous population allow for study of specific aspects of the growth and differentiation of cells, as well as the kinetics of uptake and metabolism of the parent compound. The incubation period can be chosen to correspond to the period of mammalian CNS growth spurt during which glial replication is at its peak and cellular organization and differentiation are proceeding at a rapid rate or can be chosen to span over a period of enzymatic maturation. Hence, timing of the culture relative to developmental age can be followed with respect to the vulnerability of gliogenesis to the xenobiotic. Teratological mechanisms relative to the maturation of the culture can be probed. Mature glial cultures allow for the discovery of potential mechanisms associated with neurotoxicity (e.g., electrolyte and nonelectrolyte transport, altered metabolism, etc.)

The culture model also makes it possible to study regional specialization, and can be extended to study astrocytic–neuronal interactions by coculturing astroglial and neuronal cells as two separate monolayers in the same culture dish (at a distance from each other). The system may provide information on how astrocytes respond to the neuronal environment, and vice versa, and how astrocytic homeostasis affects neuronal development and function.

Tissue cultures allow direct evaluation of the effects of toxic agents on the CNS. Circumventing metabolic degradation, known pharmacological concentration of toxins can be administered to cultures. Furthermore, toxic effects on juxtaposed cells or other organs that can interact with and buffer or exacerbate the toxic effect of the xenobiotic on the CNS can be altogether eliminated or factored in sequentially. Toxins can be easily added and withdrawn from the cultures, and long-term effects may be studied.

As previously discussed, cultured glia express a variety of receptors. However, whether the receptor phenotype observed in vitro accurately reflects the in vivo situation remains to be determined. The observed phenotype might be a function of culture conditions or inherent astrocyte heterogeneity. Perhaps more important, glial membrane receptor composition appears to be dependent upon neuron-induced differentiation. The issue of differentiation is particularly important for in vitro studies of neurotoxicity. Since glial cells and neurons promote mutual functional differentiation of each other (discussed earlier), cell types resulting from purified cultures may result in undifferentiated cells or cells with altered differentiation, making results difficult to interpret. The sensitivity of undifferentiated cells to neurotoxicants has not been assessed.

Although the use of cultured astrocytes, microglia, and oligodendrocytes in toxicity testing has emerged as a powerful tool to evaluate the responses of target cells at the cellular and molecular level, one must bear in mind some intrinsic pitfalls of culture systems. For example, cells can undergo varying degrees of differentiation. From the toxicologic viewpoint, the extent of cellular differentiation must be carefully defined, since multiple phenotypic states may exhibit different toxicologic responsiveness and the phenotypic expression of cells in culture may itself be the target of toxic insult.

While chemicals can be easily added and withdrawn from the cultures, and their effects directly probed in culture systems, caution should be used when correlating effects occurring in vitro to those which are observed in the intact animal, where additive interactions are likely to occur. One must remember several concepts:

1. A number of different, sometimes competing, processes influence the ability of a toxin to attack and destroy specific cells. Metabolism of the administered agent by a nontarget cell or tissue may be responsible for bioactivation and/or detoxification of the compound or its metabolite, affecting the vulnerability of the cells to the neurotoxin.
2. A cell culture is manyfold more homogeneous and simpler than any tissues, in particular the CNS. Removal of many cell types and barriers can facilitate diffusion or even active transport of the compound or its metabolite, limiting or enhancing toxicity by determining at which sites the toxin can reach sufficiently high concentrations to interfere with vital cellular processes.
3. The capacity of the cell to repair or replace damaged organelles or enzymes can also be critical in determining cell survival after toxic insult and may obviously depend on neighboring cells and physical barriers, which may be absent in the culture altogether. Accordingly, characteristics that are described as advantageous in particular circumstances may be described as disadvantageous in others.

Culturing of Astrocytes and Sampling of Experiments Utilized to Assess Their Function

The method for astrocytic culturing is widely used and has been extensively described. Briefly, the cerebral hemispheres of newborn rats (Sprague-Dawley) are removed, the meninges are carefully dissected off, and the tissue is dissociated using Dispase II. Cultures are essentially prepared as described by Frangakis and Kimelberg.[56] The monolayers become confluent after approximately 3 wk. Immunocytochemically, 95% of the cells stain positively for the astrocytic marker, GFAP, using a previously reported procedure.[56] Cell viability is also routinely assessed by the trypan blue exclusion method (20% v/v of 0.4% staining solution).

Confluent cultures can subsequently be loaded overnight with D-[2,3-^{3}H]-aspartic acid, and the next day the cells are continuously perfused with the compound of interest to assess aspartate release. Aspartate, a nonmetabolizable analog of glutamate, serves as a marker for the latter. Aspartate and glutamate are likely to be transported on the same carrier protein and, if there is no major compartmentalization problems, the radioactive probe used at low concentrations but high specific activity should equilibrate with the entire pool of glutamate and aspartate, labeling it uniformly.

Astrocytic volume is measured by a novel dynamic method that measures electrical resistance.[57] Briefly, the astrocytes are placed in a perfusion chamber containing a channel (channel height is 100 μm) bridged between two silver wire electrodes (approximately 5 cm in length). Leads from the silver electrodes are made of insulated copper wire, soldered to the silver with pure indium, and the connections are covered with wax. The silver electrodes are connected through a large resistor (1 MΩ) to a lock-in amplifier that supplies a 500-Hz, 5-V signal to the system. The lock-in amplifier is used because it is able to resolve small voltage changes with high noise rejection. At the 500 Hz frequency, the cell membranes are insulating and current will travel over and not through the cell monolayer. Apart from the solution in the channel, the two chambers are insulated from each other. The control bathing medium for all experiments consists of the following: 22 mM NaCl, 3.3 mM KCl, 0.4 mM $MgSO_4$, 1.3 mM $CaCl_2$, 1.2 mM KH_2PO_4, 10 mM D-(+)-glucose, and 25 mM HEPES (N-2-hydroxyethylpiperazine N'-2-ethanesulfonic acid), and 200 mM mannitol. HEPES-buffered solutions are maintained at pH 7.4 by addition of 1 N NaOH. Hyposmotic solutions are made by removing the mannitol. The replacement of part of the NaCl with mannitol in isosmotic solutions has the important feature of maintaining the same electrolyte concentration in the respective iso- and hyposmotic solutions, assuring identical conductivity properties. However, a small correction has to be made for the small decrease in solution conductance due to mannitol, which is corrected for by adding a small amount of water. It is clearly critical to balance all the experimental solutions to the same resistivity so that the resistance (and voltage) differences measured when the solutions are changed can be accounted for solely due to changes in cell volume.

As cells swell their volume increases such that the volume of the solution within the channel available for current flow decreases proportionally, resulting in an increase in measured resistance in the channel above the cells. Since $V = IR$ (where V is voltage, I is current, and R is resistance) and I is constant (500 Hz), changes in V are directly proportional to changes in R. The resting height of the astrocytic monolayer is normally about 5 μM, as determined by this method. The chamber is designed to have a height of approximately 100 μm above the cells. Since the percentage change in voltage (and resistance) is measured, a 1% change in the measurement translates to approximately 1 μm change in the average cell height of the monolayer. A recorded increase in the voltage (and thus resistance) means that the volume through the channel above the cells available for current flow has decreased by the same amount as the volume of the monolayer cell height has increased.

The electrical resistance technique offers an elegant means to study cellular mechanisms of swelling and the ensuing regulatory volume decrease (RVD). When combined with the continuous perfusion method, it offers the added feature of release measurements of preloaded radiolabeled ions and amino acids. This is a promising assay system with great potential as an in vitro tool for the study of cytotoxicity. A modification of the existing chamber with suitable optics through the cell channel could also allow the simultaneous measurement of changes in intracellular ion concentrations using fluorescent probes. Thus, by combining volume measurements with intracellular ion measurements, one could not only determine the role of ions such as calcium or potassium in RVD, but also determine how interference with such processes can impact on volume regulation and the release of endogenous substances. This methodology is applicable to studying volume regulation not only in astrocytes but any substratum-attached cell types, for most mammalian cell types, when exposed to hypotonic media, will swell and subsequently return to their normal volume. Furthermore, the technique can be utilized to screen chemicals that induce cell swelling and for the release of endogenous substances. With this method, it is not necessary to have a single confluent monolayer of cells to study swelling and release, as both multilayers of cells or less than confluent cell cultures can be studied, although the system's sensitivity would change. Finally, from the economic point of view, the system is inexpensive compared to other cytotoxic screening methods. A lock-in amplifier can be purchased for approximately $3000. The method is extremely reproducible and allows for many experiments to be run in a single day. Unlike many other methods that offer a "snapshot" in time, the electrical resistance technique combined with efflux measurements allows for continuous correlation of relative changes in cell volume and release of endogenous markers, allowing for sensitive measurements of cytotoxicity.

ASTROCYTES AS MODULATORS OF METHYLMERCURY NEUROTOXICITY

We conclude this review of astrocytic function in the normal and pathologic brain by alluding to the role of astrocytes in methylmercury (MeHg) neurotoxicity. There is indeed compelling evidence that astrocytes are involved in the etiology of heavy metal neurotoxicity. As early as

1966, Oyake et al.[58] showed that, in humans, MeHg preferentially accumulates within astrocytes. This was further confirmed by Garman et al.,[59] leading to the "sink hypothesis" and the implication that the resistance of the CNS to the development of MeHg encephalopathy is dependent upon the capacity of astroglia to take up and sequester MeHg into nontoxic "dump" sites. Although current understanding of the involvement of astrocytes in MeHg-induced pathology has been enormously extended over the last decade, many questions remain. This section details studies in neonatal rat primary astrocyte cultures on the effects of MeHg exposure on astrocytic ion, and nonelectrolyte transport, and the potential for these cells both to facilitate and protect against MeHg neurotoxicity.

A prominent feature of prenatal MeHg poisoning is a reduction in CNS mitotic activity[60] and interference with neuron migration.[61,62] Effects of MeHg on neuronal migration in culture reveal cessation of cell movement at 10 μM MeHg. Abnormalities of neuronal migration are also prominent pathological features of MeHg-affected human brains (review of Reuhl and Chang[63]). Since neurons migrate along radial glial processes[64] (also see earlier discussion), it is possible that a major effect of MeHg is damage to the astrocytes. Indeed, effects on astrocytes have been shown.

Several reported actions of mercurials on membrane systems can potentially influence gains or losses of osmolytes and therefore cell volume,[65] including extensive losses[66] of K^+, which should increase RVD, as well as increased influx[66] of Na^+, which would be expected to lead to swelling, or inhibition of RVD. Aschner et al.[67] have shown by measurement of intracellular sugar space ([^{14}C]3-O-methyl-D-glucose), that MeHg exposure leads to swelling of astrocytes. Phase-contrast microscopy data have shown that exposure of mouse astrocyte cultures to 0.8–1 μM MeHg for 30 min leads to marked swelling.[68] Rothstein and Mack[65] also found that mercurials increase swelling in isotonic conditions due to an increased Cl^- as well as cation permeability. Whether the same mechanisms are operative in astrocytes remains to be determined.

MeHg leads to a dose-dependent decrease in the uptake of both [^3H]-L-glutamate and [^3H]-D-aspartate in primary astrocyte cultures. In addition to triggering excitation *en masse* in adjacent neurons by activation of N-methyl D-aspartate (NMDA) receptors,[69] increases in [glutamate]$_o$ (both because of MeHg-induced release and uptake inhibition) can also cause increased [Ca^{2+}]$_i$ and production of CO_2 due to increased astrocytic metabolism. It is also well established that astrocytes take up glutamate by an Na^+-dependent mechanism[70] that may also be partially dependent on Cl^-.[71] Uptake of glutamate has been reported in astrocyte cultures to occur with a stoichiometry of two Na^+ to one glutamate.[72] This uptake could lead to further swelling due to cells becoming loaded with Na^+ and the diminished ability of the Na^+-K^+ pump to pump out Na^+. It has also been reported that glutamate interacts with cultured astrocytes to activate an kainate/AMPA receptor.[33] Increased Na^+ uptake could thus be due to activation of the latter. Increased Na^+ will also lead to astrocytic depolarization. Since the range most conducive to glutamate uptake is around the testing potential, astrocytic depolarization may further short-circuit glutamate uptake.

Our present understanding of MeHg toxicity clearly favors the concept that high concentrations of this organometal are cytotoxic to astrocytes, leading to a continuum of metabolic changes. Upon continuous exposure to this organometal the astrocytes exhibit progressive biochemical derangement resulting in compromised neuronal function once astrocytic control of the extracellular microenvironment becomes impaired. An important question, however, still remains. What is the cellular adaptation of astroyctes to MeHg exposure in the initial stages of low-level MeHg exposure? And it is possible that these cells can develop relative tolerance to MeHg, specifically via the amplification of metallothionein (MT) genes?

A novel kind of SH-based metal clusters that have come recently to attention are the MTs (reviewed by Kägi[73]). The mammalian forms of MT are characterized by a molecular mass of 6000–7000 kD, containing some 60 amino acid residues, among them 20 cysteines, and binding a total of 7 equivalents of metal ions.[73,74] All cysteines occur in the reduced form and are coordinated to the metal ions through mercaptide bonds, giving rise to spectroscopic features characteristic of metal thiolate complexes. Under normal conditions of chronic low-level exposure, the basally synthesized astrocytic MTs are probably sufficient to chelate most or all of the MeHg ions. Under conditions of sudden high-level exposure, the induction of MT gene transcripts may provide an additional measure of safety. An important conceptual contribution to the understanding of these faculties was the realization that the biological functions of metals and their accumulation within cells are invariably linked to the existence of specific metal-binding proteins.

Owing to their inducibility, MTs can provide astrocytes with a potential mechanism to attenuate, at least temporarily, the toxicity of MeHg. An astrocyte can be envisioned to experience several stages,[75] beginning with nonexposure, a state of grace that evidently no longer exists in nature, and ending with cell death or pervasive cell dysfunction once tolerance mechanisms have been overwhelmed. Between these extremes lies a continuum of metabolic changes consisting of initial injuries that take place at discrete molecular sites, followed by the metabolic amplification of such injuries. The toxic effects of MeHg become more pervasive until the astrocytes exhibit significant biochemical impairments, affecting the function of juxtaposed neurons. Additional MeHg exposure would presumably hasten the process. Because MeHg turnover in the CNS is very slow, the process may continue without additional exposure. During all stages, the cells may develop tolerance for MeHg, brought about by amplification of the MT genes. The astrocytes are excellent candidates for examining this concept, because they both preferentially sequester MeHg and, are immunopositive for MTs,[76] specifically the MT-I and MT-II isoforms.

We have recently investigated the ability of astrocytes to innately express MTs, as well as the ability of low-level MeHg exposure to induce MT both at the mRNA level and protein level. Astrocytes constitutively express MT mRNA, corroborating the in situ observations by Blaauwgeers et al.[76] Treatment of astrocytes with MeHg at concentrations that do not produce overt cytotoxicity increased MT mRNA expression in a time-dependent fashion. MeHg-induced MT expression was also shown by means of western blot analysis to be increased compared with controls, and this was further corroborated by immunocytochemical methods.

Although the precise significance of MeHg-induced MT expression in astrocytes will remain a topic for discussion for some time, the hypothesis that MTs serve a nonspecific protective function, limiting the intracellular concentrations of MeHg and shielding cellular structures from its harmful effects, is presently favored. That MTs potentially provide a reservoir for MeHg is supported by studies demonstrating that MeHg in the CNS preferentially accumulates within astrocytes.[58,59] Whether elevated astrocytic MT levels protect against MeHg-induced toxicity remains to be determined.

CONCLUSIONS

This it review cannot do justice to the rapid advances in experimental data and concepts now being made within the "glial" field, and this is just as applicable to astrocytes alone. In contrast to the previously emphasized support roles of astrocytes for neurons, new information now provides evidence that astrocytic contact with neurons significantly affects the morphological and functional differentiation of the latter. This reciprocity between neurons and astrocytes suggests that the morphological and physiological attributes of neurons are a product of this cell–cell interaction and vice versa. In addition, such reciprocity appears to exist with other CNS cell types such as oligodendrocytes, microglia, and endothelial cells. The wide diversity of astrocytic functions in maintaining homeostasis and the number of functions assumed by these cells are also quite large. Their potential in modulating damage and repair is also reflected in this review.

Thus it seems likely that chemicals may have a number of effects on astrocyte function, comparable to the effects reported for neuronal systems. The small amount of information currently available on the effects of chemicals makes the expansion of such studies timely and worthwhile at this juncture in view of the large number of properties that we now attribute to astrocytes and that can be experimentally examined. Thus, the large number of second-messenger systems and the effects on channels and transmitter effects on membrane electrical properties, among many others, can provide a rich field for investigations of the action of chemicals on astroglial function. Their potential in modulating damage to the CNS by MeHg (and other chemicals) and their capacity to be damaged when their own defenses are overwhelmed are also reflected in this review. Expanded investigation of the astrocytic involvement in xenobiotic-induced neurotoxicity is clearly warranted to improve our understanding of these processes. It will be some time, however, before we will know how "guilty" the astrocytes are in the etiology of chemical-induced neurotoxicity.

REFERENCES

1. Somjen, G. G. 1988. Nervenkitt: Notes on the history of the concept of neuroglia. *Glia* 1:2–9.
2. Tower, D. B. 1992. A century of neuronal and neuroglial interactions, and their pathological implications: An overview, In *Progress in brain research—Neuronal–astrocytic interactions, implications for normal and pathological CNS formation*, vol. 94, eds. A. C. H. Yu, L. Hertz, M. Norenberg, E. Sykova, and S. Waxman, pp. 3–18. Amsterdam: Elsevier.
3. Bignami, A., Dahl, D., and Rueger, D. C. 1980. Glial fibrillary acidic protein (GFA) in normal neural cells in pathological conditions. In *Advances in cellular neurobiology*, vol. 1, eds. S. Fedoroff and S. Hertz, pp. 285–310. New York: Academic Press.
4. Bruckner, G., Brauer, K., Hartig, W., Wolff, J. R., Rickmann, M. J., Derouiche, A., Delpech, B., Girard, N., Oertel, W. H., and Reichenbach, A. 1993. Perineuronal nets provide a polyanionic glia-associated form of microenvironment around certain neurons in many parts of the rat brain. *Glia* 8:183–200.
5. Kuffler, S. W., Nicholls, J. G., and Orkand, R. K. 1966. Physiological properties in glial cells in the CNS system of amphibia. *J. Neurophysiol.* 29:768–787.
6. Booher, J., and Sensenbrenner, M. 1972. Growth and cultivation of dissociated neurons and glial cells from embryonic chick, rat and human brain in flat cultures. *Neurobiology* 2:97–105.
7. Eng, L. F., Vanderhaeghen, J. J., Bignmi, A., and Gerstl, B. 1971. An acidic protein isolated from fibrous astrocytes. *Brain Res.* 28:351–354.
8. McCarthy, K. D., and De Vellis, J. 1980. Preparation of separate astroglial and oligodendroglial cell cultures from rat cerebral tissue. *J. Cell Biol.* 85:890–902.
9. Raff, M. C. 1989. Glial cell development in the rat optic nerve. *Science*, 243:1450–1455.
10. Barres, B. A., and Chun, L. L. Y. 1990. Ion channels in vertebrate glia. *Annu. Rev. Neurosci.* 13:441–474.
11. Bevan, S., Chiu, S. Y., Gray, P. T. A., and Ritchie, J. M. 1985. Presence of voltage-gated sodium, potassium and chloride channels in rat cultured astrocytes. *Philos. Trans. R. Soc. Biol.* 225:299–313.
12. Walz, W., Physiological consequences of activating serotonin receptors. In *Glial cell receptors*, ed. H. K. Kimelberg, pp. 121–130. New York: Raven Press.
13. Duffy, S., and MacVicar, B. A. 1993. Voltage-dependent ionic channels in astrocytes. In *Astrocytes, pharmacology and function*, ed. S. Murphy, p. 137. San Diego: Academic Press.
14. Bowman, C. L., Kimelberg, H. K., Frangakis, M. V., Berwald-Netter, Y., and Edwards, C. 1984. Astrocytes in primary culture have chemically activated sodium channels. *J. Neurosci.* 4:1527–1534.
15. Sontheimer, H. 1991. Astrocytes, as well as neurons, express a diversity of ion channels. *Can. J. Physiol. Pharmacol.* 70:S223–S238.
16. Sontheimer, H., Black, J. A., Ransom, B. R., and Waxman, S. G. 1992. Ion channels in spinal cord astrocytes in vitro. 1. Transient expression of high levels of Na^+ and K^+ channels. *J. Neurophysiol.* 68:985–1000.
17. MacVicar, B. A. 1984. Voltage-dependent calcium channels in glial cells. *Science* 226:1345–1247.
18. Jalonen, T. 1993. Single-channel characteristics of the large-conductance anion channel in rat cortical astrocytes in primary cultures. *Glia* 9:227–237.
19. Kimelberg, H. K., O'Connor, E., Goderie, S. K., Higman, S., and Jalonen, T. 1993. Transmitter and ion uptake in astrocytes. In *Astrocytes, pharmacology and function*, ed. S. Murphy, pp. 193–228. New York: Academic Press.
20. Kimelberg, H. K., and Frangakis, M. V. 1985. Furosemide- and bumetanide-sensitive ion transport and volume control in primary astrocyte cultures from rat brain. *Brain Res.* 361:125–134.
21. Sweadner, K. J. 1991. Overlapping and diverse distribution of Na-K ATPase isozymes in neurons and glia. *Can. J. Physiol. Pharmacol.* 70:S255–S259.
22. Newman, E. A. 1991. Sodium-bicarbonate cotransport in retinal Muller (glial) cells of the salamander. *J. Neurosci.* 11:3972–3983.
23. Chesler, M., and Chen, J. C. T. 1991. Alkanline extracellular pH shifts generated by two transmitter-dependent mechanisms. *Can. J. Physiol. Pharmacol.* 70:S286–S292.
24. Kanner, B. I. 1993. Glutamate transporters from brain: A novel neurotransmitter transporter family. *FEBS Lett.* 325:95–99.
25. Matz, H., and Hertz, L. 1990. Effects of adenosine deaminase inhibition on active uptake and metabolism of adenosine in astrocytes in primary cultures. *Brain Res.* 515:168–172.
26. Holopainen, I. 1988. Taurine and beta-alanine uptake in primary astrocytes differentiating in culture: Effects of ions. *Neurochem. Res.* 13:853–858.
27. Lee, I. S., Renno, W. M., and Beitz, A. J., 1992. Quantitative light and electron microscopic analysis of taurine-like immunoreactivity in the dorsal horn of the rat spinal cord. *J. Comp. Neurol.* 321:65–82.

28. Shain, W., and Martin, D. L. 1990. Uptake and release of taurine—An overview. In *Taurine, functional neurochemistry, physiology and cardiology*, eds. H. Pasantes-Morales, D. L. Martin, W. Shain, and R. del Rio, pp. 243–252. New York: Wiley-Liss.

29. Huszti, Z., Rimanoczy, A., Juhasz, A., and Magyar, K. 1990. Uptake, metabolism, and release of histamine by glial cells in primary cultures of chicken cerebral hemisphere. *Glia* 3:159–168.

30. Aoki, C. 1992. Beta-adrenergic receptors: Astrocytic localization in the adult visual cortex and their relation to catecholamine terminals as revealed by electron microscopic immunocytochemistry. *J. Neurosci.* 12:781–792.

31. Derouiche, A., Heimrich, B., and Frotscher, M. 1993. Loss of layer-specific astrocytic glutamine synthetase immunoreactivity in slice cultures of hippocampus. *Eur. J. Neurosci.* 5:122–127.

32. Bowman, C. L., and Kimelberg, H. K. 1987. Pharmacological properties of the norepinephrine-induced depolarization of astrocytes in primary culture: Evidence for the involvement of an alpha 1-adrenergic receptor. *Brain Res.* 423:403–407.

33. Sontheimer, H., Kettenmann, H., Backus, K. H., and Schachner, M. 1988 Glutamate opens Na^+/K^+ channels in cultured astrocytes. *Glia* 1:328–336.

34. Muller, T., Moller, T., Berger, T., Schnitzer, J., and Kettenmann, H. 1992. Calcium entry through kainate receptors and resulting potassium-channel blockade in Bergmann glial cells. *Science* 256:1563–1566.

35. Aschner, M., and Kimelberg, H. K. 1996. Astrocytes: Potential modulators of heavy metal-induced neurotoxicity. In *Toxicology of metals*, ed. L. W. Chang. pp. 587–608. Boca Raton, FL: CRC Press.

36. Rakic, P. 1990. Principles of neural migration. *Experientia* 46:882–891.

37. Rakic, P., and Siedman, R. L. 1973. Weaver mutant mouse cerebellum: Defective neuronal migration secondary to specific abnormality of Bergmann glia. *Proc. Natl. Acad. Sci. USA* 10:240–244.

38. Reichenbach, A. 1989. Glia: Neuron index: Review and hypothesis to account for different values in various mammals. *Glia* 2:71–77. 1989.

39. Hatten, M. E., Fishell, G., Stitt, T. N., and Mason, C. A. 1990. Astroglia as a scaffold for development of the CNS. *Semin. Neurosci.* 2:455–465.

40. Chuong, C. M. 1990. Differential roles of multiple adhesion molecules in cell migration: Granule cell migration in cerebellum. *Experientia* 46:892–899.

41. Stitt, T. N., and Hatten, M. E. 1990. Antibodies that recognize astrotactin block granule neuron binding to astroglia. *Neuron* 5:639–649.

42. Smith, G. M., Rutishauser, U., Silver, J., and Miller, R. H. 1990. Maturation of astrocytes in vitro alters the extent and molecular basis of neurite outgrowth. *Dev. Biol.* 138:377–390.

43. Gloor, S., Antonicek, H., Sweadner, K. J., Pagliusi, S., Frank, R., Moos, M., and Schachner, M. 1990. The adhesion molecule of glia (AMOG) is a homologue of the α subunit of the Na,K-ATPase. *J. Cell Biol.* 110:165–174.

44. Kruse, J., Keilhauer, G., Faissner, A., Timpl, R., and Schachiler, M. 1985. The J1 glycoprotein—a novel nervous system cell adhesion molecule of the L2/HNK-1 family. *Nature* 316:146–148.

45. Schachner, M. 1991. Cell surface recognition and neuron-glia interactions. In *Glial–neuronal interaction*, vol. 633, ed. N. J. Abbot, New York Academy of Science New York: pp. 105–112.

46. Chamak, B., Fellous, A., Glowinski, J., and Prochiantz, A. 1987. MAP2 expression and neuritic outgrowth and branching are coregulated through region specific neuro-astroglial interactions. *J. Neuroski.* 7:3163–3170.

47. Pollerberg, G. E., Burridge, K., Krebs, K. E., Goodman, S. R., and Schachner, M. 1987. The 180-kD component of the neural cell adhesion molecule N-CAM is involved in cell–cell contacts and cytoskeleton–membrane interactions. *Cell Tissue Res.* 250:227–236.

48. Acheson, A., and Thoenen, H. 1983. Cell contact-mediated regulation of tyrosine hydroxylase synthesis in cultured bovine adrenal chromaffin cells. *J. Cell Biol.* 97:925–928.

49. Acheson, A., and Rutishauser, U. 1988. Neural cell adhesion molecule regulates cell contact-mediated changes in choline acetyltransferase activity of embryonic chick sympathetic neurons. *J. Cell Biol.* 106:479–486.

50. Schuch, U., Lohse, M. J., and Schachner, M. 1989. Neural cell adhesion molecules influence second messenger systems. *Neuron* 3:13–20.

51. Ingraham, C. A., and McCarthy, K. D. 1989. Plasticity of process-bearing glial cell cultures from neonatal rat cerebral cortical tissue. *J. Neurosci.* 9:63–69.

52. Saneto, R. P., and De Vellis, J. 1985. Characterization of cultured rat oligodendrocytes proliferating in serum-free, chemically defined medium. *Proc. Natl. Acad. Sci. USA* 82:3509–3513.

53. Raff, M. C., Williams, B. P., and Miller, R. H. 1984. The in vitro differentiation of a bipotential glial progenitor cell. *EMBO J.* 3:1857–1864.

54. Keilhauer, G., Meier, D. H., Kuhlmann-Krieg, S., Nieke, J., and Schachner, M. 1985. Astrocytes support incomplete differentiation of an oligodendrocyte precursor cell. *EMBO J.* 4:2499–2504.

55. Aloisi, F., Agresti, C., D'Urso, D., and Levi, G. 1988. Differentiation of bipotential glial precursors

into oligodendrocytes is promoted by interaction with type-I astrocytes in cerebellar cultures. *Proc. Natl. Acad. Sci. USA* 85:6167–6171.

56. Frangakis, M., and Kimelberg, H. K. 1984. Dissociation of neonatal rat brain by dispase for preparation of primary astrocyte cultures. *Neurochem. Res.* 9:1689–1698.

57. O'Connor, E. R., Kimelberg, H. K., Keese, C. R., and Giaever, I. 1993. An electrical resistance method for measuring changes in monolayer cultures applied to astrocyte swelling. *Am. J. Physiol.* 264:c47–c48.

58. Oyake, Y., Tanaka, M., Kubo, H., and Cichibu, H. 1966. Neuropathological studies on organic mercury poisoning with special reference to the staining and distribution of mercury granules. *Adv. Neurol. Sci.* 10:744–750.

59. Garman, R. H., Weiss, B., and Evans, H. L. Alkylmercurial encephalopathy in the monkey: A histopathologic and autoradiographic study. *Acta Neuropathol.* 32:61–74.

60. Rodier, P. M., Aschner, M., and Sager, P. R. 1984. Mitotic arrest in the developing CNS after prenatal exposure to methylmercury. *Neurobehav. Toxicol. Teratol.* 6:379–385.

61. Choi, B. H., Cho, K. H., and Lapham L. W. 1981. Effects of methylmercury on human fetal neurons and astrocytes in vitro: A time lapse cinematographic, phase and electron microscopic study. *Environ. Res.* 24:61–74.

62. Choi. B. H. 1983. Effects of prenatal methylmercury poisoning upon growth and development of fetal central nervous system. In *Reproductive and developmental toxicity of metals*, eds. T. W. Clarkson, G. F. Nordberg, and P. R. Sager, pp. 473–495. New York: Plenum Press.

63. Reuhl, K. R. and Chang, L. W. 1979. Effects of methylmercury on the development of the nervous system: A review. *Neurotoxicology* 1:21–55.

64. Rakic, P. 1972. Mode of cell migration to the superficial layers of fetal monkey neocortex. *J. Comp. Neurol.* 145:61–84.

65. Rothstein, A., and Mack, E. 1991. Actions of mercurials on cell volume regulation of dissociated MDCK cells. *Am. J. Physiol.* 260:C113–C121.

66. Rothstein, A. 1970. Sulfhydryl groups in membrane structure and function. In *Current topics in membrane and transport*, eds. F. Bronner and A. Kleinzeller, pp. 135–176. New York: Academic Press.

67. Aschner, M., Eberle, N., Miller, K., and Kimelberg, H. K. 1990. Interaction of methylmercury with rat primary astrocyte cultures: Effects on rubidium uptake and efflux and induction of swelling. *Brain Res.* 530:245–250.

68. Brookes, N., and Kristt, D. A. 1989. Inhibition of amino acid transport and protein synthesis by HgCl$_2$ and methylmercury in astrocytes: Selectivity and reversibility. *J. Neurochem.*, 53:1228–1237.

69. Choi, D. W. 1988. Glutamate neurotoxicity and diseases of the nervous system. *Neuron* 1:623–634.

70. Hertz, L. 1979. Functional interactions between neurons and astrocytes 1. Turnover and metabolism of putative amino acid transmitters. *Prog. Neurobiol.* 13:277–323.

71. Waniewski, R. A., and Martin, D. L. 1986. Exogenous glutamate is metabolized to glutamine and exported by primary astrocyte cultures. *J. Neurochem.* 47:304–313.

72. Kimelberg, H. K., Pang, S., and Treble, D. H. 1989. Excitatory amino-acid stimulated uptake of ^{22}Na$^+$ in primary astrocyte cultures. *J. Neurosci.* 9:1141–1149.

73. Kägi, J. H. R. 1991. Overview of metallothionein. In *Methods in enzymology*, vol. 205, *Metallobiochemistry*, part B, *Metallothionein and related molecules*, eds. J. F. Riordan and B. F. Vallee, pp. 613–626. New York: Academic Press.

74. Dunn, M. A., Blalock, T. L., and Cousins, R. J. 1987. Metallothionein. *Proc. Soc. Exp. Biol. Med.* 185:107–119.

75. Tiffany-Castiglioni, E. 1993. Cell culture models for lead toxicity in neuronal and glial cells. *Neurotoxicology* 14:513–536.

76. Blaauwgeers, H. G., Sillevis-Smitt, P. A., DeJong J. M., and Troost, D. 1993. Distribution of metallothionein in the human central nervous system. *Glia* 8:62–70.

Chapter Twenty-one

ALTERED ANGIOTENSIN-INDUCED DRINKING AS A NONINVASIVE BEHAVIORAL BIOMARKER OF NEONATAL GLUTAMIC ACID NEUROTOXICITY IN THE RAT

Florence A. Caputo and Andrew C. Scallet

Early postnatal administration of monosodium glutamate (MSG) eventually results in stunted growth, hyperinsulinemia, reproductive abnormalities, and obesity in the adult rodent. These conditions are due to circumventricular organ (CVO) and hypothalamic damage. The circulating neurohormone angiotensin II (AII) binds to AII receptors located outside the blood–brain barrier in the hypothalamus and CVOs. Exogenous AII has been shown to result in a robust drinking response, even in water-satiated rats. Currently, few noninvasive procedures exist to determine the presence of an MSG lesion. Thus, the present study was designed to test our hypothesis that AII administration would fail to increase water consumption in MSG-treated (CVO-damaged) rats. If AII is ineffective in the presence of a MSG lesion, then damage by MSG (or other neurotoxicants) to vulnerable CVO regions unprotected by the blood–brain barrier might be inferred.

Male Sprague-Dawley pups were injected with either MSG or saline on postnatal d 1, 3, 5, 7 and 9. Drinking tests were conducted in adulthood, and prior treatment with MSG resulted in a shift to the right of the dose-response curve for AII-induced drinking. Thus, the AII-induced drinking response may be a sensitive, noninvasive method for detecting CVO/hypothalamic damage produced by MSG or other neurotoxicants.

INTRODUCTION

Numerous reports have shown that early postnatal administration of monosodium glutamate (MSG) results in various abnormalities, such as stunted growth,[17] hyperinsulinemia,[23] impairments in analgesic response,[1] reproductive abnormalities,[16,17,20–22] and obesity.[2,10,17] These conditions can be traced to damage of the hypothalamus and other brain circumventricular organs (CVOs). Specific areas known to sustain damage after neonatal MSG administration include the preoptic area (POA), the arcuate nucleus (AH) of the hypothalamus, the median eminence (ME), the area postrema (AP), and the subfornical organ (SFO).[4,14,17,18]

The hypothalamus and CVOs are of considerable interest in the area of blood pressure and body fluid homeostasis.[8,24] The principal neurochemicals involved in blood pressure and fluid

This research was supported in part by an appointment to the Postgraduate Research Program at the National Center for Toxicological Research administered by the Oak Ridge Institute for Science and Education through an interagency agreement between the U.S. Department of Energy and the U.S. Food and Drug Administration.

homeostasis are thought to activate the renin-angiotensin system (RAS).[12] CVOs, such as the SFO and organum vasculosum laminae terminalis (OVLT), as well as various hypothalamic nuclei, have been implicated in the control of angiotensin (AII) induced drinking and have been shown to contain AII receptors,[3,24–26] most of which are located outside the blood–brain barrier (BBB) where they can be acted on by circulating AII.

A number of neurochemical abnormalities have been measured in the hypothalamus (as defined and dissected according to Glowinski and Iverson[7]) and CVOs after neonatal MSG administration. Among these alterations, reductions in adrenocorticotropic hormone (ACTH) and β-endorphin-like material in the mediobasal hypothalamus, the medial preoptic nucleus, and the amygdala have been reported. Reduced hypothalamic β-endorphin levels reported by Krieger et al.[11] have been confirmed by Hong et al.[9] Thus, a decrease in β-endorphin content is a reliable neurochemical measure of hypothalamic damage due to neonatal MSG administration. AII has also been reported to cause release of ACTH and β-endorphin from the anterior pituitary.[19]

Currently, β-endorphin content provides a sensitive method for assessing MSG-induced damage to the hypothalamus. However, there are few noninvasive behavioral procedures of similar sensitivity for determining the presence of a MSG lesion. Neonatal administration of MSG is known to damage areas containing AII receptors and hypothesized to mediate AII-induced drinking responses. Therefore, the primary aim of the present study was to determine whether MSG-induced damage could be assessed by monitoring drinking responses after administration of AII. We also intended to utilize the selective lesioning properties of MSG to better characterize the role of the CVOs in AII-mediated drinking responses. Specifically, we hypothesized that AII would be an ineffective dipsogen in the MSG-lesioned rat.

METHODS

Animals and Housing

Male Sprague-Dawley pups from the colony at the National Center for Toxicological Research (NCTR) were separated, and cross-fostered randomly (8 pups/dam) on the day of birth. On postnatal day (PND) 1, half of the pups were injected with MSG, 2 mg/g sc, while the other half received saline. On PND 3, 5, 7, and 9 MSG-injected pups were given 4 mg/g sc of a 40% (w/v) solution of MSG. The saline-treated animals were further split into two groups, one receiving the traditional 0.9% sc sodium chloride (NaCl) solution, while the other half received an injection of NaCl, which was iso-osmotic with the MSG solution (2.14 M). The two saline groups were included to determine whether early exposure to solutions of differing osmolarity would impact our behavioral results. All pups with a particular dam received the same treatment to prevent unequal access to maternal milk. Pups were allowed to remain with the dam until PND 21, at which time they were singly housed in hanging wire cages in a temperature-controlled room (24 ± 2°C) on a 12:12, light:dark schedule. Food pellets (NIH 31, vitamin fortified) and distilled water were available ad libitum, except during testing sessions. Animals were also handled daily to habituate subjects and minimize the effects of handling on test days. All drinking tests were conducted between PND 91 and 131.

Drinking Tests

Acute drinking tests were conducted in the animals' home cage in the middle of the light period. During drinking tests, food was removed from the front of the cage, and the water bottle was replaced with a graduated (±0.1 ml) plastic tube with a sipper attachment. Water intake was recorded volumetrically at 15, 30, and 60 min postinjection with either AII or 0.9% saline. Animals were administered the dipsogens subcutaneously in the following order: AII 25 μg/kg, AII 100 μg/kg, and AII 50 μg/kg. Doses of isoproterenol (25 and 100 μg/kg) were included as an alternate dipsogen acting by a separate mechanism to activate the renin-angiotensin system. Drug doses to produce a dipsogenic response were based upon previous reports in the literature.[5] A minimum of 48 h was allowed between drinking tests to minimize drug carryover effects. Animals were given isotonic (0.9%) NaCl sc on separate test days before and after each new dose of drug to ensure that all water intake returned to their baseline levels prior to further drug administration.

Drugs

Angiotensin II was the acetate salt of the human sequence, and isoproterenol hydrochloride (ISOP) was the *d,l*-racemate. Both were obtained from Sigma Chemical Co., St. Louis, MO.

Statistics

Data were analyzed utilizing a two-way analysis of variance (ANOVA) with repeated measures on one factor (Sigma Stat statistical software) with the Newman-Keuls test for post-hoc comparisons. The significance level was set at $p < .05$.

RESULTS

ANOVA revealed that there was no significant difference in water intake between the pups that had received isotonic (0.9%) NaCl postnatally and those that received iso-osmotic NaCl postnatally, when 0.9% NaCl was given as the dipsogen [$F(2,19) = 0.49, p > .05$]. Therefore, the data from the two groups of NaCl-treated animals were combined into a single control group for further analysis.

Also, due to the unexpected ISOP-induced mortality (7/10 MSG and 1/10 saline subjects died after 100 μg/kg ISOP), the overall ANOVA was based on only 5 groups of dipsogens (saline; AII 25 μg/kg; AII 50 μg/kg; AII 100 μg/kg; ISOP 25 μg/kg).

ANOVA with the combined controls (control, $n = 12$; MSG, $n = 10$) revealed no significant main effect of postnatal MSG treatment [$F(1,20) = 3.44, p = .079$] on overall water intake. However, there was a significant main effect of dipsogen [$F(4,80) = 23.75, p < .001$], as well as an MSG treatment × dipsogen interaction [$F(4,80) = 4.95, p = .001$]. As predicted (Figure 1), control rats given 0.9% saline as a dipsogen drank significantly less than controls given either 50 μg/kg AII or 100 μg/kg AII subcutaneously. There was no significant difference in water intake between controls given saline as a dipsogen versus those controls given either 25 μg/kg AII or 25 μg/kg ISOP.

Animals treated neonatally with MSG and given saline as a dipsogen drank significantly less than animals exposed to MSG neonatally and given 100 μg/kg AII sc as the dipsogen. However, there was no significant difference in water intake between rats given MSG neonatally and saline as the dipsogen versus those rats exposed neonatally to MSG and given either 25 μg/kg AII, 50 μg/kg AII, or 25 μg/kg ISOP.

Water intake in control rats given 100 μg/kg AII sc as the dipsogen was significantly greater than rats given MSG neonatally and 100 μg/kg AII sc as the dipsogen. All other combinations of control rats versus those given MSG neonatally and tested with the remaining dipsogens (i.e., saline; 25 μg/kg AII; 50 μg/kg AII; and 25 μg/kg ISOP) were not significantly different. Thus, animals exposed neonatally to MSG were less responsive to exogenous administration of high doses of AII (100 μg/kg) than those exposed neonatally to saline.

DISCUSSION

Since there was such a high mortality rate in our MSG-treated rats after administration of 100 μg/kg ISOP (a dose that previously had not been lethal[5]), it is likely that some aspect of the cardiovascular system was compromised in the MSG-treated animals. ISOP is a mixed β1- and β2-adrenergic agonist, which induces vasodilation resulting in a decrease in blood pressure, sensed by the juxtaglomerular apparatus in the kidney, and results in a subsequent release of renin. ISOP is also known to bind directly to receptors located on the kidney to induce the release of renin and to receptors located on the heart to increase heart rate.[6,13] No animals died after administration of AII, which is known to increase blood pressure. Therefore, it is suspected that the mortality noted in our MSG-treated rats after ISOP administration was due to the induced hypotension, rather than the eventual hypertension resulting from activation of the RAS. In

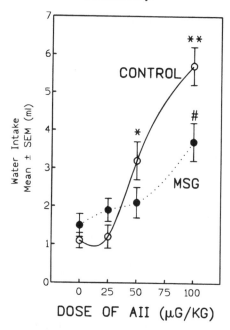

Figure 1. The effects of subcutaneous doses between 0 and 100 μg/kg of angiotensin II (AII) on cumulative 90-min water intake (mean ± SEM in ml). Asterisk indicates dose as low as 50 μg/kg of AII significantly increased water intake ($p < .05$ compared to a saline injection as dipsogen) in control rats. Hash mark (#) indicates a higher dose of 100 μg/kg AII was needed to significantly increase drinking ($p < .05$ compared to a saline injection as dipsogen) in MSG-treated rats. Double asterisk indicates a dose of 100 μg/kg AII greatly increased drinking ($p < .01$ compared to a saline injection as dipsogen) in control rats. The AII effect in control rats was also significantly greater ($p < .05$) than the effect in MSG-treated rats.

addition, all animals died in less than 5 min after administration of ISOP, a time in which ISOP is known to have its most potent hypotensive effects.[5]

Recently Millan et. al[15] have reported that the CVOs and paraventricular nucleus of the hypothalamus show AII receptor binding on PND 2 and that this level remains constant throughout development. In the present study, rats treated neonatally with MSG drank significantly less than control rats after administration of the highest dose of AII. Similarly, control rats showed a significant increase in water intake above baseline at a dose of 50 μg/kg AII, while the MSG-treated rats did not show such a significant effect. Thus, there is a diminished response to the effects of AII on water intake in animals thought to have CVO and hypothalamic lesions. These results support the hypothesis that the MSG-treated rats have a loss of AII receptors in the hypothalamus and CVOs.

The attenuated drinking response to AII administration in rats treated neonatally with MSG suggests that this response may be useful as a sensitive, noninvasive method for determining the CVO/hypothalamic damage following exposure to MSG, or perhaps to other neurotoxicants.

REFERENCES

1. Badillo-Martinez, D., Nicotera, N., Butler, P. D., Kirchgessner, A. L., and Bodnar, R. J. 1984. Impairments in analgesic, hypothermic, and glucoprivic stress responses following neonatal monosodium glutamate. *Neuroendocrinology* 38:438–446.
2. Betran, M. A., Estornell, E., Barber, T., and Cabo, J. 1992. Nitrogen metabolism in obesity induced by monosodium-L-glutamate in rats. *Int. J. Obesity* 16:555–564.
3. Bunnemann, B., Fuxe, K., and Ganten, D. 1992. The brain renin-angiotensin system: Localization and general significance. *J. Cardiovasc. Pharmacol.* 19(S6):S51–S62.
4. Burde, R. M., Schainker, B., and Kayes, J. 1971. Acute effect of oral and subcutaneous administration of monosodium glutamate on the arcuate nucleus of the hypothalamus in mice and rats. *Nature* 233:58–60.
5. Caputo, F. A., Rowland, N. E., and Fregly, M. J. 1992. Angiotensin-related intakes of water and NaCl in Fischer 344 and Sprague-Dawley rats. *Am. J. Physiol.* 262:R382–R388.
6. Duling, B. R. 1983. Integrated nephron function. In *Physiology*, eds. R. M. Berne and M. N. Levy, pp. 861–876. St. Louis: C. V. Mosby.
7. Glowinski, J., and Iversen, L. L. 1966. Regional studies of cathecholamines in the rat brain. I. The disposition of ^{3}H-norepinephrine, ^{3}H-dopamine, and ^{3}H-DOPA in various regions of the brain. *J. Neurochem.* 13:655–669.
8. Harkness, J. E., and Wagner, J. E. 1983. *The biology and medicine of rabbit and rodents*, 2nd ed. Philadelphia: Lea & Febiger.
9. Hong, H.-S., Lowe, C., Squibb, R. R., and Lamartiniere, C. A. 1981. Monosodium glutamate exposure in the neonate alters hypothalamic and pituitary neuropeptide levels in the adult. *Reg. Peptides* 2:347–352.
10. Kanarek, R. B., Meyers, J., Meade, R. G., and Mayer, J. 1979. Juvenile-onset obesity and deficits in caloric regulation in MSG-treated rats. *Pharmacol. Biochem. Behav.* 10:717–721.
11. Krieger, D. T., Liotta, A. S., Nicholsen, G., and Kizer, J. S. 1979. Brain ACTH and endorphin reduced in rats with monosodium glutamate-induced arcuate nuclear lesions. *Nature* 278:562–563.
12. Leenan, F. H. H., and McDonald, R. H. 1974. The effect of isoproterenol on blood pressure, plasma renin activity and water intake in rats. *Eur. J. Pharmacol.* 26:129–135.
13. Lefkowitz, R. J. 1974. Selectivity in beta-adrenergic responses; Clinical implications. *Circulation* 49:783–786.
14. Lemkey-Johnson, N., and Reynolds, W. A. 1974. Nature and extent of brain lesions in mice related to ingestion of monosodium glutamate. *J. Neuropathol. Exp. Neurol.* 33:74–97.
15. Millan, M. A., Kiss, A., and Aguilera, G. 1991. Developmental changes in brain angiotensin II receptors in the rat. *Peptides* 12:723–737.
16. Nemeroff, C. B., Konkol, R. J., Bissette, G., Youngblood, W., Martin, J. B., Brazeau, P., Rone. M. S., Prange, A. J., Jr., Breese, G. R., and Kizer, J. S. 1977. Analysis of the disruption in hypothalamic-pituitary regulation in rats treated neonatally with monosodium L-glutamate (MSG): Evidence for the involvement of tuberoinfundibular cholinergic and dopaminergic systems in neuroendocrine regulation. *Endocrinology* 101:613–622.
17. Olney, J. W. 1969. Brain lesions, obesity, and other disturbances in mice treated with monosodium glutamate. *Science* 164:719–721.
18. Phelix, C. F., and Hartle, D. K. 1990. Systemic glutamate induces degeneration of a subpopulation of tyrosine hydroxylase-immunoreactive neurons in the rat area postrema. *Brain Res.* 516:335–340.
19. Phillips, M. I. 1987. Functions of angiotensin in the central nervous system. *Annu. Rev. Physiol.* 49:413–435.
20. Pizzi, W. J., Barnhart, J. E., and Fanslow, D. J. 1977. Monosodium glutamate administration to the newborn reduces reproductive ability in female and male mice. *Science* 196:452–454.
21. Redding, T. W., Schally, A. V., Arimura, A., and Wakabayashi, I. 1971. Effect of monosodium glutamate on some endocrine functions. *Neuroendocrinology* 8:245–255.
22. Rodriguez-Sierra, J. F., Blaustein, J. D., Blake, C. A., Clough, R. W., and Elias, K. A. 1982. A decrease of cytosol estrogen receptors in the hypothalamus after treatment of neonatal rats with glutamate. *Exp. Brain Res.* 48:272–278.
23. Scallet, A. C., and Olney, J. W. 1986. Components of hypothalamic obesity: Bipiperidyl-mustard lesions and hyperphagia to monosodium glutamate-induced hyperinsulinemia. *Brain Res.* 374:380–384.
24. Simpson, J. B. 1981. The circumventricular organs and the central actions of angiotensin. *Neuroendocrinology* 32:248–256.
25. Song, K., Allen, A. M., Paxinos, G., and Mendelsohn, F. A. O. 1992. Mapping of angiotensin II receptor subtype heterogeneity in rat brain. *J. Comp. Neurol.* 316:467–484.
26. Van Houten, M., Schiffrin, E. L., Mann, J. F. E., Posner, B. I., and Boucher, R. 1980. Radioautographic localization of specific binding sites for blood-borne angiotensin II in the rat brain. *Brain Res.* 186:480–485.

Chapter Twenty-two

CELL CULTURES FOR SCREENING OF ANTIESTERASE COMPOUNDS

Marion Ehrich

In vitro systems have potential use for screening toxic chemicals when they contain the specific targets for the toxicants. Although specific targets have not been defined for many neurotoxicants, they have been identified for organophosphates (Ops) and carbamates, compounds that inhibit neuronal cell esterases. Of particular importance are acetylcholinesterase (AChE), inhibition of which causes acute symptoms of cholinergic poisoning in humans and animals, and neuropathy target esterase (NTE), which may be inhibited shortly after exposure to some Ops, although progressive, irreversible delayed neuropathy does not appear for weeks. Neuronal cell lines of human (SH-SY5Y) and mouse (NB42A3) origin contain both AChE and NTE. These enzymes can be inhibited by exposure to direct-acting toxicants that target these enzymes, with only those causing OPIDN capable of notably inhibiting NTE (5 of 5 from a total of 17 compounds tested at concentration of 10^{-5} M). Although there were some species differences in esterase inhibition, notable NTE inhibition was seen with the same compounds (DFP, mipafox, cyclic totyl saligenin phosphate, cyclic phenyl saligenin phosphate, triphenyl phosphite) both in the human and mouse cell lines. Direct-acting OPs that cause acute cholinergic poisoning were capable of inhibiting AChE in both cell lines. These studies indicate that neuroblastoma cells respond in a similar manner to animal tissue when exposed to antiesterase compounds.

INTRODUCTION

Cells in culture provide an in vitro alternative in the assessment of neurotoxicity, and increased use has been suggested.[1,2] This type of test system has several advantages, including the potential to screen relatively large numbers of chemicals in a relatively short period of time and with considerably less cost than if such screening were done in animal models. In addition to increased efficiency associated with toxicity studies, data could be obtained from human cells, and it is the human that is the species of interest in risk assessment. Currently, extrapolation from animal studies is needed, and species differences can be notable.

Several factors need to be considered if neurotoxicity evaluations are to be done in cell culture systems as a potential alternative and/or adjunct to studies done in animal models. As in vivo, in vitro systems should use cells of the nervous system for study (or, at least, use cell lines in

The author gratefully acknowledges the collaborative scientific association with Dr. Bellina Veronesi, U.S. EPA Health Effects Research Laboratory, Neurotoxicology Division, and the technical assistance of Linda Correll and Kent Carlson, Virginia-Maryland Regional College of Veterinary Medicine, without whom this work could not have been done. This work has been primarily supported by the U.S. Environmental Protection Agency (68D80098; 3D0919NAEX; 2D1112NAEX; 1D1381NAEX). The work included has been subjected to agency review, but it does not necessarily reflect the views of the agency, and no official endorsement should be inferred. Mention of trade names or commercial products does not consist of endorsement or recommendation for use.

which similarities with cells of the nervous system have been defined, e.g., PC12). Endpoints should identify what is toxic to the neural cells, but, most importantly, these endpoints should include markers that are unique to the nervous system. Examples of markers that are relatively unique for the nervous system include enzymes for the synthesis and degradation of neurotransmitters, receptors for neurotransmitters, and cytoskeletal proteins uniquely located in the nervous system (e.g., neurofilaments).[1]

There is a wide variety of chemical substances that target the nervous system, and toxicity can result from a number of different mechanisms. A single in vitro screening procedure in a cell culture system is, therefore, unlikely to identify all neurotoxicants. Organophosphates (OPs) and carbamates, however, are classes of neurotoxicants that have particular potential to be screened in vitro using cell culture systems because their cellular targets (esterase enzymes) have been identified. OPs and carbamates are widely used in agriculture and industry as insecticides, lubricants, and plasticizing agents. In addition, some OPs and carbamates are used as therapeutic agents and other are used as agents for chemical warfare. OPs and carbamates both have capability to inhibit cellular esterases. Of particular importance is acetylcholinesterase (AChE), the enzyme responsible for the degradation of the neurotransmitter acetylcholine. It is through inhibition of AChE that OPs and carbamates are effective as insecticides and therapeutic agents. OP- and/or carbamate-induced inhibition of AChE causes increased availability of the neurotransmitter acetylcholine and subsequent stimulation of muscarinic and nicotinic receptors, as well as acetylcholine receptors of the central nervous system. Neurotoxicity is a result of overstimulation of these receptors, with resultant bradycardia, excessive respiratory secretions, diarrhea, flaccid paralysis, and/or convulsions. Such overstimulation can be serious, as it has the potential to cause death in humans within a short time after exposure.[1]

In addition to the neurotoxicity resulting from inhibition of AChE, some OPs have capability to induce a delayed, progressive, irreversible neurophathy. OP-induced delayed neuropathy (OPIDN) occurs days to weeks after significant inhibition of another neural esterase, neuropathy target esterase (NTE, neurotoxic esterase), in susceptible animal species, including humans.[3–5] Current evaluation of the safety of esterase inhibitors, such as OPs and carbamates, is done in animal models, using biochemical, behavioral, and morphological endpoints. A primary indicator of OP and carbamate neurotoxicity is their capability to inhibit AChE. In addition, for OPs, further testing must be done to establish the potential of the chemical to cause OPIDN. The hen is the recognized animal model for such studies, primarily because ataxia associated with OPIDN is notably evident in this species.[6] Rodents also develop OPIDN, but the neuropathy is not associated with notable ataxia, and the lesions only occur in a restricted area of the spinal cord and are similar to background lesions that occur in this species.[7,8] In addition to morphological lesions, OPs are examined for their capability to cause inhibition of NTE, as inhibitions $>70\%$ precede neuropathogy in both hens and rats.[4,5,9,10]

Because the testing of antiesterase compounds in rodents and hens is time-consuming and expensive, and because the markers that indicate the potential for neurotoxic effects have been identified (AChE and NTE inhibition), it appears reasonable to suggest that cells in culture could be used as an in vitro alternative for evaluation of antiesterase compounds. There is particular advantage in use of cell culture systems for the identification of OPs that cause OPIDN, as testing in animals is costly and time-consuming. In addition, an animal species (the hen) that is not closely related to humans is being used for testing. For screening in vitro, human cells could be used.

The objectives of our studies to examine cell cultures for the screening of antiesterase compounds were: (1) to determine if cultured cells, especially those of human origin, would be useful for evaluation of antiesterase compounds; (2) to identify cell lines useful in such studies; and (3) to identify practical advantages and limitations associated with use of cell cultures for this purpose.

MATERIALS AND METHODS

Preliminary studies examined esterase activities in a variety of cell lines, including neural cells of human origin (SK-N-MC and IMR32 from the American Type Culture Collection, Rockville, MD; SH-SY5Y, a clone of SK-N-MC,[11] from Dr. T. Rowles, Virginia-Maryland Regional College of Veterinary Medicine), neural and neural-like cells of rodent origin (NB41A3 and PC12 from the American Type Culture Collection), and human lymphoblastoid cells (AHH-1 TK and MCL-5, the derivative cell line in which 5 cDNAs of the human P-450 genome had been added, gift from C. Crespi, Gentest Inc., Woburn, MA).[2]

These cell lines were grown in medium supplemented with fetal bovine serum, 10% when grown in minimal essential medium (MEM) with Earle's salts and L-glutamine and L-leucine or 15% when grown in Ham's F12 nutrient medium. Cells were seeded at 5×10^4 cells/ml and fed every 3–4 d, with harvest when 90% confluent. At that time, they were disassociated with trypsin, centrifuged, washed with phosphate-buffered saline (PBS), and resuspended in PBS at 1×10^7 cells/ml.[13–18] Esterase determinations were done spectrophotometrically in microassay,[19] with acetylthiocholine as substrate for acetylcholinesterase (AChE), phenyl valerate as substrate for carboxylesterase (CbxE, an enzyme that contributes to the degradation of OPs),[13] and phenyl valerate in the presence of mipafox and/or paraoxan as substrate for neurotoxic esterase (NTE). Cytotoxic effects were determined by loss of capability to retain neutral red stain,[14] or by capability to take up trypan blue dye.[18]

A series of OPs were examined for capability to inhibit esterases in human and mouse neuroblastoma cells (SH-SY5Y and NB41A3, respectively). For these studies, cells were harvested and resuspended in saline at 1×10^7 cells/ml before incubation for 1 h with 10^{-5} M OP added as a 100× concentrate. OPIDN-producing compounds included in the study were diisopropylphosphorofluoridate (DFP, Aldrich Chemical Co., Milwaukee, WI), mipafox (N,N'-diisopropylphosphorodiamide fluoridate, Lark Enterprises, Webster, MA), triphenyl phosphate (TPPi, ChemService, West Chester, PA), phenyl saligenin cyclic phosphate (PSP, Lark Enterprises), tolyl saligenin phosphate (TSP, Lark Enterprises), tri-*ortho*-tolylphosphate (TOTP, the protoxicant congener of TSP, Lark Enterprises), and leptophos (4-bromo-2,5-dichlorophenyl methyl phenylphosphonothionate, Chem-Services), also a protoxicant.[4,6,20] Other OPs examined for esterase inhibition included parathion (O,O-diethyl 4-nitropenyl phosphoothioate, Chem-Services) and its active -P=O congener paraoxon (O,O-diethyl 4-nitrophenyl phosphate, ChemServices), malathion [5-(1,2-dicarbethoxyethyl) O,O-dimethyl dithiophosphate, American Cyanamid, Pearl River, NY] and its active -P–O congener malaoxon, dichlorvos [O,O-dimethyl O-(2,2-dichlorovinyl) phosphate, Fermenta Animal Products, Kansas City, MO], fenthion [O,O-dimethyl O-(4-methylmercapto-3-methylphenyl)thionophosphate, ChemServices], fenitrothion (O,O-dimethyl 3-methyl-4-nitrophenyl phosphorothionate, ChemServices), and chlorpyrifos (O,O-diethyl O-3,5,6-trichloro-2-pyridyl phosphorothioate, ChemServices). Cytotoxicity was examined using a series of concentrations up to 10^{-3} M and times of exposure of at least 24 h, with mostly studies extending to 72 h.

RESULTS AND DISCUSSION

All cell lines that were examined for esterase activities (SK-N-SK, IMB32, SH-SY5Y, NB41A3, PC12, AHH TK, MCL-5) expressed activities of acetylcholinesterase (AChE), neuropathy target esterase (NTE), and carboxylesterase (CbxE), an enzyme that contributes to the detoxification of OPs.[3] Although NTE activities were relatively similar among the cell lines and relatively similar to that seen in animal (hen) tissue, there was wide variability among the cell lines in activity of CbxE and AChE. AChE activities were considerably less in all cell lines than in hen brain.[13,14,17,18] In the human neuroblastoma cell line SH-SY5Y esterase-specific activities were 9 ± 2 nmol/min/mg protein for AChE, 21 ± 3 nmol/min/mg protein for NTE, and 61 ± 8 nmol/min/mg protein or CbxE. These values were 16 ± 2, 5 ± 1, and 31 ± 4 nmol/min/mg protein for AChE, NTE, and CbxE in mouse neuroblastoma cells NB41A3, respectively. Activities of these esterases in hen brain were 187 ± 3, 26 ± 2, and 167 ± 10 nmol/min/mg protein, respectively.[13,17,21] Comparing the relationship of the activities of NTE and CbxE in cell cultures to animal tissues indicated that the proportion of NTE to total CbxE in the human SH-SY5Y cell line more closely resembled the proportion of NTE to total CbxE tissue from the hen,[21] which is the animal model for OPIDN.[6] These proportions differed from those of the mouse NB41A3 cell line and rat tissue. Human beings and hens are susceptible to both ataxia and morphological changes that occur after exposure to NTE-inhibiting OPs that cause OPIDN; rodents do not develop notable ataxia.[3,4,6,20] Exposure to relatively high concentrations of test compounds were necessary before effects, as determined using the neutral red assay or trypan blue dye exclusion, were noted. These indicators of cytotoxicity were unaltered unless exposure times exceeded 24 h and concentrations were greater than 0.5×10^{-4} M.[14,18] When comparing sensitivity of cell lines to cytotoxic effects, a species difference was noted with the neutral red assay, as we found mouse NB41A3 cells more sensitive than human SH-SY5Y cells to a series of OPs that included parathion, fenthion, and DFP.[14] Parathion and fenthion are protoxicants, and therefore require oxidation before they are capable of inhibiting AChE[3].

Screening of a variety of OPs indicated that NTE inhibition could be used to identify direct-acting OPs that cause OPIDN in animal models. Figure 1 shows this in the human cell line SH-SY5Y, as mipafox, DFP, triphenyl phosphite, PSP, and TSP all caused notable NTE inhibition. This inhibition was not seen with protoxicants that cause OPIDN (TOTP, leptophos) or with any OPs that do not cause OPIDN (parathion, a protoxicant, and its active metabolite, paraoxon; malathion and its active metabolite, malaoxon; active OP dichlorvos; and protoxicants fenthion, fenitrothion, and chlorpyrifos). This study indicated that human cells could be used to detect OPs directly capable of causing OPIDN in that species. The extent of NTE inhibition in mouse neuroblastoma cell line NB41A3 could also distinguish direct-acting OPs that cause OPIDN because NTE was also more notably inhibited by such compounds in this cell line (data not shown).

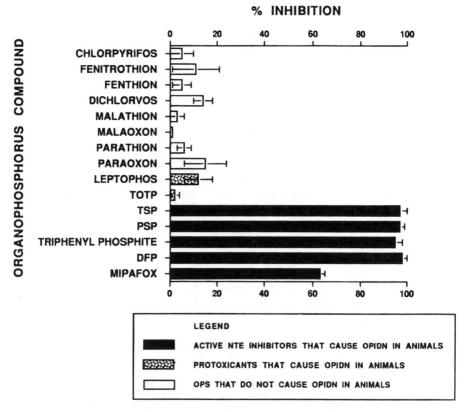

Figure 1. NTE inhibition in SH-SY5Y cells exposed to OPs. Human neuroblastoma cells (1×10^7 cells/ml in saline) were exposed for 1 h to 10^{-5} M organophosphates. DFP, mipafox, TSP, triphenyl phosphite, and PSP are active NTE inhibitors and agents that induce OPIDN in anuimal models. TOTP and leptophos are protoxicants that cause OPIDN in animal models. The protoxicant parathion and its active congener, paraoxon, malathion, malaoxon, dichlovos, chlorpyrifos, fenthion, and fenitrothion do not induce OPIDN in the hen model. Results are expressed as mean ±SEM of results from 3–7 different days on which assays were done.

One hour of incubation with 10^{-5} M direct-acting OPs (DFP, paraoxon, PSP, TSP, chloryrifos-oxon, malaoxon, TPPi) resulted in >85% inhibition of AChE activities both in human and mouse neuroblastoma cells. Mipafox, also a direct-acting OP, but more noted for capability to cause OPIDN than for capability to inhibit AChE,[8] was less effective than the other compounds listed as an inhibitor of AChE in both human and mouse neuroblastoma cells, with inhibitions generally <50%. There were significant differences in inhibition in cells of various species origin with mipafox, TPPi, and malaoxon, with human cells more susceptible to mipafox and mouse cells more susceptible to TPPi and malaoxon. AChE was generally less affected by protoxicants than by direct-acting OPs in both cell lines. The inhibition of this enzyme was greater in mouse cells exposed to the protoxicants leptophos ($p < .05$) and chlorpyrifos ($p < .1$) and greater in human cells exposed to parathion ($p < .05$). Specific inhibition (>90%) of AChE in mouse and human neuroblastoma cells with 10^{-6} M 1,5-bis-(4-allyldimethyl ammonium phenyl)-pentan-3-one dibromide (Burroughs Wellcome, Research Triangle Park, NC) indicated that true, rather than pseudo-cholinesterase, was being measured in these cells. Iso-OMPA (tetraisopropylpyrophosphoamide, Sigma Chemical Co., St. Louis, MO), a specific inhibitor of pseudocholinesterase, did not inhibit AChE activity in either human or mouse neuroblastoma cells.[16]

Conclusions from the studies just described are as follows: (1) Cells in culture have the esterases that OPs and carbamates target in vivo; (2) these target esterases (AChE and NTE) can be inhibited in cultured cells by compounds that inhibit these esterases in animal models; (3) neuroactive OPs that cause OPIDN in animal models can be distinguished by their capability to inhibit NTE in cultured cells; and (4) inhibition of esterases occurs more quickly and at lower concentrations than does uptake of neutral red or trypan blue, indicating that neurotoxicity is occurring at concentrations less than responsible for cytotoxicity in neuroblastoma cells.

REFERENCES

1. Veronesi, B. 1992. In vitro screening batteries of neurotoxicants, *NeuroToxicology* 13:185–196.
2. Office of Technology Assessment, U.S. Congress. 1992. *Neurotoxicity: Identifying and controlling poisons of the nervous system.* OTA-BA-436. Washington, DC: U.S. Government Printing Office.
3. Ecobichon, D. J. 1991. Toxic effects of pesticides. In *Casarett and Doull's toxicology, the basic science of poisons,* 4th ed., eds. M. O. Amdur, J. Doull, and C. D. Klaassen, pp. 565–622. New York: Pergamon Press.
4. Johnson, M. K. 1982. The target for initiation of delayed neurotoxicity by organophosphorus esters: Biochemical studies and toxicological applications. In *Reviews in biochemical toxicology,* vol. 4, eds. E. Hodgson, J. R. Bend, and R. M. Philpot, pp. 141–212. New York: Elsevier.
5. Lotti, M. 1992. The pathogenesis of organophosphate polyneuropathy. *CRC Crit. Rev. Toxicol.* 21:465–488.
6. Abou-Donia, M. B. 1981. Organophosphorus ester-induced delayed neurotoxicity. *Annu. Rev. Pharmacol. Toxicol.* 21:511–548.
7. Veronesi, B. 1984. A rodent model of organophosphorus-induced delayed neuropathy, distribution of central (spinal cord) and peripheral nerve damage. *Neuropathol. Appl. Neurobiol.* 10:357–368.
8. Dyer, K. R., Jortner, B. S., Shell, L. G., and Ehrich, M. 1992. Comparative dose-response studies of organophosphorus ester-enduced delayed neuropathy in rats and hens administered mipafox. *Neurotoxicology* 13:745–756.
9. Ehrich, M., Jortner, B., and Padilla, S. 1993. Relationship of neuropathy target esterase inhibition to neuropathy and ataxia in hens given organophosphorus esters. *Chem. Biol. Interact.* 87:431–437.
10. Padilla, S., and Veronesi, B. 1985. The relationship between neurological damage and neurotoxic esterase inhibition in rats acutely exposed to tri-*ortho*-cresyl phosphate. *Toxicol. Appl. Pharmacol.* 78:78–87.
11. Ross, R. A., Spengler, B. A., and Biedler, J. L. 1983. Coordinate morphological and biochemical interconversion of human neuroblastoma cells. *J. Natl. Cancer Inst.* 71:741–749.
12. Crespi, C. L., Gonzalez, F. J., Steimel, D. T., Turner, T. R., Gelboin, H. V., Penman, B. W., and Langenbach, R. 1991. A metabolically competent human cell line expressing five cDNAs encoding procarcinogen-activating enzymes: Application to mutagenicity testing. *Chem. Res. Toxicol.* 4:566–572.
13. Veronesi, B., and Ehrich, M. 1993. Using neuroblastoma cell lines to examine organophosphate neurotoxicity. *In Vitro Toxicol.* 6:57–65.
14. Veronesi, B., and Ehrich, M. 1993. Differential cytotoxic sensitivity in mouse and human cell lines exposed to organophosphate insecticides. *Toxicol. Appl. Pharmacol.* 120:240–246.
15. Ehrich, M., Correll, L., and Veronesi, B. 1994. Neuropathy target esterase inhibition by organophosphorus esters in human neuroblastoma cells. *Neurotoxicology* 15:309–314.

16. Correll, L., Carlson, K., Wilcke, J., Veronesi, B., and Ehrich, M. Examination of culture conditions on esterase activities in human and mouse neuroblastoma cells. *In Vitro Toxicol.* 8:199–207.

17. Nostrandt, A. C., and Ehrich, M. 1992. Development of a model cell culture system in which to study early effects of neuropathy-inducing organophosphorus esters. *Toxicol. Lett.* 60:107–114.

18. Nostrandt, A. C., Rowles, T. K., and Ehrich, M. 1992. Cytotoxic effects of organophosphorus esters and other neurotoxic chemicals on cultured cells. *In Vitro Toxicol.* 5:127–136.

19. Correll, L., and Ehrich, M. 1991. A microassay method for neurotoxic esterase determinations. *Fundam. Appl. Toxicol.* 16:110–116.

20. Abou-Donia, M. B., and Lapadula, C. M. 1990. Mechanisms of organophosphorus ester induced delayed neurotoxicity: Type I and Type II. *Annu. Rev. Pharmacol. Toxicol.* 30:405–440.

21. Correll, L., and Ehrich, M. 1987. Comparative sensitivities of avian neural esterases to in vitro inhibition by organophosphorus compounds. *Toxicol. Lett.* 36:197–204.

Chapter Twenty-three

MECHANISTIC NEUROTOXICITY STUDIES USING PC12 CELLS

Gary E. Isom, A. G. Kanthasamy, and J. L. Borowitz

Development of efficacious in vitro toxicological models of the nervous system has proven difficult due to the complex physiology and biochemistry of the brain. To develop an in vitro cell model for mechanistic and toxicological screening, a well-characterized neuronal system is needed. The PC12 cell line is a popular neuronal model that can be employed for neurotoxicological studies. This clonal cell line, derived from a rat pheochromocytoma, expresses a number of neuronal properties useful for in vitro studies. The cells are electrically excitable, express a variety of functional polypeptide and neurotransmitter receptors, and secrete neurotransmitters. The syntheses, storage, and secretion of neurotransmitters is well characterized in this cell line, and the cells have been used for studies of neurosecretion, calcium and potassium channels, ion handling mechanisms, and proto-oncogene expression. Hence, the PC12 cell line serves as a well-studied neuronal model useful for examining the interaction of neurotoxic compounds with basic neuronal processes. Cyanide-induced neurotoxicity has been studied in detail in this cell line. By developing a comprehensive understanding of the effect of cyanide on basic neuronal processes, this cell line can be used as an in vitro neurotoxic screen in which a series of neurochemical markers in PC12 cells were used to evaluate potential anticyanide compounds. Several compounds have been identified that inhibit the neurochemical action of cyanide in PC12 cells and may be useful in vivo as cyanide antidotes. This application demonstrates that a well characterized cell model, on which detailed basic mechanistic information is available, can be used as an in vitro toxicological screen.

INTRODUCTION

The classic treatment of cyanide intoxication is based on the ability of sodium nitrite to generate methemoglobin, a cyanide scavenger, and sodium thiosulfate, a substrate for cyanide metabolism.[1] This antidotal combination is effective when the patient is treated immediately after poisoning. However, there is a clear need for a more effective, safer antidote that can be administered in the field. The present study was initiated in an effort to develop an in vitro assay that could screen a large number of potential antidotes in a cost-effective manner and minimize the use of animals. Since the primary target organ of cyanide is the central nervous system, the strategy was to develop a more comprehensive understanding of cyanide's action on the nervous system

This work was supported in part by the U.S. Army Medical Research and Development Command under contract DAMD17-89-9033 and National Institutes of Health grant ES04140. In conducting research using animals, the investigators adhered to the Guide for the Care and Use of Laboratory Animals, prepared by the Committee on Care and Use of Laboratory Animals of the Institute of Laboratory Animals Resources, National Research Council.

and then to develop a mechanistic based screen in a clonal cell line. Validation of the assay would be based on correlating animal data with that obtained in the screen battery.

Mechanism of Action of Cyanide

Cyanide produces a rapid effect on the nervous system, with seizures and loss of consciousness occurring within seconds of exposure to a lethal concentration.[1] In the past it was well accepted that the primary biochemical lesion produced by cyanide is inhibition of cytochrome oxidase, the terminal oxidase in oxidative phosphorylation. The result is a rapid decline in the cell's energy charge and gradual impairment of all active processes within the cell.[2] In the nervous system this would result in loss of cell homeostasis and function culminating in impaired neurological function. Antidotal development in the past has been directed toward removal of cyanide from cytochrome oxidase to reactivate oxidative metabolism and then metabolize cyanide to a nontoxic metabolite.[3] The goal of therapy is to restore normal metabolic function.

A number of recent studies have questioned the classic concept that cyanide toxicity results solely from cytochrome oxidase inhibition.[4] It has been reported that cyanide lethality can occur without significant inhibition of brain cytochrome oxidase, and in isolated brain slices, cyanide-induced inhibition of neurotransmission could be reversed within seconds by washing cyanide out of the tissue, whereas the energy deficit was not immediately reversed.[5] It is apparent that cyanide produces multiple actions on the nervous system that can be viewed as potential targets for antidotes (Table 1).

Following exposure to cyanide, cytosolic free Ca^{2+} is rapidly elevated and this event appears to play a central role in cyanide-induced neurotoxicity.[6] The rise in cytosolic free Ca^{2+} occurs within seconds and is attributed to multiple actions. In PC12 cells (a rat pheochromocytoma cell), cyanide activates voltage-sensitive calcium channels (VSCC) to initiate Ca^{2+} influx that can be blocked by calcium channel blockers.[7] Additionally, in cultured primary neurons from select brain areas, cyanide can activate the N-methyl-D-Aspartate NMDA glutamate receptor resulting in stimulation of Ca^{2+} influx.[8] This may predispose to excitotoxic responses in the nervous system. In addition, the rise in Ca^{2+} results partially from the action of cyanide stimulating phospholipase C to generate inositol 1,4,5-triphosphate (IP_3).[9] IP_3 then activates a receptor on the endoplasmic reticulum resulting in release of stored Ca^{2+} into the cytosol. Concurrent with mobilization of stored Ca^{2+} and influx of extracellular Ca^{2+} is an impairment of the Ca^{2+} extrusion mechanisms that would normally maintain cytosolic Ca^{2+} levels within a physiological concentration.

Calcium ion is an important regulatory element of many cellular functions. Under normal conditions, transient increases of cytosolic free Ca^{2+} above normal levels (>100 nM) trigger intracellular Ca^{2+}-dependent processes and serve as major signaling pathways for neurons.[10] When intracellular Ca^{2+} is increased to excessive levels and homeostatic processes are unable to buffer the increase, the ion may activate in concert several critical membranous, cytoplasmic, and genomic events (Figure 1). Unregulated activation of these Ca^{2+} sensitive mechanisms can lead to dysfunction and eventually, if not controlled, to impairment of the nervous system.[11] These cyanide-induced changes in intracellular homeostasis can occur within seconds of exposure and are characterized by global secretion of neurotransmitters leading to compensated central regulation of vital functions (respiration and cardiovascular control), seizures, and loss of consciousness. If an individual survives this acute toxic insult, then cyanide can initiate neuronal death that can lead to brain damage, for example, in the basal ganglia.[12] The dopaminergic

Table 1. Neurochemical Markers of Cyanide Toxicity

Cytochrome oxidase inhibition
Activation of voltage-sensitive calcium channels
Activation of receptor-operated calcium channels
Elevation of cytosolic free calcium
Activation of intracellular calcium cascades
Inhibition of antioxidant enzymes (superoxide dismutase, catalase, glutathione peroxidase)
Peroxidation of membrane lipids
Generation of reactive oxygen species and nitric oxide

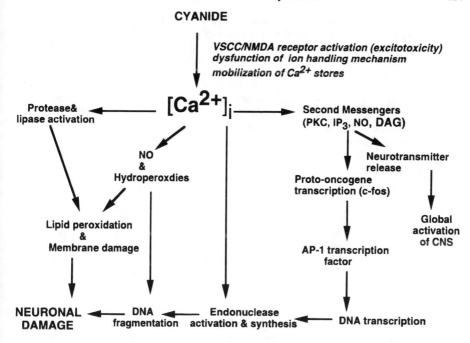

Figure 1. Proposed role of Ca^{2+} signaling in cyanide-induced neurotoxicity.

system of the striatum is sensitive to cyanide, and numerous reports describe cyanide-induced Parkinsonism following an acute intoxication.[13,14] Thus, activation of a cascade of intracellular signaling processes appears to play an important role in the neuronal injury produced by cyanide.

In Vitro Model of Cyanide Intoxication

To develop an in vitro cell model useful for mechanistic studies and toxicological screening, a well-characterized neuronal system is needed. The PC12 cell line is a popular neuronal model that can be employed for neurotoxicological studies.[15] The cell line, derived from a rat pheocyto-mocytoma, expresses a number of neuronal properties useful for in vitro studies (Table 2). The cells are electrically excitable, express a variety of functional polypeptide and neurotransmitter receptors, and secrete neurotransmitters (norepinephrine, dopamine, and acetylcholine).[16] The synthesis, storage, and secretion of neurotransmitters are well characterized in this cell line. The PC12 cell has been used for basic studies of neurosecretion, calcium and potassium channels, ion handling mechanisms, and proto-oncogene expression. Hence, the PC12 cell line serves as a well-studied neuronal model useful for examining the interaction of neurotoxic compounds with basic neuronal processes.

The response of the PC12 cell to cyanide has been well characterized in our laboratory and we have isolated subclones that are sensitive to cyanide.[1] The effect of cyanide on the PC12

Table 2. Neuron-like Properties of PC12 Cells

Electrically excitable cells
Neurosecretory cells (dopamine, norepinephrine, acetylcholine)
Express membrane-bound receptors
Functional intracellular Ca^{2+} signal cascades
Express functional Na^+, K^+, and Ca^{2+} channels

cell plasma membrane ion channels has been studied in detail, and most recently, signal transduction systems have been studied and their responses to cell injury characterized.[17] In turn, by developing a comprehensive understanding of the effect of cyanide on these processes, this cell line can serve as an in vitro model of toxicity. By using this cell line we have identified a series of neurochemical markers that can be monitored during toxicity, and quantification of these markers following cyanide exposure can be used to evaluate potential anticyanide compounds.[18] Initially the effect of cyanide on six markers of toxicity was used to develop an in vitro screen for compounds that could reverse these actions (Table 3). The goal was to identify compounds that can reverse cyanide's intracellular actions in the in vitro model and then evaluate their antidotal efficacy in an animal model.

METHODS

Culturing of PC12 Cells

PC12 cells were obtained from the American Type Culture Collection (Rockville, MD) and subclones sensitive to cyanide were isolated by the agar suspension technique coupled with morphological and biochemical screening techniques.[15] Cell were grown as monolayers attached to plastic culture flasks in RPMI 1640 medium supplemented with 10% v/v heat-inactivated horse serum and 5% v/v fetal calf serum. After 5–6 d of growth, cells were harvested and suspended in Krebs–Ringer bicarbonate solution.

Treatments

Potassium cyanide solutions were prepared just prior to use. Compounds to be screened were used at a concentration of 10 μM and were added to the cell suspensions 15 min prior to cyanide. The concentration of KCN added to the cell suspension was determined from dose-response curves for each assay and ranged from 0.05 to 5 mM. Results obtained with KCN alone were compared with those obtained using KCN plus the compound being screened. Controls were run to determine basal activity of each biochemical marker. The biochemical marker was assayed after 30 min of exposure to cyanide alone or in the present of the compound being screened. The selection of compounds to be screened was based on their known pharmacology and their potential to alter neural systems such as enzymes, ionic homeostasis, or membrane function.

Measurement of Biochemical Markers

Six biochemical markers of cyanide toxicity were measured in PC12 cells following addition of KCN either alone or in the present of potential antidotes. Based on mechanistic studies it was determined that these markers represent key intraneuronal events that are influenced by cyanide, and reversal of cyanide's effect on these markers reflects restoration of cellular function and can be used to predict antidotal potential. The ability of compounds to reverse cyanide's

Table 3. Biochemical Markers of PC12 Cells Used in the Multiple-Stage Assay for Anticyanide Compounds

Marker	Effect of cyanide
Cytochrome oxidase	Inhibits
Dopamine release	Stimulates
Cytosolic free calcium	Increases
Catalase	Inhibits
Superoxide dismutase	Inhibits
Intracellular hydroperoxide generation	Stimulates

Note. To measure anticyanide activity, the ability of compounds to reverse each action of cyanide was measured and a score of 0–10 was assigned for each assay (0, no effect, 10, 100% reversal), and a composite score (sum of all assay scores) was given to each compound.

action on each marker was graded on a scale of 0–10 in which no effect on cyanide action was graded zero and complete reversal was given a score of 10. A composite score representing the sum of each compounds action on all six assays was used to rank compounds as potential cyanide antidotes. The details of each assay have been previously published.[18]

Validation of Screen

Validation of the screen was determined by correlating the composite score of compounds identified as active against cyanide in the PC12 cells screen with the LD50 of cyanide in mice treated with the potential antidote. The LD50 values were obtained from the literature or conducted by the dose-effect analysis. Twenty-four-hour lethality was used for determining LD50s. Potency ratios were calculated for each compound by dividing the LD50 of cyanide alone into the LD50 of cyanide in mice given the antidote plus sodium thiosulfate. These studies were approved by the Purdue University Animal Care and Use Committee.

RESULTS

Fifty compounds were screened in the multiple assays and composite scores (sum of all assay scores) generated. Figure 2 illustrates the results of the top 10 compounds. The anticonvulsants, carbamazepine and phenytoin, had the highest scoring of the compounds screened and were the most effective in blocking cyanide-induced dopamine release. Of all the 39 compounds tested, only allopurinol equaled the potency of the anticonvulsants in blocking cyanide-stimulated release of dopamine from PC12 cells. None of the compounds screened significantly reversed cyanide inhibition of superoxide dismutase, whereas catalase appeared to be one of the more sensitive markers. Reversal of cyanide inhibition of catalase activity may be one of the more sensitive indicators of anticyanide action. Presently the significance of catalase inhibition in cyanide toxicity is being studied.

The in vitro screen is based on the rationale that compounds that can block the biochemical effects of cyanide in a neuronal cell model should afford protection against cyanide in an animal model. To validate the assay, correlation of the in vitro screen to the anticyanide action of the compounds in mice was conducted. Several known cyanide antidotes (naloxone, pyruvate, mercaptopyruvate, and flunarizine) scored relatively high in the in vitro screen, and effectiveness in the screen correlated with the ability of the compounds to prevent lethality in mice. When

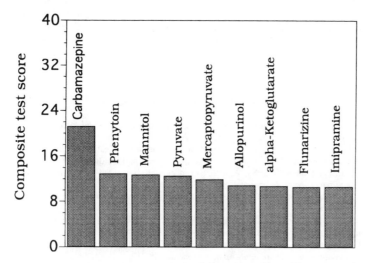

Figure 2. Composite in vitro score of potential cyanide antidotes. The compounds exhibiting the highest total scores in the six assays are presented.

the potency ratio (LD50 of cyanide divided into the LD50 of cyanide in mice pretreated with thiosulfate and the antidote) was compared to the composite scores obtained in the screening assays, a correlation coefficient of .88 ($p < .05$) was obtained. Known cyanide antidotes used in this correlation were chlorpromazine, naloxone, flunarizine, and carbamazepine.

Known cyanide antidotes that have mechanisms not operative in vitro (sodium nitrate and sodium thiosulfate) scored low in the screen as anticipated, since PC12 cells do not generate methemoglobin and have a low level of rhodanese to catalyze the metabolism of cyanide in which thiosulfate serves as a substrate. Thus the screen appears to be capable of identifying biochemical cyanide antidotes, but would not be expected to detect sulfur donors or methemoglobin formers.

DISCUSSION

This study demonstrates that by understanding the mechanism of action of a toxic compound, an in vitro screen for antidotes can be developed. The mechanistically based screen was validated by correlating in vitro assay parameters with animal data. By application of such an assay, it is projected that a large number of compounds could be screened, in turn reducing the number of animals needed for the traditional screening process. Future work will refine the screen with the objective of developing new, efficacious cyanide antidotes.

The compounds with the highest scores in the screen exhibit anticonvulsant activity in vivo. Since acute intoxication to cyanide is characterized by seizures, tremors, and loss of consciousness, these results suggests anticonvulsants or their combination with other antidotes should be evaluated in detail in animals as potential cyanide antidotes. The main anticonvulsant action of phenytoin and carbamazepine is thought to be blockade of sodium channels to inhibit high-frequency discharges around epileptic foci. Minimal disruption of normal neuronal traffic is produced by these drugs. These results suggest that cyanide may enhance sodium influx through channels responsible for high frequency discharges. In support, epileptiform discharges have been observed in guinea pig hippocampal slices after cyanide exposure in vitro.[19]

Cyanide intoxication is a complex syndrome that results from multiple actions in the central nervous system and cardiovascular system. Inhibition of cytochrome oxidase is considered to be the primary action of cyanide resulting in a lowering of the cell's energy charge.[1] Accompanying this action, a number of other events play a significant role in the toxicity. Changes in Ca^{2+} handling mechanisms appear to play a pivotal role in toxicity. Cyanide induces an increase in cytosolic free Ca^{2+} levels that functions as an intracellular transduction process to initiate a series of intracellular events contributing to the toxic syndrome.[6,17] By understanding these responses to cyanide, a mechanistically based screen assay was developed. Validation in animals indicates the assay is a good predictor of potential antidotal activity, and it is reasonable to suggest that substances which prevent cyanide-induced biochemical changes may be clinically effective cyanide antidotes.

REFERENCES

1. Way, J. L. 1984. Cyanide intoxication and its mechanism of antagonism. *Annu. Rev. Pharmacol. Toxicol.* 24:451.
2. Ballantyne, G. 1987. Toxicology of cyanide. In *Clinical and experimental toxicology of cyanides*, eds. B. Ballantyne and T. C. Marrs, p. 127. Bristol: Wright.
3. Isom, G. E., and Johnson, J. D. 1987. Sulphur donors in cyanide intoxication. In *Clinical and experimental toxicology of cyanides*, eds. B. Ballantyne and T. C. Marrs, p. 413. Bristol: Wright.
4. Petterson, J., and Cohen, S. 1985. Antagonism of cyanide poisoning by chlorpromazine and sodium thiosulfate. *Toxicol. Appl. Pharmacol.* 81:265.
5. Aitken, P., and Braitment, D. 1989. The effects of cyanide on neural and synaptic function in hippocampal slices. *Neurotoxicology* 10:239.
6. Johnson, J. D., Meisenheimer, T. L., and Isom, G. E. 1986. Cyanide-induced neurotoxicity. Role of neuronal calcium. *Toxicol. Appl. Pharmacol.* 84:464.
7. Johnson, J. D., Conroy, W. G., and Isom, G. E. 1987. Alteration of cytosolic calcium levels in PC12 cells by potassium cyanide. *Toxicol. Appl. Pharmacol.* 88:217.
8. Patel, M. N., Yim, G. K. W., and Isom, G. E. 1993. N-Methyl-D-aspartate receptors mediate cyanide-induced cytotoxicity in hippocampal cultures. *Neurotoxicology* 14:35.

9. Yang, C.-W., and Isom, G. E. 1994. Metabotropic receptor mediated inositol trisphosphate generation: Stimulation by cyanide. *Toxicologist* 14:351.
10. Kennedy, M. B. 1989. Regulation of neuronal function by calcium. *Trends Neurosci.* 12:417.
11. Nicotera, P., McConkey, D. J., Dypbukt, J. M., Jones, D. P., and Orrenius, S. 1989. Ca^{2+}-activated mechanisms in cell killing. *Drug Metab. Rev.* 20:193.
12. Kanthasamy, A. G., Borowitz, J. L., Pavlakovic, G., and Isom, G. E. 1994. Dopaminergic neurotoxicology of cyanide: Neurochemical, histological and behavioral characterization. *Toxicol. Appl. Pharmacol.* 126:156.
13. Rosenberg, N. L., Myers, J. A., and Martin, W. R. W. 1989. Cyanide-induced Parkinsonism: Clinical, MRI and 6-fluorodopa PET studies. *Neurology* 38:142.
14. Valenzuela, J., and Godoy, J. 1992. Delayed cyanide-induced dystonia. *J. Neurol. Neurosurg. Psychiatry* 55:198.
15. Isom, G. E., and Borowitz, J. L. 1993. Neural system: PC12 cell. In *Methods of toxicology*, eds. C. A. Tyson and J. M. Frazier, p. 82. San Diego: Academic Press.
16. Shafer, J. J., and Atchison, W. D. 1991. Transmitter, ion channel and receptor properties of pheochromocytoma (PC12) cells: A model for neurotoxicological studies. *Neurotoxicology* 12:473.
17. Yang, C.-W., Rathinavelu, A., Borowitz, J. L., and Isom, G. E. 1994. Activation of a calcium and pH-dependent phospholipase A_2 by cyanide in PC12 cells. *Toxicol. Appl. Pharmacol.* 124:262.
18. Borowitz, J. L., Kanthasamy, A. G., Mitchell, P. J., and Isom, G. E. 1993. Use of PC12 cells as a neurotoxicological screen: Characterization of anticyanide compounds. *Fundam. Appl. Toxicol.* 20:133.
19. Lebeda, F., VanMeter, W., and Braitmen, P. 1990. Epileptogenic and depressant effects of cyanide in the hippocampus. *Pharmacologist* 32:161.

Chapter Twenty-four

MDCK: AN EPITHELIAL CELL LINE MODEL OF THE BLOOD–BRAIN BARRIER AND ITS RESPONSE TO CHOLINESTERASE INHIBITORS

Bellina Veronesi and Marion Ehrich

A commercially available epithelial cell line, the Madin-Darby canine kidney cell (MDCK), displays various functional and enzymatic similarities to cerebral endothelial cells of the blood–brain barrier (BBB). These include electrical resistance, morphological (i.e., ultrastructurally defined tight junctions), and enzymatic activities such as acetylcholinesterase (AChE), butyrylcholinesterase (BuChE), γ-glutamyltranspeptidase (GGTP), alkaline phosphatase (APP), and superoxide dismutase (SOD). Since many of these endpoints are affected by chemical disrupters of the BBB, MDCK cells were tested for their potential to screen BBB toxicants. Confluent MDCK cells were exposed to several non-cytotoxic concentrations of the organophophorus (OP) cholinesterase inhibitors (mipafox, parathion, and paraoxon), and their effects on electrical resistance, passage of fluorescein tracers, and enzyme chemistry in confluent MDCK cells were monitored. Neither depression of resistance nor passage of fluorescein markers occurred after 48 h of exposure to non-cytotoxic (10^{-2}, 10^{-3}, 10^{-4} M) concentrations of either paraoxon or parathion. However, enzyme analysis of MDCK cells exposed to parathion or paraoxon at these doses for 24 h indicated a marked increase (650, 450, 400%) in APP activity in the absence of changes in other assayed enzymes. After 72 h of exposure to mipafox (10^{-4} and 10^{-5} M), paraoxon (10^{-4} and 10^{-5} M), or parathion (10^{-3} and 10^{-4} M), MDCK cells displayed evidence of cytotoxicity (increased lactate dehydrogenase activity). At this time point, exposure to all doses of OPs was associated with decreased levels of APP, GGTP, and SOD activities and moderate increases in BuChE activity. Although various test chemicals await trial in this model, these preliminary results suggest that permeability alterations and enzyme changes in MDCK culture might be used to evaluate chemicals that disrupt the BBB in vivo.

INTRODUCTION

The need to use cell culture models on a first-tier level of chemical testing is critical in view of the overwhelming number of untested or inadequately characterized chemicals being released into our environment. This is especially serious with neurotoxicants in view of their potential to damage central nervous system. This reasoning is shared by all concerned toxicologists, whether our thinking is driven by ethical, financial, or political reasons or their combination.

Recently, recommendations have been made to regulatory agencies of the federal government

This manuscript has been reviewed by the National Health Effects and Environmental Research Laboratories, U.S. Environmental Protection Agency, and approved for publication. Mention of trade names or commercial products does not constitute endorsement or recommendation for use.

to examine the possibility of minimizing or actually replacing animals in testing of chemicals for neurotoxicity with cell culture models.[1-3] In this regard, we have used neuroblastoma cell lines to identify and characterize organophosphorus (OP) cholinesterase inhibitors.[4,5] However, for more general identification of putative neurotoxicants, cell culture "screens" are required. In vitro "screens" are test systems that can generate data in a relatively inexpensive, rapid, and reproducible fashion relative to whole-animal testing.[6,7] By definition a screen uses cells and support media that are commercially available so that the recipes can be standardized and easily transferred for interlaboratory validation. Consequently, a "screening battery" often features commercially available cell lines and reagents.

One needed component of a screening battery for neurotoxicants is a cell culture model that simulates key features of the blood–brain barrier (BBB). This model is not meant to mimic the BBB as it exists in situ, but rather it is viewed as an isolated system that may contain similar functional and structural features of the barrier that are targeted in vivo by neurotoxicants. In keeping with the criteria of an in vitro screening battery and in view of the technical difficulties associated with isolating primary microvessel cultures (e.g., cost, speed, standardization, commercial availability etc.), an epithelial cell line (Madin-Darby Canine Kidney, MDCK) was evaluated for similarities to cerebral endothelial cells that compose the BBB. This chapter outlines the initial characterization and use of this in vitro barrier model to assess changes that occur in response to cholinesterase inhibitors.

MATERIALS AND METHODS

Cells and Media

The MDCK (CCL number 34) cell line was obtained from the American Type Culture Collection (Rockville, MD). Cells were grown in a modified Eagle's minimum Essential medium (MEM) supplemented with 10% fetal bovine serum and 1% penicillin/streptomycin (500 units penicillin and 500 μg/ml streptomycin). Cells were established in 75-cm^2 flasks at seeding densities of 1.5×10^5 cells/ml and incubated at 37°C in 95% O_2 and 5% CO_2 ambient atmosphere. At this final seeding density, MDCK cells became confluent in 4–6 d in vitro (DIV). Cells were fed every 3 d, washed in Hanks basic salt solution, and when appropriate densities were reached, trypsinized using solutions of 0.25% trypsin in 0.53 mM ethylenediamine tetraacetic acid (EDTA). Chemicals for cell cultures were purchased from Sigma Chemical Corp. (St. Louis, MO) and from Gibco Corp. (Grand Island, NY).

Enzyme Chemistry

Marker enzymes known to be present in BBB endothelial cells[8] were assayed in the MDCK cells. For enzyme chemistry analysis, cells were cultures to a population density of 1×10^7 cells/ml, pelleted, and processed according to the individual assays. Enzymes were assayed in unexposed confluent MDCK cells and those exposed to cholinesterase inhibitors at various concentrations for 24 and 72 h. All enzymes were assayed using commercially available enzyme diagnostic kits (Sigma Chemical Corp., St. Louis, MO). These included the cholinergic transmitter deactivating enzymes for acetylcholinesterase (AChE) and for butyrylcholinesterase (BuChE), the cytotoxic marker for lactate dehydrogenase (LDH), the protein transporter enzymes, for alkaline phosphatase (APP) and kit 545-A for the amino acid carrier γ-glutamyltranspeptidase (GGTP). The Coomassie Plus protein assay kit (Pierce Corp., Rockford, IL) was used to quantitate protein concentrations on the individual cell samples.

Intoxication of Barrier Cells

Parathion and paraoxon were obtained from Chem Service (Warren, PA), and mipafox was obtained from Lark Enterprise (Webster, MA). The OP cholinesterase inhibitors were dissolved in ethanol and exposed to MDCK cells in serum-free media. Cytotoxicity tests using a neutral red viability stain established EC50 values (the effective concentration producing 50% cytotoxicity) for the individual chemicals. MDCK cells were plated and grown to confluency. Cells were exposed to concentrations of EC0 to EC25 for times ranging from 24 to 72 h. Separate endpoints (electrical resistance, fluorescence tracers) were monitored to indicate permeability disruption by the test chemical.

Resistance Measurements

For resistance measurements, cells were plated at a density of 5×10^4 cells/ml in 12-mm Millicell HA inserts (Millipore Corp., Bedford, MA). Confluency was monitored visually and by measuring cultures with the Millicell-ERS electrical resistance system (Millipore Corp., Bedford, MA). Resistance measurements were made at intervals throughout the 72-h exposure period.

Fluorescence Measurements

Cells were grown in Millipore chambers and at confluency were exposed both to the test OP and a fluorescein isothionate tracer (FITC-dextran, MW 68,500, Sigma Chemical Corp., St. Louis, MO). At postexposure times ranging from 4 to 120 h, chamber inserts containing the MDCK cells, OP test agent, and fluorescein tracer were removed and the lower chamber, which contained any fluorescein leakage, was read using a Millipore Cytofluor fluorescence spectrophotometer (Millipore Corp., Bedford, MA).

RESULTS

Resistance

MDCK monolayers were grown in insert chambers and their resistance was measured daily. Resistance increased to approximately 110 ohm over a 6 DIV period. After 7 DIV, resistance began to decrease as the MDCK tight junctions became "leaky" as previously reported.[9]

Enzyme Chemistry

When cells reached 90% confluency, they were harvested and assayed for enzymes characteristic of cerebral endothelial microvessels. In keeping with its properties as a transport epithelium, MDCK contained high activities of many enzyme markers noted in cerebral endothelial cells such as the carrier enzymes APP and GGTP, AChE, BuChE and the free-radical scavenger molecule, superoxide dismutase (SOD). LDH activity was characteristically lower in control, untreated confluent MDCK cells.

Permeability Disruption by OPs

The observations that MDCK developed electrical resistance and contained a variety of enzymes similar to cerebral endothelial cells suggested that these endpoints might be used to assess the potential of cholinesterase inhibitors to disrupt its permeability since OPs are thought to disrupt the BBB in vivo.[10–13] When a chemical irritant interacts with the MDCK, one of the first physiological events is loss of the permeability barrier.[14] The tight junctions separate, leading to loss of cell contact, passage of fluorescein tracers, and depression of electrical resistance. Consequently, electrical resistance, fluorescence passage, and cellular enzyme activities were featured as endpoints to monitor OP exposure to MDCK barrier cells. Cultures were exposed for 48 h to parathion (10^{-2}, 10^{-3}, 10^{-4} M) and paraoxon (10^{-2}, 10^{-3}, 10^{-4} M), and resistance measurements were made throughout the exposure period. No significant loss of resistance was observed at any time point or concentration of OP. Similarly, no passage of fluorescein tracer was observed earlier than 72 h in MDCK cells treated with mipafox, parathion, or paraoxon at concentrations of 10^{-3} M. At 72 h, however, we and others have reported a loss of cell-to-cell contact and permeability leakage begin to occur naturally in confluent MDCK cells.[9]

Enzyme Chemistry and OPs

Separate flasks of confluent MDCK cells were exposed to parathion and to paraoxon at concentrations of 10^{-2}, 10^{-3}, and 10^{-4} M for 24 h, to 10^{-4} and 10^{-5} M mipafox for 72 h, to 10^{-4} and 10^{-5} M paraoxon for 72 h, and to 10^{-3} and 10^{-4} M parathion for 72 h. Following exposure, the cells were harvested and subjected to enzyme assays for APP, GGTP, AChE, BuChE, SOD, and LDH (as an indicator of cytotoxicity).

At 24 h postexposure, cells exposed to parathion and to paraoxon showed no evidence of cytotoxicity. Changes in enzyme activity, however, were associated with the 24-h exposure to parathion and paraoxon at concentrations of 10^{-2}, 10^{-3}, and 10^{-4} M. Slight (15–22%) depression of AChE and BuChE activities occurred at all three concentrations of parathion. Higher (35–50%) inhibitions of these esterases occurred with exposures to the more metabolically active paraoxon. This suggested a metabolic incompetence of the MDCK epithelial cells to convert protoxicant pesticides (i.e., parathion) to more neuroactive metabolites. Negligible changes in LDH and SOD activities occurred at all doses of both OPs. Significant depression of GGTP was observed in response to 10^{-2} M parathion (42%) and 10^{-2} M paraoxon (68%). A striking increase in APP activity was seen at all doses of parathion (350–335%) and paraoxon (370–600%) at 24 h of exposure. These increases occurred in the absence of cytotoxicity as evidenced by low LDH activity.

Enzyme changes in response to lower concentrations of paraoxon (10^{-4} and 10^{-5} M), parathion (10^{-3} and 10^{-4} M), and mipafox (10^{-4} and 10^{-5} M) occurred after 72 h. Increases in LDH activity ranging from 36 to 28% above controls suggested cytotoxicity from cultures treated with mipafox (10^{-4} and 10^{-5} M), from 21 to 46% above controls with paraoxon (10^{-4} and 10^{-5} M), and from 87 to 81% above control with parathion (10^{-3} and 10^{-4} M). Depressed enzyme activities occurred in GGTP, APP, and SOD for all tested OPs. GGTP activity was not affected by mipafox, but GGTP activity was depressed from 60 to 40% of control activity by paraoxon (10^{-4} and 10^{-5} M), and from 60 to 65% of control activity by parathion (10^{-3} and 10^{-4} M). APP activity was depressed from 40 to 15% by mipafox (10^{-4} and 10^{-5} M), from 75 to 70% by paraoxon (10^{-4} and 10^{-5} M), and from 54 to 38% by parathion (10^{-3} and 10^{-4} M). SOD activity was depressed from 70 to 52% by mipafox (10^{-4} and 10^{-5} M), from 75 to 65% by paraoxon (10^{-4} and 10^{-5} M), and from 80 to 63% by parathion (10^{-3} and 10^{-4} M). There was negligible effect on AChE activity and mild upregulation of BuChE activity, which probably reflected the resynthesis of the inhibited enzymes.

DISCUSSION

The BBB, by definition, is a capillary system composed of endothelial cells and astrocytes, which together act to protect and nurture the brain. Under optimal conditions, the endothelial cells are circumferentially sealed together by continuous tight junctions (i.e., zonula occludens), structures that restrict passage of most polar molecules between the bloodstream and interstitial fluid and even limit the passage of ions, organic acids, and neuroactive amino acids.[15] The endothelial cells that compose the BBB contain enzymes such as AChE and BuChE that deactivate cholinergic neurotransmitters. Chemicals transverse the BBB by distinct transporter enzymes such as GLUT1 and carriers that are protein or amino acid specific like APP and GGTP. In addition to transporters, chemicals cross the barrier in large part by their lipophility. Indeed, the importance of lipid solubility on the rate of passage of compounds such as the present OP cholinesterase inhibitors may be a primary determinant in their permeability of the BBB.

The MDCK epithelial cell line has many similarities to BBB endothelial cells, since the epithelial cell also engages in transport and barrier functions. Selective transport is a major function of kidney epithelia cells and suggested that this cell line would have many enzyme carriers similar to the BBB endothelial cells. In addition to enzyme activities, tight junctions also occur in the apical ends of the MDCK cell, effectively preventing the passage of most molecules, strengthening cell-to-cell connections, and producing cell–cell electrical resistance in confluent MDCK cultures. Both categories of endpoints were used in the present study to assess whether OP cholinesterase inhibitors cause permeability disruption or enzyme changes in the MDCK barrier cell model. The absence of permeability disruption in confluent MDCK cells exposed to mipafox, parathion, and paraoxon indicate that cholinesterase inhibitors do not disrupt junctional complexes and overtly disrupt cellular barriers at the tested doses and time points. The enzyme changes recorded after 24 and 72 h of exposure, however, indicate that OPs do transverse the barrier cells, probably by virtue of their lipophilicity. Our data support an earlier study that reported esterase inhibition produced by soman, and paraoxon does not account for BBB disruption in rats.[10] The enzyme data also indicate that MDCK cells lack robust metabolic properties, since esterase activities were only moderately inhibited in response to parathion, a metabolically inactive organophosphate. While the present study cannot link depression of AChE and BuChE with permeability disruption in MDCK, it is noted that pesticide exposure is associated with a distinct upregulation of the protein carrier APP. The significance of this striking (>600%) increase in activity after 24 h of exposure in the absence of cytotoxicity is presently unknown, but has recently been reported in MDCK cells exposed to another neurotoxicant, triethyl tin.[16]

Adopting cell culture models to screen putative neurotoxicants for hazard identification of environment chemicals has been strongly encouraged. In view of the vulnerability of the BBB to environmental chemical insult, various groups have recommended that cell culture of the BBB be incorporated into screening batteries to detect putative neurotoxicants.[3,17,18] Because of this, devising a surrogate BBB has become a focus of in vitro neurotoxicologists committed to developing "risk-relevant" screening batteries. The pilot data from this and other studies[16] suggest that the MDCK cell line be considered for such use.

SUMMARY

Many putative neurotoxicants are alleged to disrupt the blood–brain barrier (BBB) in vivo. The development of a cell culture model that simulates the barrier properties of the BBB could be useful to identify such chemicals and provide a more "risk relevant" in vitro screening battery. This study reports that a commercially available cell line, the Madin-Darby canine kidney epithelial cell (MDCK), displays several functional and enzymatic similarities to the endothelial cells of the BBB including electrical resistance and enzymatic (acetylcholinesterase, butyrylcholinesterase, γ-glutamyltranspeptidase, alkaline phosphatase) activities. This chapter further reports that OP cholinesterase inhibitors do not disrupt electrical resistance or cause fluorescein leakage in confluent MDCK cells but that enzyme changes (e.g., increases in APP activity) in the MDCK are associated with exposure to non-cytotoxic concentrations of OP cholinesterase inhibitors.

REFERENCES

1. National Research Council Committee on Neurotoxicology and Models for Assessing Risk. 1992. Commission of Life Science, pp. 1–27.
2. Interagency Regulatory Alternatives Group. 1993. IRAG Work Group Report Guidelines, pp. 1–10. November.
3. ECVAM. 1994. Report and recommendations on in vitro neurotoxicity testing. *ATLA* 22:350–362.
4. Veronesi, B., and Ehrich, M. 1993. Using neuroblastoma cell lines to evaluate insecticides' neurotoxicity. *In Vitro Toxicol.* 6(1):57–65.
5. Ehrich, M., Correl, L., and Veronesi, B. 1994. Neuroblastoma cell lines as models to predict organophosphorous induced delayed neuropathy. *Neurotoxicology* 2:309–314.
6. Veronesi, B. 1992. In vitro screening batteries for neurotoxicants. *Neurotoxicology* 13:185–196.
7. Veronesi, B. 1992. The use of cell culture for evaluating neurotoxicity, In *Target organ toxicology series. Nervous system toxicology*, eds. H. A. Tilson and C. Mitchell, pp. 21–49. New York: Raven Press.
8. Vorbrodt, A. W. 1988. Ultrastructural cytochemistry of blood-brain barrier endothelia. *Prog. Histochem. Cytochem.* 3:1–99.
9. Cereijido, M. 1984. Electrical properties of Madin-Darby canine kidney cells. *J. Cell Biol.* 2230–2235.
10. Ashani, Y. and Cartravas, G. N. 1981. Seizure-induced changes in the permeability of the blood-brain barrier following administration of anticholinesterase drugs to rats. *Biochem. Pharmacol.* 30(18):2593–2601.
11. Carpentier, P., Delamanche, I. S., Le Bert, M., Blanchet, G., and Bouchaud, C. 1990. Seizure-related opening of the blood-brain barrier induced by Soman: Possible correlation with the acute neuropathology observed in poisoned rats. *Neurotoxicology* 11(3):493–508.

12. Petrali, J. P., Maxwell, D. M., Lenz, D. E., and Mills, K. R. I Effect of an anticholinesterase compound on the ultrastructure and function of the rat blood-brain barrier: A review and experiment. *Submicrosc. Cytol. Pathol.* 23(2):331–338.

13. Sellstrom, A., Algers, G., and Karlsson, B. 1985. Soman intoxication and the blood-brain barrier. *Fundam. Appl. Toxicol.* 5:S122–S126.

14. Tchao, R. 1988. Trans-epithelial permeability of fluorescein in vitro as an assay to determine eye irritants. *In Vitro Toxicol.* 6:271–283.

15. Bradbury, M. W. B., and Lightman, S. L. 1990. The blood brain interface. *Eye* 4:249–254.

16. Veronesi, B., Carlson, K., Ehrich, M. 1996. The response of madin-darby canine kidney barrier cells to the neurotoxic metal, triethyl tin. ATLA 24:349–357.

17. Walum, E., Hansson, E., and Harvey, A. L. 1990. In vitro testing of neurotoxicity. *ATALA* 18:153–179.

18. World Health Organization. 1989. International Programme on Chemical Safety. Report of Planning Meeting: In Vitro Techniques for the Assessment of Neurotoxic Chemicals. Geneva: WHO.

PART V

ORAL/DERMAL/OCULAR
VALIDATION

Chapter Twenty-five

THE BLOOD-PERFUSED PIG EAR: A POTENTIAL IN VITRO ALTERNATIVE FOR DERMAL PERMEATION AND TOXICITY STUDIES

Piet Bruijnzeel, Jan de Lange, Govert van der Schans, and Graham Elliott

To overcome most disadvantages of current models for percutaneous penetration of drugs or toxic substances, an alternative model is proposed: the isolated pig ear perfused with autologous oxygenated blood. Previous investigations have shown that this model can be used to study skin penetration of xenobiotics for a period of at least 8–10 h. During that period, the temperature is kept at 30°C and the air humidity at 40–60%. Cell viability, vasomotor activity, ear weight, perfusion pressure, and flow hardly change. Therefore, this model allows the performance of skin penetration studies under standard criteria.

Using xylene as a model substance we have been able to demonstrate that skin penetration is determined by both the recipient phase constituents and the depots formed in the various skin compartments.

Data are presented to show that the pig ear model can also be used in studies dealing with sulfur mustard vapor intoxication of the skin. When pig ears are exposed to sulfur mustard, epidermal damage and occasional microblister formation occur. DNA–sulfur mustard adduct formation can be demonstrated in epidermal keratinocytes.

The pig ear model also allowed the measurement of transepidermal water loss (TEWL) as a measure of skin irritancy. A fairly good concordance was present with TEWL measurements obtained in human volunteers with a series of compounds with increasing dermatotoxic potency.

In summary, the whole-blood-perfused pig ear model is an alternative to in vivo animal models for studying interactions between chemicals and the skin.

INTRODUCTION

Cutaneous penetration studies in human volunteers are hampered due to the complexity of xenobiotic toxicokinetics and metabolism in vivo and due to the ethical problems associated with possible undesirable effects of the chemical under investigation. The use of animal species, such as hairless mice,[1] human skin grafted nude mice,[2] hairless rats,[3] or dogs,[4] is equally cumbersome and also has the disadvantage that species differences in metabolism, elimination, etc. prevent extrapolation of the results to humans.[5,6]

In vitro, the diffusion cell technique using human skin is most widely used to measure skin

Part of this work was financially supported by the Platform Alternatieven voor Dierproeven (Platform Alternatives for Animal Testing), Rijswijk, the Netherlands. C. Poot is acknowledged for helping to prepare the manuscript.

penetration. However, this method has some major disadvantages: (a) Only the epidermis and the upper part of the dermis are used; effects of the investigated chemicals on the dermal vascular system are ignored;[7] (b) the rate of penetration is grossly affected by the composition of the recipient medium, usually a buffer containing organic solvents, such as ethanol;[8] and (c) the flow at which the medium moves along the inner surface of the skin piece is usually arbitrarily chosen. Different flow rates have substantial effect on the amount of substance that is measured in the medium.

Pig skin resembles human skin morphologically and functionally.[9] Furthermore, when pig and human skin are compared, percutaneous absorption rates appear to be almost similar.[10,11] Riviere et al.[12] described an in vitro model for dermatotoxicity studies, using isolated perfused porcine skin flaps. Although this model is an improvement over existing models, it still has several limitations: (a) Rather time-consuming surgery is necessary to construct the skin flap; (b) during the isolation the skin alters morphologically, that is, the epidermis becomes thicker; and (c) in this model buffer is used as perfusion fluid instead of blood. Although this may be done to facilitate detection and measurement of the chemical under investigation, it is questionable whether the binding and solubility characteristics for a variety of chemicals in blood are met by using a buffer.

To circumvent these disadvantages while retaining the advantages of this approach, an alternative in vitro model for measuring skin penetration has been developed over the past few years, the blood-perfused pig ear model.[13] Preexperimental surgery is not required; the ear preparation is ready for use within 1.5 h after isolation and is perfused with autologous oxygenated blood. During perfusion, all vessels and their anastomoses are perfused with blood (Figure 1). Perfusion can be performed for a period of at least 8 h. During perfusion, consumption of glucose does not alter when it is added to the perfusing blood at a concentration of 1 μg/ml. Also, arterial and venous lactate dehydrogenase (LDH), Na^+, and K^+ concentrations remain constant over this

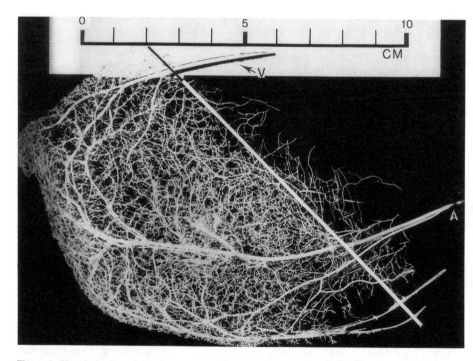

Figure 1. Vascularization of the pig ear. A cast of a pig ear vascular system was made by perfusion with dental cement. The surrounding tissue was dissolved using alkali (V, vena auricularis intermedius; A, arteria auricularis lateralis). The line indicates the cutting edge.

period. Together with vital staining of the perfused tissue, these findings indicate that the pig ear remains viable over at least 8–10 h. Since noradrenalin caused an identical dose-dependent increase in perfusion pressure at the beginning and 4–6 h after perfusion, which could be totally reversed by isoxsuprine, the vascular reactivity also remains intact.

This model has been evaluated for a number of different applications. In this chapter we describe its usefulness for predicting rates of dermal permeation in humans, in investigating parameters influencing rates of permeation, as a test system for investigating the mechanism of action of a vesicant (sulfur mustard), and for detecting the irritating potential of chemicals.

MATERIALS AND METHODS

Chemicals

All chemicals used were of analytical grade with the exception of xylene, which was a technical solution containing 11% o-xylene, 49% m-xylene, 20% p-xylene, and 19% ethyl benzene (Solvesso xylene, Exxon Chemicals Holland, Schiedam, the Netherlands). Sulfur mustard (HD) was kindly provided by Dr. H. P. Benschop (TNO Prins Maurits Laboratory). All other reagents were reagent grade.

Permeation Experiments

Cannulation and perfusion of isolated pig ears. Pig ears were prepared as described.[13] Briefly, on arrival in the laboratory, ears of healthy domestic pigs (75–100 kg) were cannulated with polythene cannulas (1.0 mm OD, 0.5 mm ID) in the vena auricularis intermedius and the arteria auricularis lateralis. Thereafter, the ears were kept in a temperature- and humidity-controlled environment (30°C, 40–60% relative humidity) and perfused with phosphate-buffered saline containing 1 mg/ml glucose and 20 U/ml heparin (PBSGH) (Figure 2). Leakages along the cutting edge were coagulated or glued (cyanoacrylate glue, Cyanolite, Permanento, Heilo, the Netherlands).

After an equilibrium period of 30 min, perfusion with filtered oxygenated autologous whole pig blood was started unless otherwise stated.

During the equilibration period, a glass ring (surface area 10.0 cm^2) was glued to the ear using the α-cyanoacrylate glue. The test solution was pipetted into the ring 15 min after beginning the perfusion and the ring was covered with a watch glass. The test solution remained present

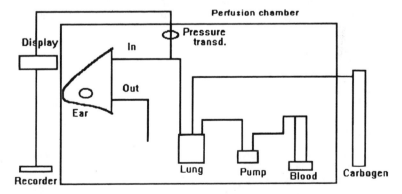

Figure 2. Schematic representation of the with full blood perfused pig ear model. After cannulation, the pig ear is placed in an incubator (perfusion chamber). Blood is oxygenated by an artificial lung and pumped through the ear. Blood samples can be collected from the outlet cannula. The air in the perfusion chamber was maintained at 30°C and a relative humidity of 40–60%. Perfusion pressure, blood flow, temperature, and relative humidity were continuously monitored.

in excess for the whole of the 4-h perfusion period. At various times thereafter, blood samples were taken for analysis of the test compound.

The penetration rate of the test compound (in steady state condition) at each time point is expressed in nanograms per minute per square centimeter and was calculated as follows:

Concentration per μl $\times$ flow rate (μl/min)/exposed area (10 cm^2)

The permeation rate for each experiment was calculated as the mean of the rates over the last 2 h of perfusion, when a plateau had been reached. During this period, the cumulative permeation curves were linear.

Quality control criteria. During the perfusion period, each pig ear must conform to the following criteria:

1. The perfusion pressure should remain between 40 and 120 mm Hg.
2. Blood flow should exceed 0.3 ml/min.
3. The weight of the pig ear should not increase more than 10% after a 4-h perfusion.
4. Glucose consumption should be at least 250 g/min/100 g tissue at the end of the experiment.

So far, 90% of the pig ear preparations made met these criteria.

We recently improved the quality control procedures by controlling the quality of the pig ear skin by histological examination of biopsies taken before and after the perfusion period. Technical and procedural modifications now allow us to perform perfusions with blood for up to 10 h.

Influence of the perfusion medium flow and composition on permeation rate using xylene as a model compound. Experiments were carried out using pigs' blood and an artificial medium containing various concentrations of albumin to investigate the influence of protein concentration on the measured permeation rate of xylene. The flow rate was kept constant.

In a second study the perfusion flow was varied from 0.2 to 1.0 μl/min. The buffer albumin concentration was constant at 4.5%.

Xylene levels in the perfusate were determined by gas chromatography as described.[14]

Influence of the stratum corneum on the rate of xylene skin penetration. The role played by the stratum corneum in the permeation of xylene was investigated by stripping ears 10 times with Scotch Magic 810 tape before (prestripping) or after (poststripping) exposure to xylene for 15 min. The perfusion period was 4 h.

The Effect of Exposing Pig Skin to Sulfur Mustard (HD) Vapor

Pig ear skin was exposed to HD vapor (1.0 cm^2, concentration about 3.5 μg/ml HD). At the end of the perfusion period ($\leq$10 h), biopsies were taken from the exposed area for examination of exposed skin by light microscopy and for the preparation of cryostat sections for immunofluorescent detection of HD–DNA adducts.[15]

Transepidermal Water Loss

Transepidermal water loss (TEWL) was measured using an Evaporimeter probe 2105. TEWL was measured 5 min before exposure and after a 4-h exposure period to the test substance. The difference in initial and final TEWL values was used as a measure of irritancy.

Statistical Methods

Nonparametric statistics were performed for comparison of the different groups. A Kruksal–Wallis test followed by a multiple comparison, according to Dunn's method, was applied. Values of $p < .05$ were considered to be significantly different.

RESULTS

Influence of the Recipient Phase on the Penetration Rate of Xylene

When performing skin penetration studies under the standard criteria mentioned, it could be shown that the rates of permeation of xylene when using whole blood and a buffer containing

4.5% albumin as recipient were all similar (± 300 ng/min/cm^2). However, when pig plasma was used, the rate of penetration became fivefold higher and when albumin was excluded from the buffer ninefold lower. Using the buffer, we found that the rate of permeation of xylene was proportional to flow (at constant protein concentration) and protein concentration (at constant flow) (Figure 3).

Influence of the Various layers of the Skin on the Penetration of Xylene

When pig ear skin was exposed to xylene for 3 periods of 5 min (each one separated by a period of 55 min), 15 min, 30 min, 60 min, or 240 min and perfused with full blood for 4 h thereafter, the following total permeation of xylene was determined: 23.2 ± 5.5 μg ($n = 5$), 29.7 ± 4.0 μg ($n = 5$), 28.2 ± 6.4 μg ($n = 6$), 48.1 ± 10.4 μg ($n = 6$), and 65.6 ± 8.3 μg ($n = 6$) (mean $\pm$ SEM). There were no differences in the total amount of xylene entering the blood after exposure periods of 3 times 5 min, 15 min, or 30 min, and between 60 min and 240 min. However, when skin was exposed to xylene for 15 min after tape stripping (10 times), the amount of xylene measured in blood over the 240-min perfusion period increased from 29.7 μg (intact skin) to 67.9 ± 15.6 μg ($n = 3$). In contrast, tape stripping after the 15-min exposure period resulted in a small decrease in the total amount of xylene permeating (22.3 ± 3.9 μg, $n = 4$). As could be deduced from histological examination of the skin, epidermal damage was maximal by 60 min. Damage appeared to be related to total exposure time, that is, 3 times for 5 min gave similar damages as 1 times for 15 min. Obviously, stripping before exposure to xylene exacerbated the dermatotoxic effects of xylene.

Blood-Perfused Pig Ear Model in Studying Sulfur Mustard Skin Damage

In human skin sulfur mustard vapor exposure induces blister formation, separating the dermal and epidermal junction. When pig ears were exposed to saturated sulfur mustard vapor for 4 min, histological examination of the skin revealed severe skin damage at the exposed side 8–10 h after exposure (Figure 4). In general, most areas showed epidermal damage reflected by damaged keratinocytes, particularly in the basal layer. Often vacuoles could be observed here and in some regions microblister formation. The skin of the other side of the pig ear did not show signs of pathology. In skin biopsies taken after exposure to HD vapor we were able to demonstrate the formation of HD–DNA adducts (Figure 5).

Measurement of Skin Irritancy by Means of Transepidermal Water Loss

The effects of various compounds on pig ear TEWL were measured after a 4-h exposure period. The data of these measurements were compared with values reported in vivo.[16] As shown in Figure 6, there appeared a fairly good concordance between these data.

DISCUSSION

Here we describe an in vitro alternative method for in vivo animal skin testing, the whole-blood-perfused pig ear model. As is illustrated, the model can be used to measure dermal penetration rates, skin dermatotoxicity and the mechanisms involved. In our opinion, this is a flexible model, and is an in vitro alternative with great potential.

Pig ears were chosen, since pig skin closely resembles human skin and pig ears are considered slaughterhouse offal. However, when quickly cannulated after removal from the pigs' heads and perfused with autologous anticoagulated blood, they proved a very useful tool for the study of skin penetration of xenobiotics. This model has a number of advantages over currently used models. Importantly, "whole" skin is used, with a structurally intact vascular system. Furthermore, the pig ear model is perfused with a very natural perfusing medium, autologous blood. The model is cheap, simple to prepare, and does not require experimental animals. The model is now well characterized. When using our exclusion criteria, we are able to obtain reproducible results. The importance of maintaining an intact skin and using the natural perfusate blood is best illustrated by the studies with xylene. In the first study, it was shown that the composition

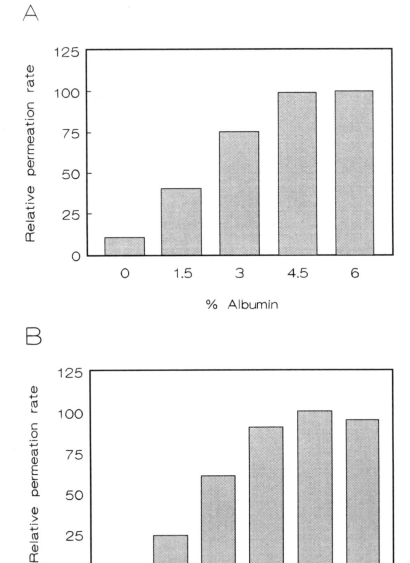

Figure 3. Influence of the recipient phase on the permeation rate of xylene in the pig ear model. (A) Effect of bovine serum albumin concentration on the measured penetration rate. (B) Effect of the perfusion flow on the measured penetration rate using buffer containing 4.5% albumin.

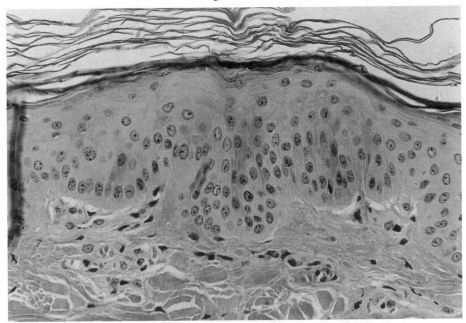

A

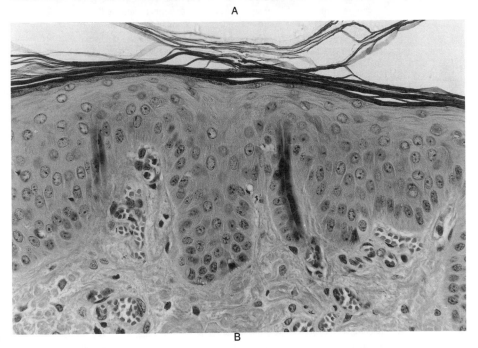

B

Figure 4. Exposure of pig ears to sulfur mustard vapor. Histological picture of skin specimens of (A) the skin area exposed to sulfur mustard vapor and (B) control skin. Pig ear skin was exposed for 4 min to saturated sulfur mustard vapor. After exposure, the pig ears were perfused with oxygenated whole blood for 10 h.

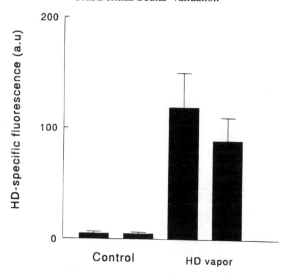

Figure 5. Illustrative example of the average FITC fluorescence for the presence of N^7-guanine monoadducts above the nuclei in the epidermis after exposure of pig skin to sulfur mustard vapor. The bars represent duplicate samples. The data presented are control (nonexposed skin) and skin exposed for 6 min to saturated HD vapor. Per data point, 100 nuclei were analyzed (± standard deviation).

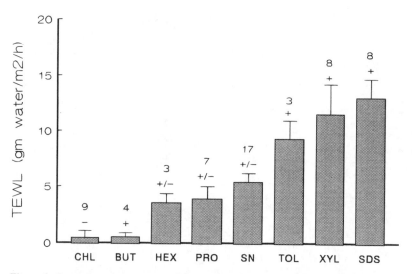

Figure 6. Concordance between transepidermal water loss measurements (TEWL) in the pig ear model and in vivo data. For a series of compounds (see text results section), the TEWL was measured in the pig ear model. The degree of irritating potential was recorded and compared with the degree of irritant potential in vivo (Guidelines of the Consumer Products Safety Commission of the European Community). Compounds were CHL, chloroform; BUT, butanol; HEX, hexane; PRO, propanol; SN, silver nitrate (5% in water or oil); TOL, toluene; XYL, xylene; and SDS, sodium dodecyl sulfate (10%). +, Designated as positive, −, designated as negative in vivo; +/−, uncertain; n, number of replicates.

of the perfusate influences the penetration rate of xylene. In particular, the relative protein concentration is important. This may not be equally important for every xenobiotic but may be a factor easily neglected or abused when designing experiments using the diffusion cell. In the second study with xylene, the influence of the presence or absence of the stratum corneum on skin penetration rate was investigated. This study made it clear that the absence or presence of this skin layer changes the barrier and depot function of the skin, and thereby the dermal permeation rate. This investigation indicates that only skin penetration studies in intact skin may have some predictive value for human skin penetration. When attempts are made to relate penetration values obtained in the pig ear model with data obtained in normal human volunteers, such a comparison is hampered by the fact that in humans few reliable penetration data have been obtained. So far, skin penetration values in the pig ear vary between 5 fold higher or lower than values obtained using volunteers. This can be an indication that the pig ear model can be used in the future to predict the skin penetration potential of a xenobiotic in the human situation. Validation studies of this type should, therefore, be encouraged in the near future, to finally have a well-developed predictive test.

A different application of the model is that it can be used to study the effectiveness of countermeasures against sulfur mustard-induced skin damage. Pig ears exposed to sulfur mustard vapor show severe skin damage (although only slight blister formation occurs) and strongly increased DNA adduct formation as measured by immunohistochemistry. Since DNA adduct formation can be quantitated, the pig ear model can be used to quantitate the effectiveness of countermeasures (e.g. protective clothing or barrier creams) against sulfur mustard-induced skin damage.

The idea that the pig ear model can also be an useful test model to predict the skin irritant potential of a xenobiotic in human skin is enforced by TEWL measurements in pig ear skin. The outcome of the irritant potential in the pig ear skin agreed fairly well with the irritating potential reported in vivo. These results can, therefore, be considered an additional argument that this test system has potential to predict effects in human skin.

Taken together, the blood-perfused pig ear model is a potential in vitro alternative for in vivo animal testing, as illustrated here in the fields of skin penetration and toxicity.

REFERENCES

1. Durrheim, M., Flynn, G. L., Higuchi, W. I., and Behl, C. R. 1980. Penetration of hairless mouse skin I: Experimental methods and comparison with human epidermal permeation by alkanols. *J. Pharm. Sci.* 69:781–786.
2. van Genderen, J. 1990. On the evaluation of a skin model: The human skin grafted nude mouse. Thesis, University of Utrecht, Utrecht.
3. Rougier, A., Lotte, C., and Maibach, H. I. 1987. The hairless rat: A relevant animal model to predict in vivo percutaneous absorption in humans? *J. Invest. Dermatol.* 88:577–581.
4. Reifenrath, W. G., Chellquist, E. M., Shipwash, E. A., Jéderberg, W. W., and Krueger, G. G. 1984. Percutaneous penetration in the hairless dog, weanling pig and grafted athymic nude mouse: Evaluation of models for predicting skin penetration in man. *Br. J. Dermatol.* 111:123–135.
5. Bond, J. R., and Barry, B. W. 1988. Limitations of hairless mouse skin as a model for in vitro permeation studies through human skin: Hydration damage. *J. Invest. Dermatol.* 90:486–489.
6. Bond, J. R., and Barry, B. W. 1988. Hairless mouse skin is limited as a model for assessing the effects of penetration enhancers in human skin. *J. Invest. Dermatol.* 90:810–813.
7. Bronaugh, R. L., and Maibach, H. I. 1985. In vitro models for human percutaneous absorption. In *Models in dermatology* vol. 2, eds. H. I. Maibach and N. J. Lowe, 178–188. Basel: Karger.
8. Scott, R. C., Dugard, P. H., Ramsey, J. D., and Rhodes, C. 1987. In vitro absorption of some *o*-phthalate diesters through human and rat skin. *Environ. Health Perspect.* 74:223–227.
9. Montagna, W., and Yung, J. S. 1961. The skin of the domestic pig. *J. Invest. Dermatol.* 43:11–21.
10. Bartek, M. J., Labudde, J. A., and Maibach, H. I. 1972. Skin permeability in vivo: Comparison in rat, rabbit, pig and man. *J. Invest. Dermatol.* 58:114–123.
11. Reifenrath, W. G., and Hawkins, G. S. 1986. The weanling Yorkshire pig as an animal model for measuring percutaneous penetration. In *Swine in biomedical research*, ed. M. E. Tumbelson, pp. 673–680. New York: Plenum Press.
12. Riviere, J. E., Bowman, K. F., Monteiro-Riviere, N. A., Dix, L. P., and Carver, M. P. 1986. The isolated perfused porcine skin flap (IPPSF) 1. A novel in vitro model for percutaneous absorption and cutaneous toxicology studies. *Fundam. Appl. Toxicol.* 7:444–453.

13. de Lange, J., van Eck, P., Elliott, G. R., de Kort, W. L. A. M., and Wolthuis, O. L. 1991. The isolated blood-perfused pig ear: A cheap animal-saving model for skin penetration studies. *J. Pharmacol. Toxicol. Methods* 27:71–77.
14. de Lange, J., van Eck, P., Bruijnzeel, P. L. B., and Elliott, G. R. 1994. The rate of percutaneous permeation of xylene, measured using the "perfused pig ear" model, is dependent on the effective protein concentration in the perfusing medium. *Toxicol. Appl. Pharmacol. Sci.* 127:298–305.
15. van der Schans, G. P., Scheffer, A. G., Mars-Groenendijk, R. H., Fidder, A., Benschop, H. P., and Baan, R. A. 1994. Immunochemical detection of adducts of sulfur mustard to DNA of calf thymus and human white blood cells. *Chem. Res. Toxicol.* 7:408–413.
16. Commission European Community Collaborative Study on relationship between in vivo primary irritation and in vitro experimental models. 1988. EC Report CEC/V/LUX/157/88.

Chapter Twenty-six

BOVINE CORNEAL OPACITY AND PERMEABILITY TEST VALIDATION AS AN ALTERNATIVE TO THE DRAIZE EYE IRRITATION ASSAY

D. Cerven and O. Moreno

The bovine corneal opacity and permeability (BCOP) assay has been proposed for use as an alternative to the Draize eye irritation assay. In this study we evaluated the in vitro scores for the BCOP assay in relation to those obtained using three abbreviated rabbit Draize eye irritation assays and the chorioallantoic membrane vascular assay (CAMVA). The products and chemicals used in this evaluation were chosen based on their Draize irritation potential and included dilutions of SDA-40 alcohols, alcohol-containing products, cosmetic products, and shampoos. Draize mean total scores ranged from 0 to 48.33. RC50 values from the CAMVA ranged from 1.0 to greater than 100 and in vitro scores from the BCOP ranged from <0 to 60.68. The data suggest that both the BCOP and CAMVA assays can be used as screens for ocular irritation potential. However, the BCOP may be more accurate at low irritancy levels.

INTRODUCTION

Both the chorioallantoic membrane vascular assay (CAMVA) and the bovine corneal opacity and permeability (BCOP) tests have been developed as alternatives to the use of laboratory animals for ocular irritation evaluations.[1-7] In the CAMVA the vascular responses of the chorioallantoic membrane (CAM) of fertile DeKalb eggs are evaluated 30 min after treatment. The RC50, the concentration that produces vascular responses in 50% of the treated eggs, is determined by probit analysis and serves as an index of ocular irritancy. The in vitro score is calculated from the responses of excised bovine corneas and consists of two parts—the opacity measurement and the permeability measurement.

MB Research Laboratories has been validating the two alternative assays. Previous evaluations[3,4] dealt strictly with the CAMVA assay. The objective of this study was to compare the BCOP test with both the CAMVA and the Draize ocular irritation assay. Four classes of materials were tested: cosmetic products, shampoos, glycols, and alcohol or alcohol-containing products.

The RC50 values and the in vitro scores were compared to the mean d 1 Draize scores from three rabbit eye irritation evaluations. Previous evaluations of CAMVA studies resulted in RC50 ranges that corresponded to the Draize classification of irritant, nonirritant, and indeterminate. Although Gautheron et al.[5] proposed irritancy levels based on BCOP in vitro scores, it was our intention to further classify the irritancy potential of the four classes of materials tested.

TEST MATERIALS

Seventeen cosmetic products were tested, including eye shadows, mascara, makeups, sun block, makeup remover, facial scrub, and blushing gel.

Ten alcohol dilutions or alcohol-containing materials were tested, including SDA-40-2, after-shave products, preshave products, and an astringent.

Three glycol products were evaluated: butylene, propylene, and hexylene glycol.

DRAIZE METHOD

Three healthy New Zealand white rabbits, free from evidence of ocular irritation and corneal abnormalities, were dosed with each product or product dilution. A dose of 0.1 ml was placed by syringe into the conjunctival sac of one eye of each animal, after gently pulling the lower eyelid away from the eye. After instillation, the lids were held together for approximately 1 s to insure adequate distribution of the test article.

Each treated eye was examined for irritation of the cornea, iris and conjunctiva on d 1, 2, and 3 following dosing. Ocular reactions were graded, according to the numerical Draize technique (Table 1).[8] Additional signs were described.

The primary eye irritation score for each rabbit was calculated from the weighted Draize scale (Table 1), and the mean total score (MTS) for each day was determined by averaging the individual primary eye irritation scores.

CAMVA METHOD

The 14-d incubation CAMVA method was selected, rather than the 10-d, because we have had more consistent results with the former.[9]

Fertile DeKalb XL strain eggs were selected for each evaluation from a larger group received from Moyer's Chicks, Quakertown, PA. The eggs were kept in incubators at 99 ± 2°F and 50–60% relative humidity. During the incubation period, the position of the egg tray within the incubator was changed daily to insure even atmospheric exposure.

On d 4 of the incubation period, the eggs were removed from the incubator and candled to determine the presence and location of the embryos. After determining the presence and marking the location of the embryo, a small hole was drilled into the narrow end of each egg, using a dentist's drill with a diamond wheel bit. Approximately 2.5 ml albumin was removed using a needle and syringe in order to lower the chorioallantoic membrane (CAM) sufficiently to prevent damage and allow an open area for treatment and examination. The hole was sealed with collodion adhesive. A rectangle window was cut, using a dental drill, and then removed with forceps. The opening was covered with transparent tape. The eggs were returned to the incubator for the remainder of the 14-d period. On d 14, the eggs were removed from the incubator, the tape peeled back, and the CAM examined for any abnormalities. Any egg with improperly developed membranes, undeveloped membranes, or any other abnormality was discarded.

Following the predose examination, a Teflon ring was gently placed on the CAM and 40 μl of the product or dilution was pipetted into the ring. The window was then resealed; the egg was numbered and returned to the incubator. After 30 ± 5 min, the eggs were removed from the incubator, and the CAM was exposed by removing the tape and portions of the surrounding shell. The condition of the CAM within the Teflon ring was examined and recorded. Vascular hemorrhage, capillary injection, and/or the presence of ghost vessels was considered a positive response. If any abnormalities were noted outside the ring, the egg was not included in the calculations. Ten eggs were used for each dilution. At least four dilutions of each product or SDA-40 were evaluated.

The percentage of CAMs responding positively to each dilution were plotted on three-cycle log-probit paper and an RC50 (the calculated concentration theoretically producing a positive reaction in 50% of the treated eggs) with 95% confidence limits was calculated, using the method of Litchfield and Wilcoxon.[10]

Table 1. Scale for Scoring Ocular Lesions

(1) Cornea:			
(A)	Opacity: Degree of density (area most dense taken for reading):		
	No ulceration or opacity		0
	Scattered or diffuse areas of opacity (other than slight dulling of normal luster), details of iris clearly visible		1[a]
	Easily discernible translucent area, details of iris slightly obscured		2[a]
	Opalescent areas, no details or iris visible, size of pupil barely discernible		3[a]
	Opaque cornea, iris not discernible through the opacity		4[a]
(B)	Area of cornea involved:		
	One quarter (or less) but not zero		1
	Greater than one-quarter, but less than one-half		2
	Greater than one-half, but less than three-quarters		3
	Greater than three quarters up to whole area		4
	SCORE EQUALS A × B × 5	Maximum Total	80
(2) Iris:			
(A)	Values:		
	Normal		0
	Folds above normal, congestion, swelling, circumcorneal injection (any or all of these or combination of any thereof), iris still reacting to light (sluggish reaction positive)		1[a]
	No reaction to light, hemoherrhage, gross destruction (any or all of these)		2[a]
	SCORE EQUALS A × 5	Maximum Total	10
(3) Conjunctivae:			
(A)	Redness (refers to palpebral and bulbar conjunctive excluding cornea & iris):		
	Blood vessels normal		0
	Some blood vessels definitely hyperemic (injected)		1
	More diffuse, deeper crimson red, individual vessels not easily discernible		2[a]
	Diffuse beefy red		3[a]
(B)	Chemosis:		
	No swelling		0
	Any swelling above normal (includes nictitating membranes)		1
	Obvious swelling with partial eversion of lids		2[a]
	Swelling with lids about half closed		3[a]
	Swelling with lids more than half closed		4[a]
(C)	Discharge:		
	No Discharge		0
	Any amount different from normal (does not include small amounts observed in inner canthus of normal animals		1
	Discharge with moistening of the lids and hairs just adjacent to lids		2
	Discharge with moistening of the lids and hairs and considerable area around the eye		3
	SCORE EQUALS (A + B + C) × 2	Maximum Total	20

Note. The maximum total score is the sum of all scores obtained for the cornea, iris and conjunctivae. From Draize et al.[8] with permission.

[a] indicates a positive response.

BCOP METHOD

The bovine eyes were received from a local supplier and transported to MB Research Laboratories in Hanks balanced salt solution in a refrigerated container. The eyes were examined within 1 h after receipt, and any eye with a cornea exhibiting evidence of vascularization, pigmentation, opacity, or scratches was discarded.

Corneas from eyes free of defects were dissected from the surrounding tissues. A 2–3 mm rim of sclera was left attached to each cornea. The dissected corneas were mounted in specially designed holders segmented into anterior and posterior chambers, which are filled separately. Each cornea was mounted allowing the epithelium of the cornea to project into the anterior chamber. The posterior chamber was filled with minimal essential media supplemented with 1%

fetal bovine serum (MEM). The anterior chamber was then filled with MEM. Each cornea was visually inspected again to insure that there were no defects. The entire holder with the cornea was submerged in a 32°C water bath and allowed to equilibrate for at least 1 h, but not longer than 2 h.

Following equilibration, the holders containing the corneas were removed from the water baths. The MEM was removed from both chambers and the chambers were refilled with fresh MEM. At this time, five corneas were selected for dosing with the test material and two were selected as controls.

Measurements of opacity through the cornea were made using an OP-KIT opacitometer produced by Electro-Design Corporation of Rion, France. At each interval, each treated cornea was scored in comparison with the two control corneas. A preexposure determination of opacity was made for each control by measuring each against the blanks supplied with the opacitometer. A preexposure determination of opacity was made for each of the 5 test corneas by measuring against each control cornea (a total of 10 determinations).

Following the pretest observations, the MEM was removed from the anterior chamber, and a volume of 0.75 ml of the undiluted test material was applied to the epithelium of each of the 5 treated corneas. The holders and corneas were then placed in the 32°C water in a horizontal position to insure contact of the test material with the cornea. After 10 ± 1 min, the test substance (or MEM in the controls) was removed from the epithelium of the cornea and the anterior chamber by washing with MEM. All holders were then refilled with fresh MEM, returned to the water bath, and incubated at 32°C for an additional 2 h.

At the end of the 2-h period, the MEM was changed again and a measurement of opacity taken comparing each of the 5 treated corneas to the 2 control corneas. Immediately following the 2-h opacity measurement, the MEM was changed in the posterior chamber of both the control and test corneas. The MEM was removed from the anterior chamber and replaced with 1.0 ml of 0.4% sodium fluorescein solution in both the treated and control corneas. Fresh holders and corneas were then returned to the 32°C water bath in a horizontal position to insure contact of the fluorescein with the cornea.

After 90 min, the fluid from the posterior chamber was removed and the amount of dye that passed through the cornea was measured as the optical density at 450 nm, using a Spectronic 20 spectrophotometer.

When the test material was a solid, it was dissolved in MEM at a 20% dilution and allowed to remain in contact with the cornea for 4 h, rather than 20 min. The opacity measurement was taken after the 4-h exposure.

When the test material was known to contain alcohol, and additional opacity measurement was taken when the test material was removed following the 10-min exposure.

The corrected mean opacity score was calculated using the control and treated cornea opacity values, as determined from the OP-KIT.

The corrected mean optical density score was calculated, using the control and treated optical density values from the fluorescein permeability analysis. The in vitro score was calculated as:

Corrected mean opacity score + 15(corrected mean optical density score).

RESULTS

The CAMVA RC50s, BCOP in vitro scores, and corresponding d 1 Draize mean total scores (MTS) are presented in Tables 2–5. The results of the Draize ocular testing were also classified for levels of irritancy, according to a modification of the original Draize interpretation, using only three animals, as follows:

Nonirritant   0 rabbits with positive scores
Indeterminate   1 rabbit with positive score
Irritant   2–3 rabbits with positive scores

The CAMVA RC50, ranged from 11 to greater than 100% for cosmetic products; 11.0 to greater than 100% for alcohol and alcohol containing materials; 0.19 to 14% for shampoos; and 7.6 to 30% for glycols.

Table 2. Cosmetic Products

Test material	Product type	Day 1 draize MTS	Draize classification	RC50 (%)	BCOP in vitro score
D-8	Eye makeup remover	0	—	100	−0.52
D-6	Mascara	0	—	>100	0.83
D-53	Nailcare powder	0	—	>100	−0.23
D-54	SPFG suntan cream	0	—	87	2.11
D-55	SPF-6 suntan cream	0	—	>100	2.23
D-50	Eye shadow	0.67	—	>100	1.07
D-51	Eye shadow	0.67[a]	—	>100	2.92
D-13	Blemish control makeup	0.67	—	30	3.65
PRODUCT 21	Powder makeup	2.00	i	>100	4.08
PRODUCT 22	Powder makeup	2.33	+	>100	4.49
D-20	Antiperspirant	4.67[a]	i	23	0.55
D-52	Eye shadow	6.00[a]	+	>100	0.81
D-4	Sun block	6.00	i	>100	0.59
D-2	Cream makeup	6.00	+	103	5.72
D-5	Facial makeup	6.67	+	>100	1.10
D-10	Blushing gel	8.67[b]	+	11	0.55
D-56	SPF-15 sun screen gel	30.00	=	18	41.35

[a] Test material remaining in rabbit conjunctiva at 24 h post dose.
[b] Red coloration of the conjunctiva may have been due to the dye in the test article and not to an irritant effect.

Table 3. Alcohol and Alcohol-Containing Materials

Test material	Product type	Day 1 Draize MTS	Draize classification	RC50 (%)	BCOP in vitro score
PRODUCT 6	After shave skin conditioner	0	—	>100	−4.25
PRODUCT 2	After shave conditioner	0	—	56	2.23
30% SDA-40-2	Aqueous dilution	0.67	—	50	6.80
PRODUCT 3	After shave	9.67	+	20	24.18
50% SDA-40-2	Aqueous dilution	11.33	+	36	15.35
PRODUCT 5	After shave	15.67	+	22	45.38
70% SDA-40-2	Aqueous dilution	16.67	+	22	22.65
PRODUCT 8	Astringent	19.33	+	16	44.28
PRODUCT 7	Preshave	23.33	+	11	26.10
100% SDA-40-2	Aqueous dilution	48.33	+	15	35.30

Table 4. Glycols

Test material	Product type	Day 1 Draize MTS	Draize classification	RC50 (%)	BCOP in vitro score
Butylene glycol	N/A	0	—	12.0	1.02
Propylene glycol	N/A	2.0	—	30.0	1.65
Hexylene glycol	N/A	16.67	+	7.6	21.45

The BCOP in vitro scores ranged from −0.52 to 41.35% for cosmetic products; −4.25 to 45.38% for alcohol and alcohol containing materials; −3.92 to 60.6% for shampoos; 1.02 to 21.45% for glycols.

Day 1 Draize mean total scores ranged from 0 to 30.0 in cosmetic products; 0 to 48.33 for alcohol and alcohol-containing materials; 0 to 18.67 for shampoos; and 0 to 16.67 for glycols. The Draize values may have overestimated the true ocular responses for D-51 and D-52 eye shadows and D-20 antiperspirant, since it was noted in the d 1 observation that the material

Table 5. Shampoos

Test material	Product type	Day 1 Draize MTS	Draize classification	RC50 (%)	BCOP in vitro score
S-4 (10%)	Shampoo aqueous dilution	0	—	5.4	−3.92
S-1 (10%)	Shampoo aqueous dilution	0.33	—	14.0	1.35
BABY SHAMPOO	Undiluted aqueous dilution	1.00	—	3.6	2.10
S-5 (10%)	Shampoo aqueous dilution	3.33	i	5.0	2.98
S-2	Shampoo—undiluted	11.67	+	0.32	10.60
S-1	Shampoo—undiluted	12.00	+	0.87	11.00
S-6	Shampoo—undiluted	12.00	+	0.99	21.83
S-3	Shampoo—undiluted	12.33	+	1.1	60.68
S-4	Shampoo—undiluted	15.00	+	1.0	13.80
S-5	Shampoo—undiluted	18.67	+	0.19	7.43

remained in the conjunctiva. The increased exposure may have resulted in elevated ocular responses. Additionally, the 8.67 d 1 Draize score for the D-10 blushing gel may have been the result of staining of the conjunctiva, rather than an erythematous response.

DISCUSSION

We conducted these evaluation to classify the irritancy potential of classes of test materials, according to their in vitro scores, using the BCOP assay. Information supplied with the Opacitometer suggested the following classification scheme:

In Vitro Score	Classification
0 to 25	Mild irritant
25.1 to 55	Moderate irritant
55.1 and greater	Severe irritant

Of particular interest was delineating the mild irritant category, that is, determining the in vitro scores that correspond to the limits of the irritant/nonirritant category of the Draize evaluations.

For cosmetic products the in vitro score, which approximates the limits of irritant/nonirritant, appears to be in the 4 to 5 units range. Although it appears from Table 2 that a number of materials would be false negatives assuring a 4 or 5 unit limit, it is likely that for two test articles, D-20 and D-52, the Draize values may be overestimations of the true irritancy potential. In both instances, the powder materials remained in the conjunctiva through 24 h. The prolonged exposure may have resulted in increased Draize mean total scores. The blushing gel, D-10, may also have been a false positive, since reddening of the conjunctiva was the only abnormal ocular effect noted in the rabbits and may have resulted from staining, rather than an erythematous reaction. The sun block, D-4, and the facial scrub, D-5, were the only other false negatives and will be reexamined in the future.

CAMVA RC50s for the cosmetic products were all above the irritant/nonirritant limit of 1–3% found for surfactants,[4] and indicated that it may be necessary to validate this study in more detail when using different chemical entities.

In the alcohol group of test materials, there were fewer Draize responses in the borderline range. The irritant/nonirritant interface for the BCOP assay appears to be in the units range of approximately 5 or 6. Previous evaluations[4] indicated the RC50 values of less than 30% corresponded to eye irritants and RC50 values greater than 40% corresponded to little or no irritation.

Among the neat shampoos, only the baby shampoo was classified as nonirritating. In addition, two aqueous shampoo dilutions were in the nonirritating category and one dilution was indeterminate. These data indicate that the irritant/nonirritant level for shampoos in the BCOP assay is between 2 and 10, but probably closer to 2. As previously published, the CAMVA RC50 limits were similar to those of surfactants,[3] where the irritant/nonirritant level was approximately 1.0.

The results observed for cosmetic products indicated the BCOP may be a better evaluation for use with products that tend to produce low levels of irritation.

REFERENCES

1. Bagley, D. M., Rizvi, P. Y., Kong, B. M., and DeSalva, S. J. 1988. An improved CAM assay for predicting occular irritation potential. In *Alternative methods in toxicology*, vol. 6, ed. A. M. Goldberg, pp. 131–138.
2. Bagley, D. M., Kong, B. M., and DeSalva, S. J. 1989. Assessing the eye irritation potential of surfactant-based materials using the Chorioallantoic Membrane Vascular Assay (CAMVA). In *Alternative methods in toxicology*, vol. 7, ed. A. M. Goldberg, pp. 265–272.
3. Cerven, D., Szivos, M., Kaminsky, M., and Moreno, O. 1991. CAMVA validation as an alternative to the Draize Ocular: Part 1; Surfactants. Poster presented at American College of Toxicology Meeting, Orlando, Fl.
4. Cerven, D., and Moreno, O. 1992. Poster presented at Society of Toxicology Meeting, Seattle, WA.
5. Gautheron, P., Dukie, M., Alix, D., and Sina, J. 1992 Bovine corneal opacity and permeability test: An in vitro assay of ocular irritancy. *Fundam. Appl. Toxicol.* 18:442–449.
6. IRAG Work Group Report. 1993. CAM-Based Assays. Draft. November.
7. IRAG Workshop on Eye Irritation Testing. 1993. Draft Report. Organotypic Models. November.
8. Draize, J. H., Woodward, G., and Calvery, H. D. 1944. Methods for the study of irritation and toxicity of substances applied topically to the skin and mucous membranes. *J. Pharmacol. Exp. Ther.* 82:377–390.
9. Cerven, D., and Moreno, O. 1993. CAMVA validation as an alternative to the Draize ocular: Part 3: 10 and 14 Day incubation CAMVA. Poster presented at the Society of Toxicology Meetings, New Orleans, LA.
10. Litchfield, J. T., Jr., and Wilcoxon, F. 1949. A simplified method of evaluating dose effect experiments. *J. Pharmacol. Exp. Ther.* 96:99.

Chapter Twenty-seven

METABOLISM OF HUMANS AND ANIMALS COMPARED BY ORGAN CULTURES

Byong Han (Paul) Chin

The purpose of this chapter is to introduce an in vitro liver explant technique reflecting in vivo metabolic processes of chemicals in animals, including humans, without resorting to the risk of dosing human beings. Since the pesticide carbaryl (1-naphthyl N-methylcarbamate) has been investigated extensively in humans and other species by many laboratories, this chemical was selected as the prototype for development of an in vitro liver explant technique. This presentation, therefore, addresses the metabolic comparison of carbaryl based on in vitro and in vivo procedures among animal species including humans. The in vitro technique was successful in generating in vivo metabolism of carbaryl in various species semiquantitatively. Also, the in vitro liver explant technique was successful for reproducing semiquantitatively in vivo metabolites of three other chemicals (ethylbenzene, methylethylbenzene isomers, and ethylcyclohexane). Therefore, this in vitro liver explant procedure provides metabolic information concerning the metabolic similarity or difference between the human and the animal without resorting to the dosing of human beings. Because this in vitro technique is species specific, it can facilitate selection of animals with a similar metabolic pattern to humans for further in-depth toxicity studies.

INTRODUCTION

This chapter reviews in vitro organ explant technique,[1-9] which offers promise as a practical method to determine the metabolism of a chemical in humans without direct human dosing and its attendant risks. Metabolites of chemicals are often responsible for toxic effects of chemicals. In-depth studies of comparative metabolism of humans and animals would then fulfill the concepts proposed by Frazer[10] in regard to selection of animals for toxicological studies: "If two or more different metabolic patterns are found in animals investigated, it becomes necessary to discover which of these patterns occurs in man. When this is known, animals with a similar pattern should be chosen for further toxicological studies."

The assumption that metabolites formed in the liver[11] would predominate in the urine made it the major organ of choice for this investigation. Its availability as a result of surgical procedure and diagnostic biopsy made its use practical.

The pesticide carbaryl (Sevin, 1-naphthyl *N*-methylcarbamate) was selected as the prototype because of the extensive metabolic studies[12-15] done in humans and other species. Any other compound with a comparable body of information on anionic metabolites would have served the purpose equally well. For the purposes of this study, the anionic metabolites were chosen for profile analysis, because they not only reflect the complex redox systems in metabolism,

Dr. Chin's presentation here represents his own professional opinions and not agency policy. This research was carried out at Bushy Run Research Center, Union Carbide Corporation, Export, PA.

but include the conjugating systems as well. The important neutral or nonconjugated materials also will be treated species by species in later studies.

The following steps are taken to select species that metabolize the test chemical like humans:

1. The test chemical is introduced by the route to be used in the chronic toxicity studies to an animal species (rat will be used as an example in the subsequent steps) and an in vivo (24-h urine sample) metabolic profile is generated by chromatographic method.
2. In vitro metabolic profiles of rat and human tissues (liver will be used as example) are generated by the same chromatographic method.
3. Compare the three metabolic profiles: rat in vivo, rat in vitro, and human in vitro.

The rationale of this approach may be best demonstrated by the following equations:

1. If rat in vivo metabolites approximate rat in vitro metabolites, and
2. If rat in vitro metabolites approximate human in vitro metabolites, then
3. Rat in vivo metabolites approximate human in vivo metabolites.

In the event that the rat metabolic profiles do not match that of humans, similar comparisons should be made on other species (mouse, hamster, guinea pig, dog, etc.). The species most closely resembling humans is the animal of choice.

METHODS

1-Naphthyl-[^{14}C]methylcarbamate ([^{14}C]carbaryl) of specific activity 5.8 μCi/mg was used. Trowell T8 medium[16] was procured from Microbiological Associates, Bethesda, MD. Organ tissues from the following species were used: 120- to 150-g male Harlan-Wistar rats, 6-kg male beagle dogs, mature male guinea pigs, and liver biopsy from a human female. In all the explant studies, 100 μg carbaryl/500 mg tissue was used. For the rat, this is roughly equivalent to an in vivo dose of 7 mg/kg body weight.

Culture Methods

Trowell T8 medium was oxygenated by passing carbogen (95% oxygen:5% carbon dioxide) at the rate of 100 ml/min through a 10-ml aliquot in a 15-ml beaker for 30 min. Aseptically procured liver was gently rinsed in oxygenated medium until free of blood. Tissue, 500 mg, was weighed on the sterilized cover of a 60 × 15 mm petri dish and then cut freehand with a number 10 scalpel blade into 2-mm cubes (approximately 80 pieces) under oxygenated medium using aseptic technique. The cubes were then transferred to an open petri dish containing 3 ml oxygenated Trowell T8 medium and placed in a 9-L vacuum desiccator. Again this entire unit was flushed with carbogen at 1.5 L/min for 30 min. The chamber was sealed and maintained at room temperature for 90 min; the labeled compound, dissolved in 5–10 μl of 95% ethanol, was then added dropwise from a 10-μl syringe, while gently swirling the dish. The dish was returned to the desiccator and again flushed with carbogen, sealed, and placed in an incubator at 37°C for the desired incubation time (18 h).

Analytical Methods

At the termination of incubation, the medium was subjected to diethylaminoethyl (DEAE) cellulose chromatography technique,[12] utilizing an ammonium formate buffer instead of Tris-HCl buffer. The formate columns were prepared by adding 6 g DEAE-cellulose to 150 ml of 0.005 N formic acid at pH 4, stirring for 15 min, and packing this slurry into a 1.5 × 24 cm column. The column was then washed with 750 ml of 0.005 N formic acid, pH 4, and equilibrated by washing with 6 L of 0.005 N ammonium formate, pH 6.5. The elution gradients for these columns consisted of 0.005–0.01, 0.01–0.05, and 0.05–0.1 N ammonium formate; 300 ml of each concentration was used per gradient. Fractions (4 ml) were collected, and every fifth fraction was analyzed by liquid scintillation counting techniques.

Table 1. Variation of In Vitro Rat Liver Metabolites of Naphthyl-[^{14}C]carbaryl

	Neutrals		Metabolites					
Rat number	(Phase I reaction products) (A & B)	dihydrodi-hydroxy-carbaryl glucuron-ide (D)	Unknown + hydroxy carbaryl glucuron-ide (E) + (F)	Naphthyl glucuron-ide (G)	Hydroxy carba-ryl sul-fate (I)	Naph-thyl sulfate (J)	Pooled fractions[a]	Percent cor-rected recovery
1	26	19	4.2	7.5	0.4	20	5.8	83
2	21	23	5.0	6.0	1.7	21	4.2	84
3	25	27	2.7	6.3	Trace	20	4.5	89
4	29	23	4.5	6.3	Trace	14	13.5	90
5	25	18	5.8	5.8	Trace	24	4.2	83
Mean	25.2	22.0	4.44	6.38		19.8	6.44	85.8
(SD)	(2.9)	3.6	(1.15)	(0.66)		(3.6)	(4.00)	(3.4)

Note. Quantity of metabolite expressed as percent of ^{14}C applied on the column. From Sullivan et al.[9] with permission.
[a] Combined fractions from areas of chromatogram not containing a distinguishable peak.

RESULTS

To examine the reproducibility of the in vitro technique, profiles of metabolites of naphthyl-[^{14}C]carbaryl obtained from livers of five male Harlan-Wistar rats are compared in Table 1. In most instances, the identity of the peak component in Table 1 is that assigned by Knaak et al.[12] The designation of major metabolites of carbaryl in this chapter was based on the chromatographic behavior and fluorescence characteristics, rather than the actual isolation and structural verification of the metabolites. If the means and standard deviation (SD) of peaks A, D, E + F, G, I, and J are considered, all peaks show good reproducibility. Variations are within the limits of experimental error. "Pooled fractions" represent the combined areas of chromatographic profiles not containing distinguishable peaks. In the case of rat number, the pooled fractions deviated markedly from the others, because of poor resolution of column peaks. This was not seriously detrimental to the overall profile analysis and can be minimized by improvement in analytical methodology.

In order to estimate the incubation time required by the in vitro method, experiments were designed utilizing rat liver to determine a practical incubation period. Results of these studies are given in Tables 2 and 3. The 18-h data are the mean values from Table 1. The 6- and 18-h times are comparable for the anionic metabolites as illustrated in Table 2. The major difference found was with the neutral fractions containing Phase I reaction products.

Percentages of unreacted carbaryl, 5,6-dihydro-5,6-dihydroxy-carbaryl (the major in vivo metabolite), ether-extractable neutrals, and of the neutrals per se are given in Table 3. The percentages of neutrals, ether-extractable neutrals, and unmetabolized carbaryl all decreased with

Table 2. In Vitro Metabolic Profiles for Various Incubation Periods

	Metabolites						
Incubation	Neutrals (Phase I reaction products) (A & B)	dihydrodi-hydroxy-carbaryl glucuron-ide (D)	Unknown + hydroxy-carbaryl glucuron-ide (E) + (F)	Naphthyl glucuron-ide (G)	Hydroxy carba-ryl sul-fate (I)	Naph-thyl sulfate (J)	Pooled fractions
3	56.4	17.1	4.2	0.9	1.4	11.0	1.9
6	38.6	21.6	10.5	4.6	15.9		3.8
18	25.2	22.0	4.4	6.4	Trace	19.9	6.4

Note. Quantity of metabolite expressed as percent of ^{14}C applied on the column. From Sullivan et al.[9] with permission.
[a] Combined fractions from areas of chromatogram not containing a distinguishable peak.

Table 3. Operational Parameters Expressed as Percentage of Carbaryl Equivalents

Incuba-tion (h)	Neutrals (Phase I reaction products)	Neutrals (Phase I reaction products) found in ether phase[a]	Unmetabo-lized carbaryl found in ether phase[a]	Carbaryl found in medium	dihydrodihy-droxycarba-ryl found in ether phase[b]
3	56	82	74.7	30	9.8
6	39	69	56.3	15	10.6
18	25	40			
			T[c]	T	56.7

Note. From Sullivan et al.[9] with permission.
[a] As percent of radioactivity recovered from a silica gel column.
[b] Based upon silica gel column chromatographic position of dihydrodihydroxycarbaryl, a major neutral metabolite, found in vivo in the rat and expressed as percent of recovered radioactivity.
[c] T, Trace quantity (less than 0.4% of the ^{14}C applied on the column).

time. Only the 18-h incubation data approach that found in vivo for any of these parameters. The major in vivo metabolite was found to increase as a percent of recovered activity with time and approached the in vivo results at 18 h. Based upon profile analysis of the medium, in all probability a 6-h incubation period is adequate for study of anionic metabolites.

Figure 1 illustrates a direct comparison of typical naphthyl-[^{14}C]carbaryl DEAE cellulose profiles for both an in vitro and in vivo study in the rat.[15] Table 4 shows the comparative metabolism of carbaryl by in vitro liver explant versus an in vivo 24-h urine sample[9] using naphthyl-[^{14}C]carbaryl. The in vitro results in the rat for naphthyl-[^{14}C]carbaryl are related qualitatively to results obtained in vivo and provide evidence for the presence of similar major and minor metabolic components, except for naphthyl sulfate. This component was produced by rat liver in vitro in approximately three times the amount found in vivo. Part of this higher level of naphthyl sulfate is caused by nonenzymatic hydrolysis of carbaryl. Nonenzymatic

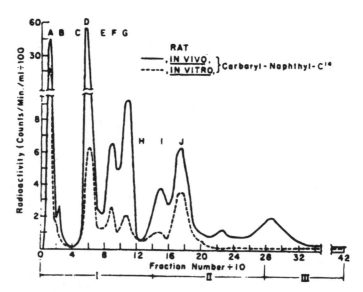

Figure 1. DEAE-cellulose chromatogram of in vivo and in vitro rat metabolites of naphthyl-[^{14}C]carbaryl. Gradient elution program: (I) 0.01 M Tris:HCl buffer, pH 7.5, to 0.05 M Tris-HCl buffer, pH 7.5. (II) 0.05 M Tris:HCl buffer, pH 7.5, to 0.1 M Tris-HCl buffer, pH 7.5. (III) 0.1 M Tris:HCl buffer, pH 7.5, to 0.5 M Tris-HCl buffer, pH 7.5. From Sullivan et al.[9] with permission.

Table 4. Comparison of In Vitro and In Vivo Metabolites of Carbaryl by Rat

	Neutrals (Phase I reaction products) (A & B)	Dihydrodihydroxycarbaryl glucuronide (D)	Metabolites					
			Hydroxy carbaryl glucuronide (E) + (F)	Naphthyl glucuronide (G)	Hydroxy carbaryl sulfate (I)	Naphthyl sulfate (J)	Total recovery[b]
In vitro	25.2	19.0	4.0	8.0	T[a]	20.0	76.20
In vivo	11.5	37.2	6.8	11.3	6.0	9.4	82.20

Note. Quantity of metabolite expressed as percent of ^{14}C applied on the column. From Sullivan et al.[9] with permission.
[a] T, Trace quantity (less than 0.4% of the ^{14}C applied on the column).
[b] Total recovery did not include fractions between peaks

hydrolysis was estimated to be 10% as determined in buffered systems at pH 7.2 and 37°C without tissue.[1] Failure to find appreciable amounts of 1-naphthol in the tissue studies from ether extracts of the neutrals indicates that this material is conjugated with either glucuronic or sulfuric acid.

Figure 2 illustrates the in vitro results obtained with naphthyl-[^{14}C]carbaryl in liver tissue obtained during surgical procedure on a 40-yr-old female, when plotted with the in vivo results of Knaak et al.[14] The qualitative agreement of the profiles is extremely good. The minor peak D, absent in vivo, was demonstrated to be a nonfluorescent metabolite in the rat.[12] The major difference in the two profiles is a substantially greater percent of naphthyl sulfate in vivo and a greater percent of naphthyl glucuronide in vitro. Reasons for this disagreement are not currently known.

Figure 3 represents the results found with studies in guinea pigs using naphthyl-[^{14}C]carbaryl. The solid line in Figure 3 represents the in vivo results, and the dashed line represents the in vitro results. All peak designations (Table 1) are the same as for the rat. In vitro results show a higher percent of unconjugated neutrals than in vivo. The major metabolite from the guinea pig under these conditions was naphthyl glucuronide from both in vivo and in vitro.

Figure 4 represents the results found with studies in dogs using naphthyl-[^{14}C]carbaryl. Qualitatively, the profiles from in vivo and in vitro studies compare favorably. Both in vivo and in vitro neutrals comprise the major metabolites accounting for approximately 50% of the radioactivity.

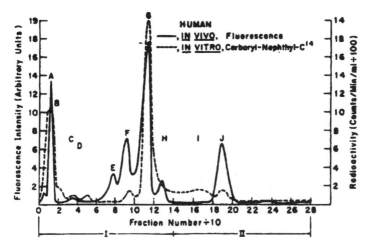

Figure 2. DEAE-cellulose chromatogram of in vivo and in vitro human metabolites of naphthyl-[^{14}C]carbaryl. Gradient elution program as in Figure 1. From Sullivan et al.[9] with permission.

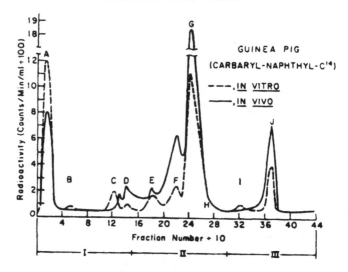

Figure 3. DEAE-cellulose chromatogram of in vivo and in vitro guinea pig metabolites of naphthyl-[^{14}C]carbaryl. Gradient elution program as in Figure 1. From Sullivan *et al.*[9] with permission.

Carbaryl metabolism in the dog is an excellent example for comparison of in vivo and in vitro techniques. Peak G in the in vivo studies of Knaak and Sullivan[13] was reported to chromatograph on DEAE-cellulose, as if it were naphthyl glucuronide (peak G), but it proved to be nonfluorescent. In the profile obtained for the in vitro metabolism of carbaryl with dog liver, the same results were obtained. Thus, the in vitro technique in this species not only gave profiles of similar character, but reproduced this particular unique metabolite.

The quantitative results obtained from the in vitro metabolism of carbaryl by liver tissues of

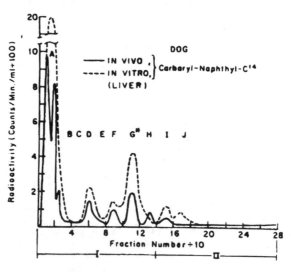

Figure 4. DEAE-cellulose chromatogram of in vivo and in vitro dog metabolites of naphthyl-[^{14}C]carbaryl. Gradient elution program as in Figure 1. From Sullivan *et al.*[9] with permission.

human, rat, guinea pig, and dog, respectively, are given in Table 5. These data are given as percent of radioactivity recovered from the column. Generally speaking, a higher percent of dose will be found in the neutral fraction from these in vitro studies than would be found in vivo in the same species. There are several factors that can contribute to this result, including the physical parameters of diffusion, a static versus a dynamic system, and time. A further complication arises from the possible interaction of the kidney and other organs with the in vivo liver metabolites. Humans metabolized a higher percent of carbaryl to neutrals than did the other species under scrutiny. Analysis showed that no more than 6% of the dose was unreacted carbaryl. The remainder of the neutrals was found to be a mixture of unknown metabolites.[9]

Based upon chromatographic and fluorometric analysis, naphthyl glucuronide was the most significant anionic metabolite from humans and the guinea pig, and a dihydrodihydroxycarbaryl glucuronide from the rat and dog.[15] The other significant anionic found in the dog was the nonfluorescent material, cochromatographing with naphthyl glucuronide as reported by Knaak and Sullivan[13] and described earlier.

DISCUSSION

Studies comparing the results of the in vitro metabolism of carbaryl with in vivo results have confirmed that the in vitro organ maintenance technique can be used to demonstrate comparative metabolism. The in vitro results closely paralleled in vivo metabolism of the compounds as derived from analysis of 24-h urine samples. The metabolic products found in vitro are species specific, and they are not dependent upon the addition of cofactor for their production. The method is qualitatively correct, but semiquantitative in its present form. In vitro profiles were reproducible, and the individual variation was not significantly different in five rat livers. The anionic metabolites were found to have an SD of 0.7–4%, depending upon the fraction analyzed. The SD as percent of ^{14}C applied to the chromatographic column was generally of the order of magnitude of the quantity present for minor metabolites, a finding that precludes quantitative comparison of the importance of differences between species. However, with major metabolites in humans, the value of the standard deviation, as determined from rat data, was such that direct quantitative comparison could be made.

There was a closer agreement between the profiles of in vitro and in vivo metabolites formed by the same species than between the profiles of different species (whether in vitro or in vivo). Thus, there is a satisfactory way of comparing the biotransformation carried out by different species, including humans. The in vitro organ maintenance technique thus can be used as a method to determine metabolism in humans utilizing radioactivity of high specific activity without direct dosing of human subjects. This technique thus facilitates the selection of animals with a similar metabolic pattern to humans for further in-depth toxicity studies.

Table 5. Comparison of In Vitro Metabolites of Carbaryl by Rat, Human, and Other Nonhuman Mammalian Livers

Species (Sex)	Neutrals (Phase I reaction products) (A & B)	Metabolites						
		Dihydrodi-hydroxy-carbaryl glucuron-ide (D)	Hydroxy carbaryl glucuron-ide (E) + (F)	Naphthyl glucuron-ide (G)	Hydroxy carba-ryl sul-fate (I)	Naph-thyl sulfate (J)	Total recovery[b]
Human (male)	66	1	1	28	T[a]	1	97
Cow (female)	41	1	3	24	0	13	82
Guinea pig (male)	26	3	6	33	2	12	82
Rat (male)	25	19	4	8	T	20	76
Dog (male)	29	26	6	19*	4	3	87
Monkey (male)	33	3	40	12	3	3	94

Note. Quantity of metabolite expressed as percent of ^{14}C applied on the column. From Sullivan et al.[9] with permission.
[a] T, Trace quantity (less than 0.4% of the ^{14}C applied on the column).
[b] Chromatographed as naphthyl glucuronide but does not fluoresce.
[c] Total recovery did not include fractions between peaks.

The in vitro technique was also applied to three other chemicals. Based on the chromatographic profile analysis of in vitro derived metabolites of ethylbenzene (EB), ethylmethylbenzene (EMB) isomers, and ethylcyclohexane (ECH) in rat and dog, the in vitro results semiquantitatively reproduced in vivo urinary metabolism of EB, EMB isomers, and ECH in the corresponding animal species.[5-8] The detailed findings will be addressed in another review.

The contributory role of other organ tissues (e.g., kidney and lung) in the total metabolism of a chemical has been evaluated using the in vitro technique.[2,3] Based upon total anionic metabolites formed from each tissue using [^{14}C]carbaryl, the quantitative tissue metabolic activity in descending order is liver, kidney, and lung. The comparative metabolic profiles from selected organs clearly show that the metabolic products found in vivo are not necessarily limited to liver-generated metabolites, but that they represent a composite of metabolites formed from the liver, the lung, and the kidney, and possibly from other organs as well. The investigation of metabolic activity of individual organs for a given compound can be important in the interpretation of toxicological effects as they relate to a target organ. The detailed findings will be addressed in another review.

REFERENCES

1. Chin, B. H., Eldridge, J. M., and Sullivan, L. J. 1974. Metabolism of carbaryl by selected human tissues using an organ-maintenance technique. *Clin. Toxicol.* 7(1):37–56.
2. Chin, B. H., Sullivan, L. J., Eldrige, J. M., and Tallant, M. J. 1979. Metabolism of carbaryl by kidney, liver and lung from human postembryonic fetal autopsy tissue. *Clin. Toxicol.* 14(5):489–498.
3. Chin, B. H., Eldridge, J. M., Anderson, J. H., and Sullivan, L. J. 1979. Carbaryl metabolism in the rat. A comparison of *in vivo, in vitro* (tissue explant) and liver perfusion techniques. *J. Agric. Food Chem.* 27(4):716–720.
4. Chin, B. H., and Sullivan L. J., 1979. Carbaryl metabolism by the selected tissue of the dog via the *in vitro* explant maintenance technique. *Agric. Food Chem.* 27(6):1419–1420.
5. Chin, B. H., McKelvey, J. A., Calisti, T. R., Kozbelt, S. J., and Sullivan L. J., 1980. Absorption, distribution and excretion of ethylbenzene, ethylcyclohexane and methylethylbenzene in rats. *Bull. Environ. Contam. Toxicol.* 24:477–483.
6. Chin, B. H., McKelvey, J. A., Calisti, L. J., Kozbelt, S. J., and Sullivan, L. J. 1980. A comparison of *in vivo* and *in vitro* (tissue explant) technique: Metabolic profile of ethylbenzene in the rats and the dogs. *Bull. Environ. Contam. Toxicol.* 25(2):241–245.
7. Chin, B. H., McKelvey, J. A., Calisti, L. J., Kozbelt, S. J., and Sullivan, L. J. 1981. A comparison of in vivo and in vitro (tissue explant) techniques: Metabolic profile of ethylcyclohexane in the rats and the dogs. *Bull. Environ. Contam. Toxicol.* 26:461–465.
8. Chin, B. H., McKelvey, J. A., Calisti, L. J., Kozbelt, S. J., and Sullivan, L. J. 1981. A comparison of in vivo and in vitro (tissue explant) techniques: Metabolic profile of methylethylbenzene in the rats and the dogs. *Bull. Environ. Contam. Toxicol.* 26:621–625.
9. Sullivan, L. J., Chin, B. H., and Carpenter, C. P. 1972. *In vitro* vs. *in vivo* chromatographic profiles of carbaryl anionic metabolites in man and lower animals. *Toxicol. Appl. Pharmacol.* 22:161–174.
10. Frazer, A. 1970. The need for more biochemical information in the field of food safety evaluation. In *Metabolic aspects of food safety*, ed. F. J. C. Roe, p. 9. Oxford: Blackwell.
11. Parke, D. V. 1968. *The biochemistry of foreign compounds*, p. 3. Oxford: Pergamon.
12. Knaak, J. B., Tallant, M. J., Bartley, W. J., and Sullivan, L. J. 1965. Metabolism of carbaryl in the rat, guinea pig, and man. *J. Agric. Food Chem.* 13:537–543.
13. Knaak, J. B., and Sullivan, L. J. 1967. Metabolism of carbaryl in the dog, *J. Agric. Food Chem.* 15:1124–1126.
14. Knaak, J. B., Tallant, M. J., Kozbelt, S. J., and Sullivan, L. J. 1968. Metabolism of carbaryl in man, monkey, pig and sheep. *J. Agri. Food Chem.* 16:465–470.
15. Sullivan, L. J., Eldridge, J. M., Knaak, J. B., and Tallant, M. J. 1970. 5,6-Dihydro-5,6-dihydroxycarbaryl glucuronide as a significant metabolite of carbaryl in the rat. Paper 6, Division of Pesticide Chemistry, presented at Joint Chemical Institute of Canada/American Chemical Society Conference, Toronto, May 24–29.
16. Trowell, O. A. 1959. The culture of mature organs in a synthetic medium. *Exp. Cell Res.* 16:118–147.

Chapter Twenty-eight

SULFUR MUSTARD-INCREASED PROTEOLYSIS IN CULTURED HUMAN CELLS

Fred M. Cowan, Clarence A. Broomfield,
and William J. Smith

The similarity between the dermal–epidermal separation and vesication produced by sulfur mustard (HD) and that produced by proteolytic cutaneous injury has fostered the hypothesis of increased proteolysis as a component of HD toxicity. In vitro exposure of human peripheral blood lymphocytes (PBL) or keratinocyte cell culture to HD is followed by increased proteolytic activity that is time and temperature dependent. The enhanced proteolysis in HD-exposed PBL at 4, 8, and 24 h agrees well with the time course of cutaneous pathology observed during HD vesication. Assay of PBL and keratinocyte HD-increased proteolysis with a panel of 10 protease substrates produced a characteristic pattern or "fingerprint" for each cell type that could be compared to the cleavage patterns of known proteases. Increased proteolysis in cell cultures may thus provide an in vitro biomarker for HD-induced pathology that might be utilized to identify both the mechanisms of action and potential treatment compounds for HD toxicity.

INTRODUCTION

Sulfur mustard (HD) is a chemical warfare blistering agent for which neither the mechanism of action nor an antidote is known. Papirmeister and co-workers[1,2] hypothesized that HD alkylates DNA, predisposing to DNA strand breakage and leading to subsequent biochemical and metabolic alterations that culminate in enhancement of proteolytic activity. This increased proteolysis has been proposed as the penultimate event in the dermal–epidermal separation and vesication that follows cutaneous HD exposure.[1,2] In vitro cell and tissue culture models such as human peripheral blood lymphocyte (PBL) cytotoxicity[3] and morphological changes in the human skin equivalent TESTSKIN[4] have been used for the investigation of HD toxicity. Enhanced proteolysis has been reported following in vitro exposure to HD in skin cultures from rabbits,[5] in PBL,[6] in epidermal keratinocytes, and in the human skin equivalent TESTSKIN.[7,8] In vitro exposure of human PBL to HD demonstrated that the increase in proteolytic activity is both time and temperature dependent.[9,10] Assay of PBL HD-increased proteolysis with a panel of 10 protease substrates produced a characteristic pattern or "fingerprint" that can be compared to the cleavage patterns of known proteases such as plasminogen activator.[9,10] HD-increased proteolysis in cell cultures of PBL and keratinocytes should facilitate characterization of the proteolytic activity and may be useful as a biomarker of HD-induced vesication.[11]

MATERIALS AND METHODS

Peptide Substrates and Reagents

The following Boehringer Mannheim Biochemicals Chromozym substrates (enzyme specificity) were used: t-PA (plasminogen activator), PL (plasmin), TRY (trypsin), TH (thrombin), PK (plasma kallikrein), X (Factor Xa), U (urokinase), GK (glandular kallikreins), PCa (Protein C), and XIIa (Factor XII). RPMI 1640 tissue culture medium (GIBCO, Grand Island, NY) was used in assays. Histopaque ($d = 1.077$), trypan blue, and tissue plasminogen activator were purchased from Sigma, St. Louis, MO. Sulfur mustard (HD, 2,2'-dichlorodiethyl sulfide) with a purity of >98% was obtained from the Edgewood Research, Development and Engineering Center, Aberdeen Proving Ground, MD. The protease inhibitors antipain, APMSF, aprotinin, bestatin, chymostatin, leupeptin, pepstatin, E-64 (1 μg/ml), ethylenediamine tetraacetic acid (EDTA, 1 μg/ml), and phosphoramidon (4 μg/ml) were obtained from Boehringer Mannheim Biochemicals, Indianapolis, IN, and the concentration of protease inhibitor incubated with assay samples was 400 μg/ml unless otherwise stated. Human keratinocyte cultures and KGM were provided by Clonetics, San Diego, CA.

Lymphocytes and Keratinocytes

PBL were collected by venipuncture from healthy normal volunteer donors under an approved human use protocol and maintained under sterile conditions. PBL were isolated by buoyant density centrifugation[6] using Histopaque and resuspended in RPMI 1640. Cell counts were done with trypan blue on a hemacytometer. Human keratinocytes were grown to 100% confluence using KGM in 24-well tissue culture plates.

Sulfur Mustard Exposure

PBL in 25-cm^2 tissue culture flasks were exposed to 5 ml of 0.05 or 0.1 mM HD. Keratinocytes in 24-well tissue culture plates at 100% confluence were exposed to 250 μl of 0.1 mM HD per well. The PBL in flasks and keratinocytes in tissue culture plates were maintained at room temperature in a fume hood for 1 h to allow venting of volatile agent and then transferred to a CO_2 incubator at 37°C for a total incubation time of from 4 to 24 h.

Chromogenic Peptide Substrate Protease Assay

Chromogenic peptide substrates, when cleaved by protease, release p-nitroaniline (pNA), producing a change in absorbance measured spectrophotometrically at 405 nm.[12] The use of these small proteolysis-sensitive peptides was adapted for protease assay by microplate reader (Bio-Rad, Richmond, CA) as previously described.[6]

Briefly, HD-exposed and untreated control PBL in cell culture were harvested by centrifugation. For assay of PBL, 50 μl of the 5-ml harvest supernate or cell pellet resuspended in RPMI containing 10^6 to 10^7 lymphocytes per 50-μl sample was added to individual wells of a 96-well flat bottom tissue culture plate. Fifty microliters of protease detection peptide substrate (2.5 mM substrate in H_2O) was added to each well, for a total volume of 100 μl (1.25 mM substrate concentration). The 96-well plates containing PBL were placed inside a CO_2 incubator at 37°C for 1 h, while PBL supernates were incubated under like conditions for 24 h.

Keratinocyte supernates (100 μl) plus 100 μl substrate and attached cells plus 125 μl KGM plus 125 μl substrate (1.25 mM) were assayed separately, and placed inside a CO_2 incubator at 37°C for 24 h. Fifty microliters of PBL and 100 μl of keratinocyte assay supernates were removed to a microliter plate to eliminate PBL or keratinocyte background, and absorbance readings were made on a microplate reader at 405 nm using media/substrate controls as blank values.

Data Analysis

All data points in the chromogenic assays for PBL were derived from quadruplicate samples, whereas keratinocyte studies, substrate "fingerprints," and protease inhibitor studies were assayed in duplicate. Data are from single experiments that are representative of other like experiments and are expressed as mean of absorbance or percent of control. Individual group significance was determined by Student's t-test and data are presented with standard errors.

RESULTS

HD-increased proteolysis in PBL was associated with the PBL and was not detected in cell culture supernates. Control and HD-exposed PBL were assayed with 1.25 mM of 10 different protease substrates: t-PA, PL, TRY, TH, PK, X, U, GK, PCa, and XIIa. HD-increased proteolysis in PBL gave a substrate hydrolysis pattern or "fingerprint" wherein the proteolysis of t-PA, PL, TRY, TH, X, PCa, and XIIa were increased (Figure 1). The degree of PBL HD-increased substrate hydrolysis varied, with TH substrate being most active. HD-exposed PBL assayed with the TH

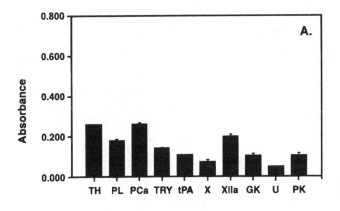

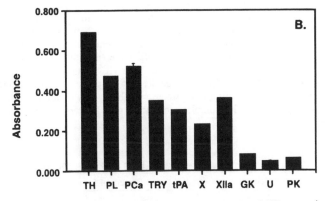

Figure 1. Patterns of substrate hydrolysis for control and HD-exposed human PBL. Patterns of substrate hydrolysis of a panel of 10 substrates: TH, PL, PCa, TRY, t-PA, XIIa, GK, U, and PK; 1.25 mM for control (A) and HD-exposed (B) human PBL showed increases in proteolytic activity resulting from HD exposure.

Table 1. Time Course of Proteolytic Activity After HD
Exposure of Human PBL

Time[a]	Percent of Control[b]
4 h	166 ± 2%
8 h	224 ± 2%
12 h	N.T.
24 h	250 ± 2%

Note. Assay of PBL proteolysis using 1.25 mM TH substrate as described in methods.

[a] Time after exposure to HD.

[b] Absorbance of HD-treated sample divided by absorbance of untreated control.

substrate showed a time-dependent increase in proteolysis above the baseline activity of unexposed controls (Table 1). Incubation of HD-exposed PBL for 24 h at 4, 20, and 37°C resulted in significant increases of proteolytic activity for the TH substrate at 20 and 37°C, but not 4°C (Table 2). The protease inhibitors antipain, APMSF, aprotinin, bestatin, chymostatin, leupeptin, pepstatin, E-64, EDTA, and phosphoramidon were incubated with assay samples and compared to untreated controls (Figure 2). Complete inhibition of sulfur mustard-increased proteolysis was achieved by antipain, APMSF, and leupeptin.

Control and HD-exposed keratinocytes were assayed with 1.25 mM of 10 different protease substrates. Keratinocytes exhibited some cell-associated increased protease activity for the X, XI, and U substrates after HD exposure. However, most proteolytic activity was for the TRY substrate and was found in keratinocyte culture supernates (Figure 3). The HD-enhanced protease "fingerprint" of PBL (Figure 1) and keratinocytes (Figure 3) for a panel of 10 substrates did not match the proteolysis patterns of tissue plasminogen activator (5 μg/ml) (Figure 4).

DISCUSSION

The hypothesis of Papirmeister et al.[1] predicts that HD alkylation of DNA leads to production of DNA strand breaks that mobilize DNA repair processes, primarily increasing activity of poly(ADP-ribose) polymerase. According to the hypothesis, activation of this enzyme, which utilizes NAD$^+$ as a substrate, results in NAD$^+$ depletion. Glycolysis becomes inhibited and the NAD$^+$-dependent hexose monophosphate shunt is stimulated, which results in release of protease. HD exposure may increase proteolysis in skin cells such as keratinocytes and/or cause increased proteolysis by activation or infiltration of inflammatory cells, potentially contributing to vesication arising at the dermal–epidermal junction.[1,2,11] In vitro exposure of human PBL to HD demonstrated that the increase in proteolytic activity is both time and temperature dependent. Increases in protease in PBL agree well with the time course of cutaneous pathology observed during HD vesication.[1] The increased protease activity in PBL after HD exposure at 37°C and the virtual lack of any increased proteolysis at 4°C demonstrate that the process is temperature dependent. Whether this is due to metabolically active protease synthesis or activation of existing protease has not yet been determined. The complete inhibition of HD-increased protease in PBL by

Table 2. Temperature-Dependent HD-Increased Proteolysis

Temperature (°C)	Percent of Control[a]
4	103 ± 4%
20	226 ± 2%
37	315 ± 2%

Note. Assay of PBL proteolysis using 1.25 mM TH substrate as described in methods.

[a] Absorbance of sample divided by absorbance of control cell

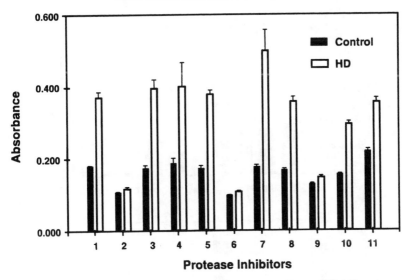

Figure 2. Effect of protease inhibitors on HD-increased protease. Human PBL 16 h postexposure to HD were assayed by chromogenic peptide substrate protease assay with Chromozym TH. Untreated control and HD-exposed PBL (1) and like samples incubated with the protease inhibitors (2) antipain, (3) bestatin, (4) chymostatin, (5) E-64, (6) leupeptin, (7) pepstatin, (8) phosphoramidon, (9) APMSF, (10) EDTA, and (11) aprotinin were assayed. Significant inhibition was seen only with (2) antipain, (6) leupeptin, and (9) APMSF.

antipain, APSME, and leupeptin but not chymostatin indicates HD-increased proteolytic activity is caused by serine protease(s) other than chymotrypsin.

A specific protease preferentially cleaves a given substrate; however, cross-reactivity with other substrates occurs. This produces an enzyme-specific pattern of multiple substrate proteolysis or "fingerprints" that can be useful for comparison to that of HD-increased protease(s).[10] For example, plasminogen activator (PA) has been proposed as a potential candidate enzyme for HD-increased proteolysis.[1] Rikimaru et al.[13] have demonstrated increased PA in HD-exposed rabbit skin. However, Lison et al.[14] have reported that PA is decreased in HD-exposed human keratinocytes. The HD-enhanced protease "fingerprint" of PBL (Figure 1) and keratinocytes (Figure 3) for a panel of 10 substrates did not match tissue PA[9] (Figure 4). This indicates that PA is not a major component of HD-increased proteolysis in these human cell cultures. However, due to the involvement of protease cascades in activation of protease, a role for tissue PA in activation of the enhanced proteolysis seen in HD-exposed cells cannot be ruled out.

HD exposure of PBL and keratinocyte cell cultures increases proteolysis in a time-dependent manner[7,9] that correlates with the ultrastructural demonstration of protease-like cleavage of adherent fibrils at the epidermal–dermal junction following HD exposure.[1] HD-increased proteolysis indicates that multiple enzymes and cell types may play a role in HD pathology. The detection of these proteolytic activities may prove useful for elucidating the mechanism(s) of HD-induced vesication. Furthermore, the use of compounds that reduce HD-increased proteolytic activity might further define the mechanisms of HD-induced cutaneous pathology and identify potential treatment compounds for HD toxicity. For example, treatment with niacinamide (10^{-3} M) 1 h after or with N-acetyl-L-cysteine (10^{-2} M) or dexamethasone (10^{-7} M) 24 h prior to HD exposure resulted in decreases of 39%, 33%, and 42%, respectively, in HD-increased protease activity in PBL.[10] Increased proteolysis in cell cultures exposed to HD provides a correlation between a measurable biochemical event and the exposure to HD. However, additional testing is required to characterize further HD-specific enhanced protease(s) and to confirm the role of proteolysis in HD-induced vesication.

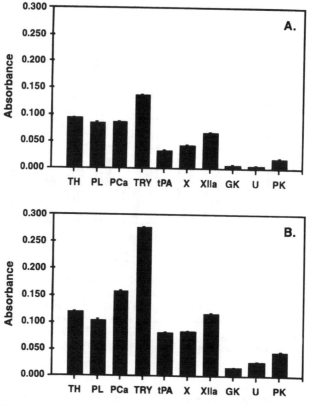

Figure 3. Patterns of substrate hydrolysis of supernates from control and HD-exposed human keratinocytes. Patterns of substrate hydrolysis of a panel of 10 substrates: TH, PL, PCa, TRY, t-PA, X, XIIa, GK, U, and PK; 1.25 mM for control (A) and HD-exposed (B) human keratinocytes showed increases in proteolytic activity resulting from HD exposure.

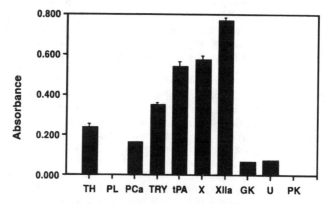

Figure 4. Patterns of substrate hydrolysis for tissue plasminogen activator. Assay of tissue plasminogen activator with a panel of 10 different protease substrates produced a characteristic pattern of reactivity that is markedly different from that generated by HD-increased protease in human PBL and keratinocytes.

REFERENCES

1. Papirmeister, B., Gross, C. L., Meier, H. L., Petrali, J. P., and Johnson, J. B. 1985. Molecular basis for mustard-induced vesication. *Fundam. Appl. Toxicol.* 5:S134–S149.
2. Papirmeister, B., Feister, A. J., Robinson, S. I., and Ford, R. D. 1991. *Medical defense against mustard gas: Toxic mechanisms and pharmacological implications.* Boca Raton, FL: CRC Press.
3. Smith, W. J., Sanders, K. M., Gales, Y. A., and Gross, C. L. 1991. Flow cytometic analysis of toxicity by vesicating agents in human cells *in vitro. J. Toxicol. Cutaneous Ocul. Toxicol.* 10:33–42.
4. Petrali, J. P., Ogelsby, S. B., and Justus, T. A. 1991. Morphologic effects of sulfur mustard on a human skin equivalent. *J. Toxicol. Cutaneous Ocul. Toxicol.* 10:315–324.
5. Higuchi, K., Kajiki, A., Nakamura, M., Harada, S., Pula, P. J., Scott, A. L., and Dannenberg, A. M. 1988. Protease released in organ culture by acute inflammatory lesions produced *in vivo* in rabbit skin by sulfur mustard: Hydrolysis of synthetic peptide substrates for trypsin-like and chymotrypsin-like enzymes. *Inflammation* 12:311–334.
6. Cowan, F. M., Broomfield, C. A., and Smith, W. J. 1991. Effect of sulfur mustard on protease activity in human peripheral blood lymphocytes. *Cell Biol. Toxicol.* 7:239–248.
7. Smith, W. J., Cowan, F. M., and Broomfield, C. A. 1991. Increased proteolytic activity in human epithelial cells following exposure to sulfur mustard. *FASEB J.* 5:A828.
8. Smith, W. J., and Gross, C. L. 1991. Early events in the pathology of sulfur mustard *in vitro*: Approaches to intervention. *Proc. NATO Panel VIII Meeting,* Grenoble, France.
9. Cowan, F. M., Yourick, J. J., Hurst, C. G., Broomfield, C. A., and Smith, W. J. 1993. Sulfur mustard-increased proteolysis following *in vitro* and *in vivo* exposures. *Cell Biol. Toxicol.* 9:269–277, 1993.
10. Cowan, F. M., Broomfield, C. A., and Smith, W. J., 1992. Inhibition of sulfur mustard-increased protease activity by niacinamide, N-acetyl-L-cysteine dexamethasone. *Cell Biol. Toxicol.* 8:129–133.
11. Cowan, F. M., and Broomfield, C. A. 1993. Putative roles of inflammation in the dermatopathology of sulfur mustard. *Cell Biol. Toxicol.* 9:201–213.
12. Friberger, P. 1982. Chromogenic peptide substrates. *Scand. J. Clin. Lab. Invest.* 42(Suppl. 162):1–98.
13. Rikimaru, T., Nakamura, Yano, T. S., Beck, G., Habicht, G. S., Rennie, L. L., Widra, M., Hirshman, C. A., Boulay, M. G., Spannhake, E. W., Lazarus, G. S., Pula, P. J., and Dannenberg, A. M. 1991. Mediators, initiating the inflammatory response, released in organ culture by full-thickness human skin explants exposed to the irritant, sulfur mustard. *J. Invest. Dermatol.* 96:888–897.
14. Lison, D., Dejardin, L., and Simon, O. 1991. Effects of sulfur mustard on plasminogen activator activity of human keratinocytes in cultures. *Ann. Med. Milit. Belg.* 5:11–15.

Chapter Twenty-nine

EVALUATION OF TWO IN VITRO HUMAN SKIN EQUIVALENTS (EPIDERM™ AND SKIN²™ MODEL ZK1300) FOR ASSESSING THE SKIN IRRITATION POTENTIAL OF PERSONAL CARE PRODUCTS AND CHEMICALS

Joanna M. Doyle, William E. Dressler, and S. R. Rachui

Living, three-dimensional human skin substrates were used to assess the relative skin irritation potential of selected chemicals and prototype shampoo formulations. Two full-thickness skin equivalent models (EpiDerm from MatTek Corp. and Skin² from Advance Tissue Sciences, Inc.) were exposed topically to the test materials for periods ranging from 15 min to 24 h. 3-(4,5-dimethylthiazol-2-4)-2,5-diphenyltetrazolium bromide (MTT) reduction was measured as the mechanistic endpoint for cytotoxicity. Relative irritancy potential was based on comparisons of the estimated time to reduce cell viability by 50% or on comparative cytotoxicity at selected time points. The objective cytotoxicity (ET50) results for the shampoos, as measured in the in vitro models, were then compared to subjective irritation results observed in vivo in a clinical repeat-application soap chamber test. The in vitro human skin equivalent models appeared versatile in categorizing or ranking materials representing a broad irritancy spectrum (i.e., chemicals). At the milder end of the spectrum, the models were able to separate the personal care products into three groupings that closely matched the in vivo groupings.

INTRODUCTION

Cosmetic products frequently undergo modification or reformulation, in order to improve performance or to enhance acceptability. Formulation changes may range from adjustments in existing component levels, to substitutions with established cosmetic ingredients, or to the introduction of new or unique materials with known safety profiles. Under many circumstances, it may be appropriate to proceed directly to clinical evaluation. In other cases, it may be more prudent, convenient, or efficient to use in vitro test systems to forecast relative dermal irritancy potential. The purpose of this study was to evaluate two promising in vitro human skin equivalent models and to compare the results obtained for shampoo formulations with clinical results obtained in a repeat application soap chamber test.

MATERIALS AND METHODS

Test Materials

Eight different prototype shampoo formulations were evaluated. The eight shampoos, including one baby shampoo, had similar pH values (range 4.7–6.5), except for one that had a pH of 9.0.

Except for the baby shampoo, which contained a nonionic surfactant, anionic surfactant levels ranged from 0.30 to 0.48 mEq/g. The shampoos were diluted 1:10 with distilled water for all assays. The shampoos represent a more limited range of dermal irritation from mild to moderate. Ten of the chemicals were selected from a published reference list by Gautheron et al.[1]; two were selected from a publication by Cottin et al.[2]

In Vitro Evaluation

Two in vitro assays were used to evaluate the shampoo formulations, EpiDerm from MatTek Corp. and Skin[2] from Advance Tissue Sciences, Inc. (ATS). The endpoint measured was cytotoxicity via MTT reduction. The chemicals were evaluated in the EpiDerm model.

MatTek Corporation's EpiDerm assay. This assay utilized a human tissue model comprised of human-derived epidermal keratinocytes cultured on permeable cell culture inserts, which allow differentiation to form a multilayered, highly differentiated model of the human epidermis. Using sterile forceps, the tissues were gently grasped by the corner, removed from the agarose, and transferred to a 6-well plate containing 0.9 ml of prewarmed assay medium per well, and incubated for 1 h at 37 $\pm$ 2°C with 5 $\pm$ 1% CO_2 before use.

All reagents were prepared according to the manufacturer's instructions. Prewarmed assay medium (9 ml, 37 $\pm$ 2°C) was placed beneath each Millicell® of the 6-well plates. One hundred microliters of the test materials (10% dilution with deionized water) and controls were pipetted in duplicate onto the EpiDerm sample. Tissues were exposed to the test materials for 1, 4, 8, and 24 h at 37 $\pm$ 2°C and 5 $\pm$ 1% CO_2. Following exposure, any test material remaining atop the EpiDerm was decanted, and the tissues were rinsed twice with approximately 100 μl phosphate-buffered saline (PBS). After the final rinse, all excess liquid was shaken from the surface of the tissue, and the insert was transferred to a clean 24-well transfer plate containing 300 μl MTT solution (1 mg/ml) per well. Plates were subsequently incubated for 3 h at 37 $\pm$ 2°C with 5 $\pm$ 1% CO_2. After incubation, the inserts were gently rinsed with PBS to remove any residual MTT solution, and the excess PBS was removed by shaking and blotting. The MTT was extracted by adding 2 ml isopropanol per well for approximately 2 h at room temperature while gently shaking. After extraction, 200-μl aliquots of extract from each well transferred to a 96-well plate and read for absorbance at 570 nm. Isopropanol was used to blank the spectrophotometer.

The mean percent MTT conversion value for each time point was plotted on the y-axis versus the exposure period on the x-axis. The MTT ET50 value, the exposure period to the test material that reduced MTT dye incorporation by 50% when compared to negative controls, was calculated from a regression analysis of the dose-response curve when feasible.

Advanced Tissue Sciences Skin[2] Model 1300/1301 MTT Assay

This assay utilized a human tissue model comprised of dermal fibroblasts cocultured on a nylon mesh with partially stratified epidermal keratinocytes. The tissues were gently grasped by the corner with forceps, removed from the agarose, and rinsed in a petri dish containing assay medium. The tissues were then transferred to 24-well plates containing 1 ml of 37 $\pm$ 2°C assay medium per well, and incubated for 1 h at 37 $\pm$ 2°C and 5 $\pm$ 1% CO_2 before use.

All reagents were prepared according the manufacturer's instructions. One milliliter of prewarmed assay medium (37 $\pm$ 2°C) was placed beneath each Millicell of the 6-well plates. Fifty microliters or milligrams of test materials (at 100% or 10% dilution with deionized water) and controls was pipetted directly onto a precut applicator pad, which was then placed directly onto the epidermal side of the tissue substrate. Tissues were exposed to the test materials for up to 24 h at 37 $\pm$ 2°C and 5 $\pm$ 1% CO_2.

After the exposure interval, the applicator pads were removed and the tissues were rinsed with prewarmed medium. The tissue was then transferred into a labeled well of a 6-well transfer plate containing 2 ml of prewarmed MTT solution (2 mg/ml), and the plates were placed in a 37 $\pm$ 2°C and 5 $\pm$ 1% CO_2 incubator for 2 h on a plate shaker at approximately 200 rpm. After incubation, the MTT solution was aspirated, and the tissues were washed twice with approximately 4 ml of Dulbecco's Phosphate Buffered Serum (DPBS). The MTT was extracted by adding 4 ml isopropanol per well for 1 h at room temperature. The plate was gently shaken at approximately

200 rpm during extraction. After extraction, 100-μl aliquots of extract from each well were transferred to a 96-well plate, diluted with an additional 100 μl, and read for absorbance at 570 nm. Isopropanol was used to blank the spectrophotometer.

The mean absorbance of each well at 570 nm was divided by the mean absorbance of negative controls at 570 nm to calculate the mean percent MTT conversion value for each exposure period to a test material. The mean percent MTT conversion value was plotted on the y-axis versus the exposure period on the x-axis. The MTT ET50 value, the exposure period to the test material that reduced MTT dye incorporation by 50% when compared to negative controls, was calculated when possible from a regression analysis of the dose-response curve. If not possible to calculate the MTT ET50 value, the mean percent MTT conversion value for 15 or 30 min was chosen.

In Vivo Evaluation

In vivo results for the shampoos were obtained experimentally in a human clinical modified repeat-application soap chamber test.

Modified Repeat-Application Soap Chamber Test[3]

Ten healthy volunteers free of chronic skin conditions, and not taking interfering medication, were qualified for this study. Test materials were diluted (10%) with distilled water and applied to randomized sites on the ventral surface of the forearm, using an occlusive Finn chamber as shown in Figure 1. Following an initial 24-h exposure, erythema, scaling, and fissuring were evaluated 20 min after patch removal. Subjects were then repatched for an additional 6 h. Readings for erythema, scaling, and fissuring were taken 6 and 24 h after patch application. Exposure continued for 3 additional days (total of 5 patch applications, an initial 24-h exposure and 4 subsequent 6-h exposures). An additional reading of erythema, scaling, and fissuring was taken after a 3-d recovery period. At each evaluation period, subjects were also asked to rate any burning or stinging they felt. Rating scales are shown in Figure 2.

Objective measurements transepidermal water loss measurements were taken at each test material site using a Servo-MED® evaporimeter prior to the first exposure (pretreatment), after the final exposure (posttreatment) and after the 3-d recovery period.[4] D-squame tape strips were placed over each test material site after all observations, and Evaporimeter readings were taken following the 3-d recovery period. Strips were then peeled off, placed on a black background, and graded for epithelial damage by comparing to a standardized scale.

RESULTS AND DISCUSSION

Table 1 summarizes the scores for posttreatment (after 5 patch applications) and recovery (after 3 d with no patches) of the 8 shampoos evaluated in the repeat-application soap chamber test. At the posttreatment reading, mean erythema scores ranged from 0.60 (for the baby shampoo) to 2.70. After the 3-d recovery period, the erythema scores substantially decreased to a range of 0.10 to 1.15 (Table 1). A different pattern was observed with the scaling/fissuring scores. On the posttreatment visit, mean combined scaling/fissuring scores ranged from 0.20 to 2.80, while on the recovery day scores ranged from 0.70 to 4.90 (Table 1). Table 1 also shows the mean Evaporimeter values for pretreatment and recovery and mean D-squame grades for recovery. The Evaporimeter values reached a peak during posttreatment with a range from 20.0 to 49.9 g/m²/h for the shampoos. Following the 3-d recovery period, Evaporimeter values returned to pretreatment value. D-squame grades ranged from 2.20 to 3.20. Three distinct classes of materials evolved from statistical analysis of these data. Figure 3 shows posttreatment and recovery rankings. Materials in separate boxes are significantly different from each other. Generally, shampoos 147 and 145 were milder than the other shampoo formulations. Shampoo 141 was the least mild in all parameters, except for fissuring on recovery day and Evaporimeter on posttreatment day. Shampoos 142 and 143 were ranked slightly milder than shampoo 141 and often placed in the same grouping as 141. Finally, shampoos 144, 146, and 140 ranked in the middle between the milder shampoos (147 and 145) and the more moderate shampoos (141,

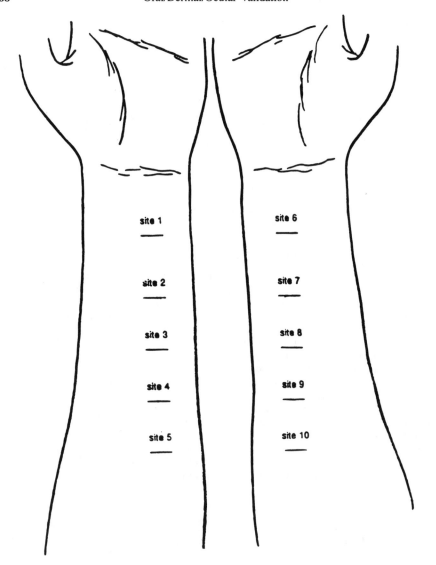

Figure 1. Site form.

142, and 143). Table 2 summarizes the results of the eight shampoos evaluated in the EpiDerm and Skin^2 models. We were not able to determine the ET50 values for the Skin^2 model, due to the variability in time-response curves. In general, the trend of the values indicates that a longer exposure time (greater than 2 h) may be needed to capture the estimated time to kill 50% of the cells. The ET50 values for EpiDerm ranged from 18.4 h (for the baby shampoo) to 2.4 h. Figure 4 shows the rankings for the shampoos based on the clinical scores (posttreatment), in vitro ET50s for EpiDerm, and 30-min viability scores for Skin^2. As determined by the clinical scores, three distinct groups are formed, with 147 and 145 being in the mildest grouping; 144, 146, and 140 being in the middle grouping; and 142, 143, and 141 in the less mild grouping. Within the groups, the ranks for shampoos tended to fluctuate for all parameters (clinical and in vitro); however, EpiDerm using the ET50s was able to group the shampoos the same as the

Erythema[a,c]
0 = No evidence
1 = Slight redness, spotty or diffuse
2 = Moderate, uniform redness
3 = Marked, uniform redness
4 = Intense redness with edema

Burning and Stinging[a]
0 = None
1 = Mild
2 = Moderate
3 = Severe

Scaling[b]
0 = No evidence
1 = Fine
2 = Moderate
3 = Severe with large flakes

Fissuring[b]
0 = No evidence
1 = Fine cracks
2 = Single or multiple broader fissures or spotty scabbing
3 = Wide cracks with hemorrhage or exudation or complete scabbing

[a] 20 minutes post-removal and 24 hours post application
[b] 24 hours post-application
[c] Scores of 0.5, 1.5, etc. used for intermediate grades

Figure 2. Rating scales for clinical evaluation.

Table 1. Clinical Scores

	Shampoo formulation							
	140	141	142	143	144	145	146	147
Posttreatment								
Erythema	1.80	2.70	2.30	2.55	1.35	1.15	1.90	0.60
Scaling	0.45	1.40	1.10	0.90	0.25	0.20	0.40	0.15
Fissuring	0.65	1.40	1.30	1.20	0.55	0.45	0.60	0.05
Scal, fiss	1.10	2.80	2.40	2.10	0.80	0.65	1.00	0.20
Eryt, scal, fiss	2.90	5.50	4.70	4.85	2.15	1.80	2.90	0.60
Evaporimeter	47.80	40.60	36.80	35.30	34.50	38.80	49.90	20.00
Recovery								
Erythemia	0.95	1.15	0.95	0.80	0.55	0.45	0.75	0.10
Scaling	1.80	2.40	2.30	2.20	1.60	0.90	1.70	0.30
Fissuring	2.00	2.50	2.20	2.60	1.60	1.10	1.90	0.40
Scal, fiss	3.80	4.90	4.50	4.80	3.20	2.00	3.60	0.70
Eryt, scal, fiss	4.75	6.05	5.45	5.60	3.75	2.45	4.35	0.80
Evaporimeter	12.10	12.90	13.20	12.20	11.90	11.20	11.80	11.00
D-Square	2.90	3.20	3.10	3.10	2.80	2.60	2.90	2.20

clinical subjective scores (both erythema and erythema/scaling/fissuring combined) and objective scores (D-squame). Skin[2] placed 4 shampoos in the correct groups based on the 30-min viability scores. The rank correlations among the assays varied slightly (Figure 5). EpiDerm showed the best correlation ($r = .86$) with the erythema rankings and a slightly lower correlation ($r = .83$) with the combined score rankings. Skin[2] showed a somewhat lower correlation ($r = .74$) with the erythema rankings and a similar correlation as EpiDerm ($r = .83$) to the combined score rangkings. The D-squame rankings showed an excellent correlation to the erythema and combined score rankings ($r = .95$ and $r = 98$, respectively), while the Evaporimeter rankings did not correlate at all ($r = .38$ and $r = .36$, respectively). The absence of a correlation of transepidermal water loss with clinical scores may reflect its utility to assess a different, but functionally important, parameter. Table 3 summarizes the results of the 12 chemicals evaluated in the EpiDerm model. Three of the chemicals (Tween 20, Tween 80, and propylene glycol) did not

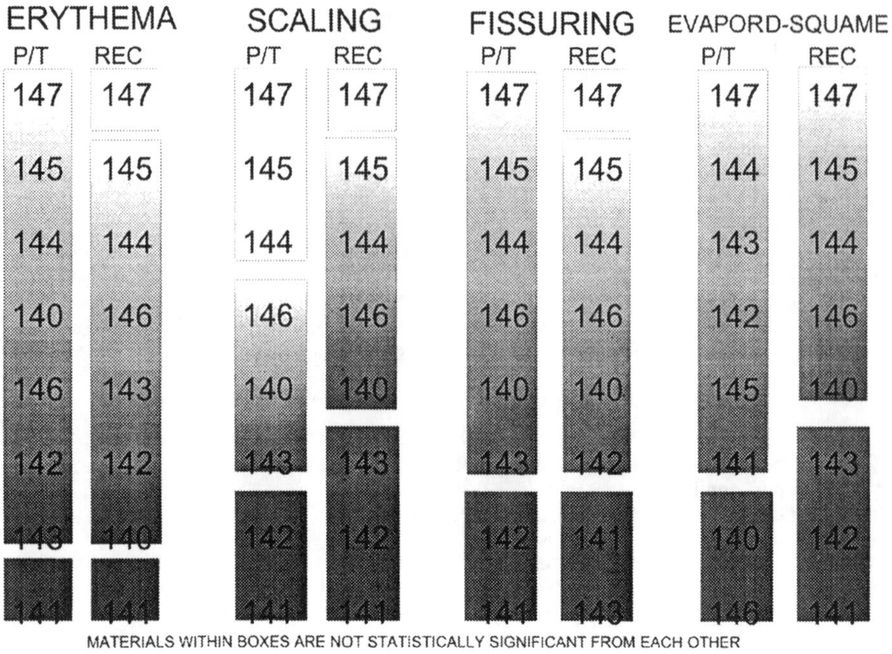

MATERIALS WITHIN BOXES ARE NOT STATISTICALLY SIGNIFICANT FROM EACH OTHER

Figure 3. Clinical groupings.

Table 2. Skin^2 ZK1300 and EpiDerm Results

Time (min)	\multicolumn{8}{c}{Shampoo formulation}
	140	141	142	143	144	145	146	147
	\multicolumn{8}{c}{Skin^2}
15 min	61.6	90.4	83.5	68.3	106.3	80.1	112.2	106.9
30 min	71.2	66.6	92.7	68.3	107.1	64.5	89.1	110.6
45 min	69.5	50.0	70.5	90.4	78.0	73.9	80.9	109.0
60 min	88.3	38.5	62.6	79.3	67.9	105.2	89.4	101.1
120 min	75.9	86.0	86.4	63.4	73.5	102.5	69.3	117.8
	\multicolumn{8}{c}{MatTek EpiDerm}
1 h	107.4	102.3	80.8	93.9	93.2	104.3	99.7	100.9
4 h	65.1	19.5	12.4	32.5	47.8	81.4	69.8	98.4
8 h	23.8	5.6	3.7	6.9	5.3	10.7	10.3	86.7
24 h	16.8	10.5	5.0	8.8	8.2	11.5	9.6	30.5
ET50	5.5	2.9	2.4	3.1	3.9	5.8	5.3	18.4

achieve ET50s by 24 h, the longest exposure time tested. This indicates a lower dermal irritation potential than the other chemicals tested. Four chemicals had very low ET50s (benzalkonium chloride at 10%, glacial acetic acid, SDS at 10%, and trichloroacetic acid at 10%), indicating a higher potential for causing dermal irritation. The rest of the chemicals had ET50s, ranging from 6.2 h to 2.3 h, except Triton X-100, which was only exposed for up to 4 h and did not achieve an ET50 within that time frame.

CONCLUSIONS

1. The clinical modified repeat application soap chamber test was useful for ranking the dermal irritancy potential of a variety of shampoo formulations, statistically categorizing them into three distinct groupings, based on subjective posttreatment and recovery scores.

RANKING - IN VITRO/IN VIVO

	IN VIVO ERYTHEMA	IN VIVO COMBINED	IN VIVO D-SQUAME	IN VITRO MATTEK	IN VITRO ATS
147	1	1	1	1	1
145	2	2	2	2	3
144	3	3	3	5	2
140	4	4	5	3	7
146	5	4	4	4	4
142	6	7	7	8	5
143	7	6	6	6	8
141	8	8	8	7	6

(MILDER ↑)

0.86

0.74

Figure 4. Dermal alternatives: shampoos.

RANK CORRELATIONS - IN VITRO/IN VIVO

IN VITRO	ERYTHEMA	COMB. SCORE	D-SQUAME	TEWL
MATTEK EPIDERM				
ET50	0.86	0.83	0.88	0.10
ATS 1300				
15 MIN	0.62	0.71	0.67	0.31
30 MIN	0.74	0.83	0.76	0.17
D-SQUAME	0.95	0.98		
TEWL	0.38	0.36		

Figure 5. Dermal alternatives: shampoos.

2. D-squame measurements showed an excellent correlation with the combined (erythema, scaling, fissuring) ($r = .98$) and erythema ($r = .95$) subjective scores. The absence of a correlation of transepidermal water loss with clinical scores may reflect its utility to assess a different, but functionally important, parameter.
3. The two commercial in vitro systems showed good but varying utility in discriminating among the materials and correlating with the clinical responses.
4. For MatTek EpiDerm, ET50 values showed a rank order correlation of .86 with the clinical

Table 3. MatTek EpiDerm Evaluation of Chemicals

Chemicals	Conc.	Time (h)						ET50
		0.25	0.5	1	4	8	24	
TCA	10%	18.1	10.8	15.6	11.7			<0.25
GAC	100%	1.0	1.1	2.0	2.8			<0.25
Triton X-100	100%	78.9	103.0	56.0	79.8			>4
IPA	100%			77.9	22.1	9.2	9.5	2.5
BAC	1%	106.6	116.5	70.0	24.9			2.3
BAC	10%	57.3	90.9	40.7	14.3			0.9
SDS	10%	45.5	54.8	48.7	14.2			0.8
Ethanol	100%			84.9	66.8	9.1	9.0	5.2
DMSO	100%			89.6	85.9	14.5	6.7	6.0
TEA	100%			80.1	65.9	37.2	10.0	6.2
Tween 80	100%			107.8	89.5	67.3	88.2	>24
Tween 20	100%			106.3	94.6	99.2	71.1	>24
Prop Glycol	100%			108.0	93.8	77.5	77.4	>24

erythema while for ATS Skin[2] the correlation was .74, which was based on a single time point (30 min) viability score, due to the variability in the time-response curves.

5. Although no direct comparative human dermal irritancy data are available on the chemicals evaluated, the groupings based on the EpiDerm ET50 values appear reasonable, based on historical use experience and published ocular irritancy categories.

REFERENCES

1. Gautheron, P., Dukic, M., Alix, D., and Sina, J. F. 1992. Bovine corneal opacity and permeability test: An in vitro assay of ocular irritancy. *Fundam. Appl. Toxicol.* 18:442–449.
2. Cottin, M., de Silva, O., Roguet, R., Catroux, P., Rougier, A., and Dossou, K. G. 1992. Investigation of a New Strategy Towards Ocular Safety Assessment, pp. 295–322. IFSCC, Yokohama, Japan.
3. Frosch, P. J., and Kligman, A. M. 1979. The soap chamber test: A new method for assessing irritancy of soaps. *J. Am. Acad. Dermatol.* 1:35–41.
4. Pinnagoda, J., Tupker, R. A., Agner, T., and Serup, J. 1990. Guidelines for transepidermal water loss (TEWL) measurement. *Contact Dermatitis* 22:164–178.

Chapter Thirty

STRATEGIES OF APPLICATIONS OF IN VITRO METHODS TO THE DEVELOPMENT OF PHARMACEUTICALS AND DEVICES

Shayne C. Gad

Pharmaceuticals and medical devices are intended to have human exposure and/or contact, and at least pharmaceuticals are intended to also have biological effects. New additions to these categories of products can both confer great benefits on society and produce significant profits for those who successfully bring them to market. But the development process for these is long and expensive, and the failure rate of candidates is high. In vitro methods can provide cost-effective, time-saving, and scientifically sound tools for assessing the safety of candidate products at early stages when effectively integrated into the development process in a manner tailored for specific development cases.

INTRODUCTION

The preclinical assessment of the safety of potential new pharmaceuticals and devices represents a special case of the general practice of toxicology possessing its own peculiarities and special considerations, and differing in several ways from the practice of toxicology in other fields—for some significant reasons.[1-4] Because of the economics involved and the essential close interactions with other activities (e.g., clinical trials, chemical process optimization, formulation development, regulatory reviews, etc.), the development and execution of a crisp and flexible, yet scientifically sound, program is a prerequisite for success. The ultimate aim of preclinical safety or biocompatibility assessment also makes them different. A good safety assessment program seeks to efficiently and effectively move safe, potential therapeutic agents or devices into, and support them through, the clinical evaluation, then to registration, and finally, to market. This requires the quick identification of those agents that are not safe so that effort (and limited resources) are not wasted on them.

Pharmaceuticals and devices are intended to have human exposure. Furthermore, pharmaceuticals are intended to have biological effects on the people that receive them. Frequently, the interpretation of results and the formulation of decisions about the continued development and eventual use of a drug are based on an understanding of both the potential adverse effects of the agent (its safety) and its likely benefits, as well as the dose separation between these two. This makes a clear understanding of dose-response relationships critical, so that the actual risk/benefit ratio can be indentified. It is also essential that the pharmacokinetics be understood and that "doses" (plasma tissue levels) at target organ sites be known.[4] Integral pharmacokinetics are essential to such a safety program—even more so now that there is wider recognition of the existence and importance of subpopulations with different metabolic competencies. As we have come to understand that pharmacogenetics underlie many of the subpopulation effects we see in both the safety and efficacy of drugs, we have also come to recognize that in vitro methods also offer some of the best and most efficient means of understanding the basis for these differences and for identifying members of specific subpopulations.

The development and safety evaluation of pharmaceuticals and medical devices have many aspects broadly or tightly specified by regulatory agencies. An extensive set of defined safety evaluation is absolutely required before a product is ever approved for market. For pharmaceuticals, regulatory agencies have increasingly come to require not only the establishment of a "clean dose" in two species with adequate safety factors to cover potential differences between species, but also an elucidation of the mechanisms underlying those adverse effects that are seen at higher doses and are not well understood. These regulatory requirements are compelling to the pharmaceutical toxicologist.[5] There is not, however, a set menu of what must be done. Rather, much (particularly in terms of the timing of testing) is open to professional judgment. Devices have tended to be more set piece in their testing approach, but are beginning to likewise require more mechanistic understanding to allow for competitive positioning in the marketplace.[6]

The discovery, development, and registration of a pharmaceutical make up an immensely expensive operation, and represent a rather unique challenge. For every 9000–10,000 compounds specifically synthesized or isolated as potential therapeutics, one (on average) will actually reach the market.[7] Each successive stage in the process is more expensive, making it of great interest to identify as early as possible those agents that are likely not to go the entire distance, allowing a concentration of effort on the compounds that have the highest probability of reaching the market. Compounds "drop out" of the process primarily for three reasons:

1. Toxicity or (lack of) tolerance
2. (Lack of) efficacy
3. (Lack of) bioavailability of the active moiety in humans

Early identification of "losers" in each of these three categories is thus extremely important,[7] forming the basis for the use of screening in pharmaceutical discovery and development. How much and which resources to invest in screening, and each successive step in support of the development of a potential drug, are matters of strategy and phasing that are detailed in a later section of this chapter. In vitro methods are now providing new tools for use in both early screening and the understanding of mechanisms of observed toxicity in preclinical and clinical studies.[2] Devices are generally less complicated in their design and in their testing procedures, and have a much lower rate of failure in the qualification and approval stages. The trend in devices, however, is for regulatory authorities to require more testing, to be more critical of results, and to take longer in the review and approval process.

The entire safety assessment process that supports new product research and development is a multistage process in which none of the individual steps in overwhelmingly complex, but for which the integration of the whole process involves fitting together a large complex pattern of pieces. In this chapter approach is proposed in which integration of in vitro test systems calls for a modification of the approach to the general product safety assessment problem. This modification can be addressed by starting with the current general case and progressing to a means for changing the process in an iterative fashion. Particularly with an understanding of mechanisms becoming increasingly important in both candidate drug selection and the design and evaluation of the relevance of findings, the integration of in vitro methodologies, particularly into the pharmaceutical safety assessment process, has become essential.

Determining what information is needed calls for understanding the way in which the device or pharmaceutical is to be made and used, as well as understanding the potential health and safety risks associated with exposure of humans who will be either using the drug/device or associated with the processes involved in making it. This is the basis of a hazard and toxicity profile. Once such a profile is established, the available literature is searched to determine what is already known. Much of the necessary information for support of safety claims in registration of a new drug or device is mandated by regulation. However, this is not the case at all for those safety studies done to (1) select candidate products or materials for development, (2) design pivotal safety studies to support registration, or (3) pursue mechanistic questions about materials and products in development.

Taking into consideration this literature information and the previously defined exposure profile, a tier approach has traditionally been used to generate a list of tests or studies to be performed based on regulatory requirements. What goes into a tier system is determined by (1) regulatory requirements imposed by government agencies, (2) the philosophy of the parent organization, (3) economics, and (4) available technology. How such tests are actually performed is determined on one of two bases. The first (and more common) is the menu approach: selecting a series of standard design tests as "modules" of data. The second is an interactive/iterative approach, where strategies are developed and studies are developed and studies are designed based both on needs and on what has been learned to date about the product.

DEFINING TESTING OBJECTIVES

The initial and most important aspect of a product safety evaluation program is the series of steps that leads to an actual statement of the problem or of the objectives of testing and research programs. This definition of objectives is essential and, as proposed here, consists of five steps: (1) defining product or material use, (2) estimating or quantitating exposure potential, (3) identifying potential hazards, (4) gathering baseline data, and (5) designing and defining the actual research program to answer outstanding questions.

Objectives Behind Data Generation and Utilization

To understand how product safety and toxicity data are used, and how the data generation process might be changed to better meet the product safety assessment needs of society, it is essential to understand that different regulatory organizations have different answers to these questions. The ultimate solution is in the form of a multidimensional matrix, with the three major dimensions of the matrix being (1) the toxicity/biocompatibility data type (lethality, sensitization, corrosion, irritation, photosensitization, phototoxicity, etc.), (2) exposure characteristics (extent, population size, population characteristics, etc.), and (3) the stage in the research and development process we are dealing with.

What is called for is a careful zero-based consideration of what the optimum product safety assessment strategy for a particular problem should be. Before formulating such a strategy and deciding what mix of tests should be used, it is first necessary to decide criteria for what would constitute an ideal (or acceptable) test system.

The ideal test should have an endpoint measurement that provides data such that dose-response relationships can be obtained. Furthermore, any criterion of effect must be sufficiently accurate in the sense that it can be used to reliably resolve the relative toxicity of two compounds that produce distinct (in terms of hazard to humans) yet similar responses. In general, it may not be sufficient to classify compounds into generic toxicity categories, such as "intermediate" toxicity, since a candidate chemical that falls in a given category yet is borderline to the next more severe toxicity category should be treated with more concern than a second candidate that falls at the less toxic extreme of the same category. Therefore, it is useful for a test system to be able to rank compounds with potentially similar uses accurately within any general toxicity category.

The endpoint measurement of the "ideal" test system must be objective. This is important so that a given compound will give similar results when tested using the standard test protocol in different laboratories. If it is not possible to obtain reproducible results in a given laboratory over time or between various laboratories, then the historical database against which new compounds are evaluated will be time/laboratory dependent. Along these lines, it is important for the test protocol to incorporate internal standards to serve as quality controls. Thus, test data could be represented utilizing a reference scale based on the test system response to the internal controls. Such normalization, if properly documented, could reduce internal variability.

The test results for any given compound should be reproducible both intrinsically (within the same laboratory over time) and extrinsically (between laboratories). If this condition is not satisfied, then there will be significant limitations on the application of the test system because it would potentially produce conflicting results. From a regulatory point of view, this possibility would be highly undesirable (and perhaps indefensible).

Alternatives to current in vivo test systems basically should be designed to evaluate the subject toxic response in a manner as closely predictive of that humans as possible while also reducing animal use and avoiding inhumane treatments.

From a practical point of view, there are several additional features of the "ideal" test that should be satisfied. The test should be rapid so that the turnaround time for a given compound is reasonable. Obviously the speed of the test and the ability to conduct tests on several chemicals simultaneously will determine the overall productivity. The test should be inexpensive so that it is economically competitive with current testing practices. And finally, the technology should be easily transferred from one laboratory to another without excessive capital investment for test implementation. It should be kept in mind that although some of these practical considerations may appear to present formidable limitations for a given test system at the present time, the possibility of future developments in testing technology could overcome these obstacles.

This brief discussion of characteristics for the "ideal" test system provides a general framework for evaluation of alternative test systems in general. No test system is likely to be "ideal." Therefore, it will be necessary to weigh the strengths and weaknesses of each proposed test system in order to reach a conclusion on how "good" a particular test is. The next section presents the basis for the specific test evaluation.

DESIGNING THE RESEARCH PROGRAM

The next step, given that no data are found from literature sources (and that it has been determined that data are needed), is to perform appropriate predictive tests. The bulk of this section addresses specifics of performing such test using in vitro models. Before considering how to design and conduct a testing program, we must first consider how the practice of safety assessment came to its current state in the employment of such tests.

To understand how product safety and toxicity data are used, and how the data-generation process might be changed to better meet the product safety assessment needs of society, it is essential to understand that different commercial and regulatory organizations have different answers to these questions. The ultimate answer is a multidimensional matrix, with the three major dimensions of the matrix being (1) the toxicity data type (lethality, sensitization, corrosion, irritation, photosensitization, phototoxicity, etc.), (2) exposure characteristics (extent, population size, population characteristics, etc.), and (3) type of commercial organization (or organizations) regulated (which we will call the "community of interest").

Communities of interest are defined by how the products are to be used, who regulates their use, and what benefits are expected for the consumer.

Medical devices and pharmaceuticals are two closely related communities. Materials of concern are agents intended as therapeutics (or medical devices) where the production worker or health care provider (doctor, nurse, or pharmacist) may have a significant chance of exposure, but the major concern is for those patients who receive or use the drug or device. The Food and Drug Administration (FDA) is the primary United States regulator.

What is called for is a careful consideration of what the optimum product safety assessment strategy would be. A framework for such a strategy is as shown in Figure 1. The components that constitute each of the data-generation tool boxes shown (screens, confirmatory tests, higher tier tests, and mechanistic evaluations) are common to all safety assessment programs in some form. But what is actually used for each of these tasks is not common to all of these programs, nor is how the judgment ovals (here labeled acceptance criterion and risk/benefit judgment) operate. The selection of these details is what constitutes the actual formulation of a strategy. Before formulating such a strategy and deciding what mix of tests should be used, it is first necessary to decide criteria for what would constitute an ideal (or acceptable) test program.

Considerations in Adopting New Test Systems

Conducting toxicological investigations in two or more species of laboratory animals is generally accepted as being a prudent and responsible practice in developing a new chemical entity, especially one that is expected to receive widespread use and to have exposure potential over human lifetimes. Adding a second or third species to the testing regiment offers an extra measure of confidence to the toxicologist and the other professionals who will be responsible for evaluating

Iterative Approach To A Tiered Product Safety Assessment

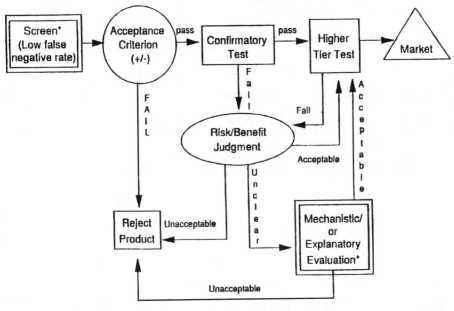

Figure 1. Points (marked by asterisks) for initial employment of in vitro tests for an iterative approach to a tiered product safety assessment. Within a tiered product safety assessment approach, it is possible to ask each question to a different degree of detail. If an early evaluation provides sufficient information, testing may be complete with relatively low expense. Conversely, it may also be determined that a more detailed (or specific) assay must be performed. Shown here is such an interactive approach, which identifies points where in vitro systems could readily be utilized in place of in vivo systems.

the associated risks, benefits, and exposure limitations or protective measures. Although it undoubtedly broadens and deepens a compound's profile of toxicity, the practice of enlarging on the number of test species, as has been demonstrated in multiple points in the literature,[8] is an indiscriminate scientific generalization. Moreover, such a tactic is certain to generate the problem of species-specific toxicoses; that is, a toxic response or an inordinately low biological threshold for toxicity is evident in one species or strain, whereas all other species examined are either unresponsive or strikingly less sensitive. The investigator confronting such findings must be prepared to address the all-important question "Are humans likely to react positively or negatively to the test agent under similar circumstances?"

Assuming that numerical odds prevail and that humans automatically fit into the predominant category, whether on the side of being safe or at risk, would be scientifically irresponsible. Far from being an irreconcilable nuisance, however, such a confounded situation can be an opportunity to advance more quickly into the heart of the search for predictive information. Species-specific toxicosis can frequently contribute toward better understanding of the general case if the underlying biological mechanism either causing or enhancing toxicity is defined, especially if it is discovered to uniquely reside in the sensitive species.

A mention of species-specific toxicoses usually implies that either different metabolic pathways for converting and excreting xenobiotics or anatomical differences are involved. The design of our current safety evaluation tests appear to serve society reasonably well (i.e., significantly more times than not) in identifying hazards that would be unacceptable in a confirmatory manner. However, the process can just as clearly be improved from the standpoints of both improving

Table 1. Rationale for Using In Vivo Test Systems

1.	Provides evaluation of actions/effects on intact animal and organ/tissue interactions.
2.	Either pure chemical entities or complete formulated products (complex mixtures) can be evaluated.
3.	Either concentration or diluted products can be tested.
4.	Yields data on the recovery and healing processes.
5.	Required statutory tests for agencies such as the Food and Drug Administration (for "pivotal" safety studies) and the European Economic Community (EEC).
6.	Quantitative and qualitative tests with scoring system, generally capable of ranking materials as to relative hazards.
7.	Amenable to modifications to meet the requirements of special situations (such as multiple dosing or exposure schedules).
8.	Extensive available database and cross-reference capability for evaluation of relevance to human situation.
9.	The ease of performance and relatively low capital costs in many cases.
10.	Tests are generally both conservative and broad in scope, providing for maximum protection by erring on the side of overprediction of hazard to humans.
11.	Tests can be either single endpoint (such as lethality, pyrogenicity, etc.) or shotgun (also called multiple endpoint), including such tests systems as a 13-wk oral toxicity study.

our protection of society and performing necessary screening and exploratory research in a manner that uses fewer animals and uses these fewer animals in a more humane manner.

In Vitro Models

In vitro models, at least as screening tests, have been with us in toxicology for some 25 years now. The last 5–10 years has brought a great upsurge in interest in such models. This increased interest is due to economic and animal welfare pressures and technological improvements.

It should be noted that, in addition to potential advantage, in vitro systems per se also have a number of limitations, which can contribute to their not being acceptable modes. Some of these reasons are detailed in Table 1–3.

At the same time, as demonstrated throughout this volume, there are substantial potential advantages in using in vitro system. These advantages of using cell or tissue culture in toxicological testing are (1) isolation of test cells or organ fragments from homeostatic and hormonal control, (2) accurate dosing, and (3) quantitation or results. It is important to devise a suitable model system that is related to the mode of toxicity of the compound. Tissue and cell culture has the immediate potential to be used in two very different ways by industry.

First, it has been used to examine a particular aspect of the toxicity of a compound in relation to its toxicity in vivo (i.e., mechanistic or explanatory studies). Second, it has been used as a

Table 2. Rationale For Seeking In Vitro Alternatives for Toxicity Tests

1.	Avoid complications (and potential confounding or masking findings) or animal and tissue/organ in vivo evaluation.
2.	In vivo systems may only assess short-term site of application or immediate structural alterations produced by agents. Note, however, that tests may only be intended to evaluate acute local effects.
3.	Technician training and monitoring are critical (particularly if the evaluation called for is subjective in nature).
4.	If our objective is either the total exclusion of a particular type of agent or the identification of agents with truly severe actions on an absolute basis (that is, without false-positives or false-negatives), in vivo tests in animals do not perfectly predict results in humans.
5.	Clearly, there are structural and biochemical differences between test animals and humans that make extrapolation from one to the other difficult.
6.	Lack of standardization of in vivo systems.
7.	Variable correlation with human results.
8.	Large biological variability between more complex experimental units (i.e., individual animals).
9.	Large, diverse, and fragmented databases that are not readily comparable.

Table 3. Possible Interpolations When In Vitro Data Do Not Predict Results of In Vivo Studies

1. Compound is not absorbed at all or is poorly absorbed in vivo studies.
2. Chemical is well absorbed but is subject to first-pass effect in liver.
3. Compound is distributed so that less (or more) reaches the receptors than would be predicted on the basis of its absorption.
4. Chemical is rapidly metabolized to an active or inactive metabolite that has a different profile on activity and/or different duration of action than the parent drug.
5. Compound is rapidly eliminated (e.g., through secretory mechanisms).
6. Species of the two test systems used are different.
7. Experimental conditions of the in vitro and in vivo experiments differed and may have led to different effects than expected. These conditions include factors such as temperature or age, sex, and strain of animal.
8. Effects elicited in vitro and in vivo by the particular case in question differ in their characteristics.
9. Tests used to measure responses will probably differ greatly for in vitro and in vivo studies, and the types of data obtained may not be comparable.
10. The in vitro study did not use adequate controls (e.g., pH, vehicle used, volume of test agent given, samples taken from sham-operated animals).
11. In vitro data cannot predict the volume of distribution in central or in peripheral compartments.
12. In vitro data cannot predict the rate constants for movement of drug agent between compartment.
13. In vitro data cannot predict the rate constants of chemical elimination.
14. In vitro data cannot predict whether linear or nonlinear kinetics will occur with specific dose of drug in vivo.
15. Pharmacokinetic parameters (e.g., bioavailability, peak plasma concentration, half-life) cannot be predicted based solely on in vitro studies. At the same time, such techniques as liver slices and specific P-450 subfraction active cell culture systems are very useful in identifying and understanding metabolically based sensitives and resistances in potential patient populations.
16. In vivo effects of chemical are due to an alteration in the higher order of an intact animal system, which cannot be reflected in a less complex system.

form of rapid screening to compare the toxicity of a group of compounds for a particular form of response. Indeed, the pharmaceutical industry has used in vitro tests systems in these two ways for years in the search for new potential drug entities.

The author has already addressed the theory and use of screens in toxicology.[3] Mechanistic and explanatory studies are generally called for when a traditional test system gives a result that is unclear or whose relevance to the real-life human exposure is doubted. In vitro systems are particularly attractive for such cases because they can focus on very defined single aspects of a problem or pathogenic response, free of the confounding influence of the multiple responses of an intact higher level organism. Note, however, that first one must know the nature (indeed, the existence of) the questions to be addressed.

Current Advances: A Mixed Battery

The current situation reflects the significant advances made in toxicology since 1985. It is very rare to see a pharmaceutical or device researched and developed with the use of other than an extensively commingled in vivo and in vitro test battery. This is reflected in the use of what may be termed a mixed test battery. The principles behind the development of these batteries are as follows.

1. Product safety assessment can not continue to be performed as it traditionally has been (on ethical, economic, or competitive grounds).
2. While there are no generally accepted in vitro test systems immediately available to completely replace all (or, indeed, any) of the in vivo testing requirements, there are test systems that can replace distinct components in vivo tests.
3. There are some steps that can be taken to move development and acceptance of additional in vitro systems along.
4. There are some modifications to current in vivo testing methods that both can and should be adopted. A current example of this would be in medical devices where a substantial portion

of the requirements under the governing regulatory agency (Tripartite on ISO) can be met with in vitro alternatives (cytogenicity, muscle cell implantation, the *Limulus* test for pyrogens, and in vitro mutagenicity assays).

Continuing Incremental Advances: How to Get Them

Clearly great progress has been made both in practices as to the conduct of safety assessment tests in intact animals and in developing an array of promising in vitro replacements, supplements, and candidates for replacement of the vivo test.

Where we would like to be is to have in place (that is, accepted and used by industry and accepted without question by regulation agencies) one or a battery of in vitro systems that would preclude or reduce the need for intact animal testing to necessary cases. And we would also like to have duplicate or unnecessary testing of materials reduced to a minimum. These goals are dictated as much by economic reasons and the need to do better science as they are by ethical and humane concerns. The efficient and effectives safety assessment/toxicology laboratory of the very near future will have as its "front door" an in vitro screening shop that will "draw" validated specific target organ screens from a library, as needed, to perform the initial go/no go evaluations on new compounds (or at least provide guidance as to where further evaluation is required). This same shop would also provide (again, from its established collection) in vitro system models to elucidate mechanistic questions later in the assessment process. Some would say that this is the current state of the art. Clearly much of the necessary library could be assembled from test systems that have been extensively evaluated and have already undergone extensive validation.[9,10]

There are two critical steps that must be taken for the eventual fulfillment of these objectives. The first of these is the acceptance of a scientific approach to the problem of safety assessment. The second is the development of an operative validation and acceptance process for new test procedures.

A scientific approach to safety assessment, such as the one presented in this chapter, does have proponents and adherents. Such an approach requires those involved in both the management and the conduct of the safety assessment process to continually question (and test) both the efficiency and the validity of their evaluation systems and processes. More to the point, it requires recognition of the fact that "we have always done it this way" is not a reason for continuing to do so. This approach asks first what is the objective behind the testing, and then it asks how well our testing is meeting this objective.

The second necessary step, which is totally absent at present, requires a collaborative process involving industrial, academic, and regulatory agencies for the validation and "acceptance" of new test systems. The general model of peer recognition leading to acceptance by the scientific community is not working in this case, as should have been expected from a situation where politics, social policy, and litigation have as much influence as science itself.

CONCLUSION

The first principle in hazard assessment is to have your real data as near as possible to the real-life situation about which you are concerned. That is, the nearer the model to human, the better the quality of the prediction of any potential hazards.

The second principle should now also be clear: To be able to translate toxicity to hazard, and to be able to manage such hazards, it is essential to know how the agent is to be used and the marketplace of which it is to be a part. It is hoped that this chapter has made these relationships clear.

Finally, alternatives of both in vitro and in vivo types are in the process of development for almost all the different endpoints of concern in safety assessment. Many of these hold great promise, and could be used as screens for many of the uses presented here or as mechanistic tools. But complete replacement is clearly not near at hand, particularly for the more complicated endpoints. How these then can (and should) be integrated into strategies for product safety assessment is the key scientific and managerial challenge for the next decade. For not only are there strong reasons making it adverse to continue where we are, but there are also the potentials for tremendous competitive advantage to those who successfully manage to integrate in vitro tools as both efficient screens and effective means of isolating and understanding the mechanistic underpinning for toxic and pathogenic processes. At the same time, each practicing toxicologist should feel both a moral and ethical compulsion to reduce the number of animals used in research and testing to the fullest extent possible, and to ensure that those that are used are maintained and used in as humane a manner as possible.

REFERENCES

1. Gad, S. C. 1988. *Product safety evaluation handbook.* New York: Marcel Dekker.
2. Gad, S. C. 1988. Principals of screening in toxicology: With special emphasis on applications to neurotoxicology. *J. Am. Coll. Toxicol.* 8(1):21–27.
3. Gad, S. C. 1988. A tier testing strategy incorporating in vitro testing methods for pharmaceutical safety assessment. *Humane Innovations Altern. Anim. Exp.* 3:75–79.
4. Meyer, D. S. 1989. Safety evaluation of new drugs. In *Modern drug research*, eds. Y. C. Martin, E. Kutter, and V. Austel, pp. 355–399. New York: Marcel Dekker.
5. Scheuplein, R. J., Schoal, S. E., and Brown, R. N. 1990. Role of pharmacokinetics in safety evaluation and regulatory considerations. *Annu. Rev. Pharmacol. Toxicol.* 30:197–218.
6. Traina, V. M. 1983. The role of toxicology in drug research and development. *Med. Res. Rev.* 3:43–72.
7. Fishlock, D. 1990. Survival of the fittest drugs. *Financial Times* 24(April):16–17.
8. Gad, S. C., and Chengelis, C. P. 1988. *Acute toxicology.* Caldwell, NJ: Telford Press.
9. Gad, S. C. 1993. Alternatives to in vivo studies in toxicology. In *General & applied toxicology*, eds. B. Ballantyne, T. Marvis, and P. Turner. New York: Macmillan.
10. Gad, S. C. 1994. *In vitro toxicology.* New York: Raven Press.

Chapter Thirty-one

A MODULAR APPROACH TO VALIDATION— A WORK IN PROGRESS

Alan M. Goldberg, Leonardo D. Epstein, and Joanne Zurlo

A modular concept to validate non-whole-animal test methods is proposed. The model follows the basic definition first suggested by Dr. John Frazier (OECD Environment Monograph 36, September 1990) that validation is the use of a test for a specific purpose. In addition, the founding principles of the model were all presented in a document by Goldberg and others. Using these first principles, the model that is developing is to pair a class of chemicals against a preidentified validation standard (for instance, human concurrent studies). Using an in vitro system, a single endpoint is measured to complete the module. The in vitro assay is then evaluated against the validation standard.

FIRST PRINCIPLES OF VALIDATION

In a 1990 OECD document,[1] John Frazier took one of the first major steps in developing an approach to validation. He defined validation as "the process by which the credibility of a candidate test is established for a specific purpose." This definition is a first principle and is the basis for the modular approach to validation. Unfortunately, most previous validation studies have not incorporated this principle, with the exception of many industrial in-house studies. The modular approach fully incorporates this definition as a guiding principle.

The second set of principles incorporated in the modular approach is the framework for validation (Figure 1) developed by a very large group of scientists representing industry, academia, and government.[2] We developed a framework for validation with three components. These components are test development, the validation itself, and acceptance of the validation as separate activities. It is important to recognize that test development can be accomplished in an academic, government, or industry laboratory. The location is immaterial. The validation methodology will require a set of resources, such as tissue banks, chemical banks, and oversight panels resulting in peer-reviewed publications. Peer-reviewed publication is a critical step within the entire validation process. The third component of validation is the acceptance of a test, as distinctly different from the validation of the test, and is generally carried out by a different group from that which conducts the validation. The validation component will be carried out by a large number of individuals, but the acceptance of the validated methods will, by necessity, be directed by the regulatory community itself; in other words the regulatory community will decide how it will use the data provided by the validation study. However, it will have a very solid scientific base from which to work.

We thank Deborah Rudacille for her editorial assistance.

Test Development

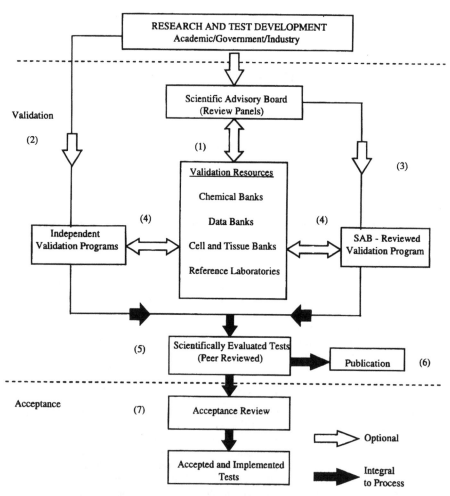

Figure 1. Framework for validation and implementation of new in vitro toxicity tests.[4] Scientific advisory board (SAB) provides oversight of validation resources, expertise and (optional) review of design/conduct of validation programs (1). Developers of tests or other parties may opt to conduct independent (2) or SAB-reviewed validation programs (3); utilization of validation resources is optional (4). Peer review (5) and publication (6) of scientifically evaluated tests are integral to the process. (7) Acceptance of a test is a separate process.

MODULAR APPROACH TO VALIDATION—THE MODEL

Based on these two basic principles, we have developed a modular approach to validation. Each module has three defined components: (1) a group of chemicals in a specific chemical class, (2) the validation standard, and (3) the in vitro assay.

At the present time, we have identified five possible validation standards: human concurrent, human historical, animal concurrent, animal historical, or structure-activity data. However, each module has only one validation standard, and it is linked to the chemical class. Once a validation standard is prespecified for an assay, along with a single endpoint, then these three components compose a module (Figure 2).

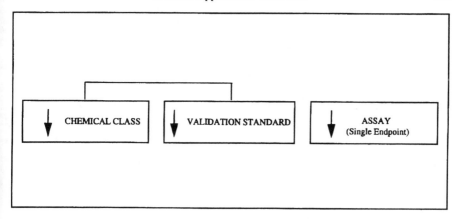

Figure 2. The validation module.

For example, if one would like to validate a skin irritation method and use a class of compounds that are mildly irritating, the validation standard might be a human concurrent study. We will pair that chemical class with the human study and then select our assay. Any assay can be used, such as cultured cells, engineered products, etc., and each of these will assess a single endpoint. However, only one assay and one endpoint are permitted per module. A very major difference between this and other validation approaches is that we do not compare one in vitro assay to another in vitro assay. We compare an in vitro assay to an in vivo endpoint, whether human or animal, concurrent or historical.

MECHANISTIC BASIS OF VALIDATION

Another issue that requires careful discussion is correlative (or phenomenologically) versus mechanistically based tests. While this issue is beyond the scope of this chapter, it is necessary to discuss it. I would like to share our conclusion as it relates to the modular approach, since both kinds of methods have to be validated. Correlative tests may be satisfactory for screening, even if they are going to give false positives and false negatives. We must accept this limitation at present. However, we believe that mechanistically based tests are essential for replacement methodology and/or regulatory use. Clearly, as this field develops, we will use nonmechanistically based tests or partially mechanistically based tests in our decision making. But mechanistically based tests are our goal.

Mechanistically based tests will give no false positives, but there will be false negatives and that is acceptable. This may be a reversal of common wisdom, but let me explain this using a graphical display (Figure 3). If the cube is a system that can respond to either the square, circle, or the triangle and if any one of these mechanisms are activated, there will be a response, so the system will respond to any one of three mechanisms and declare the agent toxic. If the assay system we develop measures only one of these responses, then it will give us a true positive every time it sees a square, but it will miss, give us false negatives, every time it sees a circle or a triangle. This leads us to the conclusion that, in the situation Figure 3 describes, one will need a battery of three individual tests, each responding to one of the mechanisms, namely, the square, the circle, or the triangle.

STAGING OF VALIDATION

An additional aspect of the modular approach is the staging of the validation protocol (Table 1). The first step is optimization of the assay. To date, we may have missed optimizing the assays that we were attempting to validate. We have tried to rush them to the marketplace to meet requests from the animal activist community, legislators, and stockholders. I believe that

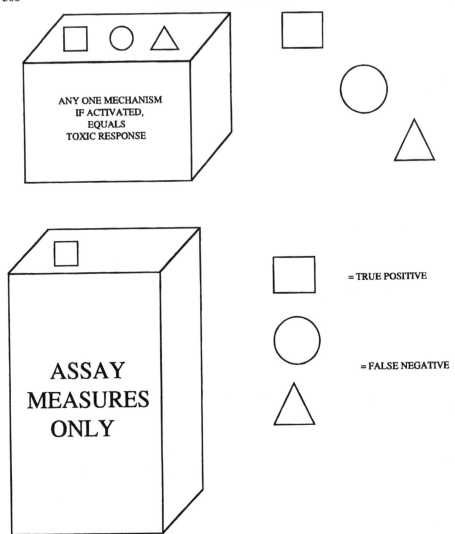

Figure 3. Mechanistic basis of toxicology assays.

Table 1. Staging of validation

1. Optimization of assay
2. Performance test
3. Validation

if we optimize the assays very carefully, we will be able to define their usefulness for specific purposes. When the assays are optimized, we will also know, because we are incorporating a statistical component into the validation from the very beginning, how many chemicals will be necessary in each group, how many replicate assays are required, and how many performance sites are necessary. With this understanding, we will then proceed to what we are calling a performance test. Each performance site must demonstrate that it can follow standard operating protocols that will include internal standards that will give positive and negative responses, as well as unknowns. Once we know the necessary number of laboratories (be it four or seven, depending on how "tightly" these assays work) we then proceed to blinded validation studies against identified chemical classes. The modular approach is a very specific process allowing an assay with a specific endpoint to be evaluated against a chemical class (or group).

The modular approach requires a statistical component and an oversight committee. We are looking for a very large multinational group from government, industry, and academia to oversee this study. What makes this study unique is that each module can be published immediately upon completion because each module is independent of others. We do not have to wait for other modules to be completed before analyzing the data. Therefore, we can provide an ongoing flow of data from this research. All studies will, again, be blinded so that once the data are collected and analyzed, only then will the blind be broken and the data shared with everyone.

One of the problems noticed in several of the other studies is the huge numbers of chemicals and the inclusion of divergent groups of chemicals.[3-8] In the modular approach, we use very small numbers of very highly defined similar chemicals for validation. We may be using as few as six to eight chemicals in any one replica. The number of replicates will depend on the variability of the assay.

I have tried to point out differences between the modular approach and other validation efforts. If one examines how methodology, in general, is accepted within the scientific community or in an individual laboratory, one sees that the exact same steps are followed as in the modular approach. The test is optimized, a number of laboratories begin to use it, it goes through further optimization, and then it begins to spread. To date, I do not think that this procedure has been generally followed with in vitro assays. We have witnessed large, very expensive studies that have failed to provide "validated tests." The modular approach may allow us to validate tests appropriately and in a reasonable time frame.

In closing, let me state that this is a work in progress. It will change and evolve. Each time we peel back one layer, the amount of detail to be evaluated is quite remarkable. I hope that we have the beginnings of an approach that will allow us to validate in vitro methodologies in a timely manner.

REFERENCES

1. Frazier, J. M. 1990. OECD Environment Monographs 36. Scientific Criteria for Validation of In Vitro Toxicity Tests. September.
2. Goldberg, A. M., Frazier, J. M., Brusick, D., Dickens, M. S., Flint, O., Gettings, S. D., Hill, R. N., Lipnick, R. L., Renskers, K. J., Bradlaw, J. A., Scala, R. A., Veronesi, B., Green, S., Wilcox, N. L., and Curren, R. D. 1993. Framework for validation and implementation of in vitro toxicity tests. *J. Am. Coll. Toxicol.* 12:1. Also published simultaneously in: *In Vitro Toxicol.* 5:1:47–44; *In Vitro Cell. Dev. Biol.* 29A:688–692; *Xenobiotica.* 23:563–572.
3. Ekwall, B., Clemendson, C., Barile, F., Calleja, M. C., Castell, J., Chesne, C., Clothier, R., Curren, R., Dierickx, P., McFarlane-Abdullah, E., Ferro, M., Fiskejo, G., Garza-Ocanas, L., Gomez-Lechon, M. I., Gulden, M., Isomaa, B., Janus, J., Kerszman, G., Kristen, U., Kunimoto, M., Karenlampi, S., Lavrijsen, K., Lewan, L., Ohno, T., Persoone, G., Roguet, R., Romert, L., Sawyel, T., Seibert, H., Shrivastava, R., Stadtlander, K., Stammati, A., Tanaka, N., Triglia, D., Valentino, M., Walum, E., Wang, X., Zucco, F., Harvell, J. D., and Maibach, H. 1993. Comparison between human skin irritancy and in vitro cytotoxicity from 77 systems for the first 12 MEIC chemicals. *First World Cong. Alternatives and Animal Use in the Life Sciences,* Baltimore, November.
4. Gettings, S. D. 1991. The CTFA Evaluation of Alternatives Program: Objectives and overview. *Proc. 2nd CTFA Ocular Safety Testing Workshop: Evaluation of In Vitro Alternatives,* eds. S. D. Gettings and G. N. McEwen, Jr., Summit, NJ, September. Washington, DC: CTFA.
5. Gettings, S. D., and McEwen, G. N., Jr. 1990. Development of potential alternatives to the Draize eye test: The CTFA Evaluation of Alternatives Program. *ATALA* 17:317–324.
5. Spielmann, H., Balls, M., Holzhutter, H. G., Kalweit, S., Klecak, G., Liebsch, M., L'Eplattenier, H. L., Lovell, W., Maurer, T., Moldenhauer, F., Moore, L., Pape, W., Pfannbecker, J. R., Potthast, J., De Silva, O., Steiling, W., and Willshaw, A. 1993. EEC/Colipa project on in vitro photoirritancy testing. *Practical In Vitro Toxicology III,* Nottingham, UK, July.
7. Spielmann, H., Gerner, I., Kalweit, S., Moog, R., Wirnsberger, T., Krauser, K., Kreiling, R., Kreuzer, H., Luepke, N. P., Miltenburger, H. G., Mulder, N., Murmann, P., Pape, W., Siegemund, B., Spengler,

I., Steiling, W., and Wiebel, F. J. 1991. Interlaboratory assessment of alternatives to the Draize eye irritation test in Germany. *Toxicol. In Vitro* 5:539–542.

8. Speilmann, H., Kalweit, S., Liebsch, M., Wirnsberger, T., Gerner, I., Bertram-Neis, E., Krauser, K., Kreiling, R., Miltenburger, H. G., Pape, W., and Steiling, W. 1993. Validation study of alternatives to the Draize eye irritation test in Germany: Cytotoxicity testing and HET-CAM test with 136 industrial chemicals. *Toxicol. In Vitro* 7:505–510.

Chapter Thirty-two

EVALUATION OF THE CORROSITEX METHOD TO DETERMINE THE CORROSIVITY POTENTIAL OF SURFACTANTS, SURFACTANT-BASED FORMULATIONS, CHEMICALS, AND MIXTURES

Virginia C. Gordon, Soheila Mirhashemi, and Rosalind Wei

A new in vitro method, CORROSITEX,* has been developed to determine the corrosivity potential of chemicals and formulations. This in vitro method assigns corrosive materials into Packing Groups I, II and III as described in United Nations (UN) guidelines or into R34, R35, and noncorrosive groups based on their ability to produce necrosis in 3 min, 1 h, 4 h, or later, respectively, on the skin of a rabbit.[1] CORROSITEX consists of two compartments: a dermal biobarrier and a chemical detection system (CDS). The dermal biobarrier has been developed using relevant target macromolecules. Test chemicals and formulations, including solids and liquids, are applied directly to the dermal biobarrier. When the chemical destroys the full thickness of this biobarrier, it is detected by the CDS, which produces a simple color change. This color change is visually observed and the time required for the color change to occur is recorded in order to assign a packing group. If no color change occurs, the chemical may be noncorrosive.

A major study of this in vitro method using 85 Department of Transportation corrosive chemicals was undertaken. CORROSITEX correctly identified 100% of these samples as corrosive or noncorrosive. In addition, this new method correctly assigned 84% of the 85 materials into the correct packing group. An initial interlaboratory study using 29 of these reference chemicals and formulations resulted in a interlaboratory reproducibility of 93%.[2]

Studies were performed on raw surfactants including all surfactant classes and blends. In these studies, 53% of the surfactants were qualified. The concordance of the in vitro results to in vivo results for corrosive and noncorrosive classifications was 93%.

Additional studies were conducted on more than 104 surfactant-based test materials. In these studies, 100% of these test samples were qualified. In the CORROSITEX system, 88% demonstrated concordance to in vivo corrosive and noncorrosive classification. Only two corrosives were underestimated and five noncorrosives were overestimated, of which four were severe irritants.

This study demonstrates the utility, reproducibility, and relevance of the CORROSITEX method to the prediction of potential dermal corrosion. The use of this in vitro test as a screen or tier approach to the current test method shows substantial promise, particularly for industrial cleaners, surfactants, and household products.

---

* Trademark of In Vitro International, Irvine, California.

INTRODUCTION

Federal legislative agencies and commercial manufacturers must consider numerous risks when developing, registering, certifying, and shipping materials that produce corrosivity. In order to evaluate the risk of dermal corrosivity, an in vivo procedure based on the Department of Transportation (DOT) Method of Testing Corrosion to Skin[1-3] is currently being used within the United States.[4]

In 1977, the United Nations printed special recommendations for class eight chemicals. The distinctions among chemicals in Packing Groups I, II and III were outlined. In subsequent years, legislative activity in Europe has increased in an attempt to classify and label potentially dangerous preparations.[5-7]

The chemical industry in Europe uses slightly different guidelines. This group bases their guidelines on European Commission[7] classifications, which state that a substance is corrosive if, when applied to intact animal skin, it produces full thickness destruction of the tissue in at least 2 of 6 animals within 4 h. If destruction occurs within 3 min, an R35 class is assigned to the test sample, If destruction occurs between 3 min and 4 h, the test sample is classified as R34.

Our extensive scientific examination of the property of skin corrosivity confirms that one cannot determine corrosivity by the pH value of a sample. In addition to the fact that pH may only be measured for aqueous samples, a study in which the pH of samples was compared to in vivo corrosivity results demonstrated very limited correlation between the two values.

A detailed study of samples that have both pH values and in vivo data out of the 1050 samples has been carried out to determine if there is a relationship between the pH value of a substance and its corrosive properties. Figure 1 shows the relationship between pH and Packing Groups for 552 test results. "NC" included all of the noncorrosive materials, and "C" included all corrosive materials (i.e., corrosive, Packing Group I, II, and III). Two important conclusions can be made from these studies:

1. The pH is not a reliable indicator of corrosivity. It has often been assumed that an aqueous substance with a pH value of less than or equal to 2.0, or greater than or equal to 11, is corrosive. The study demonstrated that this is not necessarily true. Seventy-five out of 277 samples that were considered to be corrosive according to this definition were, in reality, noncorrosive based on in vivo data. In addition, 35 out of 182 samples that would not be considered corrosive under the pH definition were actually corrosive based on in vivo data. Three of these were found to be in Packing Group 1.
2. It is impossible to assign packing group classification using pH value. This is clearly shown in Figure 1. For 127 substances that had a pH value of less than or equal to 2.0, 14 were assigned to Packing Group I, 91 to Packing Group II, 10 to Packing Group III, and 12 were

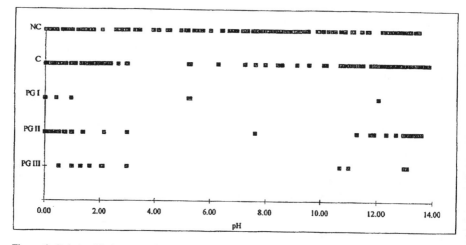

Figure 1. Relationship between pH and packing group.

found to be noncorrosive. Similar findings held for the 150 substances whose pH was greater than or equal to pH 11: One was assigned to Packing Group I, 94 to Packing Group II, 25 to Packing Group III, and 30 were found to be noncorrosive. Clearly, pH cannot be used to assign packing groups.

CORROSITEX is based on the target biomacromolecular approach. Dermal biomacromolecules have been utilized to study the potential effects of chemicals and formulations on the skin for the past 40 years. As early as 1953, Van Scott and Lyon[8] quantified an increase in exposed sulfhydryl groups of keratin when soaps and detergents were applied to the keratin. This exposure resulted from a separation of keratin chains.

Harrold[9] expanded this work to include investigation of complete formulations on keratin denaturation and separation, and in 1971, Choman[10] evaluated the swelling response of in vitro skin discs prepared from dermal calf collagen. Absorption of test samples to the stratum corneum was thoroughly investigated by Imokawa et al.,[11,12] who established a correlation between in vivo skin roughness and in vitro absorption. These studies, as well as others, established a correlation between in vivo skin roughness and in vitro absorption. These studies, as well as others, also established the relevance of studying changes in macromolecules to determine potential effects of chemicals and formulations on the skin in vivo.

The integrity of the stratum corneum and its relevance to corrosive potential has been investigated recently. Oliver and Pemberton[13] monitored electrical resistance in skin slices as a measurement of barrier integrity and as an indicator of the corrosive potential of chemicals. They showed that corrosive agents have a greater ability than noncorrosives to exert a direct physicochemical lytic action on the stratum corneum.

This effect of direct lytic action is mimicked in the CORROSITEX biobarrier when a corrosive sample produces full thickness destruction in a specified period of time. Many samples produce time-dependent changes within the biobarrier in direct proportion to their lytic action on the biobarrier. The time to produce destruction of the biobarrier is determined by the samples detection in a chemical detection system. The basic components of the CORROSITEX model are illustrated in Figure 2.

MATERIALS AND METHODS

Prequalification Test

Prior to performing the CORROSITEX test, the sample is prequalified. The sample is placed in a small amount of chemical detection system fluid. If any detectable change occurs in the

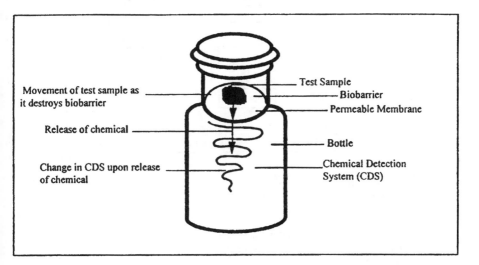

Figure 2. The CORROSITEX model.

CDS, the sample is qualified and can be run in CORROSITEX. If a sample is nonqualified it is incompatible with the CDS and must be tested as described in 49 CFR 173.136 (Figure 3).

Screening Test

Test samples are classified into categories which will determine how packing groups are assigned (Figure 3). Test samples are classified by pH changes produced in two well-defined buffers: one designed to buffer acids and another that buffers bases. The four different categories are defined as follows:

- Category A_1 substances produce a large change in pH when they are added to the acid buffer. This change in pH is indicated by a strong color change of the acid buffer solution.
- Category B_1 substances produce a large change in pH when they are added to the base buffer. This change in pH is indicated by a strong color change of the base buffer solution.
- Category A_2 substances produce little or no pH changes when added to the acid buffer, and therefore, little or no color change in the buffer solution is observed.
- Category B_2 substances produce little or no pH changes when added to the base buffer, and therefore, little or no change in the buffer solution is observed.

The CORROSITEX Assay

CORROSITEX is based on the target biomacromolecular approach, which evaluates the effect of chemicals and formulations on relevant biomacromolecules. It predicts in vivo corrosivity potential, using as an endpoint the time it takes for the chemical or formulation to produce alteration or destruction of a dermal biobarrier composed of specifically formulated solubilized

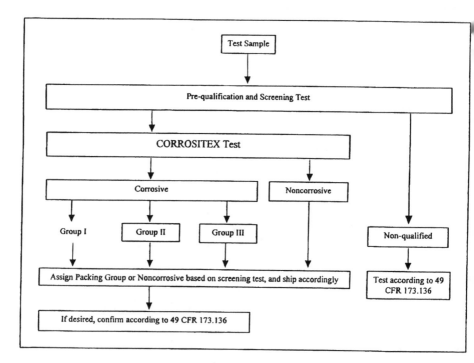

Figure 3. Tiered in vitro approach. Note that if material is corrosive to aluminum or steel at the prescribed rates, it would be shipped as a Packing Group III corrosive. The term "noncorrosive" in this context means that the substance is not skin-corrosive.

proteins. A well-defined chemical detection system (CDS) and the precisely constructed dermal biobarrier are the two key components of the CORROSITEX model. Test chemicals and formulations, including solids and liquids, are applied directly to the dermal biobarrier. When the chemical destroys the full thickness of this biobarrier, it is detected by the CDS, which produces a simple color change. This color change is visually observed and the time required for the color change to occur is recorded in order to assign a packing group. If no color change occurs, the chemical is noncorrosive.

Dermal Biobarrier

The dermal biobarrier has been developed using specifically formulated solubilized proteins. This biobarrier is prepared by coating a support with a mixture of diluent and solubilized protein. The macromolecules are gelled onto a cellulose support within a circular disc delivery system. The biobarrier is then sealed and stored at 4°C. The shelf life of the biobarrier is two weeks under these storage conditions. Prior to mixing with the diluent the shelf-life of the materials is 2 years.

Chemical Detection System

The chemical detection system (CDS) consists of multiple chemical detectors including specific ions, indicators, and other detectors that have demonstrated responsiveness with numerous classes of chemicals (Table 1). A simple, visually detectable color change of the CDS occurs when the biobarrier is altered or destroyed due to the chemical exposure. If no color change occurs, the sample is not compatible with CORROSITEX.

Table 1. Chemical and Product Classes Identified by CORROSITEX Chemical Detection System

Primary alkyl amines	Polymers
Secondary alkyl amines	Carbohydrates
Tertiary alkyl amines	Mercaptans
Aromatic amines	Polymers
Alkylamine salts	Resins
Ethoxylates	Biocides
n-Oxides	Insect powders
Quarternary ammonium salts	Pesticide classes
Oxidizing agents	Polymers
Reducing agents	Fertilizer classes
Metal salts	Propellants
Aid halides	Metal-working fluids
Acids	Organophosphates
Bases	Phosphines
Esters	Fuel additives
Anhydrides	Heavy-duty cleaners
Chloroformates	Window cleaners
Halogen derivatives	Strippers
Silanes	Degreaser/cleaners
Silicates	Light-duty cleaners
Organic solvents	Powdered cleaners
Formulated amines	Anionic surfactants
Acrylates	Cationic surfactants
Sterols	Nonionic surfactants
Hydrocarbons	Amphoteric surfactants
Carbohydrates	Surfactant blends
Mercaptans	

Assignment of Packing Groups

In the CORROSITEX system, packing group assignments are made by taking into account the category that is assigned to a sample by the screening test, and the time it takes to detect a color change in the CDS in the CORROSITEX assay.

Packing Groups I, II, or III are assigned to test samples from Category A_2, and B_2, that produce a detectable color change in the CDS between 0 and 3 min, greater than 3 min, and up to 1 h, or greater than 1 h and up to 4 h, respectively. If no color change occurs in 4 h, the chemical is classified as noncorrosive (Table 2).

Packing Group I, II, or III is assigned to test samples from Category A_1, and B_1, that produce a detectable color change in the CDS between 0 and 3 min, greater than 3 min and up to 30 min, or greater than 30 min and up to 45 min, respectively. If no color change occurs in 45 min, the chemical is classified as noncorrosive (Table 3).

RESULTS

Results of DOT Classified Corrosive Chemicals

All commercially available corrosive chemicals listed on the DOT Table 172.101 were retested. The summary is presented in Table 4. Corrosive classifications were assigned for the chemicals based on Tables 2 and 3. *In vivo* packing groups were obtained from industrial laboratories or the DOT Hazardous Material Table 172.101 of 49 CFR. When actual in vivo data was available, it was preferentially used for comparison. CORROSITEX correctly distinguished 100% of the chemicals to be corrosive or noncorrosive and also assigned correct packing groups with 84% concordance, having 9 overestimates and 5 underestimates.

Table 2. CORROSITEX Assignment of Corrosive Packing Groups for Category A_2 and B_2 Samples

Time(h:mm:ss)	Abbreviation	Classification
0:00:00–0:03:00	I	Corrosive Packing Group I
>0:03:00–1:00:00	II	Corrosive Packing Group II
>1:00:00–4:00:00	III	Corrosive Packing Group III
>4:00:00	NC	Noncorrosive

Table 3. CORROSITEX Assignment of Corrosive Packing Groups for Category A_1 and B_1 Samples

Time(h:mm:ss)	Abbreviation	Classification
0:00:00–0:03:00	I	Corrosive Packing Group I
>0:03:00–0:30:00	II	Corrosive Packing Group II
>0:30:00–0:45:00	III	Corrosive Packing Group III
>0:45:00	NC	Noncorrosive

Table 4. Summary of the 85 DOT Corrosive Chemicals Study Using New Categorization Test

	Number of chemicals	New study With screening test
Total tested	85	
Correct corrosive/noncorrosive classification (concordance)	85	100%
Correct packing group assignment (concordance)	71	84%
Higher packing group assignment (overestimates)	9	10%
Lower packing group (underestimates)	5	6%

Complete results on these chemicals are presented in Table 5. The concordance of in vitro with in vivo results was determined when specific in vivo results were available. If these results were not available, a comparison to the classification in the DOT Table 172.101 of 49 CFR was made.

Results of Double-Blind Study

This study was reanalyzed using the new screening approach. Originally a double-blind study by a third-party laboratory was performed to evaluate transferability and interlaboratory reproducibility. A summary of the reanalyzed study, including screening results, is presented in Table 6. The samples have now been categorized and the packing groups reassigned based on the screening of the test sample. No change in the high interlaboratory reproducibility was noted.

Detailed results of the 29 chemicals studied are presented in Table 7. This study was performed in a contract laboratory in Los Angeles, California.

Comparison of CORROSITEX With Screening Test to the Physicochemical Method

Using a series of acids and bases diluted to different pH and acid/alkali reserve, the physicochemical method can be compared to CORROSITEX. The physicochemical method assigns an index, based on pH and the acid/alkali reserve, to a test sample.[14] On the basis of this index, a prediction of corrosivity can be made. It is only applicable to test samples with pH >11 and pH <1.0. Many materials with a pH between 1 and 11 cannot be classified by this method. The physicochemical method does not predict packing group assignments.[14]

The in vivo results were compared to the CORROSITEX packing groups using the new screening test. For 19 chemicals studied by both methods, there was no underestimation with the CORROSITEX method (Table 8). The physicochemical method was able to assign only 15 chemicals to corrosive/noncorrosive groups, underestimated the corrosivity potential of 6 of the test samples, and overestimated the corrosivity potential of 1 of the test samples. CORROSITEX overestimated the corrosivity potential for five of the test samples with no underestimation.

Summary of 104 Household and Industrial Cleaner Field Studies from 12 Companies

One hundred and four test samples from 12 companies have been studied that are surfactant-based industrial cleaning and stripping products. Primary ingredients are acid or base components that may be blended with surfactants, solvents, metasilicates or silicates, and other ingredients. These are all complex mixtures and exhibit synergistic effects between components. This table includes screening of all test samples. A summary of these studies is presented in Table 9, and the complete results are listed in Table 10.

Fifty-nine samples of the 104 surfactant-based formulations had in vivo data. Twenty-nine formulations were corrosive in vivo and 30 formulations were noncorrosive. This study provided some of the information for assignment of categories for modified CORROSITEX times. These results are summarized in Table 11 and Figures 4 and 5.

In this study of 29 corrosive surfactant formulations, 28 were correctly identified as producing destruction or alteration of the dermal biobarrier in less than 45 min. Only one corrosive was determined to be noncorrosive. This demonstrates a high sensitivity to detection of corrosives before 45 min. This is depicted in Figure 4.

In the study of 30 surfactant formulations that were noncorrosive in vivo, only 5 exhibited destruction or alteration of the dermal biobarrier in less than 45 min. Twenty-nine of the formulations produced slow alteration of the dermal biobarrier. This is depicted in Figure 5.

These figures support the 45-min NC/C assignment time for Category B_2 and A_2 materials. The times were established with analysis of 390 Category B_2 and A_2 test samples. The complete results for these 59 surfactant-based formulations are presented in Table 12.

Raw Surfactant Study

A study of 63 raw surfactants was conducted in CORROSITEX with the use of the screening test. Only two surfactants were corrosive. One of these was not qualified and one was classified

Table 5. Corrosive Chemicals of Hazardous Material Table (49 CFR 172.101, U.S. Department of Transportation)

						100% Concordance	71	84%
						Overestimates	9	10%
						Underestimates	5	6%

No.	Chemical	U.N. Number	Chemical class	Conc.	pH of 10%	CORROSITEX time Mean	CORROSITEX time Std	Category	Packing group	DOT table	In vivo group[2]	Concordance
1	Benzyl chloroformate	1739	Acid ester	95%	2.54	>4 hours	0:00:02	A_1	NC	1	NC	1
2	Fluorosulfonic acid	1777	Acid	Pure	0	0:00:13	0:00:05	A_1	I	I		1
3	Nitric acid	2031	Acid	90%	0	0:00:34	0:00:05	A_1	I	I		1
4	Selenic acid	1905	Acid	95%	0	0:01:41	0:00:07	A_1	I	I	I	1
5	Sulfur monochloride	1828	Halogen derivative	98%	5.2	0:05:54	0:00:28	A_1	II	I	I	Under
6	Trifluoroacetic acid	2699	Acid	99%	0.75	0:04:30	0:00:12	A_1	II	I	I	Under
7	Acetic acid, glacial	2789	Acid	99+%	2.3	0:29:31	0:02:58	A_1	II	II		1
8	Acetic anhydride	1715	Anhydride	Pure	1.99	0:47:00	0:02:29	A_1	II	II		1
9	Acetyl bromide	1716	Halogen derivative	99%	~2.0	0:00:42	0:00:27	A_1	1	II		Over
10	Acrylic acid	2218	Acid	99%	2.07	0:29:00	0:00:13	A_1	II	II		1
11	Aluminum bromide. anhydrous	1725	Metal salt	98+%	1.22	0:10:30	0:00:10	A_1	II	II		1
12	Aluminum chloride	1726	Metal salt	Pure	2.92	0:16:30	0:01:53	A_1	II	II		1
13	Ammonium hydrogen fluoride	1727	Halogen derivative	98%	5.22	0:26:30	0:00:03	A_1	II	II		1
14	Ammonium hydrogen sulfate	2506	Acid	neat	0.78	0:13:00	0:02:28	A_1	II	II		1
15	Anisoyl chloride, ortho-	1729	Halogen derivative	97%	0.72	0:10:20	0:00:19	A_1	II	II		1
16	Antimony tribromide	NA 1549	Metal halide	99%	0.35	0:22:00	0:00:07	A_1	II	II		1
17	Antimony trichloride	1733	Metal halide	100%	0.3	0:04:15	0:00:00	A_1	II	II		1
18	Boron fluoride—dihydrate	2851	Reducing agent	96%	0.41	0:01:15	0:00:07	A_1	1	II	I	1
19	Boron trifluoride—acetic acid complex	1742	Reducing agent	98%	0.95	0:03:34	0:00:13	A_1	II	II	II	1
20	Bromoacetic acid	1938	Acid	99+%	1.41	0:09:30	0:00:31	A_1	II	II		1
21	Bromoacetyl bromide	2513	Halogen derivative	98+%	0	0:02:05	0:00:08	A_1	1	II		Over
22	Chloroacetic acid	1751	Acid	99+%	1.44	0:04:30	0:01:49	A_1	II	II		1
23	Chromium(III) fluoride	1756	Metal salt	97%	3.9	3:00:00	0:15:00	A_2	NC	II	NC	1
24	Cyclohexylamine	2357	Amine	99%	12.34	0:31:00	0:12:04	B_1	II	II	II	1
25	Dichloroacetic acid	1764	Acid	99+%	0.64	0:08:00	0:01:12	A_1	II	II		1
26	Dichloroacetyl chloride	1765	Halogen derivative	99+%	0.46	0:05:00	0:01:01	A_1	II	II		1
27	Dichlorophenylphosphine	2798	Acid	97%	0	0:02:00	0:00:04	A_1	1	II		Over
28	Diethylene triamine	2079	Amine	99%	12.01	0:34:00	0:00:22	B_1	II	II		1

No.	Name	ID	Type	Conc.	Value	Time 1	Time 2	Code		II	III	Under 1
29	Dimethylbenzylamine	2619	Amine	99+%	10.7	1:27:00	0:00:00	B$_2$	NC	II		under 1
30	Dimethylcarbamyl chloride	2262	Halogen derivative	98%	2.31	0:17:00	0:00:18	A$_2$	II	II	II	1
31	Dimethylcyclohexylamine 2,3-	2264	Amine	99+%	11.79	1:25:00	0:02:00	B$_1$	III	II	II	under 1
32	Dodecyl trichlorosilane	1771	Silane	98%	0.5	0:11:35	0:00:09	A$_1$	II	II	II	1
33	Ethylenediamine	1604	Amine	neat	12.13	0:19:00	0:00:30	B$_1$	II	II		1
34	Ferrous chloride tetrahydrate	NA 1759	Metal salt	pure	2.05	0:35:00	0:10:00	A$_2$	III	II	III	Over 1
35	Fluoboric acid	1775	Acid	48w+%	1.3	0:02:24	0:00:10	A$_1$	I	II	III	1
36	Formic acid	1779	Acid	96%	1.55	0:06:30	0:00:36	A$_1$	II	II		1
37	Fumaryl chloride	1780	Halogen derivative	95%	0.05	0:18:50	0:00:12	A$_1$	II	II		1
38	Hydrobenzene sulfonic acid	1803	Acid	65w+%	0.55	0:13:00	0:00:35	A$_1$	II	II		Over 1
39	Hydrogen bromide	1788	Acid	48%	0.3	0:02:39	0:00:18	A$_1$	I	II		1
40	Iodine monochloride	1792	Halogen derivative	98%	0.75	0:03:12	0:00:03	A$_2$	II	II		Over 1
41	Lithium hydroxide, monohydrate	2680	Base	98%	11.8	0:20:00	0:00:24	B$_1$	II	II		1
42	Mercaptoacetic acid	1940	Acid	97%	0.3	0:11:37	0:02:27	A$_1$	II	II		1
43	Octadecyltrichlorosilane	1800	Silane	95%	0.3	0:17:00	0:00:18	A$_1$	II	II		1
44	Octyltrichlorosilane	1801	Silane	97%	0.1	0:07:30	0:00:40	A$_1$	II	II		1
45	Phenly acetyl chloride	2577	Halogen derivative	98%	0.92	0:13:20	0:00:31	A$_1$	II	II		1
46	Phenly trichlorosilane	1804	Halogen derivative	98%	0	0:07:00	0:00:18	A$_1$	II	II		1
47	Phosphorus pentachloride	1806	Halogen derivative	98%	0	0:00:18	0:00:01	A$_1$	I	II	I	1
48	Phosphorus tribromide	1808	Halogen derivative	97%	0	0:01:00	0:00:11	A$_1$	I	II	I	1
49	Potassium hydrogen sulfate	2509	Salt	35–37%	0.85	0:21:00	0:00:16	A$_1$	II	II		1
50	Potassium hydroxide	1813	Base	Pellets	14	0:06:50	0:00:05	B$_1$	II	II		1
51	Sodium hydrogen fluoride	2439	Halogen derivative	99%	5.16	1:36:00	0:00:00	A$_2$	NC	II	NC	1
52	Sodium hydroxide, solid	1823	Base	Pellets	13.81	0:12:00	0:02:00	B$_1$	II	II		1
53	Sulfuric acid	1830	Acid	100%	0	0:01:30	0:00:04	A$_1$	I	II	I	1
54	Sulfurous acid	1833	Acid	neat	1.78	0:18:00	0:03:24	A$_1$	II	II		1
55	Tetramethylammonium hydroxide pentahydrate	1835	Base	99%	13.61	0:11:30	0:00:45	B$_1$	II	II		1
56	Thiophosphoryl chloride	1837	Halogen derivative	98%	5.81	0:10:08	0:00:23	A$_1$	II	II		1
57	Trichloroacetic acid	1839	Acid	99+%	0.74	0:11:00	0:00:21	A$_1$	II	II		1

(Table continued on next page)

317

Table 5. Corrosive Chemicals of Hazardous Material Table (49 CFR 172.101, U.S. Department of Transportation) *(Continued)*

No.	Chemical	UN No.	Type	Conc.	pH	Time 1	Time 2	Group				
58	Trichlorotoluene	2226	Solvent	99%	3.32	>4 h	NA	A₂	NC	II	NC	1
59	Triethylene tetramine	2259	Amine	60%	11.91	0:49:00	0:01:19	B₁	II	II	II	1
60	Valeryl chloride	2502	Halogen derivative	98%	0.45	0:10:40	0:00:09	A₁	II	II	II	1
61	1(2-AE)Piperazine	2815		99%	11.78	0:44:15	0:05:11	B₁	II	III	II	1
62	2,2-Amino ethoxyethanol	3055		98%	11.3	0:31:00	0:04:09	B₁	II	III	II	1
63	Benzene sulfonyl chloride	2225	Halogen derivative	neat	1.8	3:30:00	0:14:22	A₁	III	III	III	1
64	Butyric acid	2820	Acid	99%	2.15	0:55:40	0:04:20	A₁	II	III	II	1
65	Butyric anhydride	2739	Anhydride	99.2%	3.08	2:30:00	0:02:35	A₁	III	III	III	1
66	Copper(II) chloride	2802	Metal salt	97%	2.99	0:42:41	0:06:20	A₁	III	III	III	1
67	Crotonic acid	2823	Acid	99+%	2.3	1:22:25	0:00:00	A₁	III	III	III	1
68	Cyanuric chloride	2670	Halogen derivative	99%	1.72	3:40:00	0:04:05	A₁	III	III	III	1
69	Diaminopropane	2258	Solvent	99+%	12.06	0:21:36	0:00:14	B₁	II	III	I	Under 1
70	Dicyclohexylamine	2565	Amine	99%	9.57	3:30:00	0:02:17	B₁	III	III	III	1
71	Diethylaminopropylamine	2684	Amine	99+%	12.17	0:61:00	0:00:40	B₁	III	III	III	1
72	Ethanolamine	2491	Amine	99+%	11.82	0:21:41	0:00:00	B₁	II	III	II	1
73	Ethylhexylamine	2276	Amine	98%	11.98	2:45:00	0:14:21	B₁	III	III	III	1
74	Ferric chloride	1773	Metal salt	98%	3	0:21:18	0:00:59	A₁	II	III	II	1
75	Hexanoic acid	2829	Acid	99.5%	3	2:29:00	0:15:00	A₁	III	III	III	1
76	Hydroxylamine sulfate	2865	Salt	97+%	3.58	3:30:00	0:00:00	A₁	III	III	III	1
77	Maleic acid	NA 2215	Acid	99%	1.3	0:15:33	0:00:00	A₁	II	III	II	Over 1
78	Maleic anhydride	2215	Anhydride	99%	1.05	0:34:34	0:02:19	A₁	II	III	II	Over 1
79	Phosphoric acid	1805	Acid	85%	0.85	0:15:00	0:00:57	A₁	II	III	II	1
80	Propionic acid	1848	Acid	99+%	2.68	0:41:00	0:05:15	A₁	II	III	II	1
81	Sodium hydrogen sulfate	1821	Acid salt	pure	0.75	0:14:04	0:01:06	A₁	II	III	II	Over 1
82	Sodium hypochlorite with 5% available chlorine	1791	Oxidizer	5% Cl	11.65	>4 h		B₂	NC	NC	NC	1
83	Sulfamic acid	2967	Acid	99+%	0.65	0:20:55	0:01:14	A₁	II	II	II	1
84	Tetraethylenepentamine	2320	Amine	neat	11.85	1:01:00	0:00:00	B₁	III	III	III	Over 1
85	Tributylamine	2542	Amine	99+%	10.7	>4 h		B₂	NC	NC	NC	1

Table 6. Summary of Double-Blind Study Including Use of Screening Test

	New study with screening test	Original study without screening test
Interlaboratory reproducibility	93%	93%
Number of chemicals studied	29	29
Number of chemicals with identical packing group assignments	27	27

Table 7. CORROSITEX Double-Blind Study

Number	Chemical	Code	Category	Double-blind grouping	In vitro international grouping	Concordance
1	Sulfuric acid	A0002	A_1	I	I	1
2	Fluorosulfonic acid	A0032	A_1	I	I	1
3	Ethylhexylamine	A0003	B_2	III	III	1
4	Chloroacetic acid	B1123-1	A_1	II	II	1
5	Nitric acid	A0033	A_1	I	I	1
6	Sulfurous acid	B1120-6	A_1	II	II	1
7	Acetic acid, glacial	B1122-2	A_1	II	II	1
8	Valeryl chloride	B1124-3	A_1	II	II	1
9	Butyric anhydride	B1121-5	A_1	III	III	1
10	Dithiodipropionic acid	A0004	A_1	NC	NC	1
11	Butoxyethylacetate	A0001	B_2	NC[a]	NC	1
12	Dodecyl trichlorosilane	A0014	A_1	II	II	1
13	Dichloroacetyl chloride	A0025	A_1	I	II	Over
14	Dicyclohexylamine	A0022	B_1	III	III	1
15	Acetic anhydride	A0029	A_1	II	II	1
16	Acrylic acid	A0026	A_1	II	II	1
17	Hydroxybenzenesulfonic acid, 4-	A0030	A_1	II	II	1
18	Crotonic acid	A0031	A_1	II	III	Over
19	Ethylene diamine	A0011	B_1	II	II	1
20	Formic acid	B1125-4	A_1	II	II	1
21	Sodium hydroxide, solid	A0021	B_1	II	II	1
22	Pyridine	A0005	B_1	III	III	1
23	Hydroxylamine sulfate	A0027	A_2	NC	NC	1
24	Aluminum chloride	A0023	A_2	II	II	1
25	Ammonium bisulfate	A0015	A_2	II	II	1
26	Antimony tribromide	A0012	A_1	II	II	1
27	Dichloroacetic acid	A0028	A_1	II	II	1
28	Sodium carbonate	A0024	B_2	NC	NC	1
29	Potassium bisulfate	A0013	A_2	II	II	1

[a] Not enough chemical for qualification test, but the chemical has been tested and qualified in other studies.

Table 8. Comparison of CORROSITEX to Physicochemical Method

Number	Chemical	Chemical category	Concentration (%)	pH	CORROSITEX results			Physicochemical		in vivo [24]	CORROSITEX concordance to in vivo	Physicochemical concordance to in vivo
					Category	Time	Packing Group	Index	Class			
1	NaOH	Base	100	13.79	B_1	0:20:00	II	—	—	C	1	1
2	NaOH	Base	5	13.67	B_2	0:21:20	II	5	C	C	1	1
3	NaOH	Base	1	13.11	B_2	0:39:00	III	1	NC	NC	Over	—
4	NaOH	Base	0.1	12.25	B_2	>4 h	NC	—	—	C	1	—
5	KOH	Base	5	13.83	B_1	0:18:51	II	3.5	NC	NC	1	Under
6	KOH	Base	1	13.05	B_2	0:41:21	III	0.7	NC	C	Over	1
7	H_2SO_4	Acid	15	0	A_1	0:11:29	II	12.1	C	C	1	1
8	H_2SO_4	Acid	5	0.31	A_2	0:17:39	II	4.1	NC	NC	Over	1
9	HNO_3	Acid	20	0	A_1	0:05:45	II	12.4	C	C	Over	1
10	HNO_3	Acid	5	0.18	A_1	0:11:48	II	3.2	NC	C	1	Under
11	H_3PO_4	Acid	25	0.44	A_1	0:21:11	II	17.6	NC	C	1	Under
12	Acetic acid	Acid	25	1.92	A_1	0:31:28	II	3.4	NC	C	1	Under
13	Acetic acid	Acid	10	2.33	A_2	0:40:10	III	1.3	NC	C	1	Under
14	Acetic acid	Acid	1	2.89	A_2	3:00:00	NC	—	—	NC	1	—
15	Acetic acid	Acid	0.1	3.39	A_2	>4 h	NC	—	—	NC	1	—
16	HCl	Acid	25	0	A_1	0:07:35	II	27.2	C	C	1	1
17	HCl	Acid	10	0.17	A_2	0:12:30	II	10.8	C	NC	Over	Over
18	NH_3	Base	10	12.4	B_2	0:08:58	II	7.2	NC	NC	Over	1
19	Formic acid	Acid	25	1.48	A_1	0:21:40	II	17.6	NC	C	1	Under

Table 9. Summary Table of 104 Household and Industrial Cleaners in from 12 Companies

Number of samples studied	104	100%
Number of samples qualified	102	98%
Number of samples with in vivo data	58	57%
Concordance of in vitro and in vivo	51	88%
Number of samples overestimated	5	8.6%
Number of samples underestimated	2	3.4%

as noncorrosive. See a summary of this study in Table 13 on page 329. The complete results are presented in Table 14.

Some pure surfactants do not qualify in CORROSITEX. However, all surfactant-based formulations (>104) have qualified in CORROSITEX.

DISCUSSION

CORROSITEX has been used by over 200 laboratories to evaluate approximately 4000 test materials in its first phase of utilization in industry. Diverse chemicals and formulations that include liquids, solids, insolubles, and immiscibles have been studied from many major industries, including petrochemical, agrochemical, surfactant, textile, paper and pulp, electroplating, and water treatment.

Field testing and additional internal studies resulted in an enhancement of the CORROSITEX assay, referred to as the "screening test," which categorizes all test samples, whether soluble or insoluble, liquid or solid, into four categories. Two of these categories (A_1 and B_1) exhibit very high acid or base content and retain the original CORROSITEX times for assignment of Packing Groups. Two new categories (A_2 and B_2) with little or no acid or base content, are given new CORROSITEX time limits for assignment of packing groups.

Studies on chemicals, mixtures, surfactants, and surfactant formulations demonstrated excellent agreement of in vivo and in vitro packing group classification. This method has demonstrated transferability and 97% interlaboratory reproducibility. A low coefficient of variation of .045 permits categorizing chemicals and formulations within distinct packing groups.

After additional testing, 1050 CORROSITEX test results have been analyzed. Among these samples, 92% qualified and 93% of all corrosives were identified as corrosive. Additionally, 83% of the noncorrosives were correctly identified as noncorrosive. Only 5.4% underestimation was demonstrated. These underestimates represent nine different chemical classes or product types and do not appear to indicate a problem for any specific materials. These data substantiate the use of the CORROSITEX system (including the screening test) as a definitive test to determine noncorrosivity (Table 15).

CORROSITEX is highly concordant with corrosive/noncorrosive in vivo results. Of 406 corrosives samples with in vivo data, 377 (93%) were correctly identified as corrosive by CORROSITEX. Of 296 noncorrosive samples with in vivo data, 83% were identified as noncorrosives, demonstrating the ability of this in vitro method to correctly identify corrosives and noncorrosives. Only 38 test samples out of 702 samples that had in vivo data were found to underestimate. Of these 38 samples, 28 were distinct samples and the remainder were samples that had been tested in more than 1 laboratory. When taking this into account, the percent of underestimation decreases to about 4%. These underestimates do not appear to be from one single chemical class. These include petrochemical active ingredients with different vehicles, which most likely represent a single problem. They also include anhydrides, chlorides, amine sulfates, insolubles, quaternary ammonium compounds, and surfactants. Most of these 300 noncorrosives were tested because they were expected to be hazardous or potentially corrosive, which further increases the validity of this corrosive analysis.

CORROSITEX has demonstrated substantial equivalence to in vivo data in 18 major studies, in addition to a demonstrably high degree of reproducibility. This suggests that CORROSITEX can be used as a scientifically based alternative to the current test method for not only corrosive UN Packing Groups, but noncorrosive determinations as well, thus fulfilling the stated desire of industry to minimize animal testing.

Table 10. Results of Household Cleaners and Industrial Cleaners from 12 Companies

Number	Sample name	Conc. (wt%)	CORROSITEX Time, min., CDS	Category	Packing Group	DOT	Packing Group In vivo	Concordance
1	Adhesive, Company 4	neat	29.32	B_2	II	NA	ND	—
2	Adhesive, Company 4	neat	66.70	B_2	NC	NA	ND	—
3	Cleaner, Company 2	1.0	>240	B_2	NC	NA	ND	—
4	Cleaner, Company 2	10.0	>240	B_2	NC	NA	ND	Under
5	Cleaner, Company 2	neat	88.90	B_2	NC	NA	III	—
6	Cleaner, Company 2	neat	56.25	B_2	NC	NA	NC	1
7	Dish Powder 2	neat	60.95	B_2	NC	NA	NC	1
8	Cleaner, Company 1	neat	76.13	B_2	NC	NA	ND	—
9	Cleaner, Company 1	neat	167.57	B_2	NC	NA	ND	—
10	Cleaner, Company 1	neat	64.72	B_2	NC	NA	ND	—
11	Cleaner, Company 1	neat	>240	B_2	NC	NA	ND	—
12	Cleaner, Company 1	neat	16.54	B_2	II	NA	II	1
13	Cleaner, Company 1	neat	>240	B_2	NC	NA	ND	—
14	Cleaner, Company 1	neat	13.98	B_2	II	NA	II	1
15	Cleaner, Company 1	neat	11.19	B_2	II	NA	II	1
16	Cleaner, Company 1	neat	14.88	B_1	II	NA	ND	—
17	Cleaner, Company 1	neat	72.91	B_2	NC	NA	ND	—
18	Cleaner, Company 1	neat	31.48	B_2	III	NA	ND	—
19	MWF, Company 3	neat	51.06	B_2	NC	NA	ND	—
20	MWF, Company 3	neat	22.10	B_2	II	NA	II	1
21	MWF, Company 3	neat	67.20	B_2	NC	NA	ND	—
22	MWF, Company 3	neat	45.03	B_2	NC	NA	ND	—
23	MWF, Company 3	neat	47.49	B_2	NC	NA	ND	—
24	MWF, Company 3	neat	84.33	B_2	NC	NA	ND	—
25	MWF, Company 3	neat	25.50	B_2	II	NA	ND	—
26	Oil, Company 5	neat	NQ	B_2	NQ	NA	ND	—
27	Oil, Company 5	neat	NQ	B_2	NQ	NA	ND	—
28	Company 6	neat	45.61	B_2	NC	NA	ND	—
29	Company 6	neat	45.78	B_2	NC	NA	ND	—
30	Company 6	neat	37.80	B_2	III	NA	ND	—
31	Company 6	neat	32.02	B_2	III	NA	ND	—
32	Company 6	neat	35.62	B_2	III	NA	ND	—
33	Company 6	neat	37.47	B_2	III	NA	ND	—
34	Company 6	neat	35.91	B_2	III	NA	ND	—
35	Company 6	neat	36.61	B_2	III	NA	ND	—

36	Company 6	neat	35.42	B_2	III	NA	ND	—
37	Cleaner, Company 7	neat	166.18	B_2	NC	NA	ND	—
38	Cleaner, Company 7	neat	>240	B_2	NC	NA	ND	—
39	Cleaner, Company 7	neat	>240	B_2	NC	NA	ND	—
40	Cleaner, Company 8	neat	45.07	B_2	NC	NA	NC	—
41	Cleaner, Company 8	neat	48.93	B_2	III	NA	NC	1
42	Cleaner, Company 8	neat	41.17	B_2	II	NA	NC	Over
43	Cleaner, Company 8	neat	14.66	B_2	NC	NA	C	1
44	Cleaner, Company 9	neat	87.07	B_2	III	NA	ND	—
45	Cleaner, Company 9	neat	43.71	B_2	NC	NA	ND	1
46	Blend, Company 10	neat	>240	B_2	NC	NA	NC	1
47	Blend, Company 10	neat	>240	B_2	NC	NA	NC	1
48	Blend, Company 10	neat	>240	B_2	NC	NA	NC	1
49	Blend, Company 10	neat	>240	B_2	NC	NA	NC	1
50	Blend, Company 10	neat	>240	B_2	NC	NA	NC	1
51	Blend, Company 10	neat	>240	B_2	NC	NA	NC	1
52	Blend, Company 10	neat	>240	B_2	NC	NA	NC	1
53	Blend, Company 10	neat	104.1	B_2	NC	NA	NC	1
54	Blend, Company 10	neat	>240	B_2	NC	NA	NC	1
55	Blend, Company 10	neat	>240	B_2	NC	NA	NC	1
56	Blend, Company 10	neat	>240	B_2	NC	NA	NC	1
57	Blend, Company 10	neat	>240	B_2	NC	NA	NC	1
58	Blend, Company 10	neat	>240	B_2	NC	NA	NC	1
59	Blend, Company 10	neat	>240	B_2	NC	NA	NC	1
60	Blend, Company 10	neat	>240	B_2	NC	NA	NC	1
61	Blend, Company 10	neat	>240	B_2	NC	NA	NC	1
62	Blend, Company 10	neat	>240	B_2	NC	NA	NC	1
63	Blend, Company 11	neat	15.38	B_1	II	NA	I	Under
64	Blend, Company 11	neat	23.47	B_2	II	NA	II	1
65	Blend, Company 11	neat	16.40	B_1	II	NA	II	1
66	Blend, Company 11	neat	39.00	B_2	III	NA	NC	Over
67	Blend, Company 11	neat	22.46	B_2	II	NA	II	1
68	Blend, Company 11	neat	17.91	B_2	II	NA	II	1
69	Blend, Company 11	neat	24.73	B_2	II	NA	II	1
70	Blend, Company 11	neat	26.06	B_2	II	NA	II	1

(Table continued on next page)

Table 10. Results of Household Cleaners and Industrial Cleaners from 12 Companies *(Continued)*

Number	Sample name	Conc. (wt%)	CORROSITEX Time, min., CDS	Category	Packing Group	DOT	Packing Group In vivo	Concordance
71	Blend, Company 11	neat	33.38	B$_2$	III	NA	III	1
72	Blend, Company 11	neat	27.63	B$_2$	II	NA	II	1
73	Blend, Company 11	neat	31.75	B$_2$	III	NA	III	1
74	Blend, Company 11	neat	>240	B$_2$	NC	NA	NC	1
75	Blend, Company 11	neat	45	B$_2$	NC	NA	NC	1
76	Blend, Company 11	neat	24.08	B$_2$	II	NA	II	1
77	Blend, Company 11	neat	20.71	B$_2$	II	NA	II	1
78	Blend, Company 11	neat	14.67	B$_1$	II	NA	II	1
79	Blend, Company 11	neat	31.33	B$_2$	III	NA	III	1
80	Blend, Company 11	neat	23.92	B$_1$	II	NA	II	1
81	Blend, Company 11	neat	30.17	B$_2$	III	NA	III	1
82	Blend, Company 11	neat	14.67	B$_2$	II	NA	ND	—
83	Blend, Company 11	neat	>240	B$_2$	NC	NA	ND	—
84	Blend, Company 11	neat	24.38	B$_1$	II	NA	ND	—
85	Blend, Company 11	neat	136.09	B$_2$	NC	NA	ND	—
86	Blend, Company 11	neat	28.75	B$_1$	II	NA	ND	—
87	Blend, Company 11	neat	>240	B$_2$	NC	NA	NC	—
88	Blend, Company 11	neat	19.59	B$_1$	II	NA	NC	Over
89	Blend, Company 11	neat	51.00	B$_2$	NC	NA	ND	—
90	Blend, Company 11	neat	26.33	B$_2$	II	NA	II	1
91	Blend, Company 11	neat	24.94	B$_2$	II	NA	II	1
92	Blend, Company 11	neat	19.71	B$_2$	II	NA	II	1
93	Blend, Company 11	neat	26.92	B$_2$	II	NA	NC	Over
94	Blend, Company 11	neat	42.38	B$_2$	III	NA	ND	—
95	Blend, Company 11	neat	182.22	B$_2$	NC	NA	NC	1
96	Blend, Company 11	neat	168.74	B$_2$	III	NA	NC	Over
97	Blend, Company 11	neat	39.19	B$_2$	III	NA	NC	Over
98	Cleaner, Company 12	neat	17.18	B$_1$	II	NA	ND	—
99	Cleaner, Company 12	neat	18.12	B$_2$	II	NA	ND	—
100	Cleaner, Company 12	neat	21.13	B$_1$	II	NA	ND	—
101	Cleaner, Company 12	neat	132.90	B$_2$	NC	NA	ND	—
102	Cleaner, Company 12	neat	69.96	B$_2$	NC	NA	NC	1
103	Cleaner, Company 12	neat	211.19	B$_2$	NC	NA	NC	1
104	Cleaner, Company 12	neat	177.81	B$_2$	NC	NA	NC	1

Table 11. Summary of CORROSITEX Results on 59
Surfactant-Based Products with In Vivo Data

In vivo and in vitro data	59
Concordance	90%
Sensitivity to detect corrosives	97%
Sensitivity to detect noncorrosives	83%

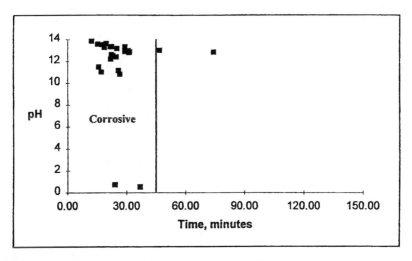

Figure 4. Surfactant formulations with in vivo corrosive designation.

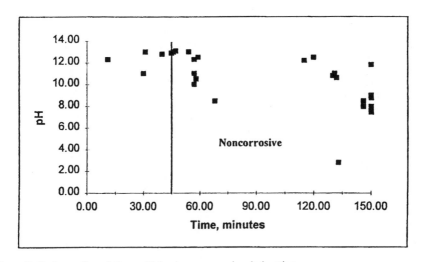

Figure 5. Surfactant formulations with in vivo noncorrosive designation.

Table 12. CORROSITEX Study of 59 Surfactant-Based Formulations with In Vivo Data

	Formulation category	Categorization	pH	Minutes	Group	In vivo	Concordance
1	Cleaner	B_1	13.57	15.50	II	C	I
2	Heavy-duty stripper	B_1	13.54	17.53	II	C	I
3	Cleaner	B_1	13.56	18.83	II	C	I
4	Stripper	B_1	13.85	12.23	II	C	I
5	Cleaner	B_1	11.00	17.27	II	C	I
6	Stripper	B_1	13.29	18.75	II	C	I
7	Degreaser/cleaner	B_1	13.64	19.65	II	C	I
8	Industrial cleaner	B_2	13.35	21.72	II	C	I
9	Cleaner	B_2	12.20	22.00	II	C	I
10	Cleaner	B_1	13.34	22.33	II	C	I
11	Stripper	B_1	12.60	22.42	II	C	I
12	Stripper	B_1	12.50	23.00	II	C	I
13	Shower room cleaner	A_1	0.72	24.13	II	C	I
14	Stripper	B_1	13.19	25.01	II	C	I
15	Stripper	B_1	11.17	25.85	II	C	I
16	Industrial cleaner	B_2	10.81	26.45	II	C	I
17	Degreaser/cleaner	B_2	12.99	30.80	III	C	I
18	Stripper	B_1	12.80	31.00	II	C	I
19	Stripper	B_2	12.85	31.50	III	C	I
20	Industrial cleaner	B_1	12.40	24.65	II	C	I
21	Industrial cleaner	B_2	12.90	29.00	II	C	I
22	Degreaser/industrial cleaner	B_2	13.34	29.01	II	C	I
23	Cleaner	A_1	0.51	36.78	III	C	I
24	Cleaner	B_2	12.83	74.17	NC	C	Under
25	Cleaner	B_2	12.97	7.50	II	NC	Over
26	Glass cleaner	B_1	12.23	14.47	II	NC	Over
27	Stripper	B_2	11.16	30.38	III	NC	Over
28	Degreaser/cleaner	B_2	13.01	32.32	III	NC	Over
29	Glass cleaner	B_2	10.76	34.67	III	NC	Over
30	Calcium carbonate	B_2	12.56	>240.00	NC	NC	I
31	Cleaner	B_2	12.70	45.20	NC	NC	I
32	Cleaner	B_2	12.64	46.40	NC	NC	I
33	Dishwasher detergent	B_2	10.87	56.00	NC	NC	I
34	Cleaner	B_2	12.18	56.40	NC	NC	I
35	Cleaner	B_2	12.67	57.50	NC	NC	I
36	Laundry detergent	B_2	10.48	57.58	NC	NC	I
37	Cleaner	B_2	8.65	66.63	NC	NC	I
38	Bathroom cleaner	B_2	12.26	113.00	NC	NC	I
39	Bathroom cleaner	B_2	12.50	122.73	NC	NC	I
40	Glass cleaner	B_2	10.79	129.70	NC	NC	I
41	Resin	B_2	10.51	131.10	NC	NC	I
42	Cleaner	A_2	2.80	139.20	NC	NC	I
43	Resin	B_2	7.89	147.07	NC	NC	I
44	Resin	B_2	8.17	188.13	NC	NC	I
45	Bathroom cleaner	B_2	9.16	197.83	NC	NC	I
46	Bathroom cleaner	B_2	9.07	200.58	NC	NC	I
47	Resin	B_2	7.96	218.62	NC	NC	I
48	Industrial cleaner	B_2	7.25	240.00	NC	NC	I
49	Cleaner	B_2	11.49	15.91	II	C	I
50	Cleaner	B_2	NA	20.46	II	C	I
51	Cleaner	B_2	NA	26.85	II	C	I
52	Cleaner	B_2	NA	32.02	III	C	I
53	Cleaner	B_2	13.02	43.43	III	C	I
54	Cleaner	B_2	12.86	46.79	NC	NC	I
55	Cleaner	B_2	12.74	53.29	NC	NC	I
56	Cleaner	B_2	NA	54.04	NC	NC	I
57	Cleaner	B_2	9.87	56.08	NC	NC	I
58	Cleaner	B_2	11.10	130.09	NC	NC	I
59	Cleaner	B_2	8.66	146.97	NC	NC	I

Table 14. CORROSITEX Study of Raw Surfactants

Number	Name	Class	% Active	Category	pH	Time	Group	In vivo[h]	Conc.
1	Cerylpyridinium Chloride	Cationic	1	A₂	6.79	>4 h	NC	NC	I
2	Sodium laureth sulfate-4 1M	Nonionic	100	A₂	5.37	>4 h	NC	NC	I
3	Sodium leuroam phoacetate/tridecyl sulfate	Blend	31.24	B₂	NA	NA	NQ	NC	—
4	Disodium sulfosuccinate	Anionic	5	A₂	5.57	NA	NQ	NC	—
5	Disodium cocamphodipropionate	Amphoteric	16	B₂	NA	NA	NQ	NC	—
6	Myriatyl myristate	Nonionic	5	A₂	.43	NA	NQ	NC	—
7	Stearyl stearac	Nonionic	3	B₂	NA	NA	NQ	NC	—
8	Ceteryl alcohol	Nonionic	5	B₂	NA	NA	NQ	NC	—
9	Glyceryl stearate	Nonionic	5	B₂	NA	NA	NQ	NC	—
10	olealkonium chloride	Cationic	55	A₂	6.7	>4 h	NC	NC	I
11	Sodium caproamphoacetate	Amphoteric	16	B₂	7.14	NA	NQ	NC	—
12	Benzalkonium chloride	Cationic	2	B₂	7.55	>4 h	NC	NC	I
13	Sodium laureth sulfate 1 M	Anionic	25.3	B₂	8.26	>4 h	NC	NC	I
14	Sodium lauryl sulfate	Anionic	29.5	B₂	7.91	>4 h	NC	NC	—
15	Sodium lauriaminodipropionate	Amphoteric	16	B₂	7.32	>4 h	NC	NC	—
16	Stearalkonium chloride	Cationic	2	A₂	4.4	>4 h	NC	NC	I
17	Stearyl alcohol, cetrimonium bromide	Cationic	3	B₂	NA	NA	NC	NC	—
18	Sodium laureth carboxylate-13	Anionic	5	B₂	NA	NA	NC	NC	—
19	Disodium caprykloamphodiacate	Amphoteric	38	B₂	8.98	>4 h	NC	NC	I
20	Cetaryl alcohol glycol stearate	Nonionic	3	B₂	7.71	>4 h	NC	NC	I
21	Sodium cocoamphopoaprionate	Amphoretic	16	B₂	NA	NA	NQ	NC	—
22	Sodium tridecyl sulfate	Anionic	29.59	B₂	7.89	NA	NQ	NC	—
23	Anionic/amphoteric blend[a]	Blend	16	A₂	7.18	NA	NQ	NC	—
24	Ammonium lauryl sulfate	Anionic	27.4	A₂	6.65	NA	NQ	NC	—
25	Sodium laureth sulfate	Anionic	27.2	B₂	7.8	>4 h	NC	NC	I
26	Sodium cocoamphoacetate	Amphoteric	36.4	B₂	8.34	>4 h	NC	NC	—
27	Amphoteric/anionic/nonionic[b]	Blend	20	B₂	8.16	NA	NQ	NC	—
28	Disodium laureth succinate	Blend	16	B₂	7.5	>4 h	NC	NC	I
29	Sulfoccinate	Anionic	5	A₂	5.69	NA	NQ	NC	—
30	Sodium cocoamphohydroxypropylsulfonate	Amphoteric	37.53	B₂	NA	NA	NQ	NC	—
31	Disodium caprylamphodipropionate	Amphoteric	38.9	B₂	8.91	2:21:41	NQ	NC	I
32	Sodium stearoamphoacetate	Amphoteric	25.8	B₂	NA	NA	NQ	NC	—
33	Cocamide DEA	Nonionic	5	B₂	9.53	>4 h	NC	NC	I
34	Anionic/nonionic blend[c]	Blend	39.67	B₂	8.94	>4 h	NC	NC	I
35	Cocamide DEA	Nonionic	5	B₂	NA	NA	NQ	NC	—

(Table continued on next page)

327

Table 14. CORROSITEX Study of Raw Surfactants (*Continued*)

Number	Name	Class	% Active	Category	pH	Time	Group	In vivo[h]	Conc.
36	Sodium detoxyethoxy acetate	Amphoteric	46.45	A_2	5.12	NA	NQ	NC	—
37	Disodium tallowiminodiproprionate	Amphoteric	16	B_2	7.25	>4 h	NC	NC	I
38	Disodium tallow glycinate	Amphoteric	1.5	A_2	5.46	>4 h	NC	NC	I
39	Mixed C8 amphocarbocylic acid	Amphoteric	28.1	B_2	NA	NA	NQ	NC	—
40	Octoxycol-33, sodium laureth sulfate	Anionic	45.8	B_2	8.05	>4 h	NC	NC	I
41	Sodium laureth sulfate 2 *M*	Anionic	35.12	B_2	8.06	>4 h	NC	NC	I
42	Betaine	Amphoteric	15	A_2	6.38	NA	NQ	NC	—
43	Anionic blead[a]	Blend	39.07	B_2	NA	NA	NQ	NC	—
44	Amphoteric/nonionic blend[e]	Blend	40.6	B_2	8.23	>4 h	NC	NC	I
45	Disodium cocoamphodiacetate	Amphoteric	16	B_2	NA	NA	NQ	NC	—
46	Disodium lauroamphodiacetate	Amphoteric	30	B_2	8.35	>4 h	NC	NC	I
47	Blend[f]	Blend	20	B_2	8.78	>4 h	NC	NC	I
48	Blend[g]	Blend	30	B_2	7.71	>4 h	NC	NC	I
49	Sodium benzyl sulfonate	Anionic	22.42	B_2	8.99	>4 h	NQ	NC	—
50	Alkyl benzene sulfonate	Anionic	91	B_2	NA	NA	NQ	NC	—
51	Sodium methyl cocoyl taurate	Anionic	10	B_2	NA	NA	NQ	NC	—
52	Alkylamine rhoxylate	Anionic	100	B_2	NA	>4 h	NC	C	Under
53	Cocodimethylanineoxide	Cationic	100	B_2	NA	>4 h	NC	NC	I
54	Dicocoalkylbenzylammonleuric chloride	Cationic	100	B_2	NA	NA	NQ	C	—
55	Alkylsulfate C12	Anionic	100	B_2	NA	>4 h	NC	NC	I
56	Aklyethersulfate 2 *M*	Anionic	100	B_2	NA	>4 h	NC	NC	I
57	Olefia sulfonate	Anionic	100	B_2	NA	>4 h	NC	NC	I
58	Alkyphosphoric acid 4 *M*	Anionic	100	B_2	NA	NA	NQ	NC	—
59	Fatty alkylethozylate	Anionic	100	B_2	NA	>4 h	NC	NC	I
60	Fatty acid monoethanolanide	Anionic	100	B_2	NA	>4 h	NC	NC	I
61	Cocoalkyltrimethylammonium chloride	Cationic	100	B_2	NA	>4 h	NC	NC	I
62	Benzyltrimethylammonium chloride	Cationic	100	B_2	NA	>4 h	NC	NC	I
63	Alkyldimethylamine oxide[h]	Anionic	100	B_2	NA	>4 h	NC	NC	I

[a] Lauryl sulfate/DEA lauraminopropionate/NA lauraminoproprionate/propylene glycol.
[b] Amphoteric/anionic/nonionic surface-active agent.
[c] Disodium cocoamphodiacete/SLS/SLES/propylene glycol.
[d] Disodium cocoamphodiacete/SLS/Hexylene glycol.
[e] Disodium cocoamphodipropionate/SLS/hexylene glycol.
[f] Not available.
[g] Disodium lauramphodiacetate/sodium trideceth sulfate/hexylene glycol.
[h] C, corrosive; NC, noncorrosive.

328

Table 13. Summary of CORROSITEX Data on 63 Raw Surfactants

Number of samples	63
Number qualified	34
Noncorrosives were noncorrosive in vitro	33
Corrosive was corrosive in vitro	0
Concordance	97%
Sensitivity to detect noncorrosives	97%

Table 15. Summary of 1050 Test Samples Evaluated in CORROSITEX

	Number	%
Total samples	1050	100%
Total qualified	965	92%
Corrosive (C) with in vivo or DOT data	406	39%
Noncorrosive (NC) with in vivo or DOT data	296	28%
Corrosive identified correctly	377	93%
Noncorrosive identified correctly	246	83%
Qualified samples with in vivo or DOT data	702	67%
Concordance with in vivo or DOT data	600	85.5%
Overestimates with in vivo or DOT data	64	9.1%
Underestimates with in vivo or DOT data	38	5.4%

References

1. DOT Hazardous Materials Table 49. 1993. CFR 172.101.
2. Report from BioTechnics, 1992. In vivo Studies on corrosives and noncorrosives. Los Angeles, CA.
3. CFR Code of Federal Regulations. 1991. Transportation Title 49, Part 173, Appendix A. Method of Testing Corrosion to the Skin.
4. United Nations. 1973. Transportation of Dangerous Goods. Orange Book. Special Recommendations Relating to Class 8, p. 173.
5. European Economic Community. 1973. European Council Directive Relating to the Classification, Packaging and Labeling of Paints, Varnishes, Inks, Adhesives and Other Products. 1977 *Off. J. Eur. Commission* 29 (L303).
6. European Economic Community. 1978. European Council Directive Relating to the Classification Packaging and Labeling of Dangerous Preparation. *Off. J. Eur. Commission* 21 (L296).
7. Organization for Economic Cooperation and Development. 1981. Acute Dermal Irritation/Corrosion in OECD Guidelines for Testing of Chemicals. Sect. 4 404. Paris: OECD.
8. Van Scott, E. J., and Lyon, A. 1953. Chemical measure of the effect of soap and detergents on the skin. *J. Invest. Dermatol.* 21:99.
9. Harrold, S. P. 1959. Denaturation of epidermal keratin by surface active ingredients. *J. Invest. Dermatol.* 32:581.
10. Choman, B. R. 1963. Determination of the response of skin to chemical agents by an in vitro procedure. *J. Invest. Dermatol.* 40:177.
11. Imokawa, G., et al. 1975. Study on skin roughness caused by surfactants. *J. Am. Oil Chem. Soc.* 52:475.
12. Imokawa, G. 1978. Cumulative effect of surfactants on cutaneous horny layer. *Contact Dermatitis* 5:357.
13. Oliver, G. J. A., Pemberton, M. A., and Rhodes, C. 1988. An in vitro model for identifying skin-corrosive chemicals. *Toxicol. In Vitro* 2:7.
14. Young, I. R., et al. 1988. Classification as corrosive or irritant to skin of preparations containing acid or base substances without testing on animals. *Toxicol. In Vitro* 1:19–26.

Chapter Thirty-three

COMPARISON STUDY OF IN VITRO AND IN VIVO RESULTS ON TEXTILE FABRIC EXTRACTS FOR ASSESSING DERMAL IRRITANCY POTENTIAL TO INDUSTRIAL WORKERS

Virginia C. Gordon, K. Harris, Howard I. Maibach, and S. Patil

In vitro alternative assays have gained acceptance due to their reduction of the number of animals used in toxicological risk assessment testing. The increased reproducibility and sensitivity of these methods permit their application to the assessment of safety in the workplace. The purpose of this study was to determine applications of an in vitro assay, SKINTEX,* as a screen to detect contaminants in dyed fabrics prior to exposing workers. In this study, dyed and undyed fabrics have been evaluated in the SKINTEX system, a standardized in vitro, two-compartment physicochemical model, to predict dermal irritation. An extraction procedure and a rapid in vitro screen were developed that identified dyed fabrics that produced worker irritation. Human clinical studies on 8 fabrics using repeat application of the extracts of fabrics for 6 d confirmed the human response to extracts of dyed fabrics identified by the SKINTEX test. Negative control materials were identified as negatives in vivo and in vitro. One fabric that produced human irritation in the human clinical study was not identified in the SKINTEX test. A concordance of 92% was observed for in vitro to in vivo results. The SKINTEX test provides a reproducible quantitative screen to assess cumulative dermal irritancy potential of dyed fabrics prior to worker exposure.

INTRODUCTION

Relevance of In Vitro Studies to the In Vivo Test Method

Many commercial products are recognized as potential sources of dermal irritation. A multitude of chemicals in the workplace and environment have been recognized as dermal irritants. Federal agencies and commercial manufacturers must consider dermal irritation risks when developing, registering, or certifying materials.

The test most widely used for predicting potential human skin irritants with an animal model was published by Draize et al.[1] Many modifications to improve inconsistent results and interpretation have been utilized. The DOT[2] (Department of Transportation) recommends an exposure

---

* Trademark of In Vitro International, Irvine, CA.

period of 4 h. Four-hour and shorter periods are recommended by the NAS[3] (National Academy of Science).

Introduction to the SKINTEX Assay System as an Example of the Target Biomacromolecular Approach

The SKINTEX system is based on the use of target biomacromolecules to predict in vivo dermal irritation. It is the first well-defined prototype assay system representing the use of target macromolecules or macromolecular structures relevant to in vivo pathways, structures, or events in the skin to predict in vivo toxic effects of chemicals and formulations. The use of target biomacromolecules provides a standardized substrate for continued analysis and database development. Changes that occur in these macromolecules upon interaction with chemicals or formulations can be quantified and used to predict in vivo toxic endpoints. This is called the target biomacromolecular approach (TBA) in in vitro toxicology.

The SKINTEX model incorporates two compartments. The first compartment is a biomembrane barrier of keratin and collagen. Materials can absorb onto or permeate through this biomembrane barrier to a macromolecular matrix. Changes in the integrity of the first compartment due to absorption of a test sample to the keratin can release dye incorporated into this biomembrane. In the second compartment, organized protein filaments are spatially arranged with collagen into a transparent matrix. Test samples that are chemical irritants alter the conformation and/or hydration of the protein filaments to produce turbidity (Figure 1). The biobarrier was designed by assessing the effects of known chemicals that bind to or alter the stratum corneum. The second compartment, including molecular mechanisms of membrane perturbation, protein conformational change, and protein hydration, was optimized by known chemicals' effects with respect to these mechanisms and dermal irritation.

MATERIALS AND METHODS

The SKINTEX Method includes a biomembrane barrier and biomacromolecular matrix.

Biomembrane Barrier

A buffered salt solution of keratin, collagen, and a dye was bound to cellulose within a plastic disc with 0.1% glutaraldehyde at 25°C for 1 h. After washing the support in distilled water, the biomembrane barriers were stored at 4°C and have a 180-d shelf-life.

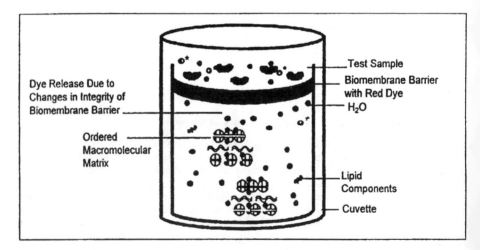

Figure 1. The SKINTEX model.

Biomacromolecular Matrix

A lyophilized powder containing globulins, collagen, glycos-aminoglycans, free fatty acids, amino acids, phospholipids, and buffer salts is rehydrated.

Procedure and Scoring

A method called the high-sensitivity assay (HSA) was used to establish the relationship between the response of known irritants and their in vivo dermal irritation. This procedure permitted testing of undiluted liquids, solids, and insolubles at three different doses. Samples were applied directly to the barrier matrix and inserted into the reagent. The absorbance at 470 nm was used to quantitate the response. A calibration system based on the irritancy of known controls of sodium lauryl sulfate from 0.1 to 2.0% was used to establish a scoring system. The net absorbance at 470 nm was read as a SKINTEX/PDII equivalent. In vitro dermal irritation classes of nonirritant, minimal, and minimal/mild corresponded directly to in vivo classes (Figure 2).

Fabric Samples

Fabric samples were supplied by a large textile manufacturer. The samples were both positive samples and negative controls, based on worker complaint records and observations. Identical fabric samples were used for both in vitro and in vivo studies.

Preparation of Extracts for In Vivo and In Vitro Protocols

A final protocol using a 37°C saline extraction of the fabric for 24 h was developed. Either 10 or 25% by mass of the fabric and saline was used to prepare extracts. Extracts were studied directly in SKINTEX HSA at 100 μl, 200 μl, 300 μl, or 400 μl. Each sample was treated the

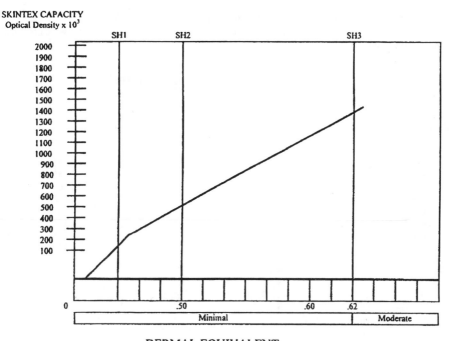

Figure 2. SKINTEX Scoring

same way. A 5 × 5 cm piece of material was placed into 3 different solutions to produce extraction fluids for testing. The three were:

1. The piece was placed into 0.9% NaCl solution for 24 h, then tested.
2. The piece was placed in 70% ethanol for 24 h, and then the solution was tested.
3. The piece was soaked for 2 h in distilled water and then sonicated for 1 h.

In Vivo Protocol

Test sample extracts after concentration were applied to the backs of 10 human volunteers with the occlusive patch test. The readings were taken after 24 h for up to 7 d of exposure and the arithmetic mean was calculated. Visual scores were read and assessed for 7 d and transepidermal water loss readings were taken on d 7.

Experimental Design

Two fabrics were studied in phase 1. One had been positive to workers and the other negative to workers. Evaluation of extraction fluids, concentration of fabric in extract, time of extraction, and extraction concentrations was made. A saline extraction procedure at 37°C with sonication was selected to optimize the relevance to the factory and human exposure conditions. In vivo tests on concentrated extracts confirmed the identity of the positive fabric.

In phase 2, extracts of 22 additional fabrics were studied in SKINTEX HSA. All fabrics were extracted at 25% by mass fabric/fluid ratio. Diverse colors of dyed fabrics were studied, representing products from several sources, different dying processes, and different records of worker complaints. A subset of positive and negative fabrics in SKINTEX was selected for in vivo human clinical studies.

RESULTS

The results obtained from in vitro studies of 22 fabrics in SKINTEX HSA are presented in Table 1. Extracts of eight of these samples were also studied in vivo. Visual scores were obtained and are presented in Table 2.

Table 1. Evaluation of Extracts of 22 Fabrics in SKINTEX HSA

Color	Sample	Net optical density change
Blue	S1984	−32
Brown	S1988	9
Brown	S1987	39
Plum	S2006	43
Maroon	S1986	53
Maroon	S2002	55
Maroon	S2005	65
Brown	S2004	75
Black	S2008	81
Black	S1956	118
Undyed	S1954	135
Green	S2007	136
Black	S2014	138
Black	S2012	141
Black	S2010	144
Green	S1985	149
Black	S1953	151
Black	S1955	158
Black	S2011	166
Black	S2003	180
Black	S2013	183
Blue	S2009	200

Table 2. Summary of Visual Scores

Number	Sample	Preparation	Mean visual score	SD
1	2013	Sonicated	0.70	±1.40
2	2014	Sonicated	0.68	±1.35
3	1953	Sonicated	0.68	±1.35
4	2008	Sonicated	0.27	±0.65
5	1986	Sonicated	0.27	±0.90
6	2008	Saline	0.64	±1.43
7	2008	Ethanol	0.68	±1.52
8	2002	Sonicated	0.68	±1.19
9	2010	Sonicated	0.50	±1.12
10	2013	Ethanol	0.91	±1.63
11	2002	Saline	0.59	±1.43
12	2002	Ethanol	0.86	±1.58
13	1986	Ethanol	0.70	±1.60
14	1986	Saline	0.18	±0.60
15	2014	Ethanol	0.73	±1.62
16	2014	Saline	0.18	±0.40
17	2010	Ethanol	0.36	±1.21
18	2010	Saline	0.09	±0.30
19	1953	Ethanol	0.64	±1.43
20	1953	Saline	0.45	±1.21
21	2013	Saline	0.09	±0.30
22	Control	Water	0.09	±0.30

A summary of in vivo and in vitro results on eight samples is presented in Table 3. The visual scores and transepidermal water loss were also recorded in the in vivo human clinical studies and are included. A comparison of in vitro results from three extraction procedures are provided for in vitro studies. Three different extraction fluids were used in the in vivo human clinical study. When additional preparations were made and studied again in SKINTEX, excellent reproducibility was observed. If sonication was used to extract the fabric, the results produced are similar to those obtained with prolonged incubations (Table 3). The in vitro and in vivo results for eight samples are compared in Table 3.

In this comparison, it is demonstrated that a good correlation is obtained for saline sonication extracts studied in vivo and in vitro. Ethanol extracts produced elevated visual responses for seven of the eight test samples in human clinical studies.

Therefore, the best method of preparing fabric extracts for in vivo human clinicals is sonication. It provided the maximum separation of positive fabric response to negative fabric response. In our opinion, the sonication procedure provided the best removal of the contaminants into the extraction fluid, and these results were used for correlation of the in vitro and in vivo scores in Figure 3. One sample that produced an elevated human response was not detected in the SKINTEX HSA test. All positives in the SKINTEX HSA test produced elevated results in human patch testing.

A washing procedure using soap or distilled water at 37°C for 4 h was applied to a positive and a negative fabric. The washing with either soap or water reduced the response of the positive fabric in SKINTEX HSA (Table 4).

DISCUSSION

In earlier studies of the SKINTEX method,[4–10] it was demonstrated that this method can detect and reproducibly quantitate dermal irritants. The current study evaluated the applicability of this in vitro method as a screen for dyed fabrics prior to exposure of workers. This study confirmed that extracts of dyed fabrics producing elevated cumulative responses in humans during human clinical studies could be detected in SKINTEX (Table 5). Furthermore, a cutoff of 1.00 absorbance units could be established for identifying potentially irritating fabrics in this study (Figure 4). In Figure 4, an established cutoff based on the 25% saline extract analysis of

Table 3. Summary of Results of In Vitro and In Vivo Study

Sample number	In vitro				In vivo					
	Saline evaluation	Repeat	1-h Sonication	4-h Sonication	Visual score			TEWL		
					Saline	Sonication	Ethanol	Saline	Sonication	Ethanol
	25%	25%	25%	25%						
1986	53	62	57	63	0.18	0.27	0.70	6.2	3.7	2.2
2008	81			110	0.64	0.27	0.68	3.6	4.4	2.2
2002	55	69	85		0.59	0.68	0.86	4.1	2.8	1.7
2010	144			140	0.09	0.50	0.36	3.9	3.9	1.9
2014	138			135	0.18	0.68	0.73	3.9	4.1	2.4
1953	151	182	183	138	0.09	0.68	0.64	2.8	4.6	2.4
2013	183			150	0.09	0.17	0.91	4.0	3.5	2.3

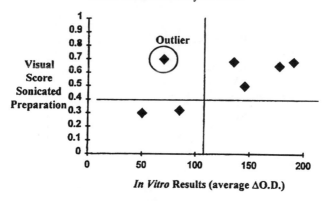

Figure 3. Correlation of in vitro and in vivo results for dermal irritancy of fabric extracts.

Table 4. Evaluation of Positive and Negative Fabrics after Washing at 37°C for 4 h

Sample	Volume	Original	After soap wash	After distilled water wash
negative	1	100	96	120
negative	2	90	84	98
positive	1	205	130	140
positive	2	192	120	98

Table 5. Summary of Fabric Extracts in In Vitro and In Vivo Studies

Sample number	In vitro, Δ OD > 100 (+) Δ OD < 100 (−)	In vivo, human response > 0.4 (+), human response < 0.4 (−)
1986	−	−
2008	−	−
2010	+	+
2002	−	+
2014	+	+
1953	+	+
2013	+	+

a dyed fabric permits selection of fabrics that have been shown in phase 1 and phase 2 studies to produce elevated response in human clinical studies.

The quality assurance procedure can be implemented at the manufacturing site. Upon receipt of new lots of dyed fabrics, a quality assurance screen can be performed. Extracts are prepared with a known positive control fabric; then test extracts and control extract are analyzed in a 24-h screen. Changes in absorbance are compared to established cutoffs for acceptance of dyed fabrics for worker processing (Figure 5).

REFERENCES

1. Draize, J. H., Woodward, G., and Calvery, H. O. 1944. Methods for study of irritation and toxicity of substances applied topically to skin and mucous membranes. *J. Pharmacol. Exp. Ther.* 82:377–90.
2. Code of Federal Regulations. 1980. Title 49, Part 173.240.
3. National Academy of Sciences, Committee for Revision NAS Publication 1138 1977. Principles for Evaluating the Toxicity of Household Substances: Washington, DC: NAS.

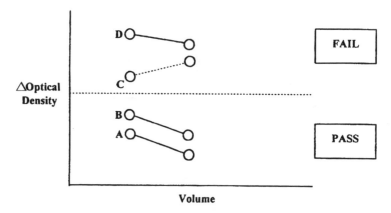

Evaluation of Dyed Fabrics: A, B = Pass   C, D = Fail

Figure 4. Quality assurance model for textile industry.

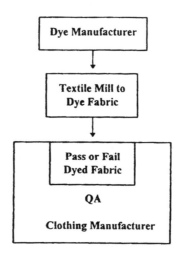

Figure 5. Practical application of quality assurance in vitro for worker safety in the textile industry.

4. Soto, R. J., and Gordon, V. C. 1991. Evaluation of an in vitro dermal irritation assay. Society of Toxicology Meeting. Seattle, WA.
5. Soto, R. J., Lake, L. K., Fell, L. A., Gordon, V. C. 1993. Mechanisms and new technology. In *In vitro toxicology,* ed. A. M. Goldberg. pp. 157–162. New York: Mary Ann Liebert.
6. Bason, M., Harvell, J., Realica, B., Gordon, V. C., and Maibach, H. I. 1992. Comparison of in vitro and human in vivo dermal irritancy data for four primary irritants. *Toxicol. In Vitro* 6:383–387.
7. Harvell, J., Bason, M., and Maibach, H. T. 1992. In vitro skin toxicity assays: Relevance to human skin. *J. Toxicol. Clin. Toxicol.* 30:359–369.
8. Harvell, J., Gordan, V. C., and Maibach, H. I. 1993. Use of Skintex™ high sensitivity assay for predictive assessments of cutaneous fatty and irritation in man. *In Vitro Toxicol.* December.
9. Khaiat, A. T., and Morgin, D. 1991. Study of 30 personal care formulations. *European Symposium,* Paris, May.
10. Kruczewski, F., and Renskers, K. 1991. Evaluation of the EXTEX method. *European Symposium,* Paris, May.

Chapter Thirty-four

VALIDATION ISSUES FOR ALTERNATIVES TESTING

Stanley B. Gross

Regulatory toxicology employs a variety of whole-animal testing procedures attempting to predict chemical hazards for humans under use conditions. Over the past several decades, alternatives to animal testing have been developed to reduce the number of animals used to meet regulatory requirements. Validation of these alternative methods is lacking. This chapter recommends conceptual approaches for the validation of various levels of testing. It attempts to define thresholds for adverse effects and differentiates between reversible alterations and irreversible disease processes.

Validation procedures should include (1) internal validation for precision, reproducibility, and reliability of methods within and between laboratories, and (2) external validation for the ability of alternatives to predict safety or toxicity in animals. External validation will include qualitative validity for yes/no decisions for the presence or absence of toxic hazard and quantitative validity to assess dose-response relationships in response to chemical exposure. The effects of using different species, routes, chemical matrices, and exposure regimens are important.

INTRODUCTION

Regulatory Toxicity Testing

The regulatory toxicologist employs a variety of animal studies in order to determine chemical safety in humans. An overview of the testing requirements, good laboratory practices, and reporting requirements has been presented by the author in a chapter published in 1981.[1] That discussion was based on U.S. Environmental Protection Agency (EPA), interagency, and international (OECD) developments at that time.

Table 1 gives a brief list of some of the testing requirements and their uses. Short-term single exposures by various routes are used for the purpose of labeling and handling requirements. Such short-term tests also evaluate irritation (eye and skin) and sensitization. Safety/risk requirements involve repeat exposures (weeks to years) for the purpose of determining no-observable-effect levels (NOELs) and target organ toxicity produced in dose-response relationships. Using safety factors or quantitative risk assessment models, these tests are used to predict safety or risk for humans, assuming humans respond in a similar manner.

Dr. Gross is a senior toxicologist/industrial hygienist in the EPA Office of Pesticides. His presentation here represents his own professional opinions and not agency policy.

Table 1. Overview of Regulatory Needs

Short-term toxicity tests	
Acute toxicity:	Oral, dermal, inhalation routes
Irritation:	Eye, skin
Sensitization:	Dermal
Safety/risk assessment (NOELs/thresholds, toxicity for)	
Subchronics:	All routes
Chronics:	All routes
Oncogenicity:	All routes
Reproduction:	All routes
Developmental:	All routes
Special (neurotoxicity, metabolism, etc.):	All routes
Variables of importance	
Routes of administration:	Including oral, dermal, inhalation
Matrix factors:	Pure compound vs. formulation/vehicles
Rate of administration:	Bolus, water or food carriers
Species:	Different metabolic transformation, kinetics, physiological handling

Note. Adapted from Gross[1] with permission. Emphasizes complexity and variability of the requirements and test systems.

The Three Rs

Proponents of the alternative tests have aimed at three uses of alternatives tests,[2,3] the "three Rs": reduction in animal use, refinement of procedures, and replacement of whole-animal procedures. Reduction in the number of animals, refinement of currently used tests and replacements for the current animal tests should only be accepted if the test can be validated as useful for the purposes sought. Validity of alternatives in predicting animal toxicity has been generally lacking. This is also true of the currently used in vivo animal testing relative to human toxicity assessment.

VALIDATION MATRIX

Figure 1 depicts relationships between different levels of testing: biochemical systems, cellular test systems and whole-animal systems.

Whole-Animal Test Systems

The body is made up of highly complex and interdependent organs and cells. The organs, tissues, and cells perform complex functions that support the viability of the whole animal and individual

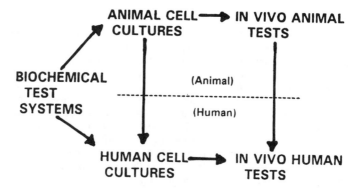

Figure 1. Validation matrix. The validation of biochemical systems progresses through cell cultures (animal or human), to animal testing, and finally to verification in humans.

cell groups. Whole animals provide interactive processes such as detoxification and excretion by the liver, storage in bone and fat, and buffering capacities of the blood, lungs, and kidneys, which are lacking in vitro cellular test systems and the biochemical alternatives.

Cellular Test Systems

Cellular test systems have provided important information on metabolism, biological control, and specialized functions at individual cell levels. Cellular systems are studied in more rigidly controlled environments of culture media but lack the extensive buffering, interactive biotransformation capacities, removal of wastes, and other biological support processes integrated within the whole animal. Cells derived from cancer cell lines over many generations often lose metabolic functions as compared with cell cultures freshly taken from animal organs. Because of this and other limitations of cellular studies, any data obtained from in vitro cell studies need to be validated in intact animals.

Biochemical Systems

Biochemical (and physical) systems recommended as alternative tests are the least physiological of the three types of test systems discussed here. Examples of biochemical systems include the CAM, TESTSKIN, EYETEX, and ARGOS diffusion method testing procedures. The biochemical systems attempt to simulate a very narrow function of the living system such as protein interaction, enzyme function, or cell membrane reactions.

Because the biochemical test systems are narrowly focused on a limited aspect of cell or animal process, it is important to assess the ability of these systems to predict each test's objectives in studies over a range of experimental variables (concentration, chemical types, etc.).

TERMINOLOGY/CONCEPTUAL FOCUS

A number of terms used in this discussion are defined here and are then discussed in the context of dose-response relationships to help refine concepts used in this chapter:

Adverse effects: These refer to changes in body or cellular function or morphology that adversely affects the ability of the body to maintain healthy function. "Health" is discussed later. The adverse effect may be a reversible alteration (see next) or an irreversible change (disease).

Alterations: Reversible changes in measurable parameters of bodily or cellular function (biochemical, physiological, behavior). These changes may or may not be relatable to a recognized disease complex and are often seen as isolated and unexplainable findings in animal studies, reversed when the exposure is terminated.

Disease: Nonreversible abnormal condition of the body or cells based on objective measures of function (biochemical, physiological, and/or morphological). The condition should be part of a recognized disease complex and not just part of an alteration.

Dose response: Changes in the condition or status of an organism with increasing internal exposure. In Figure 1, the condition of the organism goes from normal (adaptive homeostasis), through alterations, disease, and finally death.

Exposure: Herein refers to internal exposure of an organism to a chemical (see *marker of exposure*) at the cellular levels to differentiate external exposures to chemicals in the environment (water, air, food, etc.) without knowing how much of that agent may have been absorbed into the body.

Health: Herein refers to normal longevity, development, function, and processes of disease ("normal disease" discussed later) characteristic of that group of organisms (based on age, sex, species, climatological, laboratory conditions). Health and disease are usually discussed in whole animals. The concept should carry over to observations made on cells in culture, relative to growth, development, reproduction, etc.

Homeostasis: State of being in healthy balance (adaptive homeostasis) in which the organism (cells or body) is able to maintain normal health.

Markers of effect: Refers to a variety of objective measures in cells or animal tissues that can be quantitatively correlated to adverse effects to a toxic chemical within the whole organism.

For hazard assessment in humans, the marker should be assessed by noninvasive techniques such as a biochemical changes in the blood or urine or a physiological measurement (such as nerve conduction).

Markers of exposure: Refers here to measurable signs of internal dose such as blood and urinary levels of the chemical or metabolites or adducts of the chemical with receptors and that can be quantitatively related to overall internal dose. For human hazard assessment, the marker of exposure should be assessable by noninvasive techniques.

Maximum tolerable dose: Dosage level just above a threshold overriding adaptive homeostasis in which objectively measurable alterations in function (reversible) are observed. The maximum tolerable dose is intended to produce only minor alteration and not to produce irreversible effects (disease)—dosing level in a cancer testing study, for example, in which the animal's defense mechanisms (especially metabolic) are not compromised.

Threshold dose: The dose level of a chemical above which a reversible adverse effect (alteration) begins to occur and below which the organism is in adaptive homeostasis. Thresholds are seen in whole-animal and cellular systems and are often considerably higher than the experimentally chosen no-observable-effect dose levels used in experimental animal studies.

Validity: The ability of a toxicity test system (biochemical, cellular or animal) to predict the presence or absences of adverse effects in the next complex level of testing, eventually relating to health or toxicity in humans.

DOSE-RESPONSE CONSIDERATIONS

Whole Animal Systems

Figure 2 depicts a classical concept of dose response that is used here to define a number of endpoints important to toxicological assessment and validation. The figure depicts a *threshold*

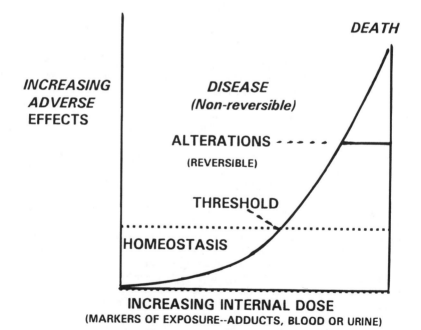

Figure 2. Dose-response relationships. As dose increases through the homeostasis range, it passes through the threshold dose to a reversible range and finally through irreversible damage. The curve applies to whole animals for acute to repeat exposures and to cell responses in culture.

dose below which any responses to a chemical exposure remains at a level which does not adversely effect the health of the organism. Below this threshold, the organism maintains a state of healthy balance (*adaptive hemeostasis*) and is able to maintain normal health. Normal *health* is characterized by normal growth and development and normal biological function based on physiology, biochemical and behavior performance, normal reproductive capability, and normal longevity and spontaneous disease incidence.

Alterations and Disease

Immediately above the threshold dose level on the response curve (Figure 2) is an area of reversible alterations that are often seen in low-dose treatment groups. Such alterations are often biochemical, psychological, or physiological changes but still can lead to normal health. These alterations have been observed in experimental studies when the chemical exposures were terminated. At the higher dose levels represented in Figure 2, the organism experiences irreversible damage or death. Disease will express itself morphologically (grossly or histopathologically), biochemically (urine, blood, tissue), or physiologically (strength or sexual function).

Cellular Test Systems

The dose-response relationships of Figure 2 also apply in concept to dose-response relationships of in vitro cellular studies. Cells survive at or below toxic thresholds to reproduce, metabolize, and maintain morphological integrity. Altered cells metabolize differently and may not reproduce or function in other normal ways. Abnormal morphological changes are seen in losses of organelles and dysplasia of nucleus and/or cytoplasm, and usually lead to death (lysis, crenation, etc.).

Biochemical/Physical Test Systems

These test systems vary considerably in process and format, and it is difficult to generalize how these systems will be related to the cellular and whole-animal studies in dose-response relationships.

VALIDATION OBJECTIVES

Validity

Validity relates to the degree to which a test system measures what it purports to measure.

Internal validity: Relates to the intra- and interlaboratory accuracy, precision, and the sensitivity of the method when used by various investigators and laboratories over time.

External validity: Relates to the ability of the testing methods (alternatives, cellular studies, and/or animal studies) to predict safety or hazard to chemical exposures in humans under use conditions.

Qualitative relationships: Qualitative results in alternatives studies relate to yes/no results relative to the presence or absence of toxicity. The use of alternatives as screens would serve this purpose; however, all screens are run at prescribed dose levels and may produce problems involving false negatives or false positives. These tests will generally involve the use of correlation techniques for validation.

Quantitative relationships: Quantitative (dose-response) relationships are used throughout acute, subchronic, and chronic tests in animals. Dose-response relationships are also an integral part of in vitro cellular testing (such as mutagenicity testing) where thresholds and dose-response levels are evident. These tests will generally involve the use of regression models that evaluate increasing effects with increasing exposures.

Proofs of External Validation?

Although there are epidemiological "proofs" for infectious epidemiology (Koch's postulates), proof in chemical epidemiology is not so straightforward. There are a number of approaches that might be useful:

Data-Bank Chemicals

It has been suggested that comparison testing be made using chemicals from an International Reference Chemical Data Bank.[4] These chemicals have been chosen to represent a variety of different types of chemicals; however, it is not clear how such data-bank studies would be used to establish validity of alternative tests for whole animals or humans.

Pharmaceuticals

Drug development requires studies in both animals and humans. Theoretically, it should be possible to use drugs studied extensively in humans as test agents in the alternative tests and to compare the dose-response findings in animals using biomarker investigations.[5]

Occupational Monitoring

Perhaps the best possible validation opportunities will derive from the validation of alternatives using studies in chemical workers or pesticide applicators. Registrants provide extensive research from animal studies that might be used to test for markers of internal exposure and markers of effects.[5] The identification of markers will need to be developed from animal studies and correlated in animal and in vitro tests.

DISCUSSION

Focus on Humans

Because different species differ between themselves and from human metabolism, kinetics and genetics, nutrition, morphology, and a host of other differences, data derived from alternative tests and whole animals studies should be validated in humans, especially if the human exposure considerations are compelling. One also needs to recognize that there are important biological differences in responses within different human populations.

Alterations, Disease, Homeostasis, and Thresholds

Animal and cellular testing procedures rarely examine the reversibility of adverse effects. Humans are not normally constantly exposed to the same environmental chemicals over extended periods of time. Humans usually have recovery periods between exposures. Therefore this discussion has noted the need to recognize reversible adverse effects.

Homeostasis, thresholds, alterations, and disease production need to be examined with respect to routes and chemicals that are related to human exposures using species that are as similar to humans as feasible. Thresholds and other aspects of the dose-response curves need to determined, rather than arbitrary uses of low-dose exposure test groups, since typical NOELs often are much lower than threshold concentration and therefore introduce unrealistically narrow margins of safety.

Spontaneous "Normal" Disease

Disease is a part of life. All organisms that live long enough eventually develop spontaneous diseases during normal life that appear to be part of normal aging, normal stress, and normal wear and tear of living. In experimental animal studies, "normal disease" (cancer, diabetes, nephropathy, etc.) incidences are represented by disease seen in the control animals. It is important to quantitatively determine if the increase of disease due to a chemical exposure is an increase or only part of normal disease variation. A variety of clinical and laboratory observations in controls and treated animals is evaluated statistically to determine if the treated animals are different from the "normal" control animals. "Normal" disease incidences in humans can be difficult to determine, especially in small population samples. Hopefully the use of exposure markers and effect markers in humans will help to overcome some of the problems of chemical hazard assessments.

Toward Validation

Alternatives validation is a goal and will probably be an ongoing process over some time. Four approaches toward validation were proposed under Validation Objectives. Several issues need to be addressed:

Mechanisms of action: Mechanisms at the biochemical and cellular level need to be verified in the whole animal, human, and cellular systems.

Markers of exposure: Markers of exposure need to be developed using various concentrations of the agent, evaluating metabolites, adducts, and the like using different routes and concentrations in order to study kinetic relationships. Although a number of markers have been discussed in the literature, the dose-response relationships to exposure have not been quantitatively established.

Markers of effect: Markers of effect (clinical chemistry alteration, morphology, physiology, etc.) can only be useful in safety assessment and exposure standard setting if these effect markers are related quantitatively to exposure (dose-response relationships).

Verification in humans: Ultimately, markers at the cellular level will need to be assessed at the whole animal level and the animal markers validated in humans using noninvasive techniques.

Practical Note

The application of these recommendations is costly and could comprise complex research projects. As a practical note, validation procedures may need to be reserved for those chemicals that serve important purposes to society and that involve widespread human exposures. Such assessments may need to be applied only to chemicals which project excessive hazards from routine toxicity and exposure assessments. Chemicals that do not appear highly toxic or have very limited exposures may not need such full validation in humans.

References

1. Gross, S. B. 1981. Regulatory guidelines for inhalation toxicity testing. In *Proceeding of the Inhalation Toxicology and Technology Symposium,* ed. B. D. J. Leong, pp. 279–294. Ann Arbor, MI: Ann Arbor Science.
2. Rowan, A. N. 1984. *Of mice, models, and men: A critical evaluation of animal research.* Albany, NY: State University of New York Press.
3. Organization for Economic Cooperation and Development. 1990. *Scientific criteria for validation of in vitro toxicity tests.* OECD Environment Monograph No. 36. OECD: Paris, France.
4. Henderson, R. R., Bechtold, W. E., Bond, J. A., and Sun, J. A. 1989. The use of biological markers in toxicology. *CRC Crit. Rev. Toxicol.* 20:65–82.
5. FRAME. 1991. Animals and alternatives in toxicology: Present status and future prospects (The Second Report of the FRAME Toxicity Committee). *Toxic Subst.* 8:403.

Chapter Thirty-five

INTRA- AND INTERLABORATORY REPRODUCIBILITY OF EPIDERM, AN IN VITRO MODEL FOR DERMAL IRRITANCY TESTING

M. Klausner, P. J. Neal, C. L. Cannon, J. Kubilus, R. D. Curren, and J. W. Harbell

An in vitro model of the human epidermis, EpiDerm, cultured from normal human epidermal keratinocytes (NHEK), was introduced by MatTek Corporation in April 1993. Using highly controlled tissue culture techniques, weekly batches of EpiDerm are produced for dermal irritancy testing, percutaneous absorption studies, and basic skin research. Histology, sterility, and the toxicological behavior are rigorously monitored on each batch. Histological evaluations show EpiDerm to be a highly differentiated skin-like structure that is very uniform within an individual batch and between batches. Over the first 13 mo of commercial production, random sterility checks at MatTek have shown no contamination and a single customer only once reported evidence of contamination. The toxicological behavior, monitored using the MTT effective time-50 assay (ET50), appears highly reproducible: the average coefficient of variation (CV) for exposure to the negative control (ultrapure water) was 6.46% and the average CV for exposure to the positive controls (1% Triton X-100 and 1% SDS) over a range of exposure times was 8.42%. Lot-to-lot MTT values for the negative control had a CV of 12.5% (n = 26 batches) and the ET50s for Triton X-100 and SDS had CVs of 13.9% and 21.1%, respectively. The average ET50 measured at MatTek for Triton X-100 was 8.63 ± 1.20 h (n = 26 batches), which compared closely to results at Microbiological Associates, Inc., which reported an average ET50 of 8.14 ± 0.79 h (n = 13 batches). Thus, EpiDerm appears to be highly reproducible both structurally and functionally and hence should be useful for toxicology and other in vitro skin-related studies.

INTRODUCTION

Reproducibility from individual sample to sample as well as from lot to lot is an extremely important characteristic of any toxicological system. For toxicological experiments to be meaningful, identical toxicological exposures should give a reproducible response (sample to sample) in the toxicological model. In addition, in order to compare the relative toxicity of compounds or materials over a long time period, clearly a reproducible (lot to lot) system that can be used in any technically proficient laboratory is required. For a cell culture based toxicological system such as EpiDerm (registered trademark of MatTek Corporation, Ashland, MA), sterility must be maintained so that bacterial or viral agents do not affect toxicological results obtained with the model.

In order to assess whether EpiDerm meets these criteria, the first 59 EpiDerm production batches (13 mo) have been monitored for sterility, histology, and toxicological behavior. The current study reports results for all batches, which were assessed using the MTT [3-(4,5-dimethyl-thiazole-2-yl)-2,5-diphenyl tetrazolium bromide] effective time-50 (ET50) protocol, and compares results of MatTek's internal quality control laboratory to those of an independent contract testing laboratory. Toxicological characterization of the remaining batches utilized the MTT effective concentration-50 assay (EC50) and results were recently reported at a Society of Toxicology meeting.[1]

MATERIALS AND METHODS

Weekly batches of MatTek's in vitro skin model, EpiDerm, are produced using highly controlled procedures. From each production batch, a 24-well kit is chosen at random for quality control testing and packaged in an identical manner to all product that is shipped for sale. This EpiDerm kit is stored for 20–22 h at 4°C (to simulate shipping conditions) and then used as follows: 1 sample is taken for histology evaluation, 2 are used for sterility testing, and the remaining 21 wells are used for end-use toxicological evaluation. For most batches, MTT EC50 assays are performed to insure sample-to-sample and lot-to-lot reproducibility. In addition, many lots have recently been characterized using the MTT ET50 assay. The MTT ET50 and other procedures are next described.

Histology

The EpiDerm samples are fixed in 10% formalin and cut from Millicell inserts using an 8-mm-diameter dermal punch and cuticle scissors. Following dehydration in a graded series of ethanol, samples are paraffin embedded, sectioned, and hematoxylin and eosin (H&E) stained. Light microscopy is performed using a Nikon Diaphot fitted with Hoffman modulation optics.

Sterility

All EpiDerm samples are monitored using phase-contrast microscopy throughout the production process to ensure that sterility is not compromised. EpiDerm is packaged under sterile conditions and shipped in hermetically sealed plastic wrapping. Two samples from the randomly chosen, packaged and stored EpiDerm kit are used for sterility control purposes. One sample is placed in antibiotic containing assay medium and the other in antibiotic-free assay medium. Both samples are returned to the incubator for 1 wk and monitored for any evidence of contamination. Recently, an additional sterility check has been instituted in which the 24-well plate filled with agarose gels (on which the EpiDerm samples are shipped) is also returned to the incubator and monitored over a 1-wk period for contamination.

Toxicological Behavior

The 21 remaining wells from the randomly chosen, packaged and stored EpiDerm kit are used to assess the toxicological reproducibility of EpiDerm. For the MTT ET50 assay, 1% solutions of two common surfactants, sodium dodecyl sulfate (SDS) and Triton X-100, along with the negative control, ultrapure water (>10 Mohm), are applied to triplicate samples of EpiDerm for time periods up to 16 h at 37°C. For the positive controls, three timed exposures of the positive controls are applied in triplicate to the apical surface (stratum corneum side) of EpiDerm for the following exposure times: SDS, 0.5, 1.0, and 3.0 h; Triton X-100, 2.0, 4.0, and 16.0 h.

The MTT ET50 protocol is described in detail in the protocol entitled MTT Effective Time-50 (ET50) Protocol, available from the authors or MatTek Corporation. Briefly, after exposure of the test materials is complete, the material is washed from the EpiDerm sample using at least 3 rinses of 0.5 ml phosphate-buffered saline (PBS). The EpiDerm samples are then loaded with 1 mg/ml MTT in Dulbecco's modified Eagle's medium (DMEM) for 3 h at room temperature. Following the MTT loading, the EpiDerm samples are again rinsed with PBS and the reduced MTT is extracted overnight using isopropyl alcohol (IPA) at room temperature in the dark. In order to minimize evaporation of the IPA, the 24-well plate containing the EpiDerm samples is placed in a plastic bag and sealed. The reduced MTT is quantified using a Molecular Devices (Menlo Park, CA) plate reader at 570 nm with a background subtract at 650 nm. Optical densities (OD) for the test materials are compared to the negative control values (ultrapure water) to determine the percent viability. The percent viability was calculated according to:

$$\text{Percent viability} = 100 \times OD(\text{test material})/OD(\text{water}) \tag{1}$$

The ET50 is then determined by interpolating between 2 exposure times that result in MTT viabilities above and below 50%. A sample dose-response curve and the interposed ET50 are shown in Figure 1.

RESULTS

Histology

Figures 2–5 shows the histology from lots 246–250, 262–266, 272–276, and 282–286, respectively. In all histology micrographs, one can see a basal cell layer with large nuclei, a spinous layer with somewhat flattened cells and fewer (smaller) nuclei, a granular layer well populated with keratohyalin granules, and a stratum corneum consisting of highly flattened, enucleated cells.

Sterility

For the 59 batches produced between April 1993 and May 1994, none of the internal MatTek sterility checks from either the antibiotic-containing or antibiotic-free media were positive. During this time period, thousands of EpiDerm cultures were shipped to over 70 customers, both domestic and international. In total, a single customer once reported evidence of contamination in a limited number of the agarose gels upon which EpiDerm is shipped.

Toxicological Behavior

Toxicological data for the first 39 EpiDerm production batches utilizing the EC50 protocol was previously presented. Table 1 presents data on 26 batches for which MTT ET50 data were also collected. Included in the table are the following:

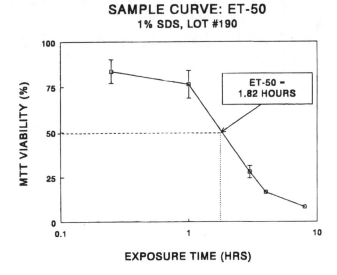

Figure 1. Sample time-response curve for 1% SDS graphically depicting the determination of the effective time 50 (ET50) value.

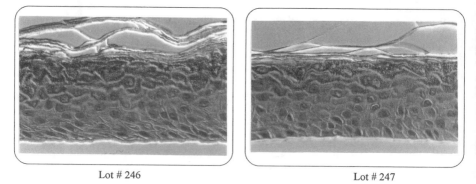

Lot # 246   Lot # 247

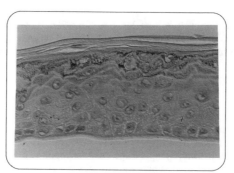

Lot # 248

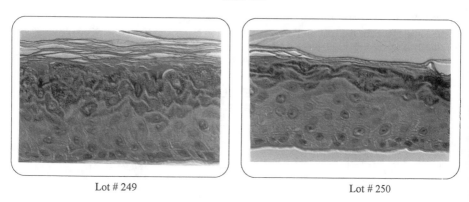

Lot # 249   Lot # 250

Figure 2. Hematoxylin and eosin stained histological cross sections of randomly chosen samples from EpiDerm lots 246–250.

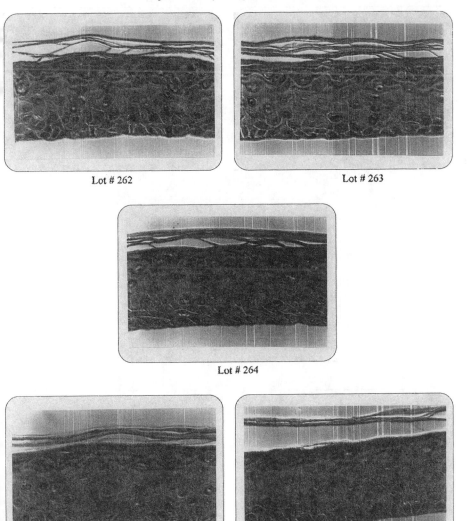

Figure 3. Hematoxylin and eosin stained histological cross sections of randomly chosen samples from EpiDerm lots 262–266.

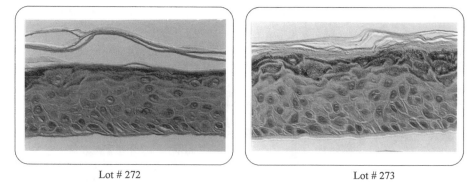

Lot # 272 Lot # 273

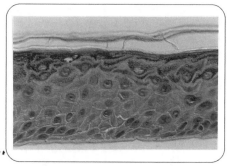

Lot # 274

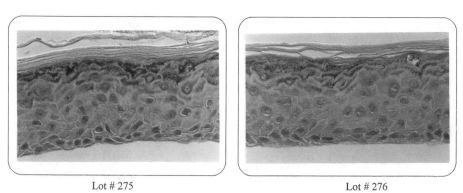

Lot # 275 Lot # 276

Figure 4. Hematoxylin and eosin stained histological cross sections of randomly chosen samples from EpiDerm lots 272–276.

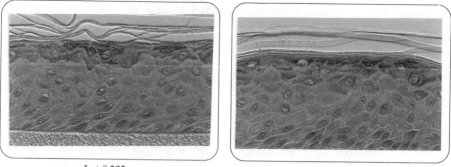

Lot # 282

Lot # 283

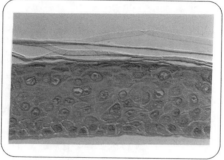

Lot # 284

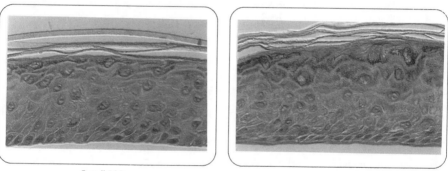

Lot # 285

Lot # 286

Figure 5. Hematoxylin and eosin stained histological cross sections of randomly chosen samples from EpiDerm lots 282–286.

Table 1. EpiDerm ET50 Results: MatTek Corporation

Sample	Ship date	Lot number	H₂O (OD)	H₂O CV (%)	EXP CV (%)	Tri-ton (h)	SDS (h)
1	06-Sep-93	270	1.509	11.76	8.52	9.62	1.76
2	13-Sep-93	271	1.114	5.22	7.12	10.29	2.16
3	27-Sep-93	273	0.854	14.48	9.81	12.41	2.23
4	04-Oct-93	274	1.425	9.48	12.75	8.95	1.05
5	18-Oct-93	276	1.126	11.92	7.24	9.92	1.82
6	25-Oct-93	277	1.281	3.28	10.38	9.45	2.41
7	01-Nov-93	278	1.234	6.43	9.78	9.79	1.53
8	08-Nov-93	279	1.266	6.23	8.87	8.87	2.01
9	15-Nov-93	280	1.469	1.40	6.98	—	1.98
10	22-Nov-93	281	1.406	13.25	10.10	8.13	1.93
11	29-Nov-93	282	1.429	8.99	12.00	8.11	1.47
12	06-Dec-93	283	1.258	6.97	5.74	9.45	2.11
13	13-Dec-93	284	1.362	1.62	8.17	—	1.78
14	27-Dec-93	286	1.300	8.77	8.25	8.29	1.99
15	10-Jan-94	288	1.541	5.88	7.63	7.86	1.70
16	17-Jan-94	289	1.302	3.04	6.15	8.81	1.93
17	24-Jan-94	290	1.619	0.48	8.32	8.03	1.64
18	31-Jan-94	291	1.478	6.03	8.54	8.19	3.06
19	07-Feb-94	292	1.538	4.37	5.15	8.27	1.87
20	04-Apr-94	298	1.615	3.38	7.88	6.66	1.40
21	11-Apr-94	299	1.642	6.42	8.54	8.11	1.44
22	18-Apr-94	500	1.367	3.94	6.04	7.85	1.43
23	25-Apr-94	501	1.353	4.54	4.92	7.98	1.96
24	02-May-94	502	1.300	13.34	7.67	7.31	1.43
25	09-May-94	503	1.475	4.04	14.01	7.28	1.69
26	16-May-94	504	1.391	2.62	8.25	7.48	1.86

Note. Key: H₂O (OD), MTT reduction negative control water; H₂O CV (%), coefficient of variation (CV) for negative control; EXP CV (%), average CV for dose-response curves of positive control; Triton X-100 (1%): ET50 values (h); SDS (1%): ET50 values (h).

1. H_2O (OD): The negative control (ultrapure water) MTT response, in optical density units (OD).
2. H_2O CV (%): The coefficient of variation (CV) for the negative control.
3. EXP CV (%): The average of the CVs for the SDS and Triton X-100 dosing experiments, 3 doses for each compound, $n = 3$.
4. Triton (%): The ET50 value determined for Triton X-100 using 2-h, 4-h, 16-h, and 24-h exposures, $n = 3$.
5. SDS (%): The ET50 value determined for SDS using 0.5-h, 1-h, and 3-h exposures, $n = 3$.

These data are presented graphically in Figure 6 and averages are given in Table 2. ET50 values for 1% Triton X-100 determined at Microbiological Associates are shown in Figure 7 and data are given in Table 3.

DISCUSSION

Using strict quality control procedures, rather good reproducibility has been observed over the first 59 production batches. An advantage of the EpiDerm system is that the skin is cultured using completely defined media, thus avoiding the use of serum, which can often introduce inconsistencies in a cell culture system due to its variable nature.

For the EpiDerm lots here reported upon, the CV for the negative control and the entire dosing experiments with the 2 positive controls averaged 6.46% and 8.42%, respectively; that is, well to well, an EpiDerm kit is highly reproducible for a biological system. The lot-to-lot consistency of EpiDerm is best illustrated by the reproducible histology (Figures 2–5) and the low variability of the negative control MTT value (CV = 12.5%, $n = 26$ batches); that is, the EpiDerm product from the vantage point of the number and level of actively metabolizing cells is highly reproducible

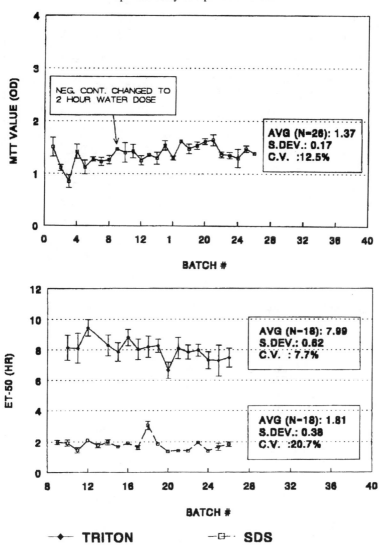

Figure 6. Results of MTT assay showing (top) MTT values (OD at 570–650 nm) following exposure of EpiDerm to the negative control (ultrapure water) and (bottom) interpolated ET50 values (h) following exposure to 1% Triton X-100 or 1% SDS for various times.

Table 2. EpiDerm ET50 Averages: MatTek Corporation

	H₂O (OD)	H₂O CV (%)	EXP CV (%)	Triton (h)	SDS (h)
Average (*n* = 26)	1.37	6.46	8.42	8.63	1.83
SD	0.17			1.20	0.39
CV (%)	12.50			13.90	21.10

Note. Key: H₂O (OD): optical density (OD) for negative control, MTT assay; H₂O CV (%): average coefficient of variation (CV) for negative control; EXP CV (%): average CV for dose response curves of positive controls; Triton X-100 (1%): ET50 values (h); SDS (1%): ET50 values (h).

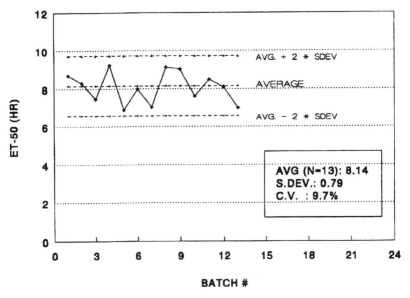

Figure 7. MTT ET50 assay results for 1% Triton X-100 at Microbiological Associates.

Table 3. EpiDerm ET50 Values for Triton X-100:
Microbiological Associates

Sample	Lot number	ET50 (h)
1	256	8.83
2	266	8.30
3	267	7.71
4	269	9.29
5	272	7.07
6	275	8.25
7	276	7.10
8	285	8.97
9	286	9.09
10	287	7.65
11	290	8.53
12	501	8.08
13	502	7.00
Average (h)	8.14	
SD ($n = 13$)	0.79	
CV (%)	9.72	

over numerous production batches. Regarding the toxicological behavior of positive control compounds such as SDS and Triton, the CVs for the computed ET50 values are in the range of 10–20%. Some variability was introduced prior to lot 280 since at this point negative control exposures of 2 h were begun instead of the previously used 16-h exposure. In addition, interlaboratory reproducibility was rather good: For Triton X-100, MatTek had an average ET50 of 8.63 ± 1.2 h ($n = 26$ lots) compared with Microbiological Associates whose average ET50 was 8.14 ± 0.79 h ($n = 13$ lots). In both laboratories, the scatter of the ET50 results was below 15%.

CONCLUSIONS

The histology of EpiDerm cultures has been shown to be consistent and reproducible over the first 13 mo of production.

Over the first 59 EpiDerm production batches (13 mo), samples retained at MatTek in antibiotic-containing and antibiotic-free assay media have not once shown signs of contamination. Over this same time period, a single customer once reported evidence of contamination in a limited number of the agarose gels upon which EpiDerm is shipped.

EpiDerm's toxicological behavior has been highly reproducible within individual EpiDerm kits (well to well); CVs for the negative and positive controls have averaged 6.46% and 8.46%, respectively, for the 26 batches here reported upon.

EpiDerm's toxicological behavior using the MTT ET50 assay has been highly repeatable over a significant number of production batches ($n = 26$); the CV for the negative control MTT response has been 12.5% and for the positive controls 13.9% and 21.1% for Triton X-100 and SDS, respectively. Note that some variability was introduced due to a change in the negative control dosing.

Interlaboratory reproducibility of EpiDerm's toxicological behavior correlates rather nicely. MTT ET50 results for Triton X-100 averaged 8.63 ± 1.2 ($n = 26$ batches) and 8.14 ± 0.79 ($n = 13$ batches) for the MatTek and Microbiological Associates toxicology laboratories, respectively.

REFERENCE

1. Harbell, J. W., Southee, J. A., Klausner, M., Neal, P. J., Kubilus, J., and Cannon, C. L. 1994. Inter- and intralaboratory reproducibility of a 3-dimensional human EpiDerm model-EpiDerm™. Toxicologist, 14: abstr. 350.

Chapter Thirty-six

PRIMARY HUMAN HEPATOCYTES AS AN IN VITRO TOXICOLOGY SYSTEM

Albert P. Li, Dale J. Beck, Linda J. Loretz, Lilly Xu,
Asenath Rasmussen, Jill C. Merrill,
and Donald L. Kaminski

Human cells and tissues, especially primary isolates, can serve as experimental systems useful for understanding human metabolism, genetics, and biochemical pathways. It is our premise that information gained from these human in vitro systems used together with data generated from laboratory animals should improve the accuracy of human risk assessment.

The liver is both a major organ for xenobiotic metabolism and a common target organ of toxic chemicals. Human hepatocytes are, therefore, a relevant toxicological system. In our laboratory, we have developed a consistent source of human liver surgical specimens for research, and a highly reproducible procedure for isolating viable human hepatocytes. These freshly dissected tissues, isolated with minimal ischemic time, consistently yield hepatocytes with high (over 80%) viability. Using these cells, we have developed assays for drug metabolism and multiple toxicological endpoints including cytotoxicity, P-450 induction, protein and RNA synthesis, and peroxisome proliferation.

Our results using specific environmental and industrial toxicants show that data obtained from human hepatocytes are useful (1) in predicting human drug metabolic fate and hepatotoxicity, (2) in the selection of an appropriate animal species for pharmacological and toxicological evaluation, and (3) as a tool for the mechanistic evaluation of toxicity.

INTRODUCTION

Accurately predicting human toxicity based on data obtained using experimental systems may be one of the most challenging goals in toxicology. In classical toxicology, these experimental systems are whole-animal systems involving several mammalian species. More recently, mechanistically based toxicity assays are being developed that use tools in cell and molecular biology. It is now a common belief that with a thorough understanding of the mode of action of a toxicant, one can more accurately predict its human toxicity at physiologically relevant doses and exposure regiments.

In vitro toxicological systems allow such mechanistic evaluation of toxicant actions. Using these in vitro systems, experimental conditions can be readily controlled. Studies can be designed that evaluate multiple variables without being as cost-prohibitive as studies involving whole animals. In addition, one can use experimental systems of human origin, so that the interactions of toxins with human biochemical and genetic elements can be directly studied.

In our laboratory, we concentrate our research in toxicology using primary human hepatocytes. Hepatocytes have long been believed to be a relevant toxicological system, as the liver is the major organ for xenobiotic metabolism and often the target organ for drug and industrial chemical toxicity. Species-specific variation in hepatic metabolism is believed to be a major determinant of species-specific difference in response to toxicants. A major drawback with human hepatocytes is the availability of human livers for research.

Because of the close working relationship between clinicians and researchers in our institute, we are able, with full Institutional Review Board approval, to routinely obtain human surgical wastes for research. We have developed a highly reproducible method for the isolation and culturing of human hepatocytes from liver fragments. We have applied human hepatocytes in various disciplines of research including drug metabolism,[1,2] toxicology,[3] gene therapy,[4] and artificial liver.[5] We report here an overview of the application of human hepatocytes in toxicology.

MATERIALS AND METHODS

Source of Livers for Hepatocyte Isolation

Rat livers were obtained from adult male Fischer 344 rats (8–12 wk; Charles River, Portage, MI), which were individually housed in stainless steel wire-mesh cages and exposed to a 12-h light/dark cycle. Purina certified rat chow 5002 and water were provided ad libitum. Human hepatocytes were isolated from surgical wastes obtained from patients undergoing liver surgery. The use of human materials for research was in compliance with legal and ethical considerations and was approved by the Human Tissue Use Committee, St. Louis University Medical School.

Hepatocyte Isolation and Culture

Hepatocytes were isolated using the biopsy procedure of Green et al.[6] with some modifications.[7–9] The procedure involves a two-step collagenase (0.5% w/v, type I) perfusion technique. The isolated cell population has over 80% viability as assessed by trypan blue exclusion. Rat livers were removed from the animals and used immediately (within 1 h). Human liver samples were used within 4 h of surgical removal. Following isolation, the hepatocytes were cultured in 6-well tissue culture plates (well diameter 35 mm, Costar, Cambridge, MA) precoated with type I rat tail collagen (Kletzien et al.[10]). Cells were plated at a density of approximately 1×10^6 trypan-blue-excluding cells per well, in 2 ml of Waymouth 752/L medium supplemented with 11.2 mg/L alanine, 12.8 mg/L serine, 24 mg/L asparagine, 2 mg/L fatty acid poor bovine serum albumin, 0.168 mg/L aminolevulinic acid, 5 mg/L oleic acid, 5 mg/L d,l-tocopherol, 0.393 mg/L dexamethasone, 7.9 mg/L d-thyroxine, 0.03 mg/L glucagon, 20 U/L insulin, and 84 mg/L gentamicin (Green et al., 1981[6]), and incubated at 37°C with 5% CO_2/95% air at high humidity. After a 2-h attachment period, the plating medium was removed, the attached cells were washed twice with prewarmed phosphate buffered saline (PBS) to remove nonadherant cells, and fresh medium was replenished.

P-450 Induction

P-450 mixed-function oxidase induction (MFO) was studied by measuring 7-ethoxycoumarin O-deethylase (ECOD) activity based on the method of Edwards et al.[11] This method measures the dealkylation of 7-ethoxycoumarin (7-EC) to 7-hydroxycoumarin (7-HC). Following a 24-h culture period, hepatocytes were treated with hexabromobiphenyl (HBB) or solvent control (dimethyl sulfoxide, DMSO). The final HBB concentration ranged from 1×10^{-9} to 1×10^{-5} M, with the final DMSO concentration of 1% (v/v) in all cases including the DMSO control. Cells were exposed to HBB for 24–96 h before they were used for the measurement of ECOD activity. After the appropriate exposure time, the medium was removed and cells were washed twice with PBS. Briefly, the hepatocytes were incubated with PBS containing 100 μM 7-EC for 90 min. Cells were then detached from the culture plate by scraping with a rubber policeman. Detached cells and supernatant were removed and sonicated to release the intracellular metabolites. The sulfate and glucuronide esters of 7-HC were deconjugated by incubation with crude betaglucuronidase. The presence of 7-HC was determined by fluorescence following extraction into diethyl ether and back extraction into 0.2 M glycine/NaOH buffer at pH 10.4. Pure 7-HC was used as a standard, and after extraction, to correct for recovery. Protein concentration of the homogenate was determined using the Pierce adaptation of the Bradford method[12] using bovine serum albumin (fraction V) as standard. Each ECOD measurement was determined using triplicate plates. The statistical significance of the data was analyzed using a one-sided Dunnett's t-test using a significant probability level (p) of <.05. HBB was obtained from the National Toxicology Program, Research Triangle Park, NC. All other chemicals were obtained from Sigma Chemical Co. (St. Louis, MO) unless otherwise indicated.

Induction of Peroxisomal Enzymes

Hepatocyte cultures were isolated and plated in culture medium. After a 2-h attachment period, the plating medium was removed, and the attached cells were washed twice with prewarmed (37°C) phosphate-buffered saline (PBS) to remove nonadherant cells prior to the addition of fresh medium. After another 24 h of incubation, fresh media containing the test compounds were added. The test compounds were dissolved in DMSO and added to the medium. The final concentration of DMSO was 1% (v/v). After a 48-h incubation period the test compounds were removed and the cells were washed twice with PBS. Cells were stored attached to the tissue culture dishes at −70°C prior to analysis. Storage time did not exceed 14 d. Peroxisome beta-oxidation activity was determined by assaying for cyanide-insensitive palmitoyl coenzyme A (CoA) oxidation activity based on the procedure of Small et al.[13] The frozen cells were harvested by scraping with a rubber policeman in 1 ml of ice-cold KCl/Tris-HCl buffer (0.154 M/50 mM at pH 7.4). The scraped cells were further sonicated for 20 s to form a homogenate. Protein concentration of the homogenate was determined using the Pierce adaptation of the Bradford method.[12] Palmitoyl CoA oxidase activity was expressed as nanomoles per minute per milligram protein. The statistical significance of the data was determined using Student's t-test. Clofibrate was obtained from Sigma Chemical Co. (St. Louis, MO). Di(2-ethylhexyl) phthalate (DEHP) was obtained from the National Toxicology Program. Lactofen was synthesized in Monsanto Company.

Drug Metabolism

[14]C-labeled SC-42867 and SC-51089 (specific activity 11.3 mCi/mmol and 2.0 mCi/mmol) were studied in rat and human hepatocytes. Methods and details of this study have been previously reported.[2]

Uridine Incorporation

Incorporation of [3H]uridine was used to monitor the effect of a test compound and its metabolites on protein synthesis in hepatocyte cultures. Human and rat primary hepatocytes were isolated and cultured following the method already outlined. Cultures were grown on six-well tissue culture plates on a substrate of rat tail collagen in the presence of Waymouth 752/1 medium (supplemented) with [3H]uridine (0.5μCi/mL) and containing a test compound or a structural analog. Cells were harvested and processed for scintillation counting at 24 h. [3H]Uridine incorporation was measured as radioactivity associated with trichloroacetic acid (10%, v/v) precipitated materials.

RESULTS

Yield and Viability of Hepatocytes Isolated from Human Liver Surgical Samples

Over the past 5 yr, we have isolated human hepatocytes from over 100 liver surgical specimens in our laboratory. During this time we have established a highly reproducible method for the isolation and culture of primary human hepatocytes. Viability is routinely at or above 80%, with average yields of approximately 50–100 million cells per 10–15 grams of liver. We have found that samples weighing less than 10 g are usually more difficult to perfuse and have greater variability in the number of hepatocytes obtained (Table 1).

Drug Metabolism Comparing Two Pharmaceutical Candidates Using Rat and Human Hepatocytes

In collaboration with the laboratory of Dr. Yves Vanderberghe, we have studied the metabolic fate of two structurally similar compounds (SC-42867 and SC-51089) following incubation with rat and human hepatocytes.[2] Human hepatocytes were found to be active in aromatic hydroxylation, N-dealkylation, N-oxidation, glucuronidation, and sulfation. For SC-42867, similar metabolites were found in human and rat hepatocyte incubates. In the case of SC-51089, however, while N-oxidation was observed for both rat and human, many other substantial interspecific differences were observed. Two pathways, N-dealkylation and deacylation, were observed only in rat hepatocytes, while aromatic hydroxylation and direct glucuronidation of SC-51089 were observed only in human hepatocytes (Figure 1).

Toxicity of a Pharmaceutical Candidate in Rat and Human Hepatocytes

Primary human hepatocyte cultures may prove to be important tools enabling accurate evaluation of potential human hepatotoxins. A pharmaceutical (compound X) that demonstrated no apparent hepatotoxic consequences when tested on several species in vivo was found to show human hepatotoxicity during clinical trials. Following this unexpected result, uridine incorporation was measured using rat and human primary hepatocyte cultures exposed to compound X. We found uridine incorporation to be substantially inhibited in human hepatocytes, but not in rat hepatocytes, following treatment with compound X (Figure 2).

P-450 Induction by Polybrominated Biphenyls in Rat and Human Hepatocytes

Polybrominated biphenyls (PBB) are environmental pollutants with known human exposure.[14] They are also a known inducer of cytochrome P-450 MFO in laboratory animals. Their P-450-inducing effects in human are not yet established. Using ECOD as an endpoint for P-450 MFO activity, we evaluated the effects of PBB in rat and human hepatocytes. PBB was found to be a potent P-450 inducer in rat hepatocytes, with significant induction observed at 10^{-8} M and higher concentrations. In human hepatocytes, significant induction was observed at 10^{-6} M and 10^{-5} M for one individual, and only at 10^{-5} M for another. Our results, therefore, suggest that humans are less sensitive than rats towards the P-450-inducing effect of PBB (Figure 3).

Table 1. Examples of Yield and Viability of Hepatocytes Isolated from Human Liver Surgical Waste Samples Using the Optimized Collagenase Perfusion Procedure

Donor		Weight (g) of perfused sample	Viability (% dye exclusion)	Yield of dye-excluding cells ($\times 10^6$)
Age (yr)	Gender			
34	M	13	86	69
83	M	19	90	78
33	M	5	86	48
73	M	8	92	13
66	M	18	85	53
64	F	42	90	10
60	F	29	97	600
49	F	13	94	88
49	F	14	81	56
72	F	13	94	110

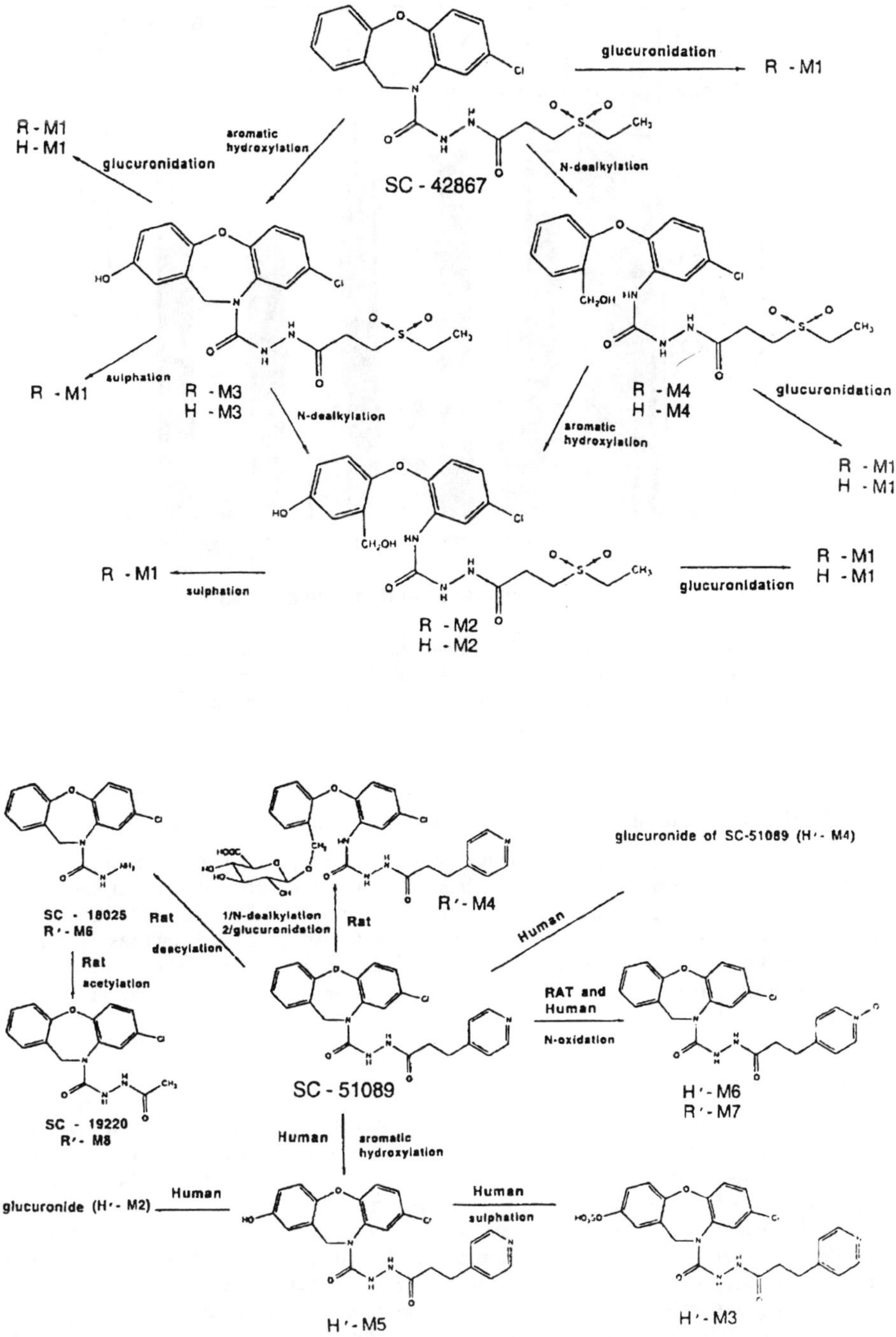

Figure 1. Metabolic pathways of (top) SC-42867 and (bottom) SC-51089 as determined following incubation of the compounds with human and rat hepatocytes. H designates human metabolites and R designates rat metabolites. Adapted from Lee et al.[2] with permission.

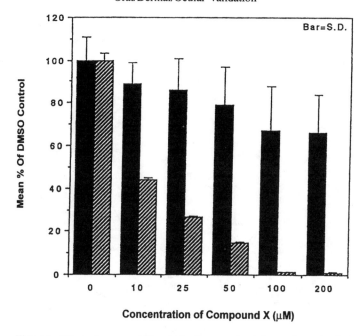

Figure 2. Effects of compound X on uridine incorporation in human (cross-hatched bars) and rat (black bars) hepatocytes. Compound X was a pharmaceutical candidate found to be hepatotoxic during human clinical trials, while no apparent hepatotoxicity was found in rats in the preclinical toxicological studies.

Induction of Peroxisomal Proliferation in Rat and Human Hepatocytes

Peroxisome proliferators—agents that induce peroxisomal enzymes and the number of peroxisomes—are known hepatocarcinogens in rodents.[15] As a step toward furthering our knowledge on the toxicity of these agents in humans, we compared the response of rat and human hepatocytes to several known proliferators: the hypolipidemic clofibrate, the plasticizer diethyl hexyl phthalate (DEHP), and the herbicide lactofen. While significant induction was observed in rat hepatocytes for these known inducers, no significant induction was observed in human hepatocytes (Tables 2 and 3).

DISCUSSION

The in vitro experimental liver systems available include cell-free preparations such as postmitochondrial supernatant and purified microsomes as well as liver slices and primary hepatocytes cultured as suspensions, or as attached cultures. For the evaluation of drug metabolism, useful information can be obtained with all the previously mentioned systems. For toxicity studies, however, we believe that the attached cultures are the most useful, due to the fact that the viability of the hepatocytes does not deteriorate as in slices or suspension cultures. This enhanced degree of viability is especially important when enzyme induction is the toxicity endpoint, as it usually requires several days for enzyme induction to occur. It is for this reason that we use attached hepatocytes when toxicity endpoints are measured in our laboratory. We believe that primary hepatocytes maintained as attached cultures are an extremely powerful tool in toxicology, since drug metabolism, toxicity, molecular and cell biology, and mechanistically relevant biochemistry can be studied in the same system.

Progress in the use of human hepatocytes in toxicology has been hampered because of the difficulty in obtaining human livers for research. We painstakingly cultivate a collaborative

Rat Hepatocytes

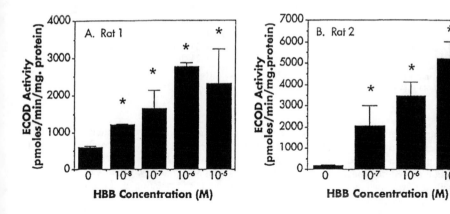

Human Hepatocytes

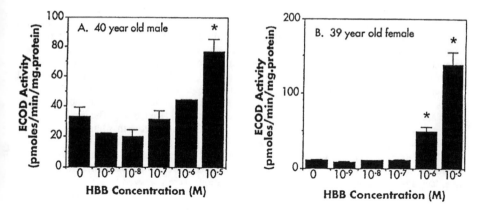

Figure 3. Polybrominated biphenyl (PBB) induction of P-450 mixed-function oxygenase (MFO) in human and rat hepatocytes. P-450 MFO was measured as 7-ethoxycoumarin O-deethylase (ECOD) activity. Asterisks represent data that were found to be statistically different ($p < .05$) from uninduced controls. Error bars represent standard errors of the mean.

Table 2. Effect of Peroxisome Proliferators on Palmitoyl CoA Oxidase Activity in Cultured Rat Hepatocytes

Treatment	Palmitoyl CoA oxidase activity (nmol/min/mg protein)[a]
DMSO control	3.72 ± 0.66
Clofibrate (1 mM)	7.18 ± 0.83[b]
DEHP (1 mM)	6.23 ± 0.02[b]
Lactofen (0.1 mM)	7.01 ± 0.32[b]

[a] Mean values for DMSO control and clofibrate calculated from four replicates. DEHP and lactofen values were calculated from two replicates.

[b] Values that are significantly different from control values ($p < .01$).

Table 3. Effect of Peroxisome Proliferators on Palmitoyl CoA Oxidase Activity
in Cultured Human Hepatocytes

Treatment	Palmitoyl CoA oxidase activity (nmol/min/mg protein)[a]
DMSO control	0.22 ± 0.015
Clofibrate (1 mM)	0.25 ± 0.010
DEHP (1 mM)	0.27 ± 0.005
Lactofen (0.1 mM)	0.24 ± 0.035

Note. Human hepatocytes were isolated from a 35-yr-old, female, Caucasian donor.
[a] All mean values calculated from two replicates.

environment between clinicians, especially surgeons, and laboratory researchers so surgical specimens are routinely sent to our institute for research. Recently we were able to sustain a supply of human liver specimens at the frequency of approximately one per week. Our hepatocyte isolation procedures consistently yield hepatocytes with high viability. Because of our extensive experience, we now have a virtually 100% success rate in the isolation of viable human hepatocytes from surgical specimens.

Our results illustrate the usefulness of cultured human hepatocytes in several important areas of toxicology, as follows.

Selection of Animal Species for Human Drug Metabolism and Toxicity Evaluation

While we fully appreciate the multiple factors involved in species–species differences in chemical toxicity, we believe that hepatic drug metabolism plays a key role and should be one of the primary factors to be considered in the selection of an appropriate animal model. The classical approach has been to select several commonly used animal species, (usually rat, mouse, and dog) for toxicological studies. We believe that human hepatocytes can be used as a tool to aid in evaluating which animal species would be the most relevant models for human toxicity. One approach might be to incubate the chemical to be studied with hepatocytes from multiple animal species, including human, and compare the resulting kinetics parameters and metabolite profiles. The animal species yielding results most similar to human would therefore be more likely to be an appropriate model for the human for pharmacokinetics and toxicology. The results obtained in this way with the compounds SC-42867 and SC-51089 demonstrate that human hepatocytes are competent in both phase I oxidation and phase II conjugation. Comparison of metabolic profiles of these chemicals using rat and human hepatocytes suggests that the rat is a good model of human for SC-42867 but not for SC-51089. For SC-51089, pathways unique to rat (e.g., acylation) and human (e.g., direct glucuronidation) were observed.[2]

Evaluation of Human Hepatotoxicity for Chemical Apparently Nonhepatotoxic in Laboratory Animals

It is not uncommon for a pharmaceutical candidate to be found hepatotoxic in humans during clinical trials, although no such hepatotoxicity was observed in the preclinical toxicology studies with laboratory animals. This has always been a difficult phenomenon to explain, and the results could have a significant impact on the pharmaceutical development process. We propose that human hepatocyte cultures can be used as a tool to evaluate the mechanism and potential health significance of the observed hepatotoxicity, and, additionally, for the screening of structural analogs for a nonhepatotoxic replacement. Our results with compound X, a hepatotoxic pharmaceutical candidate in the human, showed that the compound inhibited uridine incorporation in human hepatocytes but not in rat hepatocytes. These results were consistent with the in vivo findings and therefore pave the way for subsequent mechanistic studies (e.g., inhibition of RNA polymerase as the potential mechanism of action) and provide a screening assay for structural analogs of X available as potential nonhepatotoxic replacements.

Evaluation of Human Toxicity for "Nongenotoxic" Animal Carcinogens

Some potent animal carcinogens have no apparent genotoxic effects as measured using conventional genotoxicity assays. A majority of such agents, termed nongenotoxic carcinogens, are found to be enzyme inducers. For instance, halogenated aromatic hydrocarbons such as dioxins, polychorinated biphenyls, and PBB are potent P-450 inducers; clofibrate and structural analogs are inducers of peroxisomal proliferation. As a first step toward understanding the carcinogenic potential of these agents in human, we evaluated the enzyme induction effects in rat and human hepatocytes. Using PBB and a variety of rodent peroxisomal inducers, we found human hepatocytes to be less responsive than rat hepatocytes to the enzyme induction effects. Our results with PBB—that rat hepatocytes were highly inducible while human hepatocytes were less sensitive to induction—are consistent with in vivo data observed in rats,[16] and the limited available information from human in vivo.[17] Our results with peroxisome proliferators are also consistent with the known rodent–primate differences in response to these agents.[18,19] While such results do not have a direct link with toxicity, they illustrate a difference between human and rat hepatocytes that can be further studied, and hopefully will lead to a better understanding of the human carcinogenicity of these agents.

Besides the previously mentioned applications in toxicology, we are also currently conducting research in the use of human hepatocytes in drug interaction studies. We believe that the human hepatocyte culture system will be proven to be an essential experimental system in the evaluation of human toxicity of chemical toxicants, and will definitely aid the development of nonhepatotoxic human drugs.

References

1. Kane, R. E., Tector, J., Brems, J. J., Li, A. P., and Kaminski, D. 1991. Sulfation and glucuronidation of acetaminophen by cultured hepatocytes reproducing in vivo sex-differences in conjugation on Matrigel and Type 1 collagen. *In Vitro Cell. Dev. Biol.* 27A:953–960.
2. Lee, K., Vandenberghe, Y., Herin, M., Cavalier, R., Beck, D., Li, A., Verbekes, N., Lesne, M., and Roba, J. 1994. Comparative metabolism of SC-42867 and SC-51089, two PGE$_2$ antagonists, in rat and human hepatocyte cultures. *Xenobiotica* 24:25–36.
3. Li, A. P. 1994. Primary hepatocyte culture as an in vitro toxicological system. In *In vitro toxicology,* ed. S. Gad, New York: Raven Press. pp. 195–220.
4. Li, A. P., Myers, C. A., Roque, M. A., and Kaminski, D. L. 1991. Epidermal growth factor induction of DNA synthesis in primary cultures of human hepatocytes. *In Vitro Cell Dev. Biol.* 27A:831–833.
6. Green, C. E., Segall, H. J., and Byard, J. L. 1981. Metabolism, cytotoxicity, and genotoxicity of the pyrrolizidine alkaloid senecionine in primary cultures of rat hepatocytes. *Toxicol. Appl. Pharmacol.* 60:176–185.
7. Loretz, L. J., Li, A. P., Flye, M. W., and Wilson, A. G. E. 1989. Optimization of cryopreservation procedures for rat and human hepatocytes. *Xenobiotica* 19:489–498.
8. Loretz, L. J., Wilson, A. G. E., and Li, A. P. 1988. Promutagen activation by freshly isolated cryopreserved rat hepatocytes. *Environ. Mol. Mutagen.* 12:335–341.
9. Li, A. P., Roque, M. A., Beck, D. J., and Kaminski, D. L. 1992. Isolation and culturing of hepatocytes from human livers. *J. Tissue Culture Methods* 14:139–146.
10. Kletzien, R. F., Pariza, M. W., Becker, J. E., Potter, V. R., and Butcher, F. R. 1976. Induction of amine and transport in primary cultures of adult rat liver parenchymal cells by insulin. *J. Biol. Chem.* 251:3014–3020.
11. Edwards, A. M., Glistak, M. L., Lucas, C. M., and Wilson, P. A. 1984. 7-Ethoxycoumarin deethylase activity as a convenient measure of liver drug metabolizing enzymes: Regulation in cultured rat hepatocytes. *Biochem. Pharmacol.* 33:1537–1546.
12. Bradford, M. M. 1976. A rapid and sensitive method for the quantitation of microgram quantities of protein utilizing the principle of protein–dye binding. *Anal. Biochem.* 72:248–254.
13. Small, G. M., Burdett, K., and Connock, K. J. 1985. A sensitive spectrophotometric assay for peroxisomal acyl-CoA oxidase. *Biochem. J.* 227:205–210.
14. Carter, L. 1976. Michigan PBB incident. Chemical mix-up leads to disaster. *Science* 192:240–243.
15. Cohen, A. J., and Grasso, P. 1981. Review of the hepatic response to hypolipidemic drugs in rodents and assessment of its toxicological significance to man. *Food Cosmet. Toxicol.* 19:585–605.
16. Dent, J. G., Netter, K. J., and Gibson, J. E. 1976. The induction of hepatic microsomal metabolism in rats following acute administration of a mixture of polybrominated biphenyls. *Toxicol. Appl. Pharmacol.* 38:237–249.

17. Lambert, G. H., Humphrey, H., and Schoeller, D. 1987. The effects of polybrominated biphenyls (PBB) on the human cytochrome P-450 system (P450). *Pediatr. Res.* 21:A258.
18. Elcombe, C. R., and Mitchell, A. M. 1986. Peroxisome proliferation due to di(2-ethylhexyl)phthalate (DEHP): Species differences and possible mechanisms. *Environ. Health Perspect.* 70:211–219.
19. Foxworthy, P. S., and Eacho, P. I. 1986. Conditions influencing the induction of peroxisomal beta-oxidation in cultured rat hepatocytes. *Toxicol. Lett.* 30:189–196.

Chapter Thirty-seven

REVIEW OF THE UP-AND-DOWN METHOD FOR ACUTE TOXICITY DETERMINATION

Robert L. Lipnick, Joseph A. Cotruvo, Richard N. Hill,

Robert D. Bruce, Katherine A. Stitzel, Arthur P. Walker,

Ih Chu, Michael J. Goddard, Larry M. Segal,

Janet A. Springer, and Roy C. Myers

The up-and-down procedure (UDP), fixed-dose procedure (FDP), and conventional LD50 tests were compared to determine their consistency in chemical hazard classification for acute oral toxicity according to the European Economic Community (EEC) system. For 23 of 25 cases, there was consistent classification between the UDP versus the conventional LD50 results; 16 of 20 cases for the FDP versus the conventional LD50; and 7 of 10 cases for the UDP versus the FDP. The UDP needed only 6–10 animals of one sex (fewer than either the LD50 or FDP). Available literature indicates that the sexes are usually comparable in their acute toxicity responses and that females are often more sensitive than males when acute toxicity differences exist, thus obviating the need for both sexes to be tested in most cases. Unlike the FDP, the UDP also estimates an LD50, thus providing data directly applicable to all current hazard classification systems based upon acute oral toxicity.

INTRODUCTION

Increasing interest is being generated in reducing animal usage in toxicity testing. With respect to acute oral toxicity testing, several experimental methods have been described in the literature to obtain quantitative toxicity values that can be used for evaluating the acute hazards of chemicals and for providing hazard classifications. The most commonly employed procedure for acute toxicity quantitation has been the estimation of the LD50, such as that described in the OECD Test Guidelines.[1] An alternative to the conventional acute oral toxicity test, the fixed-dose procedure (FDP), was recently adopted by OECD as a means of somewhat reducing the number of animals in the test and avoiding lethality as an endpoint.[2] In addition, the results of another fixed-dose test procedure called the acute-toxic-class method have now been published,[3,4] and following the results of an international validation study,[5] are now under review. This method has also been adopted by OECD.[6] This present undertaking reviews available literature on the application of the up-and-down acute toxicity testing procedure (UDP) for acute toxicity testing

The authors dedicate this chapter to the memory of Dr. Robert D. Bruce (1931–1995), who adapted the up-and-down method to acute toxicity testing and actively promoted its use.

Adapted from ref. 5.

and presents existing studies where the results of the UDP could be compared with those from the conventional OECD acute toxicity method and the FDP.

METHODOLOGY

Data on 35 substances were gathered from four sources in the published literature as shown in Table 1. A review was performed on these data to assess the relationship of the up-and-down procedure (UDP) and two, the conventional LD50 and the FDP.[7] This presentation summarizes the results from that review. The UDP for acute rat oral toxicity testing is based upon the protocol proposed by Bruce.[8,9]

Data for 20 substances tested both by the conventional LD50 (1981/1987 OECD Test Guide-

Table 1. Test Materials Included in This Review

Code	Material
van den Heuvel et al. (1990)[10] and *Yam et al. (1991)[12]	
A*	Nicotine
B*	Na pentachlorophenate
C	Ferrocene
D	2-Chloroethyl alcohol
E*	Sodium arsenite
F	Phenyl mercury acetate
G*	p-Dichlorobenzene
H*	Fentin hydroxide
J*	Acetanilide
K	Quercetin dihydrate
L*	Tetrachlorvinphos
M*	Piperidine
N*	Mercuric chloride
P	1-Phenyl-2-thiourea
R*	4-Aminophenol
T	Naphthalene
U	Acetonitrile
W	Aldicarb (10%)
X	Resorcinol
Y	Dimethyl formamide
Bruce (1987)[13]	
1	Ingredient
2	Laundry detergent
3	Ingredient
4	Laundry detergent
5	Laundry detergent
6	Shampoo
7	Flavor
8	Caffeine
9	Potassium hydroxide
10	Dishwashing detergent
Bonnyns et al. (1990)[14]	
I	Barium acetate
II	Barbital
III	Coumarin
IV	Allyl heptanoate
V	Diquat

Note. Materials A–Y were tested by van den Heuvel et al[10] (conventional method), and those marked by an asterik were also tested by Yam et al.[12] (up-and-down method). Tests of materials 1–10 were reported by Bruce.[13] Tests of materials I–V were reported by Bonnyns et al.[14] From Lipnick et al.[7]

lines) and the FDP (see their Annex 1) were obtained from the study by van den Heuvel et al.[10] The conventional tests were performed in a single laboratory using both male and female Sprague-Dawley rats. The FDP tests were performed in 31 different laboratories using rats of both sexes with the choice of strain of rat left to the testing laboratory. Van den Heuvel et al.,[10] as well as the original study reports for the conventional tests were consulted to perform the analyses. Only conventional method test results for females have been included here for the sake of comparability with the UDP results, although both sexes were tested in the original van den Heuvel study. LD50 results for females for three of the substances were not present in the original van den Heuvel paper. These calculations were performed by the current authors using the Spearman–Kärber method[11] as part of this analysis.

Ten of the chemicals reported by van den Heuvel et al.[10] were also tested for acute toxicity by the UDP using female Sprague-Dawley rats.[12] Independently, data on both conventional and UDP studies were conducted on 10 additional chemicals in male or in female Sprague-Dawley rats.[13] For the conventional studies conducted by Bruce,[8,9] the data were evaluated by probit analysis with the exception of one chemical (test material 2) where the dose response for lethality was not suitable; the LD50 for this chemical was estimated by the Thompson moving average method.[11]

Data on five more substances were obtained from parallel testing using the conventional European Economic Community (EEC) acute toxicity test method in both sexes of Sprague-Dawley rats and by the UDP in females only.[14] From the conventional EEC method tests, again, only the results for females were used in this analysis since the UPD tests were conducted using females. LD50 values were estimated as described in the previous paragraph with the exception of one substance (chemical II), for which data were not amenable to probit analysis (Tables 1 and 2). For this substance, an evaluation by the Spearman–Kärber method[11] was performed.

RESULTS

There is an excellent linear correlation between the LD50 values estimated from the conventional tests and the corresponding ones using the UDP (Figure 1). The average number of animals used in the UDP is lower than that from the other two testing methods.

Animal usage numbers in the FDP do not include "sighting" studies now described in the OECD test guideline, although results from these animals were used as an aid to choosing doses both in the conventional acute toxicity tests and UDP studies. Two of the 10 conventional LD50 tests were limit tests and used only 10 animals; the remaining 8 tests used 30 animals each. For those 10 substances for which test data were available using all 3 methods, the conventional method averaged 26 total animals (males and females combined); the FDP method averaged 15.9 animals (males and females combined) per test; and the average for the UDP method was 7.6 (single sex only). Most of the time, the FDP tests employed either 10 or 20 animals total. Table 2 shows the consistency of classification based upon data from the conventional LD50, FDP, and UDP according to the EEC system for these 35 substances.

DISCUSSION

Acute Toxicity

Figure 1 shows that for the 25 diverse substances for which appropriate data were available, there was excellent agreement between the LD50 values estimated by the conventional and UDP methods, with the exception of one chemical (substance N, $HgCl_2$). The conventional study for mercuric chloride gave an LD50 value of 160 mg/kg, while the UDP gave an LD50 value of 12 mg/kg. The LD50 value cited in Gosselin et al.[15] for oral exposure to the rat is 37 mg/kg. Thus, there appears to be some anomaly associated with acute toxicity tests conducted on this compound.

Classification

The classifications (Table 2) of test materials by the conventional LD50 and the UDP agree except for substance N, $HgCl_2$, as described earlier, for which the UDP data resulted in the more

Table 2. Classification of Test Materials by Different Testing Methods

Test material	Sex	Conventional	Up-and-down	Fixed-Dose[a]
		van den Heuvel et al. (1990)[10] and Yam et al. (1991)[12]		
A	F	Toxic	Toxic	Toxic
B	F	Harmful	Harmful	Harmful
C	F	Harmful		Unclassified
D	F	Toxic		Toxic
E	F	Toxic	Toxic	Toxic
F	F	Toxic		Toxic
G	F	Unclassified	Unclassified	Unclassified
H	F	Toxic	Toxic	Harmful
J	F	Harmful	Harmful	Unclassified
K	F	Unclassified		Unclassified
L	F	Unclassified	Unclassified	Unclassified
M	F	Harmful	Harmful	Harmful
N	F	Toxic	Very toxic	Toxic
P	F	Toxic		Toxic/very toxic
R	F	Unclassified	Harmful	Harmful
T	F	Unclassified		Unclassified
U	F	Unclassified		Unclassified
W	F	Very toxic		Very toxic
X	F	Harmful		Harmful
Y	F	Unclassified		Unclassified
		Bruce (1987)[13]		
1	M	Unclassified	Unclassified	
2	F	Unclassified	Unclassified	
3	M	Unclassified	Unclassified	
4	M	Unclassified	Unclassified	
5	F	Unclassified	Unclassified	
6	F	Unclassified	Unclassified	
7	F	Unclassified	Unclassified	
8	M	Harmful	Harmful	
9	M	Harmful	Harmful	
10	F	Unclassified	Unclassified	
		Bonnyns et al. (1990)[14]		
I	F	Harmful	Harmful	
II	F	Harmful	Harmful	
III	F	Harmful	Harmful	
IV	F	Harmful	Harmful	
V	F	Harmful	Harmful	

Note. The classification scheme is based on the ranking system used in the European Commission Directive (83/467/ EEC, 1983) as described in the van den Heuvel paper[8]: very toxic = LD50 < 25 mg/kg; toxic = LD50 of 25–200 mg/ kg; harmful = LD50 of 200–2000 mg/kg; and unclassified = >2000 mg/kg body weight. From Lipnick et al.[7]
[a] Classification assigned most often, based on data from both sexes.

stringent classification, and substance R (4-aminophenol), where the conventional LD50 test in females only indicated the material would not be classified but both the UDP and the FDP found the material to be harmful.

The FDP data yielded a different classification than the conventional method in four cases: substances C (ferrocene), H (fentin hydroxide), J (acetanilide), and R (4-aminophenol). In three of these cases (C, H, and J), the FDP results gave a less stringent classification than the classical or UDP. These discrepancies are explained in the van den Heuvel paper[10] as due to a problem with the classification method for the classical method (C and J) and the apparent ability of animals given lower doses to recover in the case of substance H.

In one case (substance R) the FDP, like the UDP, gave a more stringent classification than the conventional LD50. The FDP classification for substance P(1-phenyl-2-thiourea) was deter-

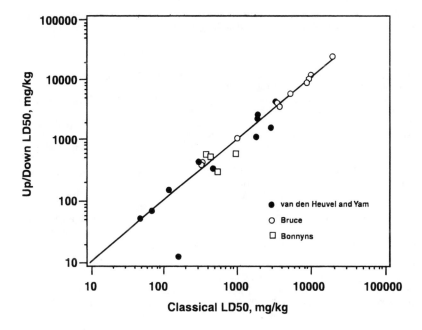

Figure 1. Correlation between conventional and UDP LD50 values. From Lipnick et al.[7]

mined to be very toxic by 12 laboratories, toxic by 12 laboratories, and harmful for 2 laboratories; it was classed toxic by the conventional method.

Interestingly, published and recently reviewed validation work on the acute-toxic-class (ATC) method[4,16] indicate that for six of the eight chemicals in common with those reviewed in this study, hazard classifications made by the ATC method and FDP method would be the same.

Animal/Endpoint Considerations

The number of required animals was considerably lower than that of conventional methods (by half or less) or the FDP. The use of females only further reduces animal use and appears to be justified based on examination of tests done by the conventional LD50[8,17-21]. Females appear to be generally more sensitive where sex differences are found. In contrast to the FDP and UDP, where 64–74% showed toxic signs[12], 93% of animals used in conventional methods showed such effects. Thus, the potential for use of non-lethal endpoints could be considered and it would appear that both the UDP and FDP are refinements to the conventional method.

Applicability of Data

The conventional acute toxicity test and the UDP both provide an estimate of the LD50 while the FDP does not. The data from the UDP and conventional acute toxicity testing are applicable to any hazard classification system, whereas the FDP is specifically designed to yield data for the assignment of a hazard classification according to the EEC system. However, the OECD FDP protocol incorporates a sighting study, which aids in the generation of data that are applicable to other classification systems. On the other hand, an estimate of the LD50 is often helpful beyond its use in classification, such as in helping to set doses for toxicity studies of longer duration and the comparison of acute toxicity by different routes of administration and direct comparison of toxicity of a number of chemicals. Each of these uses is reasonably well met by the UDP. It is recognized that the UDP, unlike the conventional method, cannot be used for generating dose-response slopes, should that be desired.

References

1. Organization for Economic Cooperation and Development. 1987. Guideline for the Testing of Chemical Substances—No. 401: Acute Oral Toxicity. Paris: OECD.
2. Organization for Economic Cooperation and Development. 1992. Guideline for Testing of Chemicals—No. 420: Acute Oral Toxicity—Fixed Dose Method. Paris: OECD.
3. Roll, V. R., Riebschläger, M., Mischke, U., and Kayser, D. 1989. Neue Wege zur Bestimmung der akuten Toxizität von Chemikalien. *Bundesgesundheitsblatt* 32:336.
4. Schlede, E., Mischke, U., Roll, R., and Kayser, D. 1992. A national validation study of the acute-toxic-class method—an alternative to the LD_{50} test. *Arch. Toxicol.* 66:455.
5. Schlede, E., Mischke, U., Diener, W., and Kayser, D. 1994. The international validation study of the acute-toxic-class method (oral). *Arch. Toxicol.* 69:659.
6. Organization for Economic Cooperation and Development. 1996. Guidelines for the testing of chemicals—No. 423: Acute oral toxicity—acute-toxic-class method. Paris: Author.
7. Lipnick, R. L., Cotruvo, J. A., Hill, R. N., Bruce, R. D., Stitzel, K. A., Walker, A. P, Chu, I., Goddard, M., Segal, L., Springer, J. A., and Myers, R. C. In press. Comparison of the up-and-down, conventional LD50 and fixed dose acute toxicity procedures. *Food Chem. Toxicol.*
8. Bruce, R. D. 1985. An up-and-down procedure for acute toxicity testing. *Fundam. Appl. Toxicol.* 5:151.
9. American Society for Testing and Materials. 1987. Standard Test Method for Estimating Acute Oral Toxicity in Rats. Designation: E 1163-87. Philadelphia: ASTM.
10. van den Heuvel, M. J., Clark, D. G., Fielder, R. J., Koundakjian, P. P., Oliver, G. J. A., Pelling, D., Tomlinson, N. J., and Walker, A. P. 1990. The international validation of a fixed-dose procedure as an alternative to the classical LD_{50} test. *Food Chem. Toxicol.* 28:469.
11. Finney, D. J. 1971. *Probit analysis,* 3rd ed. London: Cambridge University Press.
12. Yam, J., Reer, P. J., and Bruce, R. D. 1991. Comparison of the up-and-down method and the fixed dose procedure for acute oral toxicity testing. *Food Chem. Toxicol.* 29:259.
13. Bruce, R. D. 1987. A confirmatory study of the up-and-down method for acute toxicity testing. *Fundam. Appl. Toxicol.* 8:97.
14. Bonnyns, E., Delcour, M. P., and Vral, A. 1990. Up-and-Down Method as an Alternative to the EC-Method for Acute Toxicity Testing. Brussels: Institute of Hygiene and Epidemiology, Ministry of Public Health and the Environment. IHE project 2153/88/11.
15. Gosselin, R. E., Smith, R. P. and Hodge, H. C., eds. 1984. *Clinical toxicology of commercial products,* 5th ed., Section III, p. 262. Baltimore: Williams & Wilkins.
16. Organization for Economic Cooperation and Development. 1994. Ad Hoc Expert Meeting: Acute-Toxic-Class Method. Berlin, January 26–28.
17. Weil, C. S., Carpenter, C. P., and Smyth, H. F. 1953. Specifications for calculating the median effective dose. *Am. Ind. Hyg. Q.* 14:200.
18. Muller, H., and Kley, H. P. 1982. Retrospective study on the reliability of an "approximate LD50" determined with a small number of animals. *Arch. Toxicol.* 51:189.
19. Schutz, E., and Fuchs, H. 1982. A new approach to minimizing the number of animals used in acute toxicity testing and optimizing the information of test results. *Arch. Toxicol.* 51:197.
20. DePass, L. R., Myers, R. C., Weaver, E. V., and Weil, C. S. 1984. An assessment of the importance of the number of dosage levels, number of animals per dosage level, sex and method of LD50 and slope calculation in acute toxicity studies. In *Acute toxicity testing: Alternative approaches,* ed. A. M. Goldberg, pp. 139–153. New York: Mary Ann Liebert.
21. U.S. Environmental Protection Agency. 1991. Comparison of Male and Female Rat Oral and Dermal LD50 Values in OPP's One-Liner Database. Prepared for Office of Pesticide Programs by Clement International Corporation, U.S. EPA, Washington, DC.

Chapter Thirty-eight

SKIN PARTITIONS AS A SCREEN FOR DERMAL PERMEABILITY

D. R. Mattie and James N. McDougal

Octanol/water partition coefficients (PC) are used as a measure of the ability of a chemical to enter skin. Tissue partitions are used in physiologically based pharmacokinetic (PBPK) models. A technique was developed for measuring a skin:air PC with rat skin for use in PBPK models. Skin:air and skin:saline PCs measured for volatile chemicals correlated with permeability constants, while octanol/water PCs did not. Although stratum corneum:air PCs appear to work better in PBPK models, a skin:air or skin:saline PC allows for a rapid screen of the ability of a chemical to penetrate skin.

INTRODUCTION

Various methods have been used to measure the potential of a chemical to penetrate through the skin. The permeability constant of a chemical is a measure of a chemical's ability to cross the skin. Permeability constants are used to predict the absorption rate or flux of a chemical. The partition coefficient (PC) of a chemical in skin is an important parameter for determining the permeability constant.

Skin:air PCs for volatile chemicals have been used in physiologically based pharmacokinetic (PBPK) models to describe the dermal penetration of these chemicals.[1,2] The skin:air PCs were calculated, not determined experimentally.

Various experimental methods have been reported in the literature for determining PC values for skin. One method uses the octanol/water PC as a surrogate for partitioning between the skin (octanol phase) and the environment or vehicle (water phase).[3,4] Although the octanol/water PC has been used extensively in estimating dermal penetration, it is not a true representation of the process of chemical interaction with the skin.

Surber et al.[5] measured stratum corneum (SC)/water and SC/isopropyl myristate PC values. In their study, PC values were determined as a function of equilibration time, initial concentration of drug in the vehicle, delipidization of stratum corneum, and source and preparation of stratum corneum. The PCs were considered as predictors of percutaneous penetration for the purpose of conducting dermal risk assessments.[5]

The headspace method, developed by Sato and Nakajima[6] and modified by Gargas et al.,[7] has been extensively used in this laboratory for determining PCs of a variety of biological

The animals used in this study were handled in accordance with the principles in the Guide for the Care and Use of Laboratory Animals, prepared by the Committee on Care and Use of Laboratory Animals of the Institute of Laboratory Animal Resources, National Research Council, Department of Health and Human Services, National Institutes of Health Publication 86-23 (1985), and the Animal Welfare Act of 1966, as amended.

tissues. However, the methodology was not adequate for measuring skin PC due to the difficulties inherent in homogenizing skin.

The purposes of this study were to (1) develop an in vitro method to test chemicals for the potential for dermal penetration, and (2) develop skin partition coefficients for PBPK dermal models.

MATERIALS AND METHODS

The following chemicals were purchased for the determination of skin:air partition coefficients: dibromomethane, perchloroethylene, trichloroethylene, benzene, hexane, toluene, m-xylene, styrene, and methyl chloroform from Aldrich Chemical Company (Milwaukee, WI), methylene chloride and carbon tetrachloride from Fisher Scientific (Columbus, OH), halothane from Halocarbon Labs, Inc. (Hackensack, NJ), and isoflurane from Anaquest (Madison, WI).

The skin was collected for PC determination from male Fisher 344 rats (Charles River Laboratories) between 8 and 16 wk old. The species chosen was based on the database that exists for inhalation and dermal exposure in this laboratory. Rats were group housed (three per cage) in clear plastic cages with wood chip bedding. Water and feed (Purina formula 5008) were available ad libitum. The ambient temperature was maintained at 22 $\pm$ 2°C and light was regulated on a 12-h light/dark cycle (starting at 0600 h). Skin from control rats in other studies was also used for PC determinations.

The dorsal skin of a rat was clipped using an electric clipper immediately after euthanasia with carbon dioxide. After collecting the skin, the hypodermis was removed, the skin was cut into 1 by 0.5 cm strips with a razor blade, and the pieces were placed on the walls of scintillation vials without saline. Sample vials containing skin and their corresponding empty reference vials were incubated for 10 min at 32°C using a vortex evaporator to warm the skin samples and vials. After reaching 32°C, the caps were briefly removed to vent any built up pressure. A volume of air was then removed from each sample and reference vial equal to the volume of chemical vapor to be injected into the vial from a standard air bag at 10,000 ppm. Separate sets of samples were incubated for different periods of time (1, 2, 3, 4 h) to determine the time to equilibration for each chemical. A volume of chemical vapor (0.5 ml from the 10,000 ppm air bag) was injected into sample and corresponding reference vials. Each time point had a minimum of four sample and four reference vials. The vials were incubated with vortex mixing action. At each time point already listed, 1.0 ml of vapor from a reference vial was sampled on a gas chromatograph with a flame ionization detector. The corresponding sample vial was analyzed after the reference vial under the same conditions. After measuring the amount of chemical as area counts from all of the reference and sample vials in a set, sample vials were compared versus corresponding reference vials using the following equation modified from Gargas et al.[7]:

$$PC = \frac{\text{(reference area cts) (vial volume)} - \text{(test area cts) (vial volume} - \text{sample volume)}}{\text{(test area cts) (sample volume)}}$$

After determining the time to reach equilibration, sufficient samples were analyzed at that time point to ensure an accurate skin:air partition coefficient.[8]

After developing the technique for determining a skin:air PC using dibromomethane, the procedure was used for perchloroethylene, trichloroethylene, benzene, hexane, toluene, m-xylene, styrene, methyl chloroform, methylene chloride, carbon tetrachloride, halothane, and isoflurane. Between 16 and 24 samples were measured to determine skin:air partition coefficients for each of these chemicals.

A t-test was used to determine the effect of size of skin on PC values. To determine the equilibration time and compare the effect of different concentrations, PC data was compared by a one-way analysis of variance. Fresh skin versus frozen skin was compared by t-test. Linear regression and correlation for comparing PC values versus permeability constants and octanol/water PC values were determined using the line fit procedure in RSI on a VAX computer (BBN Software Products Corporation, Cambridge, MA). The level of significance was accepted at $p < .05$.

RESULTS

There was no statistical difference between minced skin and strips of skin (Table 1). There was no significant difference between the skin:air PC values determined at 203, 102, and 41 ppm concentrations (Table 1). There was no statistical difference between fresh and frozen skin (Table 1).

The skin:air PC values for selected volatile organic chemicals are shown in Table 2. Approximately 19 samples were analyzed for each chemical.

The octanol/water PC values given by Leo et al.[12] and the corresponding skin:air PC values for 11 of the chemicals of Table 2 are shown in Table 3. There is no correlation ($r^2 = .09$) between the octanol/water PC values and skin:air PC values (Figure 1).

Permeability constants were available for none of the chemicals for which skin:air PC values were measured in this study.[1,2,9] The permeability constants and their corresponding skin:air PC values are shown in Table 4. There was good correlation ($r^2 = .93$) between permeability

Table 1. Skin:Air Partition Coefficients for Dibromomethane Comparing Minced Versus Strips of Skin, with Values Determined at 41, 102, and 203 ppm Concentrations, and for Frozen Versus Fresh Skin

Frozen strips, 203 ppm ($n = 10$)	Fresh strips, 203 ppm ($n = 12$)	Fresh minced, 203 ppm ($n = 10$)	Frozen strips, 102 ppm ($n = 15$)	1/2 Fresh, 1/2 frozen strips 41 ppm ($n = 14$)
68.3 ± 3.1	61.7 ± 4.3	61.8 ± 1.8	67.2 ± 5.5	59.4 ± 4.6

Note. Values are mean ± SE.

Table 2. Skin:Air Partition Coefficients for Selected Volatile Organic Chemicals

Chemical	Skin:air PC (± SE)	n	Equilibration time (h)
Perchloroethylene	41.5 ± 1.2	16	4
Trichloroethylene	31.8 ± 1.5	19	4
Benzene	34.5 ± 1.9	19	4
Hexane	1.9 ± 0.1	18	4
Toluene	43.0 ± 1.8	16	4
Xylene	50.4 ± 1.7	24	2
Styrene	91.9 ± 6.8	20	3
Methylene chloride	13.6 ± 0.5	17	2
Carbon tetrachloride	12.4 ± 0.6	24	4
Methyl chloroform	10.8 ± 0.6	18	4
Halothane	10.6 ± 0.7	17	3
Isoflurane	4.5 ± 0.3	16	6

Table 3. Skin:Air Partition Coefficients for Organic Versus Octanol/Water

Chemical	Skin:air PC (± SE)	Octanol/water PC[11]
Hexane	1.9 ± 0.1	446.7
Methyl chloroform	10.8 ± 0.6	309.0
Carbon tetrachloride	12.4 ± 0.6	676.1
Methylene chloride	13.6 ± 0.5	17.8
Trichloroethylene	31.8 ± 1.5	263.0
Benzene	34.5 ± 1.9	134.9
Perchloroethylene	41.5 ± 1.2	1380.4
Toluene	43.0 ± 1.8	537.0
Xylene	50.4 ± 1.7	1445.4
Dibromomethane	68.3 ± 3.1	43.7
Styrene	91.9 ± 6.8	891.3

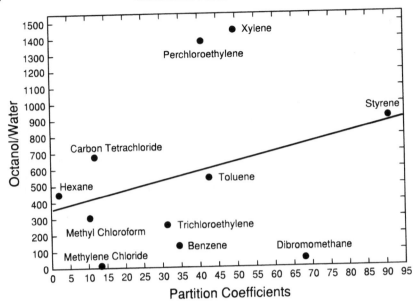

Figure 1. Comparison of skin:air partition coefficients with octanol/water PC values.

Table 4. Skin:air Partition Coefficients for Organic Chemicals Versus Permeability Constants

Chemical	Skin:air PC (± SE)	Permeability[1,2,9] (mm/h)
Styrene	91.9 ± 6.8	17.53
Dibromomethane	68.3 ± 3.1	12.19
Xylene	50.4 ± 1.7	7.23
Toluene	43.0 ± 1.8	7.21
Perchloroethylene	41.5 ± 1.2	6.68
Benzene	34.5 ± 1.9	1.52
Halothane	10.6 ± 0.7	0.45
Hexane	1.9 ± 0.1	0.31
Isoflurane	4.5 ± 0.3	0.25

constants and skin:air PC values (Figure 2). When octanol/water PC values were compared to the permeability constants (minus the octanol/water for isoflurane), the correlation was poor ($r^2 = .04$).

If a saline:air or saline:water PC value is determined for a chemical, a skin:saline or skin:water PC value can be calculated for the chemical by dividing the skin:air PC value by the saline:air or water:air PC value. Comparison of octanol/water PC values with skin:saline PC values (Table 5) resulted in a poor correlation ($r^2 = .20$).

DISCUSSION

Intact whole-thickness skin was placed on the glass surface in vitro with the stratum corneum exposed to the chemical vapor with the same orientation as in vivo conditions. The data show that skin strips give values comparable with minced tissue. This technique avoids the requirement to homogenize skin, mince skin, or separate the stratum corneum. Skin can be obtained from control rats or quality control rats. Skin can also be stored frozen for up to 1 wk.[8]

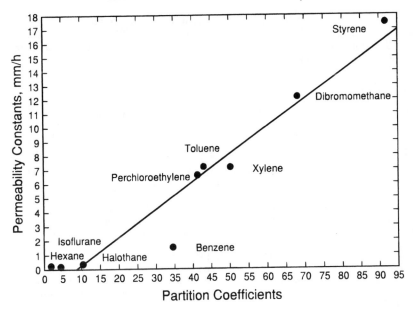

Figure 2. Comparison of skin:air partition coefficients with permeability constants.

Table 5. Skin:Saline Partition Coefficients for Organic Chemicals Versus Octanol/Water

Chemical	Skin:saline PC	Octanol/water PC[12]
Styrene	1.9 ± 0.1	891.3
Hexane	10.8 ± 0.6	446.7
Perchloroethylene	12.4 ± 0.6	1380.4
Xylene	13.6 ± 0.5	1445.4
Toluene	31.8 ± 1.5	537.0
Benzene	34.5 ± 1.9	134.9
Halothane	41.5 ± 1.2	533.4
Dibromomethane	43.0 ± 1.8	43.7

The skin:air PC values were compared to both octanol/water PC values and permeability constants. Octanol/water PC values have been used as a qualitative measure of skin permeability. Skin:air PC values for the chemicals tested showed a correlation with permeability constants, but did not show as good a correlation with octanol/water PC values. Octanol/water PC values for the volatile organic chemicals examined in this study appeared to be poor indicators of the solubility of these chemicals in skin. No single bulk solvent, such as octanol, precisely mimics the solvent properties of the stratum corneum transport barrier.[10] In addition the skin:air PC values were determined for chemicals with poor water solubility. The predictive ability of octanol/water PC values is most likely lower for these volatile chemicals because octanol/water PC values are based on water representing the vehicle or environmental medium. The data in this study suggest that skin:air PC values are a better indicator of the relative skin permeability for the volatile chemicals examined in this study. Skin:saline PC values would be representative of permeability into skin from an aqueous environmental medium. Determining a skin:air PC or skin:saline PC is proposed as an initial screen to identify the potential for skin absorption of volatile chemicals with unknown permeability constants.

In addition to indicating potential permeability, skin partition coefficients are necessary for developing the dermal compartment in a physiologically based pharmacokinetic (PBPK) model.

The skin:air PC is essential for the rate equation in the dermal compartment describing the uptake of chemical from air into the skin. A comparison of skin:air PC versus stratum corneum:air PC revealed that stratum corneum:air PCs are better values in the rate equation of the skin compartment of PBPK models.[11]

CONCLUSIONS

This method provides a screening technique for predicting skin penetration of volatile chemicals. This method is not adequate for determining skin PCs for PBPK dermal models.

References

1. McDougal, J. N., Jepson, G. W., Clewell, H. J. III, MacNaughton, M. G., and Andersen, M. E. 1986. A physiological pharmacokinetic model for dermal absorption of vapors in the rat. *Toxicol. Appl. Pharmacol.* 85:286–294.
2. McDougal, J. N., Jepson, G. W., Clewell H. J. III, Gargas, M. L., and Andersen, M. E. 1990. Dermal absorption of organic chemical vapors in rats and humans. *Fundam. Appl. Toxicol.* 14:299–308.
3. Bronaugh, R. L., and Congdon, E. R. 1984. Percutaneous absorption of hair dyes: Correlation with partition coefficients. *J. Invest. Dermatol.* 83:124–127.
4. Kasting, G. B., Smith, R. L., and Cooper, E. R. 1987. Effect of lipid solubility and molecular size on percutaneous absorption. *Pharmacol. Skin* 1:138–153.
5. Surber, C., Wilhelm, K. P., Maibach, H. I., Hall, L. L., and Guy, R. H. 1990. Partitioning of chemicals into human stratum corneum: Implications for risk assessment following dermal exposure. *Fundam. Appl. Toxicol.* 15:99–107.
6. Sato, A., and Nakajima, T. 1979. Partition coefficients of some aromatic hydrocarbons and ketones in water, blood, and oil. *Br. J. Ind. Med.* 36:231–234.
7. Gargas, M. L., Burgess, R. J., Voisard, D. E., Cason, G. H., and Andersen, M. E. 1989. Partition coefficients of low-molecular-weight volatile chemicals in various liquids and tissues. *Toxicol. Appl. Pharmacol.* 98:87–99.
8. Mattie, D. R., Bates, G. D., Jr., Jepson, G. W., Fisher, J. W., and McDougal, J. N. 1994. Determination of skin:air partition coefficients for volatile chemicals: Experimental methods and applications. *Fundam. Appl. Toxicol.* 22:51–57.
9. McDougal, J. N., Jepson, G. W., Clewell, H. J., III, and Andersen, M. E. 1985. Dermal absorption of dihalomethane vapors. *Toxicol. Appl. Pharmacol.* 79:150–158.
10. Anderson, B. D., and Raykar, P. V. 1989. Solute structure-permeability relationships in human stratum coreum. *J. Invest. Dermatol.* 93:280–286.
11. Mattie, D. R., Solscheid, J. A., Clewell, H. J., III, McDougal, J. N., and Jepson, G. W. 1994. Permeability constants determined by PBPK models for vapor, neat, and aqueous forms of volatile organic chemicals. *Toxicologist* 14:185.
12. Leo, A., Hansch, C., and Elkins, D. 1971. Partition coefficients and their uses. *Chem. Rev.* 71:525–616.

Chapter Thirty-nine

REDUCTION OF ANIMAL UTILIZATION IN DERMAL TOXICOLOGIC STUDIES

Ronald G. Menton, J. A. Blank, T. H. Snider,
C. T. Olson, and D. W. Korte, Jr.

Battelle's Medical Research and Evaluation Facility evaluates developmental drugs for their effectiveness as potential decontaminants or topical skin protectants. Several approaches are utilized to reduce the number of animals required to conduct statistically valid dermal toxicity tests. Endpoint refinement has been accomplished through replacement of quantal responses with continuous responses, yielding more precise measurements, which results in smaller sample size requirements. Novel statistical designs such as stagewise dose allocation, crossover designs, and group sequential stopping rules are also employed to reduce animal usage. This chapter discusses the application of these methods in dermal toxicity tests at our laboratory.

REPLACING QUANTAL ENDPOINTS WITH CONTINUOUS ENDPOINTS

Battelle's Medical Research and Evaluation Facility (MREF) evaluates developmental drugs and other chemical substances for their effectiveness as potential decontaminants, topical skin protectants, or treatment therapies to mitigate toxic effects associated with chemical threat agents. In the past, skin decontaminants for the treatment of organophosphorus compounds (OP) exposure were experimentally evaluated using lethality as an endpoint. The information content of quantal data is minimal: The presence or absence of a particular response provides little information on the strength of that response. This lack of sensitivity is manifested statistically as a large standard deviation relative to the magnitude of the estimated proportion. Since the standard deviation of an estimated proportion for a quantal response depends on the proportion responding, it cannot be reduced in the same way as the variability of a continuous response by using a more precise measurement.

The minimum sample size required to note a statistical difference between two sample means is proportional to the variance of the measured response. Therefore, reduced animal usage can be achieved though the use of a more precise measurement for a continuous response, as shown in Table 1. On the other hand, the minimum sample size to compare two sample proportions depends on the proportion responding for each study group.

Acetylcholinesterase (AChE) inhibition occurs following acute OP intoxication; therefore, monitoring erythrocyte AChE activity following OP exposure is an attractive replacement for lethality for evaluating the effectiveness of candidate decontaminants. Table 2 displays results for experiments in rabbits based on lethality and AChE inhibition. Increased precision in the estimate of the protective ratio (PR) based on AChE inhibition was obtained with 267 fewer animals than required in the lethality studies. The estimated PRs based on lethality and enzyme inhibition were comparable.

Table 1. Minimum Sample Sizes Required to Achieve 90% Power for Noting a Statistical Difference at 5% Significance Level Between Two Samples Based on One-Sided Hypothesis Test for Continuous and Quantal Responses

			Sample 2	
	Sample 1	$\mu_2 = 0.6$	$\mu_2 = 0.75$	$\mu_2 = 0.90$
Continuous response[a]	$\mu_2 = 0.50, \sigma = 0.50$	430	70	28
	$\mu_1 = 0.50, \sigma = 0.25$	109	18	8
			Sample 2	
	Sample 1	$P_2 = 0.6$	$P_2 = 0.75$	$P_2 = 0.90$
Quantal response[b]	$P_1 = 0.50, \sigma = 0.50$	445	71	25

[a] Based on standard normal theory for comparing two sample means via a one-sided t-test.[1]
[b] Based on exact table given in Casagrande and Pike.[2]

MORE EFFICIENT STATISTICAL DESIGNS

The goal of the experimental planning and design process is to help ensure that the right types and amounts of data will be collected to meet study objectives. Efficient designs attempt to maximize information content of data through:

• Reducing or eliminating extraneous sources of variation
• Focusing on the most informative pieces of data

Crossover designs are employed at Battelle in pharmacokinetic and/or pharmacodynamic studies to mitigate the variability from subject to subject. In a crossover design, the same subject is tested on several occasions, with each subject serving as a random block. Crossover designs also are employed to evaluate topical skin protectants (TSPs) for vesicants in rabbits using lesion area ratio (LAR) as the endpoint. The experimental design for this program provides for:

• Baseline adjustment
• Within-animal comparisons between six TSPs tested concurrently
• Within-animal comparisons between candidate TSP and concurrent standard TSP
• Between-animal comparisons between each candidate TSP and the historical database for standard TSP
• Significant reduction in animal usage

Screening a set of six candidate TSPs requires only 24 animals, providing 24 replicates for each candidate TSP and the standard TSP. Parallel testing in independent groups of animals requires 168 animals, accompanied by an expected loss in sensitivity due to between animal comparisons.

Table 2. Effect of Standard and Candidate Treatments on Toxicant-Induced Enzyme Inhibition and Lethality in the Rabbit

TX[a]	MID[b] or MLD[f]	LL[c]	UL[d]	n	PR[e]	Slope (SE)
		Enzyme inhibition				
Standard	0.005[b]	0.003	0.006	38	—	1.28 (0.21)
Candidate	0.089[b]	0.073	0.106	37	17.8	1.78 (0.23)
		24-h Lethality				
Standard	0.031[f]	0.020	0.103	136	—	2.73 (0.79)
Candidate	0.708[f]	0.567	0.814	206	22.8	3.79 (0.64)

[a] Treatment.
[b] Median inhibitory dose (mg/kg).
[c] Lower 95% confidence limit boundary.
[d] Upper 95% confidence limit boundary.
[e] Protective ratio (MLD or MID of treated rabbits/MLD or MID of control rabbits).
[f] Median lethal dose (mg/kg), MLD.

Figure 1 presents the reduction in the number of animals achieved through the use of a crossover design. Furthermore, additional reduction in animal usage was accomplished using a *two-tier screen:*

- There were 91 candidate TSPs evaluated in vitro.
- Of these, only 36 were evaluated in vivo.

STAGEWISE ADAPTIVE DOSE ALLOCATION

Advanced efficacy evaluations of dermal decontaminants are often conducted at Battelle through the use of dose-response studies. The *experimental design* of a dose-response study refers to:

- Number of dosage levels
- Dosage levels themselves
- Number of animals tested at each dose

Rather than testing all of the animals against predetermined dosage levels, the *stagewise approach* to the experimental design of a dose-response study[3,4] iteratively selects dosage levels based upon results of previous stages. Figure 2 outlines the steps involved in application of the stagewise approach.

The stagewise approach to dose allocation is similar to the up-and-down method[5,6] in that:

- Experiments are conducted in a series of stages, rather than all at once.
- Doses for the next experiment are based on experimental results, not set in advance.

The stagewise approach and up-and-down method are dissimilar in that:

- The stagewise approach supports dosing of multiple animals in each stage.
- Dose selection is not as rigid (one step up or down) with the stagewise approach.

The stagewise approach is being used at Battelle for dermal dose-response studies using both quantal and continuous endpoints. As shown in Table 3, application of the stagewise approach has been effective in reducing the number of animals utilized and in producing more successful experiments.

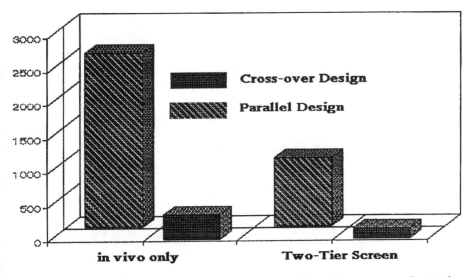

Figure 1. Reduction in number of animals required for screening of 91 candidate treatments using two-tier approach and crossover design.

DESIGN PROCESS DURING EXPERIMENT

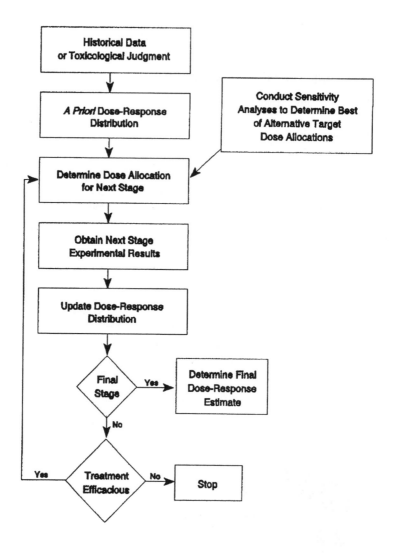

Figure 2. Stagewise adaptive dose allocation. Reprinted with permission from Feder et al.[4]

Table 3. Successful Use of Stagewise Approach to Dose Allocation in Rabbit Dose-Response Studies

Dose Response	Planned number of study groups	Planned number of animals	Actual number of animals	Comment
Enzyme inhibition	1	50	50	Even though a priori estimates of dose range were incorrect, desired precision was obtained.
Enzyme inhibition	3	150	118	Desired precision was obtained with fewer animals and study was terminated.
Enzyme inhibition	3	150	116	Desired precision was obtained with fewer animals and study was terminated.
Enzyme inhibition	3	150	125	Desired precision was obtained with fewer animals and study was terminated.

SUMMARY

Reduced animal utilization for dermal toxicity tests has been accomplished at Battelle by replacing quantal endpoints with more precise continuous responses and by implementing efficient statistical designs to generate better data. The effort needed to apply these steps at other laboratories is minimal compared to the considerable savings in animal utilization.

References

1. Bain, L. J., and Engelhardt, M. 1987. *Introduction to probability and mathematical statistics.* Boston: Duxbury Press.
2. Casagrande, J. T., and Pike, M. C. 1978. An improved approximate formula for calculating sample sizes for comparing two binomial distributions. *Biometrics* 34:483–486.
3. Feder, P. I., Hobson, D. W., Olson, C. T., Joiner, R. L., and Matthews, M. C. 1991. Stagewise, adaptive dose allocation for quantal response dose-response studies. *Neurosci. Biobehav. Rev.* 15:109–114.
4. Feder, P. I., Hobson, D. W., Olson, C. T., Joiner, R. L., and Matthews, M. C. 1992. Statistical design considerations for stagewise, adaptive dose allocation in dose response studies. In *Biopharmaceutical sequential statistical applications,* ed. K. Peace. p.p. 37–86, New York: Marcel Dekker.
5. Bruce, R. B. 1985. An up-and-down procedure for acute toxicity testing. *Fundam. Appl. Toxicol.* 5:152–157.
6. Bruce, R. B. 1987. A confirmatory study of the up-and-down method for acute toxicity testing. *Fundam. Appl. Toxicol.* 8:97–100.

Chapter Forty

COMPUTERIZED IN VITRO TEST FOR CHEMICAL TOXICITY BASED ON *TETRAHYMENA* SWIMMING PATTERNS

David A. Noever, Helen C. Matsos, Raymond J. Cronise,
Loren L. Looger, Rachna A. Relwani,
and Jacqueline U. Johnson

An apparatus and method for rapidly determining chemical toxicity has been evaluated. The toxicity monitor includes an automated scoring of how motile biological cells (Tetrahymena pyriformis) slow down or otherwise change their swimming patterns in a hostile chemical environment. The device, called the motility assay apparatus (MAA), is tested for 30-s determination of chemical toxicity in 20 aqueous samples containing trace organics and salts. With equal or better detection limits, results compare favorably to in vivo animal tests of eye irritancy, in addition to agreeing for all chemicals with previous manual evaluations of single-cell motility.

INTRODUCTION

For pollution monitoring, chemical testing, and pharmaceutical approval, existing whole-animal procedures are expensive, time-consuming, and increasingly restricted by federal law. Thus a combination of public pressure and high costs has stimulated the $3 billion chemical testing market to look for alternatives to whole animal research.

In collaboration[1] with Avon, Inc., Silverman[1,2] demonstrated that hostile chemicals could change the swimming behavior of single biological cells (*Tetrahymena*) in a controlled and reliable way. For 21 chemicals and pharmaceuticals, he found equal or better results for the toxic response of single cells compared to alternative whole-animal tests (e.g., FDA's Draize rabbit eye test). His method relied on two lab technicians performing a subjective evaluation of swimming behavior and scoring their opinions of regular versus irregular swimming patterns. Subsequent industrial interest has focused on finding more reliable and rapid ways to improve the toxicity evaluation.

Other experiments[3,4] have demonstrated that for many (*Tetrahymena*) cells suspended in shallow culture dishes, the cells rapidly (20 s) aggregate to give a characteristic signature pattern (polygonal net). The honeycombed patterns change repeatedly when chemicals alter the culture media (water), and using image analysis of the aggregation patterns, chemical toxicity could be scored accordingly. This advance took away the capital investment in microscopes and technician time required by Silverman's test,[1] but nevertheless demanded an extended time for culturing cells to high enough densities (million cells/ml). The assay's aim was to make the advantages of the single-cell method more widely accessible to smaller labs or for field tests where microscopic observation and individual cell counting might prove impractical.

While these innovative alternatives using single biological cells have shown promising results when compared to animal tests, they generally have suffered from a nonuniform procedure for scoring toxicity. Either microscopic observation of cell swimming patterns[1] has required subjective and time-consuming scoring by two lab technicians or, alternatively, macroscopic observation of cell swimming patterns[5] has required lengthy culture preparation. Industrial labs have therefore sought a more rapid and low-cost device for implementing single-cell monitoring on a wide scale.

Here we design and evaluate an automated method for computer-aided scoring of single-cell responses; 20 chemicals consisting of organics and salts are examined using *Tetrahymena* as the test organism. Changes in cell swimming velocity serve as the test's monitor, while computerized cell tracking provides the nonsubjective evaluation. The method differs from previous approaches in its relative speed, reliability, and operator ease. In several minutes, multiple chemicals can be tested as they act either alone or synergistically.

MATERIALS AND METHODS

Organisms and culture conditions

The ciliate *Tetrahymena pyriformis* (American Tissue Type Collection, Bethesda, MD) were grown in (autoclaved) 2% proteose–peptone yeast medium.[6] The organisms were cultivated axenically in a temperature-controlled (22°C) clean room (Class III). The protists were grown in 1-L glass containers without additional gassing or agitation.

Tetrahymena pyriformis was pursued as a target organism because its chemical sensitivity has been well characterized previously.[7] Its short generation times and thoroughly investigated biology make it what one researcher[8] called a "biochemical star." As a result, for more than 40 years, *T. pyriformis* has been the organism of choice[7] for assaying carcinogens, insecticides, fungicides, petroleum products and organics, mycotoxins, antimetabolites, and heavy metals.

Laboratory Preparations

Instructions for lab preparations of cell cultures include: (1) Transfer freeze-dried *Tetrahymena* cells into rehydration fluid vial; (2) incubate 10 min at 35–37°C; (3) decant entire constituents into empty petri dish with either a dilution blank or previously measured concentration of chemicals (Figure 1).

Determination of Pattern Formation

For direct comparison with computerized scoring of single-cell swimming, macroscopic aggregation patterns.[3–5,9] were also monitored at the same chemical dosages. Cell suspensions were prepared as dense, shallow cultures (3.2×10^5 cells/ml, culture depth 4 mm). Assuming typical cell parameters (20–50% g carbon/g dry weight, 80% water content by weight, and cell specific gravity of 1.05 μg/cm^3), this cell population corresponds approximately to 1 μg carbon/m^3.

Vertical migration and bioconvection patterns of the ciliate were determined in a rectangular polystyrene flask ($33 \times 77 \times 15$ mm inner dimensions). Since average pattern dimension was 1–2 mm, the effect of container dimensions on pattern formation was minimal. Different sized flasks did not affect either characteristic pattern size or overall morphology.

The flask was placed on a clear stage and illuminated (4000 lux, Edmund Scientific, Rockaway, NJ, light meter) using two collimated incandescent beams angled at 45°. A continuously cooling fan maintained thermal control of the light source; each lamp was remotely placed on a gooseneck wand and focused using 24-cm optical fibers. Thermal convection was not observed either in nonmotile (dead) cells of *T. pyriformis* or with 0.1-mm aluminum flakes in water.

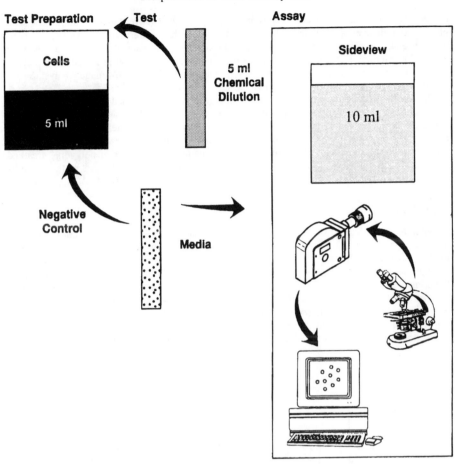

Figure 1. Schematic of assay procedure. A 5-ml sample of *Tetrahymena* cells (density 2.5 × 10³/ml) is diluted with 5 ml yeast media and test chemical at the desired concentration; 0.1 ml of the 10 ml preparation is placed on a 100-μm observation chamber, videotaped under microscopic observation, and then analyzed for cell tracking parameters (velocity and number of cells motile).

IMAGE ANALYSIS

Single Cells

Component parts of the signal detection system for single cells include: (1) compatible computer with printer; (2) two high-resolution black-and-white video monitors with black-and-white (b/w) video camera; (3) compatible microscope with phase-contrast or dark-field optics and objectives; and (4) 100 μm deep observation chamber. A live or videotaped image of 50 or more single cells of *Tetrahymena* is centered and delivered into the computer. The image is analyzed for cell identification and, as applicable, *Tetrahymena* concentration, motile velocity, and linearity data. A hard-copy printout of test results can be made or optionally stored as data as ASCII files. The assay device is able to recognize 50-μm swimming cells and to distinguish them from other biologicals based on their size, luminosity, and motion.

Aggregation Patterns

For comparison with single-cell results, aggregation patterns were evaluated and reported for identical chemical conditions. The image of bioconvection patterns was recorded by a b/w camera (Nikon FM-2, lens, Medical Nikkor 120 mm) mounted above the observation flask. The photographic images were digitized by manually tracing their pattern boundaries (e.g., regions of high relative organism density), then scanned (Albaton 300S scanner, Sacramento, CA) with a spatial resolution of 512 × 512 pixels. The digital images were further analyzed for geometric parameters of aggregation patterns using a main image analysis program (Image Analyst, Sacramento, CA) written in the computer language C.

The outline and position of each pattern (polygon) were determined using a chain coding algorithm and analyzed spatially as a best-fitted centroid. For each polygon, the geometry was stored in the form of area, perimeter, and average radius (arbitrary pixel units), as well as the number of polygonal sides, then calibrated (normalized) to the average value for all polygons. As the pattern changed with chemical addition, the geometric measures of polygonal area and perimeter were plotted as a function of cell sides. The physical significance[10] of these results has been discussed elsewhere under the heading of statistical crystallography.[5]

RESULTS

The potential importance of single-cell swimming changes and chemical detection has been discussed previously.[2,3,8] We therefore consider here the computer-scored effects of chemical loading on single-cell swimming and compare these results using geometric analysis on lab simulations, which can include this aggregation mechanism for scoring chemical toxicity. Thus the comparative framework for chemical detection involves four different tests: (1) the present computerized scoring of single-cell swimming; (2) manual scoring of single cell swimming; (3) monitoring of many cells macroscopically through their chemically hindered aggregation patterns (bioconvection)[3,4]; and (4) traditional whole-animals in vivo tests.

Twenty chemicals were tested for irritancy. Dosages are reported for organics (alcohols,

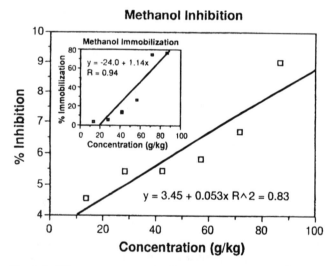

Methanol Inhibition

Figure 2. Effect of chemical addition on *Tetrahymena* swimming patterns, test results in aqueous media as a function of methanol concentration between 0 and 100 g/kg: Percent inhibition is the calculated reduction in swimming (forward) velocity, $P = 100(v - v_c/v)$, where, v_c is the control velocity with no chemical addition, and v is the measured velocity with methanol. Percent immobilization is the calculated reduction in the number of cells swimming, $P = 100 (n - n_c/n)$, where n is the control number of motile cells with no chemical addition and n is the measured number with methanol.

ketones) as well as salts. To compare different assay results, we adopt the scoring formalism developed by Silverman.[1] Tolerated doses are found based on whether a particular applied chemical yields 10% (low dose) or 90% (high dose) of the cells immobile. In this way, a direct comparison is feasible between lab technician scoring of abnormal swimming versus computerized cell tracking. Additionally, test results for the aggregation assay supplement this comparison, but instead of rendering a percentage of motile cells, the disappearance of macroscopic aggregation pattern signals the tolerated chemical dose. More toxic dosages disperse pattern formation by reducing cell mobility. All assays are effectively measuring cell swimming, whether the endpoint is direct single-cell trajectories or the overall indirect indicator of cell aggregation.

As a function of chemical concentration, a representative organic (methanol, Figure 2) and salt (dimethyl sulfoxide, DMSO, Figure 3) are tested using the computerized assay. The curve of concentration (μg/kg) generally follows an increasing trend for both the percent of cells immobilized and the percent of swimming inhibition. Higher concentrations generally react biologically to hinder cell movement. No saturation effect at high concentration (up to 100 μg/kg) appears in the *Tetrahymena* system. A summary for all the chemicals is shown in Table 1 for organics and salts and classified graphically by chemical family (Figure 4) and rank order toxicity (Figure 5)

To evaluate the assay results, Figures 4 and 5 compare toxic thresholds for previously developed assays. Both the computerized and aggregation assays were carried out on identically grown cultures. Lab technician scoring was evaluated directly from previous results[7] and compared with standard in vivo results. A comprehensive report for five representative chemicals is shown in Figure 6. The enlarged shaded region indicates that a lower average dose can be evaluated

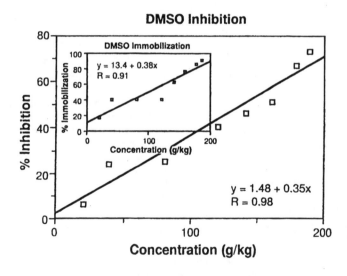

Figure 3. Effect of chemical addition on *Tetrahymena* swimming patterns, test results in aqueous media as a function of methanol concentration between 0 and 100 g/kg. Percent inhibition is the calculated reduction in swimming (forward) velocity, $P = 100(v - v_c/v)$, where v_c is the control velocity with no chemical addition, and v is the measured velocity with DMSO. Percent immobilization is the calculated reduction in the number of cells swimming, $P = 100(n - n_c/n_c)$, where n_c is the control number of motile cells with no chemical addition and n is the measured number with DMSO.

Table 1. Rank Order Toxicity for 20 Organics and Salts from Computerized Assay

Chemical	10% Motile	90% Motile (HTD)	Computer (ATD)	Rank order	Silverman
Ethylene glycol	1.000	17.500	18.500	1	11.000
Ethanol	5.310	18.800	24.100	2	13.000
Isopropanol	78.000	22.500	30.300	3	
Methanol	1.000	38.900	39.900	4	
Dimethyl sulfoxide (DMSO)	1.000	46.500	47.500	5	9.300
3-Methyl 2-butanone	18.900	40.000	58.900	6	
Isobutyl acetone	1.000	79.400	71.400	7	19.300
Methyl isobutyl ketone	13.800	58.300	72.100	8	
2-Methyl 1-propanol	1.000	78.000	79.000	9	
Methyl ethyl ketone	34.800	55.900	90.700	10	60.000
Acetyl acetone	31.200	122.000	153.000	11	
Butanol	33.000	170.000	203.000	12	
Bleach	44.600	346.000	391.000	13	
Diethylanoamine	120.000	284.000	404.000	14	
2-Octanone	250.000	308.000	558.000	15	
Nonanol	178.000	801.000	979.000	16	
1-Pentanol	321.000	687.000	1,008.000	17	
Heptanol	694.000	2,250.000	2,944.000	18	
2-Methyl 1-butanol	963.000	2,275.000	3,238.000	19	
Hexanol	2,000.000	13,000.000	15,000.000	20	

Note. Toxicity scores shown as the tolerated dose (dilution factor) which immobilized (a) d_{high}, 90% of the swimming cells (high dose); (b) d_{low}, 10% of the swimming cells (low dose); (c) the average dose as the reciprocal sum of the high and low dose ($1/d_{avg} = 1/d_{high} + 1/d_{low}$). Rank orders shown for 20 organics (alcohol, ketones, ethers, esters) and salts.

for toxic detection using the computerized assay compared to aggregation methods. The computer scoring method likewise signals positively at lower doses compared to scoring by the lab technician method (see Figure 7).

The most illustrative comparison between different methods can be constructed using a simple three-outcome score (see Table 2). For dilution factors of 0–100%, if a chemical reaction (toxic response) ccurs only for high (0–30%) dilutions, then the chemical is scored as mild. Alternatively for medium dosages (30–60% dilutions), a reaction indicates moderate toxicity. Finally for low dosages (greater than 60% dilution) then the chemical toxicity scores as severe. To evaluate an average tolerated dose, reciprocal dilutions are summed for high and low values that deliver toxic reactions, with the high dose leaving 10% of cells mobile and the low dose leaving 90% of cells mobile. The computerized assay delivers these averages in an automated fashion and final results are shown in Figure 8.

DISCUSSION

Using computerized scoring of cell motility, the present method differs from previous approaches in its speed (just 10 min from refrigeration to incubation to computerized evaluation of chemical toxicity), its ease of use (as easy as aqueous transfer), and its laboratory stability (several months shelf-life). Using computerized evaluation provides a documented report of toxicity in a labor-free (completely automated) and low-cost (pennies per test) apparatus.

Among the advantages of the motility assay apparatus (MAA) are: (1) instant results in a ready-to-use quality-controlled system of microorganisms;[11] (2) quantitative reporting that delivers a specific range of swimming changes upon chemical addition; (3) ease of use that requires only push-button effort to give documented toxicity evaluation and reporting; (4) real economy (Table 3), eliminating biological growth periods of several days (no more trial-and-error dilution of

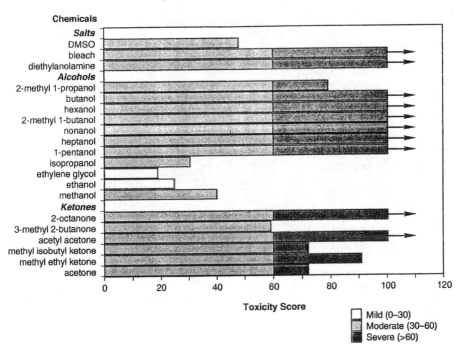

Figure 4. Toxicity scores arranged by chemical families for computerized assay results. Dilution factors (*x*) of 1:*x* that immobilized 10% and 90% of the motile cells are reciprocally summed in agreement with Silverman. Chemicals that immobilize for dilutions less than 30-fold are mild. 30 to 60-fold are moderate, greater than 60-fold are severe. Arrows indicate severe toxicity, which immobilized at trace composition for dilutions greater than 60-fold in yeast media.

suspensions to achieve desired cell counts, thus transforming lengthy technician scoring into a single objective result); (5) safety that minimizes technician handling and exposure to potentially hazardous chemicals; and finally (6) reliability, including high enough speed evaluations to make many repetitions of results realistic to perform.

Alternative applications of the MAA include: (1) an alternative to Draize rabbit eye test for cosmetic testing; (2) research tool for pollution monitoring in organic and heavy metal detection; (3) chemical safety data for federal monitoring; and (4) a standardized test for (a) growth promotion, (b) bacteriostatis, (c) effectiveness testing of antimicrobial preservatives and disinfectants, (d) microbial limit tests, and (e) media quality control in biotechnology, cleanroom testing, clinical, environmental, food and beverage, industrial, pharmaceutical, and cosmetic tests.

To summarize, the present results surveyed three alternative embodiments for testing chemical toxicity on single-cell swimming behavior. The alternatives gave results similar to existing in vivo results when adapted to a three-tiered scoring scheme (mild, moderate, and severe). In all chemicals tested (both organics and salts), the computerized assay gave equal or lower thresholds for detecting toxicity (reported as dosages that immobilize a percentage of cell activity). Given the potential time- and money-saving possibilities of an automated method, the computerized assay should receive further consideration as a scientifically competitive evaluator of chemical toxicity.

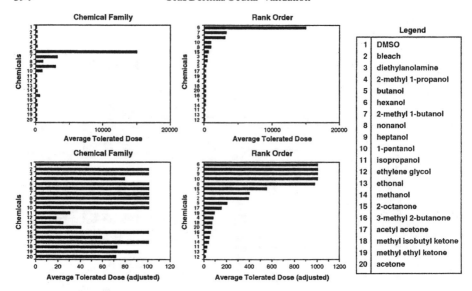

Figure 5. Toxicity scores for 20 organics and salts arranged by chemical family and rank order from computerized assay. Results shown as average tolerated doses with (lower) adjusted orders indicated in bottom graphs showing the finer details of chemical comparisons (e.g., thresholded higher toxicity like hexanol shown at arbitrary cutoff at 100 or 1000.)

Table 2. Comparison of Irritancy Rankings (Mild, Moderate, Severe) Among the Four Assay Methods

Chemical	Score			Irritancy			
	Computer	Aggregation	Silverman	Computerized	Aggregation	Silverman	In vivo
N-Butanol	203.000	168.000	64.000	Severe	Severe	Severe	Moderate
Ethanol	24.100	38.000	13.000	Mild	Mild	Mild	Mild
Ethylene glycol	18.500	29.000	11.000	Mild	Mild	Mild	Mild
Methyl ethyl ketone	90.700	111.000	71.000	Severe	Severe	Severe	Moderate?
Acetone	71.400	30.000	19.300	Moderate	Mild	Mild	Moderate

Note. Results refer to single-cell swimming behavior of *Tetrahymena* scored with cell tracking (computerized assay), microscopic method using lab technicians (Silverman), aggregation patterns (bioconvection assay). Single-cell results are compared to standard Draize tests (in vivo) as reported in Silverman.

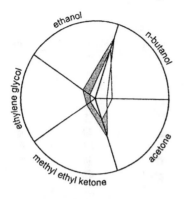 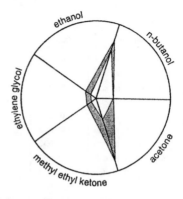

Figure 6. Graphical comparison of assay sensitivity for *Tetrahymena*. The circle perimeter correspond to an average tolerated dilution of 100% (no chemical), and the central point to 0%. The shaded region (polygon) indicates that computerized results (larger polygon) have equal or better dose discriminiation compared to models of either swimming aggregation (Noever) or lab technician (Silverman). The exception is a more sensitive aggregation test for acetone.

in vivo / in vitro	Mild	Moderate	Severe
Mild	0	0	1
Moderate	0	0	3
Severe	5	2	1

Figure 7. Graphical comparison of assay sensitivity for *Tetrahymena* versus in vivo rabbit irritancy. Three test outcomes (mild, moderate, and severe) are shown as a matrix. In vitro refers to the number of counts for the standard 20 chemicals that score in that test rating (e.g., mild). Ideal correspondence between in vivo and in vitro results would fill the central diagonal with chemicals but leave the nondiagonal elements equal to zero. Since the matrix results generally fill the higher columns and lower rows (a "bottom-heavy" matrix), the in vivo tests can be understood to give a more sensitive assay.

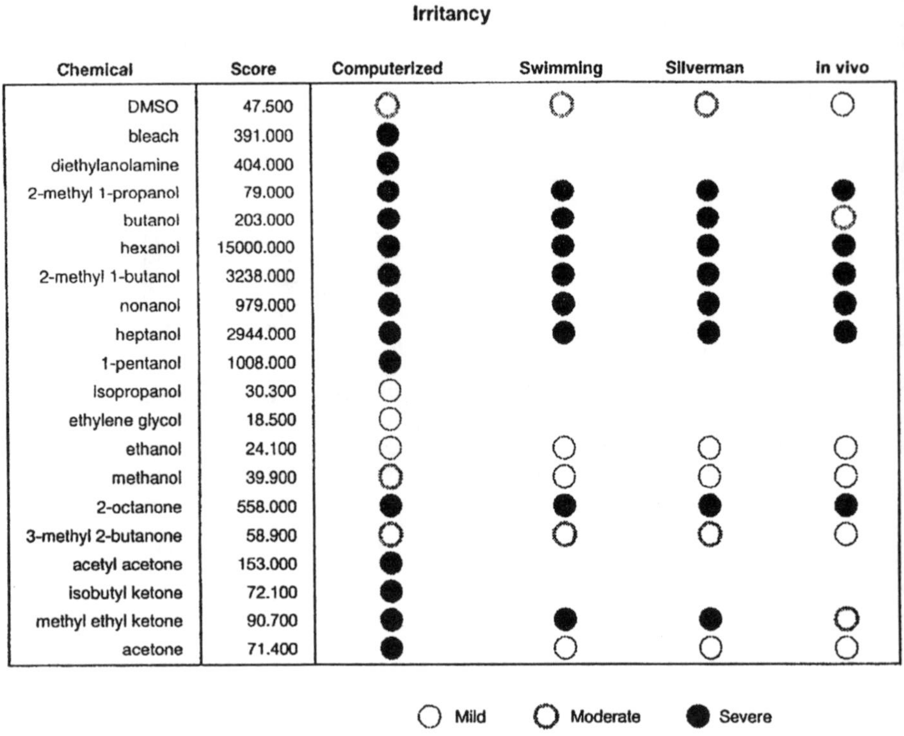

Irritancy

Chemical	Score	Computerized	Swimming	Silverman	In vivo
DMSO	47.500	○	○	○	○
bleach	391.000	●			
diethylanolamine	404.000	●			
2-methyl 1-propanol	79.000	●	●	●	●
butanol	203.000	●	●	●	○
hexanol	15000.000	●	●	●	●
2-methyl 1-butanol	3238.000	●	●	●	●
nonanol	979.000	●	●	●	●
heptanol	2944.000	●	●	●	●
1-pentanol	1008.000	●			
isopropanol	30.300	○			
ethylene glycol	18.500	○			
ethanol	24.100	○	○	○	○
methanol	39.900	○	○	○	○
2-octanone	558.000	●	●	●	●
3-methyl 2-butanone	58.900	○	○	○	○
acetyl acetone	153.000	●			
isobutyl ketone	72.100	●			
methyl ethyl ketone	90.700	●	●	●	○
acetone	71.400	●	○	○	○

○ Mild   ○ Moderate   ● Severe

Figure 8. Summary comparison for assay methods from the 20 chemicals. Toxicity scored as mild, moderate, and severe. Score reported as average tolerated dose for computerized assay with *Tetrahymena.* Identical performance for all assays would correspond to similar rankings in a single row.

Table 3. Cost Comparison Between In Vivo and In Vitro Tests for Labor Time Only in Assessing Chemical Irritancy

	Cost and time savings	
	Conventional method (in vivo)	Motility assay
Preparation time	months to days (2 to 3 days)	10 min
Analyst performance time[a]	22.5 min	0.5 min
Materials		
Supplies	2.50	0.05
Culture	8.00	8.00
Labor[b]	9.45	0.21
Total	19.95	8.26

[a] Based on performance times of similar tasks as cited in Working Time Units Catalog (Department of Labor, 1992).[12]
[b] Assume analyst salary, benefits, and overhead of $25 (U.S.)/hour.

References

1. Silverman, J., and Pennisi, S. 1987. Evaluation of *Tetrahymena thermophila* as an in vitro alternative to ocular irritation studies in rabbits. *J. Toxicol. Cutaneous Ocul. Toxicol.* 6:33–42.
2. Silverman, J. 1983. Preliminary findings on the use of protozooa (*Tetrahymena thermophila*) as models for ocular irritation testing in rabbits. *Lab. Anim. Sci.* 33:56–59.
3. Noever, D. A., and Matsos, H. C. 1991. A bioassay for monitoring cadmium based on bioconvective patterns. *J. Environ. Sci. Health* A26:273.

4. Noever, D. A., 1991. Fractal dynamics of bioconvective patterns. *J. Phys. Soc. Jpn.* 60:3573–3581.
5. Noever, D. A. 1991. Evolution of bioconvection patterns in variable gravity. *Phys. Rev.* A44:4491–4501.
6. Starr, R. C., and Zeikus, J. A. 1987. UTEX Culture Collection. *J. Phycol. (Suppl.)* 23:39.
7. Hill, D. L. 1972. *The biochemistry and physiology of* Tetrahymena. New York: Academic Press.
8. Roberts, R. O., and Berk, S. G. 1990. Development of a protozoan chemoattraction bioassy for evaluating toxicity of aquatic pollutants. *Tox. Assess.* 5:279.
9. Noever, D. A. 1991. Fractal patterns in bioconvecting cells of *Euglena gracilis. J. Phys. Soc. Jpn.* 59:276–280.
10. Weaire, D., and Rivier, N. 1984. Soaps, cells and statistics. *Contemp. Phys.* 25:73–91.
11. Nillson, J. R. 1989. *Tetrahymena* in cytotoxicology. *Eur. J. Protist.* 25:2–21.
12. U.S. Department of Labor. 1992. Working time units catalog U.S. Government Printing Office DOL-2789. Washington, DC, p. 671.

Chapter Forty-one

RENAL ALTERATIONS FOLLOWING SUBLETHAL MERCURY TOXICITY: A FISH MODEL FOR AQUATIC ENVIRONMENTAL CONTAMINATION

R. Reimschuessel and C. M. Gonzalez

Although attempts have been made to reduce mercury point-source discharges, many contaminated sites still contain elevated mercury levels. Mercury is extremely toxic to aquatic animals and bioaccumulates through the food chain. We are currently studying the effect sublethal levels of mercury have on the kidneys of fish. Goldfish were given intraperitoneal injections of 12 μg/g mercury(II) chloride. Fish were sacrificed at 1, 4, 14, and 21 d following injection. Prior to sacrifice fish were given intraperitoneal injections of bromodeoxyuridine (BrdU) to label DNA-synthesizing cells. Tissues were preserved in 10% neutral buffered formalin. Within 24 h, the proximal tubules had undergone extensive swelling and necrosis. Within 4 d the tubular epithelium had sloughed off the basement membrane. A regenerative epithelium of flattened basophilic cells began to repopulate the damaged nephrons at this point. Within 14 d entirely new nephrons formed from basophilic cell clusters located in the interstitium, totally independent from the preexisting injured nephrons. These nephrons continued to develop through 21 d. BrdU labeling was extensive in these new nephrons, indicating rapid cell proliferation. The formation of new nephrons following renal injury is a response unique to fish and is not seen in mammalian models of renal injury. Since the development of new nephrons occurs several weeks following the toxic event, it can serve as a biomarker for sublethal nephrotoxic agents intermittently released into the environment.

INTRODUCTION

The regenerative capacity of the mammalian kidney following nephrotoxicant-induced injury is well documented.[1] The denuded basement membrane is repopulated by migration and proliferation of the remaining cells. A mature cuboidal epithelium develops from flattened basophilic cells, which migrate along the intact basement membrane, divide, and differentiate into the various segments of the nephron.

Compensatory renal hypertrophy following unilateral nephrectomy involves primarily hypertrophy of the tubular epithelium in the remaining kidney. There is only minimal epithelial-cell hyperplasia.[2] Neither regeneration nor compensatory hypertrophy in mammals includes the formation of new nephrons.

The present study characterizes the regenerative response of the goldfish kidney to a nephrotoxic dose of mercuric chloride.

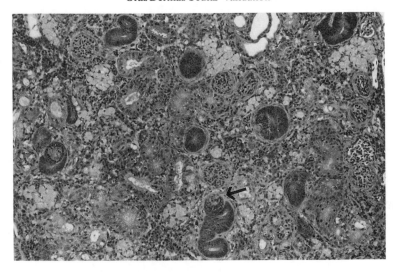

Figure 1. Goldfish kidney, 14 d following mercuric chloride administration (12 μg/g) Note the deeply staining developing tubules with narrow lumens. A developing glomerulus can be seen at one end of the longest tubule pictured. (Hematoxylin and eosin, ×160.)

METHODS

Goldfish (4–6 in) were given a single intraperitoneal (ip) injection of mercury(II) chloride (12 μg/g). Fish were sacrificed 1, 4, 14, and 21 d postinjection. Four hours prior to sacrifice they received bromodeoxyuridine (BrdU, 100 mg/kg ip). Kidneys were removed and fixed in 10% phosphate-buffered formalin. Tissues were embedded in paraffin and sections were stained with hematoxylin and eosin. Immunohistochemistry localized cells that had incorporated BrdU in S phase.[3]

RESULTS

During the first days postinjection, massive necrosis occurred in the proximal tubules. Tubules were dilated and contained cell debris with pyknotic nuclei. Within the first week following the injection injured tubules remained dilated but their lumens were clear of debris. The denuded basement membrane is covered by a flattened, basophilic epithelium. This response is similar to that of the mammalian kidney.

Two weeks following the injection, numerous basophilic tubules developed (Figure 1). These arise from small basophilic cell clusters similar to renal vesicles of mammalian embryos. The tubules penetrate into the existing collecting ducts. Mitotic figures and large numbers of bromodeoxyuridine-stained nuclei were present in these developing nephrons.

CONCLUSIONS

Increasingly investigators have recommended histopathologic examination of fish tissues for lesions caused by environmental contaminants.[4,5] The presence of developing nephrons in mature wild fish may serve as a biomarker for nephrotoxic compounds, such as mercury, in the aquatic environment.

References

1. Toback, G. F. 1992. Regeneration after acute tubular necrosis. *Kidney Int.* 41:226–246.
2. Fine, L. 1986. The biology of renal hypertrophy. *Kidney Int.* 29:619–634.

3. Reimschuessel, R., Bennett, R. O., May, E. B., and Lipsky, M. M. 1990. Renal tubular cell regeneration, cell proliferation and chronic nephrotoxicity in the goldfish (*Carassius auratus*) following exposure to a single sublethal dose of hexachlorobutadiene. *Dis. Aquatic Organisms* 8:211–224.
4. Malins, D. C., McCain, B. B., Landahl, J. T., Myers, M. S., Krahn, M. M., Brown, D. W., Chan, S. L., and Roubal, W. T. 1988. Neoplastic and other diseases in fish in relation to toxic chemicals: An overview. *Aquatic Toxicol.* 11:43–67.
5. Hinton, D. E., Lantz, R. C., Hampton, J. A., McCuskey, P. R., and McCuskey, R. S. 1987. Normal versus abnormal structure: Considerations in morphologic responses of teleosts to pollutants. *Environ. Health Perspect.* 71:139–146.

Chapter Forty-two

A NONLETHAL, ANESTHETIZED CANINE MODEL USED TO REDUCE THE NUMBER OF ANIMALS REQUIRED TO EVALUATE THE EFFECTIVENESS OF PRETREATMENT COMPOUNDS CHALLENGED WITH TOXIC CONCENTRATIONS OF CYANIDE

J. A. Vick, M. T. Marino, L. D. Brown, A. Kaminskis, J. von Bredow, and T. Brewer

Acute cyanide intoxication leads to a momentary increase in both the rate and the amplitude of respiration, followed by a sudden cessation of respiration leading to death in the untreated casualty. The most common model used to study acute cyanide poisoning has been the administration of a lethal intravenous bolus of either sodium or potassium cyanide. This model has proven to be extremely reproducible and represents the most severe challenge for evaluating new forms of prophylaxis or therapy. Inhalation of cyanide leads to a similar onset of toxic symptoms and is automatically controlled by the rate and depth of breathing. This cyanide-induced halt in respiration also stops the absorption of the cyanide, leading to a well-defined, consistent endpoint as to the amount of cyanide absorbed. Regardless of the amount of cyanide in the ambient air, the casualty can only absorb cyanide while still breathing. Therefore, a slow intravenous infusion of cyanide, continued only until respiratory arrest, should reach the same experimental level of cyanide intoxication. Anesthetized dogs infused with sodium cyanide until respiratory arrest provided the basis for the development of a useful, reusable animal test model. Survival of the animal was assured by treatment with hydroxylamine 20 mg/kg intramuscular, 30 s after respiratory arrest. The amount of cyanide required to produce respiratory arrest (1.2 ± 0.06 mg/kg) as well as the corresponding blood cyanide levels (3.7 ± 0.5 μg/ml) was consistent in repeat trials of the same animal and between animals of the same species. Pretreatment with 5 mg/kg sodium nitrite produces 3.0 ± 0.2% methemoglobin, which doubles the amount of cyanide required to produce respiratory arrest. Using respiratory arrest as a surrogate endpoint provides a nontraumatic, reproducible model to estimate the lethal level of cyanide in each dog as well as defining the protective index of potential pretreatment and antidotal compounds.

INTRODUCTION

The potential of intoxication by cyanide remains a major problem for military forces and civilian poison control centers.[1-3] The inhalation of hydrogen cyanide as a chemical warfare agent and the inhalation of cyanides emanating from fires continues to be a realistic concern that must be met with adequate prophylaxis and therapy. The evaluation of effective concepts of pretreatment or therapy is dependent upon the ability to monitor cyanide intoxication and the reversal of intoxication in an appropriate animal model.

Acute cyanide intoxication leads to a momentary increase in the rate and amplitude of respiration followed by a very sudden halt in respiration.[4,5] The halt in respiration is followed by a fall in heart rate and blood pressure, which rapidly fade to cardiac arrest, if spontaneous respiration is not reinitiated through the rapid application of an effective cyanide antidote.

The inhalation of hydrogen cyanide leads to a similar acute onset of toxic signs, which is controlled by the rate and depth of respiration.[6] The cyanide-induced halt in respiration also stops the continued inhalation of cyanide, leading to a well-defined, consistent endpoint of the amount of cyanide absorbed. Regardless of the abundance of cyanide in the ambient air, the victim can only absorb cyanide during respiration. The halt in respiration is correlated with the blood level of cyanide required to induce respiratory arrest. A slow intravenous infusion of cyanide, which is continued only until respiratory arrest is achieved, should define the same limit of cyanide intoxication.

The system developed in the current study of cyanide intoxication utilizes a slow intravenous infusion of cyanide, which is halted as soon as respiration stops. In this animal model a lethal dose of cyanide is defined as the amount of cyanide that must be infused to cause respiratory arrest.

The halt in respiration provides a well-defined endpoint of cyanide intoxication. The halt in respiration occurs several minutes before the animal would succumb to the cyanide-induced cardiovascular collapse. The time interval between cyanide-induced respiratory arrest and cyanide-induced cardiovascular collapse provides sufficient time to administer specific therapy that will ensure recovery and survival of the animal model.

The certainty of recovery of the animal model after intoxication by lethal concentrations of cyanide by the rapid administration of specific therapy encourages the possibility of repeat exposure of the same animal to the same infusion of cyanide. The repeat exposure of the same animal under identical conditions will provide a more reliable comparison of the effectiveness of various forms of therapy. The repeat exposure of the same animal to toxic levels of cyanide followed by recovery also leads to a significant reduction in the total number of animals required to provide an accurate evaluation of the effectiveness of a new pretreatment or antidote.

METHODS

Adult beagle dogs (9–12 kg) anesthetized with pentobarbital (32 mg/kg iv) were intubated and fitted with a pneumotachometer for the recording of respiration. Intravenous catheters (venocath) were placed in the jugular vein for the collection of blood samples and in the saphenous vein for the infusion of cyanide solutions. Blood samples were monitored for total cyanide levels[7] and methemoglobin activity (Radiometer, OSM-3 modified for canine blood).

Intravenous infusion of cyanide was carried out at a rate of 0.7 mg/kg/min until respiratory arrest occurred; therapy was applied 0.5 min after the onset of respiratory arrest. Therapy consisted of an intramuscular injection of hydroxylamine hydrochloride (20 mg/kg), and pretreatment comprised an im injection of 5 mg/kg sodium nitrite administered 30 min before exposure to sodium cyanide. The duration of respiration during the infusion of cyanide was monitored and calculated from physiological recordings.

RESULTS

When cyanide is infused to anesthetized dogs at a constant rate of 0.7 mg/kg/min there is a consistent increase in the rate of respiration, which continues for 103 s and is followed by a sudden halt in respiration. Respiratory arrest is correlated with a whole blood cyanide concentration of 3.7 μg/ml. The halt in respiration is reversed within 3 min following the intramuscular injection of 20 mg/kg hydroxylamine hydrochloride, leading to the resumption of respiration as illustrated in one dog in Figure 1.

When the treated animal is provided a 1-wk recovery period and then the same animal is reexposed to the same intravenous infusion of sodium cyanide, the subsequent exposure requires

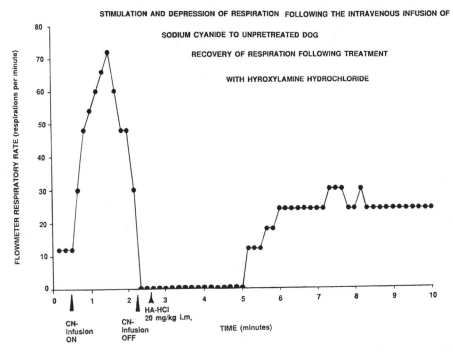

Figure 1. Increase in the rate of respiration is initiated within seconds after the introduction of cyanide, followed by as sudden decline and halt in respiration. The cyanide infusion is terminated within 5 s after respiratory arrest. Hydroxylamine hydrochloride therapy is injected intramuscularly 30 s after the termination of cyanide infusion. Spontaneous recovery of respiration occurs in less than 3 min.

a similar duration (105 s) of the 0.7 mg/kg/min infusion of sodium cyanide to induce respiratory arrest. In 12 control experiments the respiratory arrest dose of sodium cyanide was 1.21 ± 0.06 mg/kg.

Pretreatment of the animal with 5 mg/kg sodium nitrite im induces a minimal amount of methemoglobin (3.0%), which is able to sustain respiration for a longer period of cyanide infusion and to double the period of cyanide administration before the onset of respiratory arrest.[8,9] The increased period of cyanide administration resulted in a greater blood cyanide concentration (13.2 μg/ml) as shown in Figure 3. The enhanced duration of respiration in the presence of methemoglobin pretreatment is shown in the same animal in Figure 2. In 8 animal trials the respiratory arrest dose of sodium cyanide was increased to 2.45 ± 0.37 mg/kg by pretreating the animals with 5 mg/kg of sodium nitrite.

Methemoglobin pretreatment provides protection of the animal model against cyanide intoxication. Figure 3 illustrates the whole-blood level of cyanide in the control animal (open circles) and the blood cyanide levels (filled diamonds) in the same animal pretreated with 5 mg/kg of sodium nitrite. The elevated blood level of cyanide is due to the increased administration of cyanide associated with the increased duration of respiration in the presence of 3.0% methemoglobin.

The enhanced duration of respiration in the presence of methemoglobin pretreatment and the increased amount of cyanide infused to induce respiratory arrest can be used to develop a "protective ratio." Methemoglobin pretreatment at only 3.0% can provide a protective ratio of 2.0.

DISCUSSION

Acute cyanide intoxication has most often been modeled through the bolus intravenous administration of a lethal amount of sodium or potassium cyanide. This system provides the most reproduc-

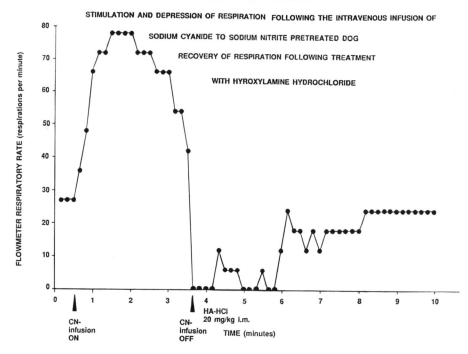

Figure 2. Effect of methemoglobin pretreatment on the duration of respiration during the infusion of cyanide solution to the same animal shown in Figure 1. The duration of respiration was double the control period and allowed twice as much cyanide to be administered before cyanide infusion was terminated.

ible effects and represents the most severe challenge to any new form of prophylaxis and therapy. Only the most rapidly acting methemoglobin formers have demonstrated the ability to save animals that have been intoxicated by a bolus injection of cyanide.

Cyanide intoxication by inhalation should be correlated with the duration of respiration. When respiration is arrested as a result of the inhalation of a toxic agent, the administration of the toxic agent should cease. The slow intravenous infusion of a solution of sodium cyanide until respiration ceases provides a more realistic approach to modeling the inhalation of cyanide and provides an exact endpoint in each individual animal. In contrast, the bolus intravenous administration of the same toxic dose of cyanide unrelated to the toxic effects of cyanide leads to a requirement to utilize the final irreversible lethal event as the sole indicator of toxicity.

Respiratory arrest during the intravenous infusion of cyanide provides a definite endpoint to stop cyanide infusion. The respiratory arrest endpoint is a surrogate endpoint for a known lethal event. The respiratory arrest endpoint can be used to initiate and evaluate the effectiveness of candidate antidotes.

The sodium cyanide infusion has been carried out repeatedly in the same animal, leading to a consistent respiratory arrest response and a consistent recovery of the animal following therapy with a methemoglobin-forming compound. The respiratory arrest response is consistent within each animal and between animals.

The model provides a nonlethal, nontraumatic approach in an anesthetized canine model to approximate a normally lethal event. The nembutal-anesthetized animals do not endure convulsions, and recovery from anesthesia is not delayed as a result of the exposure to cyanide.

Treatment of cyanide intoxication required only the temporary formation of methemoglobin with hydroxylamine,[9] no additional therapy with sodium thiosulfate was required to ensure complete recovery.

The model demonstrates the effectiveness of methemoglobin pretreatment by allowing the

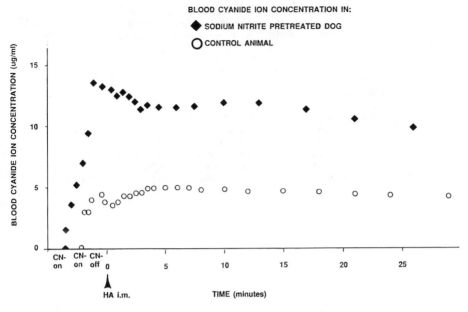

Figure 3. Blood cyanide ion concentrations during the infusion of cyanide in the unpretreated control animal and during the infusion of cyanide to the same animal pretreated with the methemoglobin-forming compound sodium nitrite.

animal to breathe longer and to endure greater levels of cyanide before respiratory arrest occurred. The same rate of recovery of the animal occurred following therapy when the animal was pretreated with a methemoglobin-forming compound.

The efficacy of a pretreatment or antidote is often defined as a ratio between the LD50 of the toxic agent in the control animal and the LD50 in an animal protected by a pretreatment regimen or an animal resuscitated by an antidote. Most improved concepts of lethality estimation focus on a reduction in the number of animals required to provide a realistic LD50 estimate. The animal model proposed in this presentation provides a reduction in the total number of animals required and a refinement in an endpoint that does not lead to the lethality required in the classical LD50 and other modified LD50 estimates.[10]

The repeated exposure of the same animal to the respiratory arrest infusion of cyanide and resuscitation with therapy demonstrates within-animal reproducibility. Utilization of the same animal for multiple trials reduces the total number of animals required for each pretreatment evaluation.

CONCLUSION

A nontraumatic, nonlethal, repeated-testing, anesthetized canine model has been developed to approximate cyanide toxicity and to evaluate the effectiveness of new pretreatment regimens.

The nonlethal model demonstrates refinement of the classical and alternative lethal LD50 estimates. The repeated testing capability of the model provides a marked reduction in the total number of animals required to evaluate new pretreatments and antidotes.

References

1. Clark, C., Campbell, D., and Reid, W. 1981. Blood carboxyhaemoglobin and cyanide levels in fire survivors. *Lancet* 1:1332–1335.
2. Wolnik, K., Fricke, F., Bonnin, E., Gaston, C., and Salzger, R. 1984. The Tylenol tampering incident— Tracing the source. *Anal. Chem.* 56:466–474.

3. Gander, T. J. 1987. *NBC: Nuclear, biological and chemical warfare.* New York: Hippocrene.

4. Klimmek, R., Fladerer, H., and Weger, N. 1979. Circulation, respiration, and blood homeostasis in cyanide-poisoned dogs after treatment with 4-dimethylaminophenol or cobalt compounds. *Arch. Toxicol.* 43:121–133.

5. Comroe, J. M. 1974. *Physiology of respiration,* pp. 57–94. Chicago: Year Book.

6. Ballantyne, B. 1984. Comparative acute toxicity of hydrogen cyanide and its salts. *Proc. Fourth Annu. Chemical Defense Bioscience Rev.* ed. R. Lindstrom. pp. 47–63. Aberdeen, MD: U.S. Army Medical Research Institute of Chemical Defense.

7. Groff, W. A., Kaminskis, A., and Coccinell, S.A. 1985. Simultaneous determination of methemoglobin and total hemoglobin by a continuous-flow method. *Clin. Toxicol.* 23:133–163.

8. Klaassen, C. D. 1995. In *The pharmacological basis of therapeutics,* eds. A. G. Gillman, T. W. Rall, A. S. Nies, and P. Taylor, 8th ed., p. 1630. New York: Pergamon Press.

9. Kruazyna, R., Krusyna, H., and Smith, R. 1982. Comparison of hydroxylamine, 4-dimethylaminophenol and nitrite protection against cyanide poisoning in mice. *Arch. Toxicol.* 49:191–202.

10. Salem, H. 1995. *Animal test alternatives: Refinement, reduction, replacement.* New York: Marcel Dekker.

Chapter Forty-three

CONFOCAL MICROSCOPY AND CALCIUM IMAGES OF KERATINOCYTES EXPOSED TO SULFUR MUSTARD

Robert J. Werrlein, J. S. Madren-Whalley,

S. D. Kirby, and M. A. E. Mol

Human epidermal keratinocytes (HEK) were grown on glass coverslips as primary cultures in a medium containing low levels of extracellular calcium (0.15 mM). Cultures preloaded with the Ca²⁺ chelator and fluorescent probe Indo-1AM were subjected to image analysis using a Meridian ACAS-570 laser cytometer. Images were obtained from control populations and populations exposed to 400 μM sulfur mustard in low (0.15 mM) and high (1.02 mM) calcium buffers. Results indicate that (1) HEK cells loaded differently with Indo-1AM depending on their relative state of differentiation and (2) acute simultaneous exposure to sulfur mustard and high calcium altered intracellular calcium activity and selective permeability of the plasma membrane.

INTRODUCTION

Incremental changes of extracellular calcium, even changes as small as 0.02 mM, can rapidly alter intracellular calcium activity and profoundly influence growth and differentiation of mouse and human keratinocytes.[1-4] It is, therefore, interesting that calcium gradients exist in the epidermis[5,6] and that differentiation of keratinocytes in vivo may be closely linked to those gradients.[7] Ion-capture cytochemistry and particle probe analysis of the skin indicate that the lowest concentrations of extracellular calcium are detected at the level of the basal cells, and that calcium concentrations become progressively higher in the suprabasal layers. When keratinocytes are grown to confluence in culture medium with <0.1 mM calcium and intentionally challenged with concentrations of calcium >1.0 mM, they undergo an early 2- to 2.5-fold increase in intracellular free calcium[8] with subsequent changes in phenotypic expression of cell-specific proteins and plasma membrane markers.[9,10] Since epidermal calcium gradients can be disrupted by acetone and lesions of the skin,[11] it seems reasonable to ask whether cellular response to sulfur mustard can be affected by the calcium microenvironment. In the following study of human epidermal keratinocytes, calcium images were recorded by confocal microscopy and analyzed to determine the effects of sulfur mustard (HD) on basaloid cells exposed in the presence of low and high concentrations of extracellular calcium.

MATERIALS AND METHODS

Cell Cultures

Human epidermal keratinocytes (HEK) from mammary tissues were cocultured on glass coverslips with feeder layers of 3T3 mouse fibroblasts lethally pretreated with 4 μg/ml mitomycin

C. During the first week in culture, their medium was a 3:1 mixture of Dulbecco's Modified Eagle's Medium (DMEM) and Ham's F-12 supplemented with 5% FCS, 0.1 nM cholera toxin, 0.4 μg/ml hydrocortisone, 10 ng/ml epidermal growth factor, and 50 μg/ml gentamicin sulfate. On d 7, the feeder layer was removed by vigorous aspiration. HEK cultures were subsequently maintained on serum-free keratinocyte growth medium (Clonetics, San Diego, CA) containing 0.15 mM calcium. All media and additives, unless otherwise stated, were obtained from the Sigma Chemical Co., St. Louis, MO.

Control and Experimental Cultures

Cultures selected for exposure to sulfur mustard served as their own controls. In low-calcium experiments, HEK were overlaid with 1.5 ml of Krebs/HEPES buffer (pH 7.3) containing 0.15 mM CaCl$_2$ plus NaCl (110 mM), MgSO$_4$ (1 mM), KCl (5.4 mM), KH$_2$PO$_4$ (0.44 mM), NaH$_2$PO$_4$ (35 mM), glucose (5 mM), L-glutamine (2 mM), and HEPES (25 mM). For high-calcium experiments, cultures were overlaid with phosphate-buffered saline (PBS) (pH 7.3) containing 1.02 mM CaCl$_2$.

Loading Cells with Indo-1AM

Keratinocyte cultures were washed twice with prewarmed (35°C) Ham's F-12 (without serum and without phenol red). Cells were then overlaid with a loading solution containing 1 μM Indo-1AM (Molecular Probes, Eugene, OR) in 2 ml PBS with Ca^{2+} and Mg^{2+} salts and were incubated for 1 h at 35°C in a humidified atmosphere of 5% CO$_2$ and air. Unincorporated (excess) dye was removed from the culture by washing the cells twice with prewarmed Ham's F-12 (as described earlier).

Mustard Exposures

Cultures were 10–14 d old when loaded with Indo-1AM and subjected to mustard exposure. Supernatant from the control culture (1.5 ml) was removed to a glass container and mixed with 300 μl sulfur mustard (2400 μM). That mixture was immediately returned to the parent culture at a volume and concentration of 1.8 ml and 400 μM, respectively. Cells were exposed to sulfur mustard for 5 min at room temperature and were subsequently washed twice with PBS containing no calcium. HEK cultures were then overlaid with the appropriate high- or low-calcium buffer (1.5 ml) before subjecting them to postexposure image analysis.

Image Analysis

Cultures loaded with Indo-1AM were placed on the scanning table (Figure 1) of a Meridian ACAS-570 interactive laser cytometer (Meridian Instruments, Inc., Okemos, MI). Specimens were brought into focus by manual adjustment, then moved by X-Y stepper motor through the optical axis and scanned with a 355 nm line from a 5-W argon laser. Excitation and emission spectra for Indo-1 were separated by dichroic beam-splitting mirrors. Emissions from the unbound, Ca^{2+}-free Indo-1 (485 nm) were directed to detector 1, and emissions from the Ca^{2+}-bound Indo-1 (405 nm) were directed to detector 2.

Data Analysis

Images generated during the initial 10 min of each scan period were analyzed for changes in the fluorescent emissions of Ca^{2+}-bound Indo-1 (detector 2) and Ca^{2+}-free Indo-1 (detector 1). The ratios of detector 2:detector 1, that is, the calcium ratios, were analyzed and compared between experiments to determine early, postexposure effects of sulfur mustard on intracellular free calcium in the presence of low (0.15 mM) and high (1.02 mM) extracellular calcium concentrations. Slopes of the average fluorescent emissions and calcium ratio curves have been expressed as mean $\pm$ SEM. The number of samples per experiment (n) varied from 16 to 47. Results subjected to t-tests were considered significant with $p < .05$

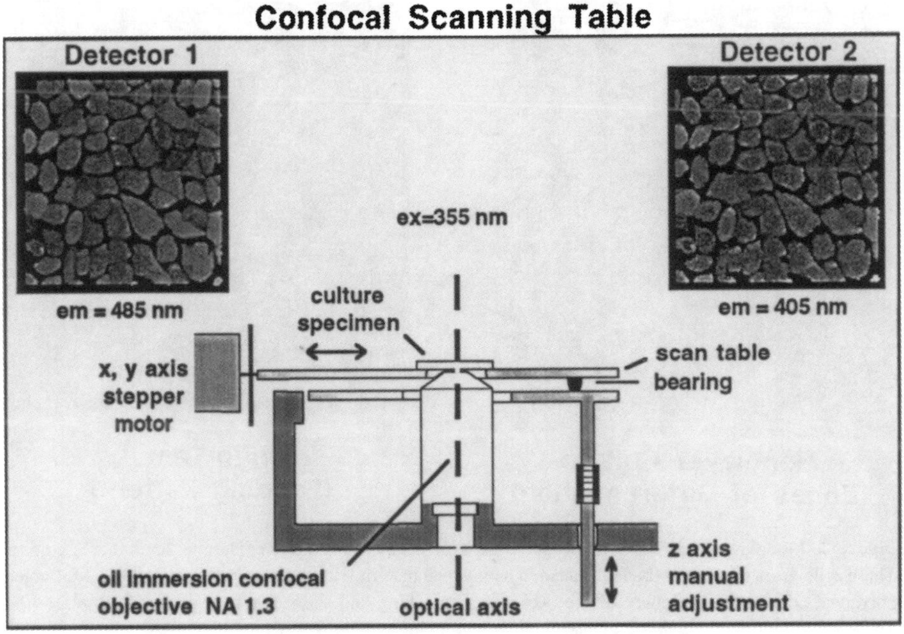

Confocal Scanning Table

Figure 1. Calcium images were produced by confocal laser microscopy using a Meridian ACAS-570 laser cytometer. Each culture of HEK cells, preloaded with 1 μM Indo-1AM, was moved by an X-Y stepper motor and scan table through the optical axis of a high numerical aperture objective lens. Fluorescent emissions produced by excitation with a 355 laser line were separated by dichroic beam splitting mirrors. Emissions of 485 nm from calcium-free Indo-1 were directed to detector 1, and emissions of 405 nm from calcium-bound Indo-1 were directed to detector 2.

RESULTS

HEK populations were observed by phase microscopy (Figure 2) to be confluent or nearly confluent on the day of experimentation. Each monolayer contained colonies and gradations of differentiated cells that varied in size and shape. HEK seed cells, which formed the core of each colony, grew in low-calcium medium to produce islands of small, compressed cells that gradually spread and gave rise to larger, polygonal cells at the periphery of converging colonies. Only the larger cells in these differentiated populations loaded with Indo-1AM. As shown (Figure 2), brightly fluorescing cells had an average long and short axis that measured 39 $\times$ 21 μm and a surface area that was approximately 800 μm^2. Poorly labeled smaller cells, located within the boundaries of the fluorescing cells, measured 33 $\times$ 16 μm with an average surface area of approximately 500 μm^2.

When HEK were maintained in a low-calcium buffer, the Ca^{2+}-bound and Ca^{2+}-free forms of Indo-1 were well contained in both the control and HD-exposed populations (Figure 3). All images had discrete margins and obvious boundaries, and each cell appeared separate and distinct from its neighbor. There were no obvious changes in morphology or calcium images following exposure to sulfur mustard. However, sulfur mustard did produce some small but measurable effects in the emissions of Ca^{2+}-free and Ca^{2+}-bound Indo-1. There was a significant ($p < .05$) decrease in the average fluorescent emissions per cell immediately after a 5-min exposure to 400 μM HD (Figure 4). The decrease was greater for detector 1 than detector 2, and produced a concomitant small increase in calcium ratios, that is, detector 2:detector 1 ratios. The latter could be due to a small increase in free calcium (Ca^{2+}-bound Indo-1) or to a decrease in Ca^{2+}-free Indo-1, or both. Decreased emissions did not occur in the unscanned areas of control populations prior to HD exposure. Precautions were taken to protect cultures from photobleaching

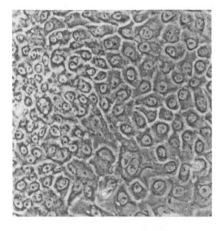
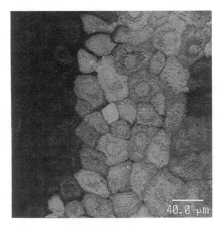

Monolayer Culture
(Zones of Differentiation)

Indo-1am
(Loading Pattern)

Figure 2. Monolayer at left is a phase photograph of a 12-d-old human epidermal keratinocyte culture. These cells, from mammary tissues, loaded in an unequal pattern with the calcium probe Indo-1AM. Larger, polygonal cells at the periphery of seed colonies had a long and short axis that averaged 39 × 21 μm. These cells were located in zones that were brightly fluorescent. Smaller cells, located within the seed colonies, measured 33 × 16 μm and did not readily incorporate the fluorescent probe.

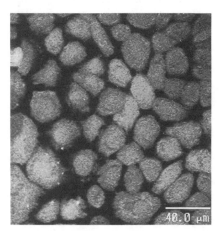
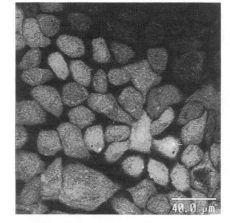

Untreated Control
Population

HD - Exposed
Population

Figure 3. HEK cells maintained in a low-calcium buffer showed no obvious change in their fluorescent, intracellular calcium images or correspondingly in their cell morphology following sulfur mustard exposure. Each image was well defined and separate from its neighbors. Cells were loaded with 1 μM Indo-1AM.

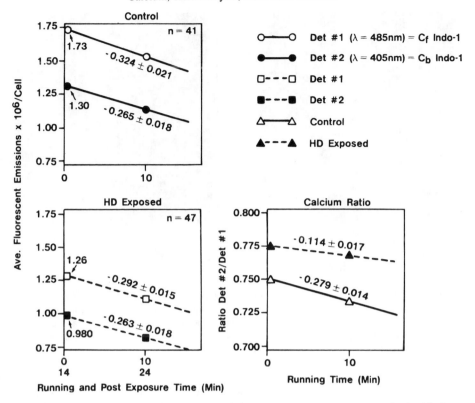

Figure 4. Sulfur mustard (400 μM) had small but significant effects on HEK cells maintained in low-calcium (0.15 mM) buffers. Compared to the control, the HD-exposed population showed a significant (p < .05) 27% decrease in the average fluorescent emissions from intracellular calcium-free C_f Indo-1 (detector 1) and a corresponding 25% decrease from calcium-bound C_b Indo-1 (detector 2). Sulfur mustard produced a concomitant small increase in detector 2:detector 1 calcium ratios. Calcium ratio analyses of detector 2:detector 1 emissions also showed that mustard caused the slope of the HD-exposed population to become less negative than that of the control population. Running and postexposure time (0–10; 14–24 min) included only images scanned during the initial 10 min of analysis.

during HD exposure by performing exposures in a light-tight container and in a darkened room. To allow for photobleaching and associated decreases in fluorescent emissions, which did occur during calcium imaging, results obtained from a series of repeated laser scans were always subjected to calcium ratio analysis.

Ratios were plotted as a function of the "running time" for analysis (10 min) and reflect the average slope (mean ± SEM) for the constituent cells (control, $n = 41$; HD-exposed, $n = 47$) of the populations analyzed. The results (Figure 4) indicate that in addition to the decrease in average fluorescent emissions and the increase in detector 2:detector 1 ratios, mustard also caused the slope of the exposed population to become less negative than that of the control population. While absolute values varied, similar changes (p <.05) were recorded in 3 replicate low-calcium experiments.

When HEK cells, maintained in low-calcium buffer, were acutely subjected to PBS, a high-calcium (1.02 mM) buffer, there was an early and obvious change in morphology (Figure 5). High calcium caused images of control populations to become larger, their shapes more polygonal, and cell margins more crowded. Despite the change in morphology, however, images retained their discrete margins and cells appeared as separate, easily analyzed units throughout a full 30-

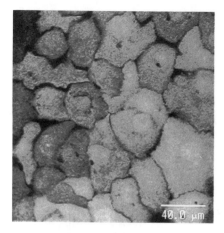

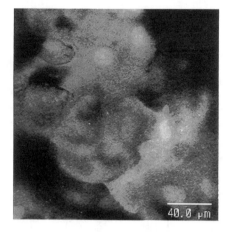

Untreated Control Population

HD - Exposed Population

Figure 5. The HEK control population (left) was acutely exposed to high-calcium PBS buffer (1.02 mM). The cells underwent a dramatic early change in size and morphology, but were able to contain the low-molecular-weight probe Indo-1 during a full 30-min study period. When exposed to 400 µM sulfur mustard (right), there was an early postexposure discharge of Indo-1, loss of cell definition, and an apparent change in the selective permeability of plasma membranes.

min study period. By contrast, HEK acutely exposed to sulfur mustard and to high calcium (1.02 mM) concentrations lost cell definition. Immediately following exposure, the Indo-1 probe was discharged or leaked from preloaded cells, and the resulting spread of fluorescence obscured their image margins. Leakage was so rapid that within the 7 min it took to locate cells on the scanning table, calcium images were blurred and discrete cells could no longer be identified. As a result, populations acutely exposed to mustard and high calcium had to be analyzed by use of superimposed polygons, drawn to approximate the shapes of underlying cells.

Comparison of high and low calcium results (Figure 6 vs. Figure 4) show that the average fluorescent emissions from Ca^{2+}-bound and Ca^{2+}-free Indo-1 became two to three times greater when HEK were acutely subjected to a high-calcium buffer. Concomitant exposure to sulfur mustard and to high calcium (Figure 6) produced a substantial, early decrease in the average number of fluorescent emissions. Detector 1 (Ca^{2+}-free Indo-1) showed a 21% decrease as the average postexposure fluorescence fell from 4.37 to 3.46 $\times$ 10^6 emissions per cell. Detector 2 (Ca^{2+}-bound Indo-1) showed a smaller 8.5% drop in fluorescence and an average decrease from 4.12 to 3.77 $\times$ 10^6 emissions per cell. The disproportionate decrease in detector 1 emissions caused detector 2:detector 1 ratios, that is, calcium ratios, to become greater than 1. Given the visible, postexposure discharge of Indo-1 from HEK (Figure 5), it is possible that calcium ratios greater than 1 reflect a substantial release of Indo-1 into an extracellular environment containing a concentration of free calcium that would favor Ca^{2+}-bound (405 nm) emissions.

DISCUSSION

Epidermal basal cells in vivo exist in a low physiological calcium environment that favors proliferation, limits differentiation, and resembles the extracellular conditions of our culture system. Ion-capture cytochemistry[5] and particle-probe analysis[6] show that increasing calcium gradients are maintained in the suprabasal layers of the skin, and that established gradients can be disrupted by chemical lesions.[11] That information lends itself to one of the most fascinating questions of sulfur mustard damage, namely, why basal cells are the specific targets of vesicating lesions. The results from our experiments may provide a clue and partial explanation to that

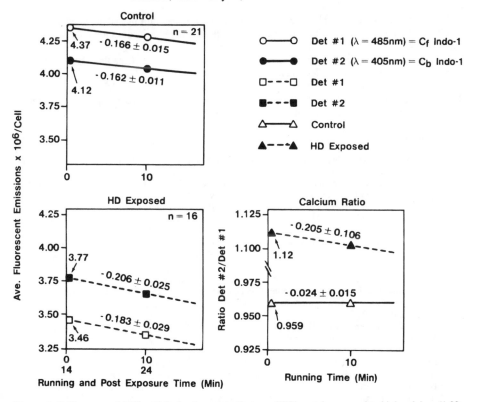

Figure 6. Sulfur mustard (400 μ*M*) had substantial effects on HEK acutely exposed to high-calcium (1.02 m*M*) buffers. In the control, average fluorescent emissions/cell were 2.6 × 7 emissions in low-calcium buffers (see Figure 4 controls). In the HD-exposed population, mustard caused a 21% decrease in the average fluorescent emissions per cell as recorded by detector 1, but only an 8% decrease in emissions recorded by detector 2. In calcium ratio analyses of the HD-exposed cells, detector 2:detector 1 ratios were >1.0 which reflects the disproportionate decrease of detector 1 emissions relative to detector 2 and the substantial leakage or discharge of Indo-1 from these cells. Mustard caused the slope of its calcium ratio curve to become negative relative to that of the control population. Running time and postexposure time included images scanned during the initial 10 min of analysis.

puzzle. We know, for example, that sulfur mustard penetrates the permeability barrier of the skin. It is interesting to speculate that mustard may disrupt calcium gradients as it passes through the epidermis and thereby cause basal cells to be acutely exposed both to sulfur mustard and to increased calcium concentrations. If basal cells then respond to this simultaneous challenge in vivo as our keratinocytes did in culture, they might alter the selective permeability of their plasma membrane and discharge or release small endogenous molecules as efficiently as HEK cells released Indo-1 (MW = 1010). Response to adverse Ca^{2+}–HD stimulation could, therefore, increase solute concentration and osmotic pressure in the extracellular spaces. Changes in selective permeability might also alter cytoskeletal organization as well as cell to cell or cell to substrate adhesion. Such events could contribute to the HD-induced mechanisms that force separation of basal cells from their basal lamina and initiates the process of vesication. This scenario may provide a useful working hypothesis for additional studies, but will require further tests and evaluation for its validation.

CONCLUSIONS

In medium containing 0.15 m*M* calcium, human epidermal keratinocytes produced monolayers that were capable of limited differentiation.

Sulfur mustard effects on HEK cells maintained in a low-calcium buffer included a decrease in Ca^{2+}-free and Ca^{2+}-bound Indo-1 fluorescence and an increase in detector 2:detector 1 calcium ratios.

In monolayer cultures, keratinocytes showed patterns of Indo-1AM loading that varied with their relative size and may reflect their state of differentiation.

When acutely exposed to both sulfur mustard and high (1.02 mM) calcium concentrations, HEK released stores of Indo-1, which altered calcium images and indicates a potential alteration in selective permeability of their plasma membranes.

References

1. Hennings, H., Michael, D., Cheng, C., Steinert, P., Holbrook, K., and Yuspa, S. H. 1980. Calcium regulation of growth and differentiation of mouse epidermal cells in culture. *Cell* 19:245–254.
2. Pillai, S., Bikle, D. D., Mancianti, M., Cline, P., and Hincenbergs, M. 1990. Calcium regulation of growth and differentiation of normal human keratinocytes: Modulation of differentiation competence by stages of growth and extracellular calcium. *J. Cell Physiol.* 143:294–302.
3. Kruszewksi, F. H., Hennings, H., Yuspa, S. H. and Tucker, R. W. 1991. Regulation of intracellular free calcium in normal murine keratinocytes. *Am. J. Physiol.* 261:C767–773.
4. Pillai, S., and Bikle, D. D. 1991. Role of intracellular free calcium in the cornified envelope formation of keratinocytes: Differences in the mode of action of extracellular calcium and 1,25-dihydroxyvitamin D_3. *J. Cell Physiol.* 146:94–100.
5. Menon, G. K., Grayson, S., and Elias, P. M. 1985. Ionic calcium reservoirs in mammalian epidermis: Ultrastructural localization by ion-capture cytochemistry. *J. Invest. Dermatol.* 84:508–512.
6. Forslind, B. 1986. Particle probe analysis in the study of skin physiology. *Scanning Electron Microsc.* 3:1007–1014.
7. Yuspa, S. H., Kilkenny, A. E., Steinert, P. M., and Roop, D. R. 1989. Expression of murine epidermal differentiation markers is tightly regulated by restricted extracellular calcium concentrations in vitro. *J. Cell Biol.* 109:1207–1217.
8. Sharpe, G. R., Gillespie, J. I., and Greenwell, J. R. 1989. An increase in intracellular free calcium is an early event during differentiation of cultured human keratinocytes. *FEBS Lett.* 254(1,2):25–28.
9. Ziboh, V. A., Isseroff, R. R., and Pandy, R. 1984. Phospholipid metabolism in calcium-regulated differentiation in cultured murine keratinocytes. *Biochem. Biophy. Res. Commun.* 122(3):1234–1240.
10. Tang, W., Ziboh, V. A., Isseroff, R., and Martinez, D. 1988. Turnover of inositol phospholipids in cultured murine keratinocytes: Possible involvement of inositol triphosphate in cellular differentiation. *J. Invest. Dermatol.* 90:37–43.
11. Menon, G. K., Elias, P. M., Lee, S. H., and Feingold, K. R. 1992. Localization of calcium in murine epidermis following disruption and repair of permeability barrier. *Cell Tissue Res.* 270:503–512.

Chapter Forty-four

INHERITED AND ACQUIRED ENZYME DEFECTS IN MULTIPLE CHEMICAL SENSITIVITY

Patricia P. Wilcox

It appears reasonable that common genetic enzyme variants could be a factor in chemical sensitivity syndrome (multiple chemical sensitivity[MCS], environmental illness). Members of a chemically sensitive family and a group of unrelated volunteers with chemical sensitivities have been tested for three enzymes sometimes implicated in adverse drug reactions: N-acetyltransferase (NAT), erythrocyte glucose 6-phosphate dehydrogenase (G6PD), and erythrocyte pyruvate kinase (PK). Results of these tests showed: (1) The distribution of acetylation (NAT) phenotype and genotype in 13 family members and 16 unrelated volunteers did not differ from that expected for the normal population; (2) tests of 5 family members and 10 other volunteers for G6PD deficiency, a common cause of drug-induced and chemically induced hemolytic anemia, showed no systematic deviation from expected values; and (3) when the same 15 individuals were tested for PK, another enzyme associated with hemolytic anemia, high-substrate PK values were not different from those in the normal population. The mean of low-substrate PK in both patient groups was, however, significantly below the average for healthy controls; no one was above average. Mean low-S PK activity ± standard deviation (in U/g Hb) was as follows: family (n = 5), 2.10 ± 0.50; other volunteers (n = 10), 2.33 ± 0.56. Compare results of a 1992 normal value study by the same laboratory (n = 30): mean 3.58 ± 1.32, median 3.0, range 2.0–6.8. The data suggest that multiple chemical sensitivity syndrome is frequently caused by individual variations in PK enzyme kinetics, leading to a heightened susceptibility to damage caused by PK inhibitors and other agents that affect the behavior of PK-related glycolytic enzymes. It would be extremely useful to have an in vitro test for PK inhibition by selected chemical agents, both as a diagnostic tool for MCS patients and as a means of identifying chemicals that might be unexpectedly toxic to a sizeable segment of the population.

INTRODUCTION

Multiple chemical sensitivity syndrome (MCS)—also called environmental illness, sick building syndrome, and possibly chronic fatigue syndrome, fibromyalgia, and Gulf War syndrome—has become increasingly visible of late; MCS appeared explicitly in the program of the Society of Toxicology annual meeting for the first time this year (1994).[1] Relatively few patients have a formal diagnosis of MCS, but some researchers think that 15% or more of the U.S. population may be affected.[2]

OBJECTIVE

The current study was a "fishing expedition" aimed at discovering whether a few well-known and easily tested enzyme variants in the human population might turn out to be strongly correlated with an exaggerated tendency to react badly to environmental chemical exposures.

Table 1 MCS Triggering Agents (Partial List)

Triggering agent	Probable chemical culprits
Dry-erase whiteboard markers	n-Butyl acetate with methyl isobutyl ketone
Lacquer/lacquer thinner	n-Butyl acetate, methyl isobutyl ketone, toluene, xylene, other toxic solvents
Hobby glues	n-Butyl acetate, other toxic solvents
Telephones	Acrylonitrile-styrene-butadiene (ABS) plastic
Computers	Acrylonitrile-styrene-butadiene (ABS) plastic
Certain photocopy toners and copies	Styrene-butadiene toners, ethylbenzene
Carpets	Styrene-butadiene rubber, no-stain coatings
Carpet glues	Toluene and other toxic solvents
Upholstered furniture	Urethane foam (isocyanates), no-stain coatings
Auto interiors	Urethane foam (isocyanates), no-stain coatings, styrene-butadiene rubber and plastic
Fabric stores	No-iron, no-stain, no-pill, waterproof, and flame-retardant finishes; sizing, resin coatings, dyes; isocyanates(?)
Polyurethane varnish	Isocyanates
Carbonless copy and fax paper	Phenolic resins (e.g., bisphenol A); formerly sometimes contained isocyanates or PCBs
Printing inks, papers	Aromatic hydrocarbons in ink oil, resin coatings, antioxidants; toluene (rotogravure process)
Drugs	Oral contraceptives, beta blockers, beta agonists, dimethyl compounds, general anesthesia (sodium pentothal?), preservatives and "inactive" ingredients
Food and drug additives	Monosodium glutamate (MSG), benzoic acid, benzoates, parabens, para-aminobenzoic acid (PABA), polysorbates, sorbates, sorbitol, antioxidants (BHA, BHT, tBHQ), isopropyl alcohol, chlorobutanol, ethylene oxide
Perfumes, colognes, natural plant oils	Oil of bergamot/orange oil/d-limonene, eucalyptus oil, benzoic acid, n-butyl compounds, solvents
Insecticides	Chlorpyrifos, pyrethrins (chrysanthemums) and pyrethroids, synergists (piperonyl butoxide), and many others
Herbicides	Glyphosate, polysorbates, isopropyl compounds, etc.
Cleaning products	2-Butoxyethanol and other glycol ethers, isopropyl alcohol, citrus oil (d-limonene), terpenes, phenols, etc.
Fresh paint	Solvents, fungicides
Mold, yeast	Mold toxins (e.g., aflatoxin, trichodermin) and metabolites (e.g., 2,3-butanedione)
Gasoline	tert-Butyl antioxidants
Radiator/boiler additives	Sodium nitrite, hydrazine (?)
Processed meats	Nitrites
Diesel exhaust/fossil fuel power plant emissions	Nitrites, including butyl nitrite

MATERIALS AND METHODS

We recruited a group of volunteers with hypersensitivities to a characteristic list of chemicals, with reactions ranging from acute attacks (asthma, migraine, vomiting, seizures, panic attacks) to long-term, chronic, and in some cases, disabling conditions. The majority of these people did not have a formal diagnosis of MCS (not surprising, since at present there is no formal case definition for the disorder), but they all tended to report problems with some of the environmental agents listed in Table 1. Participants were asked to fill out a short questionnaire describing adverse reactions to chemicals, personal and family health history, and ancestry. They signed statements of informed consent, and donated specimens of urine, hair follicles, and (in some cases) blood to be analyzed for a selected set of enzymes known to affect drug and chemical metabolism. Specimens were shipped to several commercial and research laboratories for analysis.*

* Acetylation studies were performed by E. Furman, M. Doll, and R. Ferguson in D. W. Hein's laboratory at the University of North Dakota. P. E. Harvey, MD, and several commercial laboratories assisted with other enzyme studies.

Acetylator Phenotype and Genotype

Urine (collected 2–6 h after drinking a caffeinated beverage) and DNA from hair follicles for 29 chemically sensitive individuals were analyzed by a research team at the University of North Dakota[3] for *N*-acetyltransferase (NAT) phenotype and genotype.[4]*

Erythrocyte G6PD and PK Assays

A smaller group of volunteers participated in the blood enzyme study. This group included 15 people, about half men and half women. Five of these were members of three generations of a family with mild- to severe chemical sensitivities; the other 10 were unrelated individuals, mostly in their late 30s or early 40s and of Northern European descent (but, surprisingly, 4 of the 10 turned out to have some Native American ancestry). Volunteers went to a local hospital or commercial medical lab with a doctor's order for quantitative glucose 6-phosphate dehydrogenase (G6PD) and pyruvate kinase (PK) assays. Results of these assays were: (1) a single value for G6PD enzyme activity for each participant (since these were done by several different laboratories, we normalized each result to obtain a number ranging from 0.0 for the laboratory's quoted normal low value to 1.0 for the laboratory's normal high value) and (2) two points ("high substrate" and "low substrate" values) from the curve of PK enzyme activity versus phosphoenol-pyruvate (PEP) concentration for each participant (all done by a single laboratory).†

RESULTS

Acetylation phenotype and genotype, G6PD activity, and the high-substrate end of the curve for red blood cell PK activity versus substrate concentration in our 15 chemically sensitive individuals were no different from values that would be expected for the population as a whole. However, the average PK activity at the low-substrate end of the curve was substantially below the value previously obtained by the same laboratory for 30 normal healthy controls (historical controls), as shown in Figure 1. Of the people we tested 100% were below the average low-substrate PK for controls. This pattern—normal high-substrate activity but reduced low-substrate activity—is typically caused by mutations that subtly alter the geometry of binding sites for substrates or cofactors of the enzyme.[4]‡ Might a similar picture result from chronic exposure to chemicals that block PK binding sites?

DISCUSSION

The discovery of altered PK enzyme kinetics in chemically sensitive individuals makes sense for two major reasons. First, many of the adverse effects typically reported by these individuals (Table 2) are things that would logically occur as a result of disruption of glycolytic energy metabolism. Second, many of the agents reported to cause these effects (Table 1) are known to directly or indirectly inhibit PK in various tissues of various organisms, although few of these agents have, to date, been systematically tested for their effects on PK activity in humans, let alone PK-deficient humans.

---

* About 50% of people in the United States are homozygous slow acetylators; the rest are heterozygous or homozygous rapid acetylators. Each group has its own set of problems with various drugs and chemicals.[5]

† Approximately 5% of humans have red blood cells deficient in G6PD, and are therefore highly susceptible to chemically induced hemolytic anemia; there is a well-known and rather lengthy list of drugs and chemicals that must be avoided by G6PD-deficient individuals.[6] In the United States the occurrence of PK deficiency—which accounts for roughly half the known cases of hereditary nonspherocytic hemolytic anemia world wide—is 1–2% at birth, but a larger number of people become PK deficient later in life, sometimes in response to chemical exposures such as chemotherapy.[7] Although adverse drug and chemical effects in PK deficiency have not been systematically studied, there are reports of adverse reactions to aspirin,[8] oral contraceptives,[9] and anesthesia in PK-deficient humans, and various chemical agents—e.g. sodium nitrite—have been found to cause profound PK depletion in other mammals.[10] Red blood cell (PK-R) and liver (PK-L) isozymes are encoded by a single gene on chromosome 1; muscles, white blood cells, platelets, and brain cells contain two other isozymes, PK-M1 and PK-M2, encoded by another gene, on chromosome 15.[11]

‡ Note that the numerical value of low-substrate PK, as well as the sensitivity of the test to specific types of enzyme mutations, is strongly dependent on the substrate concentrations chosen by the test laboratory. The laboratory doing the blood tests described in this chapter used the high-substrate PEP concentration recommended by Beutler (1984),[12] but a low-substrate PEP concentration 1.5 times higher than Beutler's.

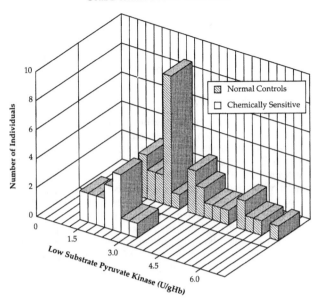

Figure 1. Low-S PK enzyme activity for 15 MCS patients (front) and 30 controls (back).

Table 2 Common Health Problems in MCS Patients and Families

Problem area	Examples
Thyroid-related disorders	Hashimoto's thyroiditis, Graves' disease, thyroid hormone resistance, attention deficit/hyperactivity disorder
Indications of abnormal K^+ (potassium ion) transport	Cardiac arrhythmias, impaired short-term memory, transient elevation of serum potassium after chemical exposure
Respiratory, etc.	Asthma, emphysema, sarcoidosis, chronic bronchitis, "sinus trouble"
Glucose metabolism	Diabetes (IDDM, NIDDM), abnormal glucose tolerance
Ethanol metabolism	Alcoholism/alcohol intolerance
Rheumatological	Rheumatoid arthritis, osteoarthritis, systemic lupus erythematosus, Sjögren's syndrome, mixed connective tissue disease, inflammatory bowel disease.
Other organs	Chronic (autoimmune?) hepatitis, kidney damage (glomerulonephritis), gallbladder disease
Neurological	Migraine, panic disorder, sleep disorders, chronic fatigue, depression, bipolar disorder, schizophrenia, abnormal EEG, epilepsy, neuromuscular disorders, peripheral neuropathy, "back trouble"
Birth defects, esp. skeletal abnormalities	Spina bifida occulta, scoliosis, congenital hip dysplasia
Hematologic abnormalities	Heavy rouleau formation 1 h after chemical exposure, elevated and fluctuating reticulocyte counts (high 2.5 d after chemical exposure), blood clotting disorders, elevated triglycerides with low HDL (Frederickson's type IV hyperlipoproteinemia), abnormal T-cell counts, multiple autoantibodies
Drug hypersensitivities	(See Table 1)

Symptoms and Their Relationship to PK

PK is a key enzyme in a sort of "metabolic switching circuit" at the downstream end of the glycolytic pathway. PK converts PEP to pyruvate—which is used for fuel and for amino acid synthesis—and adenosine diphosphate (ADP) to adenosine triphosphate (ATP), using Mg^{2+} and K^+ as cofactors. To a lesser extent, PK also converts other nucleotide diphosphates (GDP, UDP) to the corresponding triphosphates (GTP, UTP). ATP (under the control of a GTP-containing protein) is the precursor of cyclic adenosine monophosphate (cAMP), an important regulatory molecule. PK is allosterically activated by fructose 1,6-bisphosphate (FDP). FDP acts like a "wake-up signal" from phosphofructokinase (PFK) at the upstream end of the glycolytic pathway. PK activity (in some organisms, at least) is decreased by high concentrations of certain amino acids, like alanine, glutamate, and phenylalanine. Inhibition of PK activity causes the accumulation of 2,3-bisphosphoglyceric acid (2,3-DPG), which in turn signals PFK to shut down and also, in humans, alters the oxygen affinity of hemoglobin.

Alterations in PK enzyme kinetics can act in at least four ways to cause some of the ill effects observed in MCS patients, as listed in Table 2:

1. Membrane potassium channels depend on glycolytic ATP produced from ADP by the reaction catalyzed by PK. Impaired potassium channel functioning, caused by below-normal PK activity and the resulting ATP deficit, might explain the cardiac arrhythmias[13] and impaired short-term memory[14] frequently experienced by MCS patients.
2. Pyruvic acid, produced by PK from phosphoenolpyruvate, is the principal fuel for mitochondria in the central nervous system. In some portions of mammalian brain (e.g., the cat cerebellum) pyruvate flux is not much above the critical limit; interrupting the supply results in ataxia,[15,16] a symptom frequently experienced by people with chemical sensitivities.
3. Alteration of PK enzyme kinetics can result in changes of enzyme specificity toward ADP, GDP, and UDP, which would potentially alter the ratio of ATP to GTP,[17] and thus, interfere with transmembrane signaling processes involving G proteins (GTP-binding proteins). (See Stryer,[18] pp. 978 ff.) Shortage of glycolytic ATP also interferes with the capacity to rapidly synthesize its metabolite cyclic AMP (cAMP), a key component in the "fight or flight" reaction; cAMP deficiency could account for many of the symptoms experienced by chemically sensitive individuals.
4. Under the influence of FDP, PK changes back and forth from a tetrameric form, with high PK activity, to a monomer that has very low PK activity but has high binding affinity for triiodothyronine (T3).[19–21] Interference with PK activity will thus have a direct impact on thyroid function, and may explain the high incidence of thyroid disease in MCS patients and their relatives.

Triggering Agents and Their Relationship to PK Activity

Many of the agents that trigger symptoms in our study population are known to affect PK enzyme activity, either directly or indirectly:

1. MSG (glutamate) and polysorbates are known PK inhibitors in several species.[22–24] One survey estimated that 25% of people experienced hypersensitivity reactions to glutamate,[25] a percentage roughly in the same ballpark as the 15% of the population estimated to have chemical sensitivities.[2] A series of papers in the *Annals of Allergy*[26,27] describes a "BHA, BHT, tween 80 (polysorbate 80) intolerant" type of intrinsic asthma with a "deficit of beta adrenergic reserve" (that is, of reserve capacity to synthesize cAMP—see earlier discussion under Symptoms). This sounds like a description of our PK-deficient chemically sensitive group.
2. Benzoic acid, sorbic acid, and several well-known neurotoxins alter the functioning of the glycolytic pathway, in part by preventing formation of FDP, an allosteric activator of PK.[29,29]
3. Styrene and ethylbenzene produce benzoic acid (discussed earlier) as a major metabolite, and phenylglyoxal as a minor metabolite.[30,31] Phenylglyoxal inhibits PK by binding to arginine residues at active sites of the enzyme.[32] Arlien-Søborg[30] described a plastic boat factory in

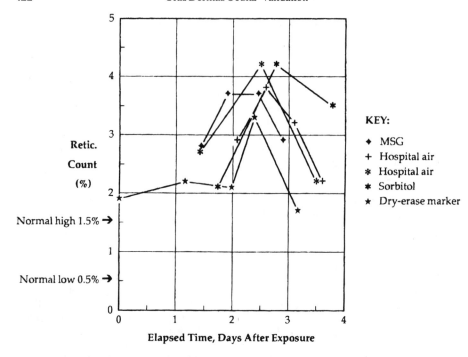

Figure 2. Reticulocytosis in a typical MCS patient after low-level chemical exposures

which 50% of styrene-exposed workers had left their jobs within the first year or two because of health problems—perhaps these were individuals with less-than-average low-substrate PK activity.

4. n-Butyl compounds will likely be oxidized to 2,3-butanedione analogs by the phenobarbital-inducible cytochrome P-450s (known to be induced by, e.g., methyl isobutyl ketone and xylene[33]). 2,3-Butanedione (and some of its analogs) can inhibit PK by binding to essential arginine residues.[34] 2-Butoxyethanol (another n-butyl compound) causes elevated reticulocytes in aging rats,[35] with a time history similar to the response of a PK-variant human exposed to n-butyl acetate in dry-erase markers (Figure 2). Methyl n-butyl ketone, a known neurotoxin, has been observed to inhibit PFK, which would reduce the supply of FDP, an allosteric activator of PK.[29] n-Butyl alcohol, which can be produced as a metabolite of n-butyl acetate [36] or of n-butyl esters (such as the herbicides in Agent Orange), is neuotoxic to rats.[37]

5. The widely used herbicide glyphosate kills plants by interfering with the PEP binding site on the plant enzyme 5-enoylshikimate 3-phosphate synthase (EPSPS)[38]; given the large number of chemically sensitive individuals reporting adverse encounters with glyphosate, and our discovery of altered PK enzyme kinetics in many chemically sensitive individuals, it might be a good idea to see if glyphosate blocks PEP-binding sites of human PK. Glyphosate is normally sold as the isopropylamine salt,[38] which has the dimethyl structure characteristic of drugs with beta-adrenergic activity. (Note: Other MCS triggers like pyrethrin/pyrethroids, isopropyl alcohol, and bisphenol A also contain a dimethyl group.) An additional possible source of trouble with glyphosate is that its formulations typically contain ethomeen T/15, which is a polyoxyethylene compound closely related to polysorbates (see item 1).

6. Sodium nitrite causes profound PK depletion in rabbits, and hemolytic anemia (due to PK deficiency?) in rats.[10] Processed meats, radiator additives, and power plant/diesel emissions can trigger MCS symptoms—possibly because they all contain PK-inhibiting nitrites.

CONCLUSIONS AND RECOMMENDATIONS

Red blood cell enzyme tests and an analysis of MCS symptoms and their inciting agents support the hypothesis that "multiple chemical sensitivity syndrome" describes errors of metabolism in the glycolytic pathway, very often involving the enzyme pyruvate kinase, which controls the downstream end of glycolysis and is known to be highly polymorphic in humans. Genetic PK variants can lead to an exaggerated susceptibility to chemical interference; on the other hand, bioaccumulation of a sufficient quantity of a PK-inhibiting agent would be expected to cause similar adverse effects even in the absence of a genetic problem. In other words, MCS is an acquired disease caused by chemical exposure; but it is also an inherited disease, in the sense that individuals with certain genetic PK variants will have a higher probability of being damaged by certain chemicals, or will suffer damage at a lower dose, than will other individuals exposed to the same chemicals.

Anyone involved in evaluating the toxic effects of environmental chemicals, or in diagnosing and treating patients with MCS and related disorders, would benefit from the availability of an in vitro test to screen chemicals for their effects on PK activity in human cells. It would make sense to start with red blood cells and possibly white blood cells donated by individuals known to have "nonstandard" forms of PK. Once such tests are available, it should be relatively simple to screen chemicals (such as those listed in Table 1) for PK-inhibiting properties, and to screen MCS patients' blood cells for susceptibility to known PK inhibitors. This would allow us to identify cases of MCS and related neurological and autoimmune disorders that represent PK-deficient individuals reacting to chemicals that exacerbate their enzyme deficiency, and to screen out other types of chemically sensitive patients without PK enzyme problems who need to be evaluated for other problems not addressed by the present study, such as defects of mitochondrial energy metabolism.

ADDENDUM

PK enzyme kinetic studies recently completed by Drs. Lakomek and Schröter[39] (also see ref. 40) confirm that several of the chemically sensitive individuals at the low end of the scale for low-S PK in the present study do, indeed, have erythrocyte PK enzymes that show mixed cooperativity and other features characteristic of PK-deficient heterozygotes. Sequencing of the red blood cell PK genes for these individuals is in progress and one of them has already been found to have a point mutation at the PK locus on chromosome 1.

Several physicians have recently found that many of their chemically sensitive patients have abnormal levels of various enzymes or metabolic intermediates (porphyrins) associated with heme biosynthesis.[41] This is consistent with my observation that MCS symptoms are associated with chemical exposures that a) interfere with red blood cell pyruvate kinase, and b) cause upregulation of cytochrome P450 enzyme expression. Interference with pyruvate kinase causes hemolysis, which is followed by an increase in erythropoiesis to replace lost red blood cells (as shown by increased reticulocyte counts $2^1/_2$ d after exposure—see Figure 2). Synthesis of red cells consumes heme, an essential component of hemoglobin. Cytochrome P450 synthesis also requires heme. Their combined effects could easily lead to temporary metabolic bottlenecks and abnormal levels of heme pathway enzymes and intermediates—that is, porphyrins and related compounds. A classic example of this effect is phenobarbital, a porphyrinogenic drug that is both a cytochrome P450 inducer[42] and a pyruvate kinase inhibitor.[43]

References

1. Rodgers, K., and Sikorski, L. E. 1994. Roundtable: The question of multiple chemical sensitivity. *Toxicologist,* 14(1):140.
2. National Research Council, Board of Environmental Studies and Toxicology. 1987. *Workshop on Health Risks from Exposure to Common Indoor Household Products.* Washington, DC: National Academy of Sciences, July 1.
3. Furman, E. J. 1993. *N-acetylation in American Indians and Other People with Diabetes Mellitus.* Master's thesis, The University of North Dakota.
4. Beutler, E. 1993. Personal communication.

5. Weber, W. W., and Hein, D. W. 1985. N-acetylation pharmacogenetics. *Pharmacological Reviews,* 37:25–79.
6. Beutler, E. 1983. Glucose 6-phosphate dehydrogenase deficiency. In *The Metabolic Basis of Inherited Disease,* eds. J. B. Stanbury, J. B. Wyngaarden, D. S. Frederickson, J. L. Goldstein, and M. S. Brown, 5th ed., pp. 1629–1653. New York: McGraw-Hill.
7. Valentine, W. N., Tanaka, K. R., and Paglia, D. E. 1989. Pyruvate kinase and other enzyme deficiency disorders of the erythrocyte. In *The Metabolic Basis of Inherited Disease,* eds. C. R. Scriver, A. L. Beaudet, W. S. Sly, and D. Valle, 6th edition, pp. 2341–2365. New York: McGraw-Hill.
8. Glader, B. E. 1976. Salicylate-induced injury of pyruvate-kinase-deficient erythrocytes. *N. Eng. J. Med.* 294(17):916–918.
9. Kendall, A. G. 1977. Red cell pyruvate kinase deficiency: Adverse effect of oral contraceptives. *Acta Haematol.* 57(2):116–120.
10. Violante, A., Cianetti, A., Ordine, A., and Peruzzi, G. 1973. Azione mielotossica sperimentale del sodio nitrito e sua interferenze su alcune attivita enzymatiche eritrocitarie [Myelotoxic experimental action of sodium nitrite and its interference on several enzyme activities]. *Q. Sclavo Diagnos. Clin. Lab.* 9(4):893–905.
11. Miwa, S., Kanno, H., and Fujii, H. 1993. Concise review: Pyruvate kinase deficiency: Historical perspective and recent progress of molecular genetics. *Am. J. of Hematol.* 42:31–35.
12. Beutler, E. 1984. *Red cell metabolism: A manual of biochemical methods,* 3rd ed. Orlando, FL: Grune & Stratton.
13. Weiss, J. N., and Lamp, S. T. 1987. Glycolysis preferentially inhibits ATP sensitive K^+ channels in isolated guinea pig cardiac myocytes. *Science* 238:67–69.
14. Etcheberrigaray, R., Ito, E., Oka, K., Tofel-Grehl, B., Gibson, G. E., and Alkon, D. L. 1993. Potassium channel dysfunction in fibroblasts identifies patients with Alzheimer disease. *Proc. Nat. Acad. Sci. USA* 90(17):8209–8213.
15. Reynolds, S. F., and Blass, J. P. 1976. A possible mechanism for selective cerebellar damage in partial pyruvate dehydrogenase deficiency. *Neurology,* 26:625–628.
16. Kark, R. A., and Becker, D. M. 1981. Multiple genotypes, multiple phenotypes, and partial defects. *Muscle Nerve,* 4:31–40.
17. Valentine, W. N., Paglia, D. E., Nakatani, M., and Brockway, R. A. 1987. Erythrocyte pyruvate kinase (PK): The variable significance of "nucleotide specificity" in the characterization of mutant variants. *Am. J. Hematol.* 26:353–356.
18. Stryer, L. 1988. *Biochemistry,* 3rd ed. New York: W. H. Freeman.
19. Hauser, P., Zametkin, A. J., Martinez, P., Vitiello, B., Matochik, J. A., Mixson, A. J., and Weintraub, B. D. 1993. Attention deficit-hyperactivity disorder in people with generalized resistance to thyroid hormone. *N. Eng. J. Med.* 328(14):997–1001.
20. Ashizawa, K., Willingham, M. C., Liang, C.-M., and Cheng, S.-y. 1991. In vivo regulation of monomer-tetramer conversion of pyruvate kinase subtype M2 by glucose is mediated via fructose 1,6-bisphosphate. *J. Biol. Chem.* 266(25):16842–16846.
21. Popescu, N. C., and Cheng, S.-y. 1990. Chromosomal localization of the gene for a human cytosolic thyroid hormone binding protein homologous to the subunit of pyruvate kinase, subtype M2. *Somatic Cell Mol. Genet.* 16(6):593–598.
22. Lin, M., Turpin, D. H., Plaxton, W. C. 1989. Pyruvate kinase isozymes from the green alga, *Selenastrum minutum* II. Kinetic and regulatory properties. *Arch. Biochem. Biophys.* 269(1):228–238.
23. Ozawa, S., Ozawa, K., and Nakanishi, N. 1990. [Studies on pyruvate kinase from pig dental pulp and brain.] *Meikai Daigaku Shigaku Zasshi* 19(2):185–196. (Published in Japanese.)
24. Yanagi, S., Sakamoto, M., Takahashi, S., Hasuike, A., Konishi, Y., Kumazawa, K., and Nakatano, T. 1985. Enhancement of hepatocarcinogenesis by sorbitan fatty acid ester, a liver pyruvate kinase activity-reducing substance. *J. Natl. Cancer Inst.* 75(2):381–384.
25. Reif-Lehrer, L. 1976. Possible significance of adverse reactions to glutamate in humans. *Fed. Proc.* 35(11):2205–2211.
26. Fisherman, E. W., and Cohen, G. N. 1974. Alpha-beta-adrenergic imbalance in intrinsic-intolerance rhinitis or asthma. *Ann. Allergy* 33:86–101.
27. Fisherman, E. W., Rosset, D., and Cohen, G. N. 1977. Serum triglyceride and cholesterol levels and lipid electrophoretic patterns in intrinsic and extrinsic allergic states. *Ann. Allergy* 38:46–53.
28. Burlini, N., Pellegrini, R., Facheris, P., Tortora, P., and Guerritore, A. 1993. Metabolic effects of benzoate and sorbate in the yeast *Saccharomyces cerevisiae* at neutral pH. *Arch. Microbiol.* 159:220–224.
29. Spencer, P. S., Sabri, M. I., Schaumburg, H. H., and Moore, C. L. 1979. Does a defect of energy metabolism in the nerve fiber underlie axonal degeneration in polyneuropathies? *Ann. Neurol.* 5(6):501–507.
30. Arlien-Søbørg, P. 1992. *Solvent neurotoxicity.* Boca Raton, FL: CRC Press.

31. Engström, K. M. 1984. Urinalysis of minor metabolites of ethylbenzene and *m*-xylene. *Scand. J. Work Environ. Health* 10(2):75–81.

32. Berghäuser, J. 1977. Modifizierung von Argininresten in Pyruvat-Kinase [Modification of arginine residues in pyruvate kinase]. *Hoppe-Seylers Z. Physiol. Chem.* 358(12):1565–1572.

33. Abou-Donia, M. B., Hu, Z., Lapadula, D. M., and Gupta, R. P. 1991. Mechanisms of joint neurotoxicity of *n*-hexane, methyl isobutyl ketone and *o*-ethyl *o*-4-nitrophenyl phenylphosphonothioate in hens. *J. Pharmacol. Exp. Ther.* 257(1):282–289.

34. Kilinç, K., and Özer, N. 1984. Irreversible inactivation of human erythrocyte pyruvate kinase by 2,3-butanedione. *Arch. Biochem. Biophys.* 230(1):321–326.

35. Ghanayem, B. I., Blair, P. C., Thompson, M. B., Maronpot, R. R., and Matthews, H. B. 1987. Effect of age on the toxicity and metabolism of ethylene glycol monobutyl ether (2-butoxyethanol) in rats. *Toxicol. Appl. Pharmacol.* 91(2):222–234.

36. Groth, G., and Freundt, K. J. 1991. Blood alcohol under the presence of *n*-butyl acetate. *Blutalkohol* 28(3):166–173.

37. Schulze, G. E. 1988. 2,4-D-*n*-butyl ester (2,4-D ester) induced ataxia in rats: Role for *n*-butanol formation. *Neurotoxicol. Teratol.* 10:81–84.

38. Devine, M. D., Duke, S. O., and Fedtke, C. 1993. *Physiology of herbicide action.* Englewood Cliffs, NJ: Prentice-Hall.

39. Lakomek, M., and Schröter, W. 1994. Personal communication.

40. Lakomek, M., Neubauer, B., van der Lühe, A., Hoch, G., Winkler, H., and Schröter, W. 1992. Erythrocyte pyruvate kinase deficiency: Relations of residual enzyme activity, altered regulation of defective enzymes and concentrations of high-energy phosphates with the severity of clinical manifestation. *Eur. J. Haematol.* 49:82–92.

41. Baker, G. P. 1995. Porphyria and MCS overlap symptoms—another chemical connection. *Townsend letter for doctors* (911 Tyler St., Port Townsend, WA 98368-6541), July 1995, 72–73.

42. Kappas, A., Sassa, S., Galbraith, R. A., and Nordmann, Y. 1995. The porphyrias. In *The metabolic and molecular bases of inherited disease,* eds. C. R. Scriver, A. L. Beaudet, W. S. Sly, and D. Valle, 7th edition, pp. 2103–2159. New York: McGraw-Hill.

43. Yanagi, S., Sakamoto, M., and Nakatano, T. 1986. Comparative study on pyruvate kinase activity-reducing action of various promoters of hepatocarcinogenesis. *Int. J. Cancer* 37(3):450–464.

Chapter Forty-five

AN IN VITRO METHOD FOR DETECTING TOXICANTS BY CHANGES IN THE PATTERN OF POLARIZED LIGHT SCATTERED FROM BACTERIA

B. V. Bronk, Zhao Z. Li, J. Czégé, and W. P. Van De Merwe

A rapid new technique for measuring size changes of bacteria resulting from their response to chemicals in their liquid environment is described. The angular function associated with the Mueller matrix ratio, S34/S11, for scattering of polarized light from bacterial suspensions has been shown to be a sensitive measure of the diameter of rod-shaped cells. When various environmental changes affecting the bacteria occur, there are easily discernable changes in the graph of this function versus angle, which can be seen within a few minutes. One example is described, a shift up of the nutritional environment of Escherichia coli *cells, which displaces the locations of the maxima in this graph toward smaller angle within 5 min. A method for using changes in the rate of the peak shifts to determine the effect of toxicants on cell growth of bacteria is described.*

INTRODUCTION

The response of various organisms to chemicals in the environment has been a classic indicator of the presence of products that are harmful to humans. While higher organisms have often been used in the past, the use of single-celled organisms for this purpose has been attempted in the past decade and is now well established as an alternate means of testing for toxicants. In the case of protozoans, measurement of the swimming movement of a population of *Tetrahymena* gives a rapid and sensitive assay.[1] Bacteria have been used both in axenic cultures and in complex heterogeneous cultures such as sludge, with a variety of methods to assay for toxicity.[2] Usually the presence of a toxicant is monitored by the decrease in some measurable function of the bacteria. Some examples are the reduction of light produced by a species of luminescent marine bacteria; growth of bacterial populations monitored by optical density; microscopic estimation of lengths of filamentous bacteria; inhibition of respiration; and reduction of heat production. All of these are discussed and reviewed in ref. 2. Bacterial measurements such as these may be used as an indicator to monitor for the presence of toxicants as well as a means for investigating the toxic mechanism.

In the present report we present a new and very sensitive measure of bacterial growth in which changes may be observed both rapidly and with high sensitivity. The new method has been used to demonstrate rapidly observable changes after nutritional shifts in a bacterial growth medium,[3] heat treatment,[4] ultraviolet (UV) exposure, and germination of spores.[5] The changes we are discussing are shifts in the graph of a particular angular function obtained from polarized light scattering. In an example to be discussed later in this chapter, a nutritional upshift of growth medium for *Escherichia coli* cells causes changes in the graph that indicate a rapid increase of diameter for these cells. This experiment is given as an example producing a measure that can be used to show the presence of toxicants.

EXPERIMENTAL METHOD

We provide here a very brief overview of how polarized light scattering may be used to monitor rapid changes in the growth properties of bacterial cells. In the next section we present an example of a measurement and then we describe how the procedure may be modified to measure the effect of toxicants.

The use of the Stokes vector to characterize polarized light and the accompanying 4×4 matrix (Mueller or Stokes matrix) that describes scattering of polarized light from any scatterer is well known to optical physicists.[6] The experimental procedures used to measure any one of the 16 Stokes matrix elements are described in detail in ref. 1, as are the mathematics of the Stokes vector and matrix. A description with specific biological applications is given in the review.[4] We do not repeat the mathematics in this brief discussion except to point out that for a scattering system with sufficient symmetry (e.g., a suspension of similar cylindrically symmetric bacteria in liquid suspension) most of the matrix elements become very small or vanish. Each of the elements remaining is a function of the angle of observation, theta, with the forward direction of the laser beam illuminating the scatterers as shown in Figure 1. Theta varies between zero and 180 degrees.

We have found that the graph of a particular ratio of two of the matrix elements, namely, S34/S11 versus angle, is quite reproducible for given experimental conditions[7] and at the same time rather sensitive to the growth conditions of the bacteria studied.[8] The scattering system we are describing here is a liquid suspension of bacteria contained in a cylindrical scattering cuvette. The concentration of bacteria in suspension is kept sufficiently low (optical density at 600 nm less than 0.1) that there is a single scattering event for each photon, and thus the ratio S34/S11 is independent of the exact concentration.

EXPERIMENTAL EXAMPLES

Typical examples of the graphs of S34/S11 versus angle are shown in Figure 2 for two different strains of the bacteria *Escherichia coli* in the early log phase stage of growth. The K12 strain

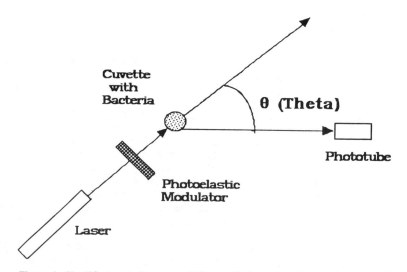

Figure 1. Simplified scattering setup. Various optical elements (e.g., polarizers) and electronic components (e.g., lock-in amplifier) are omitted for simplicity.

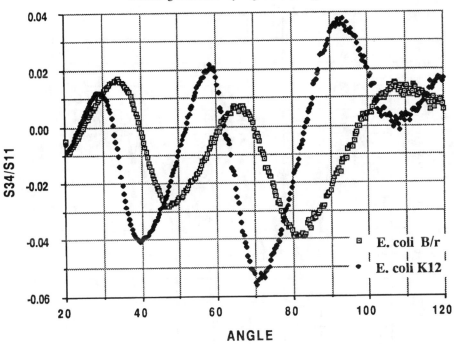

Figure 2. Comparison of graphs of S34/S11 for two different strains of *Escherichia coli* bacteria in log-phase growth. The strain with the larger diameter (K12, solid diamond) has its maxima shifted toward smaller angle compared to the strain with the smaller diameter.

has average length ~6.4 ± 1.5 μm and average diameter ~1.05 ± 0.05 μm. The B/r strain has average length ~2.5 ± 0.5 μm and average diameter ~0.92 ± 0.05 μm. (See ref. 10 for details of the measurements.) Numerous experiments[8] and calculations[9] have shown that for randomly oriented rod-shaped bacteria in liquid suspension the S34/S11 graph is insensitive to changes in cell length, but rather sensitive to changes in diameter. Thus the variation between the two graphs in Figure 2 is primarily due to the difference of about 0.1 μm between their average diameters.

In Figure 3 we show a timed sequence of graphs of S34/S11 versus angle for a particular experiment performed with *E. coli* K12 bacteria grown in a rich medium. The protocol for these experiments was as follows: The bacteria were grown overnight (~19 h) starting from low density in Luria broth (LB); an inoculum was then diluted into fresh medium at an optical density (OD) at 600 nm of about 0.03 and grown ~6 h at 37°C to late log or early stationary phase; the cells were spun down with a table-top centrifuge, washed once in phosphate-buffered saline (PBS) at pH 7, and then spun down again and resuspended at an OD < 0.1 in PBS.

Immediately following these steps, concentrated LB (2×) was added to an equal volume of the cell suspension at a temperature of 37°C. This is time zero for the sequence of scattering curves. The cells were then allowed to grow at 37°C in the cuvette with occasional stirring between scattering measurements, which were taken at various intervals up to 30 min after this nutritional upshift. The times indicated are the mid-epoch of a measurement, which takes about 3 min for the phototube to be scanned through angles between 20 and 120 degrees. The progression of a the second maximum of Figure 3 is shown as a function of time after upshift in medium in Figure 4. The steady progression with time shows that the bacterial cells are rapidly increasing their diameters when they are shifted from a poor to a rich medium. The diameter of these

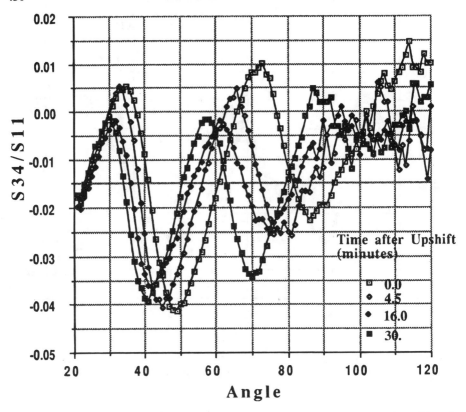

Figure 3. Graphs of the scattering function S34/S11 versus scattering angle, theta. *Escherichia coli* bacteria were grown to late log phase, washed, and then resuspended in fresh broth at 37°C at time zero. Shift of second peak (~70 degrees at $t = 0$) to smaller angles indicates that the upshift of nutritional medium causes a rapid increase of diameter, which is observable within the first 4 min by this method.

bacteria in LB medium can vary by up to ~20%,[8] which, as Figures 3 and 4 indicate, is quite adequate to give easily observable quantitative changes within the first few minutes.

APPLICATION

One method of applying this technique to obtain a rapid assessment of the effect of a toxicant on a particular strain of bacteria would require the following simple modification of procedure just described. Bacteria would be prepared for an upshift experiment as discussed in the previous section. The putative toxicant would be added in various doses to the concentrated (2×) nutrient prior to the upshift. The upshift experiment would be repeated for increasing doses either until a substantial decrease in the magnitude of the slope of the graph corresponding to Figure 4 was observed, or until a dose was reached that showed high toxicity according to other assays. A change (decrease) in the magnitude of this slope has been shown (data not shown) to be easily observed when the temperature is lowered from 37°C to room temperature during the upshift, so we may conclude that the slope is indeed sensitive to environmental conditions. Tests with toxicants remain to be carried out in the laboratory, but the easily observable movement of peaks during experiments such as this example indicate that there is a great deal of promise in the method.

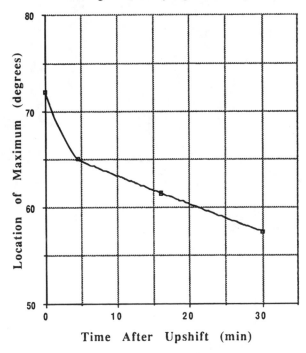

Figure 4. Position of second maximum (Figure 3) versus time after upshift.

ADDENDUM

Since submitting this chapter, experiments by Li, Bronk, and Czégé have verified that metal ions at near-toxic concentrations reduce the peak shift in graphs such as those of Figure 3.

References

1. Silverman, J., and Penisi, S. 1987. Evaluation of *Tetrahymena thermophila* as an in vitro alternative to ocular irritation studies in rabbits. *J. Cupreous Ocul. Toxicol.* 6:33–42.
2. Liu, D., and Dutka, B. J., ed. 1984. *Toxicity screening procedures using bacterial systems.* Drug and Chemical Toxicology Series. New York: Marcel Dekker.
3. Van De Merwe, W. P., Li, Z. Z., Bronk, B. V., and Czégé, J. 1995. Polarized light scattering from bacteria for rapid analysis of size changes following nutritional shift-up. In press.
4. Bronk, B. V., Van De Merwe, W. P., and Huffman, D. R. 1992. Polarized light scattering as a means of detecting subtle changes in microbial populations. In *Modern techniques for rapid microbiological analysis,* ed. W. Nelson, pp. 171–197. New York: VCH.
5. Van De Merwe, W., and Bronk, B. V. 1993. Polarized light scattering as a means of detecting heat and UV-induced changes in bacteria and bacterial spores. *SPIE Proc., Proc. Static and Dynamic Light Scattering in Medicine and Biology* 1884:202–206.
6. Bohren, C. F., and Huffman, D. R. 1983. *Absorption and scattering of light by small particles.* New York: Wiley.
7. Van De Merwe, W. P., Huffman, D. R., and Bronk, B. V. 1989. Reproducibility and sensitivity of polarized light scattering for identifying bacterial suspensions. *Appl. Optics* 28:5052–5057.
8. Bronk, B. V., Van De Merwe, W. P., and Stanley, M. 1992. An in-vivo measure of average bacterial cell size from a polarized light scattering function. *Cytometry* 13:155–162.
9. Bronk, B. V., Druger, S. D., Czégé, J., and Van De Merwe, W. P. 1995. Measuring diameters of rod-shaped bacteria in vivo with polarized light scattering. *Biophys. J.* 69:1170–1177.

Chapter Forty-six

ATTAINING A RATIONAL REFINEMENT AND REDUCTION IN THE USE OF LIVE ANIMALS: STUDIES ON CYANIDE TOXICITY

Edward U. Maduh, Steven I. Baskin, and Harry Salem

This chapter is a case study on the application of the three R's to the pharmacological and toxicological assessment of cyanide. By refinement, maximal data are obtained from each animal, thus reducing the number of animals utilized, and the use of anesthesia and noninvasive measurement techniques reduces pain. The experimental design includes the use of nuclear magnetic resonance (NMR) to study the effects of intravenously administered sodium cyanide (NaCN) in anesthetized miniature swine. This technique permits the acquisition of repeated measurements in each animal. Biochemical correlates of cyanide toxicity were determined by analyzing time-course changes in high energy phosphates. These studies demonstrated that at nonlethal doses of NaCN, high-energy intermediates are reduced and gradually return to near preinjection levels. Initial effects of cyanide may be by direct neuronal involvement rather than a later metabolic effect. There is no recovery following lethal doses. These observations suggest a loss of cellular energy as an important correlate of cyanide cytotoxicity. Using this technique, with multiple cyanide administrations in the same animal, potential anticyanide therapies or other pharmacological interventions can be developed with a minimum of experimental animals.

Alternatives to animal testing entail the three R's of refinement, reduction, and replacement. Refinement is defined as the acquisition of maximal data from each animal in the experimental set, minimizing or eliminating pain and discomfort. This chapter is a case study on the application of these principles to the pharmacological and toxicological assessment of cyanide. By refining the techniques to obtain maximal data from each animal in a noninvasive manner, a rational approach to developing appropriate antidotes is described in which the number of animals is reduced from what would have been required in the classical study design.

Cyanide is one of the most rapidly acting chemical poisons known. It is also very widely distributed in the environment, creating multiple incidences for accidental as well as intentional exposures. Industrially, cyanide is found in a variety of applications that range from the manufacturing of paper, plastics, and nylon products, to metal plating, and chemical synthesis. Indeed, the potential liberation of and poisoning by gaseous HCN from burning materials represents a major concern in both domestic and industrial fires, to the extent that some clinical settings frequently treat fire victims for cyanide toxicity. Inherently, cyanide poisoning is a life-threatening emergency as death can be quite rapid, usually in the first hour after exposure. The classic mechanism of toxicity has been established as the inhibition of the terminal oxidase of the mitochondrial electron transport chain, cytochrome oxidase (aa_3), as a principal molecular target for cyanide action.[1-3] With high doses, other enzyme systems may be affected by cyanide.[4-6]

Because cyanide acts so rapidly, there is little time to obtain detailed analysis of biochemical alterations from acute poisonings as they occur in the intact organism in a noninvasive manner. Pharmacologically, detailed understanding of the time course of cyanide effects in the intact organism is critical to developing a more rational basis for antidote selection. This is because criteria for assessing treatment progress may be achieved utilizing this in vivo cyanide model. A nuclear magnetic resonance (NMR) spectroscopic surface coil tuned to ^{31}P resonance[7,8] can analyze the time course of changes in high-energy phosphate metabolism indices, phospho-monoester (PME), inorganic phosphate (P_i), phosphodiester (PDE), phosphocreatine (PCr), and adenosine triphosphate (α-, β-, γ-ATP). This chapter describes our recent experience utilizing NMR spectroscopy to study cyanide toxicity in vivo. With the following experimental design it is possible to obtain repeated measurements of biochemical entities in the same animals on a timely basis without killing the experimental animal. Phosphorus energy parameters were analyzed in the brain of miniature swine before and after intravenous (iv) injections of NaCN. As fewer animals were employed to obtain optimal data, this technique can go a long way toward achieving a rational balance in the refinement and reduction of live animals in scientific experimentation.

MATERIALS AND METHODS

All data presented were generated in male Yucatan micropigs (6–10 kg) purchased from Charles River Laboratory (Wilmington, MA). The animals were housed in individual (4 × 6 ft) pens with water ad libitum. Food (Purina 5084) was provided twice a day. The cages were placed across from one another so that visual contact among the animals was not obstructed at any time. The room was maintained on a 12-h light/dark cycle with temperature at 20–22°C and 50 ± 10% relative humidity.

The NMR system used for ^{31}P data acquisition was a 4.7-tesla, 33-cm horizontal-bore magnet (Spectroscopy Imaging Systems, Sunnyvale, CA). A two-turn solenoidal RF coil, 6 cm in diameter, was used for acquiring phosphorus spectra, each of which contained 50 acquisitions. There is an active shield gradient that produces a maximum of 20 G/cm gradient field with a rise time less than 290 μs from 0 to 98% gradient. The radio frequency, gradient, and data acquisition were operated from a Sun SPARC II workstation (Sun Microsystems, Sunnyvale, CA) connected to a Sun 3/160 computer.

To noninvasively examine pertinent biochemical correlates of cyanide toxicity in vivo, this study was designed to analyze time course changes in high-energy phosphates of pig brain subsequent to NaCN iv injection using ^{31}P NMR spectroscopy.[7] Anesthesia was provided by inhalation of isoflurane, 3–4% for induction and 1.5–2% for maintenance. In each experiment, the anesthetized animal was placed in a plastic cradle and positioned in the core of the NMR magnet. The ^{31}P RF coil was placed immediately on top of the head of each animal, after which a period of 5–10 min was allowed for electrode stabilization and for adjustment of the magnetic field homogeneity. After stabilization, control ^{31}P NMR measurements (10 baselines) were recorded (spectral width = 3000 Hz) using a nonselective 90° RF pulse to excite the nuclei. A repetition time of 1.2 s was utilized. After the 10 baseline (control) spectra were recorded for each animal, NaCN (2.5 or 7.1 mg/kg) was administered iv. Subsequently, post-NaCN images were determined every minute from the time of injection through a 60-min period, or until the animal died.

This experimental approach followed a repeated measure design. Statistical inferences were based on results of repeated-measure analysis of variance with the Newman–Kuels post hoc comparisons.[5] Differences were accepted as significant if $p < .05$.

RESULTS AND DISCUSSION

Timely changes in cell energy profile of swine brain were analyzed before, during, and after cyanide intoxication using ^{31}P NMR spectroscopy. P_i peaks increased with the greater dose of NaCN injected, whereas PCr peaks declined. With the 2.5 mg/kg dose, there was a gradual recovery of the spectra toward pre-NaCN profiles and 5/5 animals in this group survived. In contrast, no post-NaCN ^{31}P spectral peak recovery was detected in the 7.1 mg/kg group and

0/5 animals survived. Domination of the spectra by the P_i peaks is indicative of NaCN-induced histotoxic hypoxia, which, as expected, can be a consequence of cytochrome oxidase (aa_3) inhibition.[7] Therefore, bioenergetics parameters were derived from the data by calculating ratios of the high-phosphate metabolites relative to P_i peak intensity.[7]

There were marked alterations in the PCr/P_i ratios, which exhibited significant time dependency, $p < .01$. With the 2.5 mg/kg dose, there was a biphasic response showing initial reduction and gradual recovery to near pretreatment control values. All five animals in this group lived. All 5 animals that received 7.1 mg/kg NaCN died in the course of the experiment, with accompanying domination of the ^{31}P phosphorus spectra by P_i, and PCr/P_i peak intensity ratios continually less than the pre-NaCN values.

Since the three α-, β-, and γ-ATP peaks exhibit different relaxation times, the individual peaks were accrued to obtain a better estimation of total ATP disappearance.[8] Calculations of PCr/ATP ratios also show dose-related changes across time with the 2.5 mg/kg group that elicited a mean PCr/ATP ratio greater than that attained by the 7.1 mg/kg group. The changes in PCr/ATP ratios elicited by the 2.5 mg/kg dose of NaCN displayed time-related transiency qualitatively similar to that observed for PCr/P_i ratios.

A dose-related response shows increased diffused cytotoxicity. The 7.1 mg/kg dose shows the greater effect, which is consistent with the fact that this dose produced 100% mortality under these conditions. The global pattern is suggestive of effects on the brain vasculature.

Analysis of in vivo cyanide intoxication, as it occurs in the Yucatan micropigs, shows that for nonlethal exposure, high-energy intermediates are rapidly reduced and gradually recover to near normal. A lethal dose of NaCN allows no recovery of high-energy phosphate intermediates in ATP and PCr. Lethally treated animals, but not the surviving group, displayed significant accumulation of the P_i peak accompanied by the disappearance of ATP and PCr peaks. ^{1}H-NMR spectra data suggest in vivo structural changes are diffuse and may be related to vascular alterations. This study allows for the development of rational cyanide therapies utilizing real-time in vivo analysis. The present data demonstrate that when a nonlethal dose (e.g., 2.5 mg/kg) of NaCN is involved, the loss of metabolic energy may be reversible. These observations would suggest loss of cellular energy as an important correlation of cytotoxicity of CN. This data also suggest that the change in the metabolic process occurs over the course of minutes, is gradual, and may not be rapid enough to account for some of the neural events that occur following cyanide administration. The rapid events may be results of a direct neural action of cyanide, perhaps as its anionic form.

This experimental approach has allowed monitoring of the phosphorus energy metabolites and calculations of the pertinent bioenergetics ratios[7] in whole animals, before, during, and after lethal or nonlethal NaCN injections. Since the same animal can be monitored over time repeatedly in the same experiment, future studies of this type should allow for the development of rational novel compounds as potential anticyanide therapies or other pharmacological interventions. For example, in another study, the utility of this approach has been further characterized by testing the interaction of H-7, a pharmacologic inhibitor of protein kinase C, with NaCN in the whole animal. Compared to non-pretreated controls, both the micropigs[7] and pigeons[8] were better able to survive NaCN challenge when pretreated with H-7.

CONCLUSION

It is concluded that this in vivo model not only can be useful in studying potential antidotes against cyanide, but with appropriate controls also can be broadly applied in toxicological as well as pharmacological testing.

References

1. Way, J. L. 1984. Cyanide intoxication and its mechanism of antagonism. *Annu. Rev. Pharmacol. Toxicol.* 25:451.
2. Solomonson, L. P. 1981. Cyanide as a metabolic inhibitor. In *Cyanide in biology*, eds. Vennesland B., Conn, E., Knowles, C. J., Westley, J., and Wissing, F. New York: Academic Press.
3. Maduh, E. U., and Baskin, S. 1994. Protein kinase C modulation of rhodanese-catalyzed conversion of cyanide to thiocyanate. *Res. Commun. Mol. Pathol. Pharmacol.* 86:155.

4. Chance, B. 1989. What are the goals of magnetic resonance research? *NMR Biomed.* 2:179.
5. Zai, J. H. 1984. *Biostatistical analysis,* 2nd ed. Englewood Cliffs, NJ: Prentice-Hall.
6. Maduh, E. U., Porter, D. W., and Baskin, S. I. 1993. Calcium antagonist: A role in the management of cyanide poisoning? *Drug Safety* 9:237.
7. Maduh, E. U., Nealley, E. W., Song, H., Wang, P. C., and Baskin, S. I. 1995. A protein kinase C inhibitor attenuates cyanide toxicity in vivo. *Toxicology* 100:129.
8. Maduh, E. U., Nealley, E. W., and Baskin, S. I. 1995. Prophylactic administration of H-7, an inhibitor of protein kinase c, improves the survivability of cyanide intoxication. *Toxicologist* 15:168.

Chapter Forty-seven

INTEGRATION OF ALTERNATIVE TESTS INTO A TOXICOLOGY RESEARCH PROGRAM

Sidney Green and Saura C. Sahu

Alternative tests have been a part of the Food and Drug Administration (FDA) approach to toxicological research since the early 1970s. The integration of these tests into a more traditional toxicology program really began in the 1980s. The Division of Toxicological Research in the FDA's Center for Food Safety and Applied Nutrition has a number of research branches into which these tests have been incorporated. Use of these tests has been for the purpose of rapidly identifying potential toxicants for further testing and to examine potential mechanisms of action. There has been little effort devoted to using these tests as substitutes for the animal in determining hazard/risk. The lack of application of these tests to the hazard/risk arena can be readily appreciated given the uncertainty associated with their validation. One dilemma has evolved in the field of alternative testing, and it is, how to encourage the continued development of these tests and at the same time caution developers to use more explicit endpoints—endpoints that can be correlated with effects in whole animals. Finally, it is recognized that the development of alternative tests can be a daunting task, and as such we may need to find ways to make it less burdensome for research scientists. One manner of easing the arduousness of the task is to seek more interdisciplinary approaches. Such an approach could draw together those with expertise in alternative methodologies, traditional toxicology testing, risk assessors, and regulatory toxicologists. A consortium of such individuals from academia, government, and industry could plan a multidisciplinary approach to a given area, share information as it is developed, and provide a report describing the alternative test strategy and its application to screening mechanisms as well as regulatory decision making. Such an approach could assist not only in the continued progress of alternative tests but also in better acceptance of these tests by the scientific community.

DEFINITION OF ALTERNATIVE TESTS

Alternative tests, within the context of the Food and Drug Administration (FDA) Division of Toxicological Research research program, are defined to include in vitro, various ex vivo, and in vivo tests. The in vitro tests are used primarily as rapid screens for toxicity or to study potential mechanisms of toxicity, although under highly selective circumstances they may be used to replace animal studies. Ex vivo tests generally involve an in vitro assessment of cells, tissues, organs, or embryos obtained from animals treated with a chemical(s) of interest. In vivo alternative tests typically involve test strategies that enable, in comparison with traditional regulatory toxicology studies, a reduction in animal usage, enhanced humanitarian treatment of animals, or more rapid generation of study results. The judicious use of various computer

---

modeling techniques and structure–activity relationships (SAR) for predicting pharmacokinetic parameters and toxicity, respectively, also is considered as alternative testing for application in an integrated toxicology research program.

CURRENT APPROACH OF ONE RESEARCH PROGRAM

The Division of Toxicological Research within the Food and Drug Administration Center for Food Safety and Applied Nutrition is divided into four branches, each of which has scientific expertise in one or more subdisciplines of toxicology. The broad objective of each branch is to conduct research designed to provide information in support of the center's regulatory components. These research efforts include: (a) evaluation and implementation of various in vitro test systems as well as evaluation of various test strategies composed of in vitro and in vivo components; (b) the conduct of classical regulatory toxicology studies (e.g., Segment I and II teratology studies); and (c) studies designed to contribute to an ability to more precisely interpret toxicity data, thereby reducing the uncertainties in risk assessments. The latter studies include, but are not limited to, investigation of mechanism(s) of toxicity; development of data to support pharmacokinetic and pharmacodynamic modeling or to improve predictions based on SAR, and evaluation of factors that may influence the toxic response to a given chemical or class of chemicals (e.g., interspecies comparisons, dosing regimen, intermittent exposure). Although each branch conducts some research that is independent of the other branches, there is a concerted effort to integrate research results obtained from various branches and, where possible, to integrate research efforts across branch lines as well as with other efforts in the center/agency.

In Vitro Toxicology Branch (IVTB)

Among the branches, scientists within the IVTB have a clear mandate to evaluate alternative tests through the conduct of research using isolated and cultured cells, tissues, organs, and embryos as alternatives or supplements to whole-animal toxicology testing. The research of this branch is broadly divided among (a) efforts intended to enable rapid screening of natural toxicants, (b) studies designed to either define the mechanism(s) of various toxicants or to evaluate the ability of dietary components to modulate toxicity, and (c) macromolecular effects on biochemical parameters.

Screening of Natural, Food-Related Toxicants (e.g., Fumonisins, Chaparral, L-Tryptophan)

Although three primary cell culture systems (i.e., chick embryo neural retinal cells, hepatocytes, and endothelial cells) have been under development and evaluated in various screening applications, current efforts are focused on development and application of endothelial cell cultures, derived from porcine vasculature, to study the effects of inflammatory mediators and antioxidants. The specific endpoint measurements include neutral red release (cell viability), prostaglandin E_2 release, and changes in the cell adhesion molecule (CAM) receptors. When standardized in vitro culture conditions have been defined, the work will be extended to include cultures of human endothelial cells.

Mechanism(s) of Toxicity/Dietary Modulation of Toxicity

Rat embryos, excised on gestation 9 and cultured for 48 h, are used to identify serum nutritional factors related to chronic human miscarriage, evaluate dietary modulation of radical-induced congenital heart defects, and study the mechanisms of embryotoxicity of *Fusarium moniliforme* components (e.g., aminopentol derived from alkaline hydrolysis of fumonisin B1). Serum collected from women with chronic miscarriage is used as the culture medium for organogenesis-staged rat embryos. In collaboration with physicians at the Georgetown University School of Medicine, the ability of the sera to sustain normal embryonic growth and development is assessed by both in vitro addition of amino acids and in vivo supplementation of the women with amino acids. Correlations are made between the ability of nutrients to correct deficiencies in the serum and to lead to successful pregnancies. This research is of direct relevance to the center's initiatives in women's health issues and alternative test systems, and may provide a cost-effective, reasonably short-term test to evaluate various dietary factors that may be altered as part of a medical program to ameliorate human reproductive failure due to chronic, spontaneous miscarriage.

Given the ability to culture rodent embryos in serum from species besides the rat (e.g., human or bovine), information can be obtained on potential species differences with respect to the embryotoxic potency of a given compound. Unfortunately cultured rat embryos demonstrate a high incidence of spontaneous heart malformations that may be linked to the formation of free radicals in the culture medium. Thus, additional efforts are ongoing to evaluate the incidence of heart defects following modulation of various nutrient levels thought to be essential to the generation and scavenging of free radical in the culture media.

The rodent embryo culture system also is being used to determine the embryotoxic hazard of aminopentol and to study its potential mechanism of action. In addition to the rodent embryo culture, aggregate cultures of chick embryo neural retinal cells (CERC) provide an in vitro system to measure events critical to embryonic development such as cell aggregation, growth, and differentiation. Because the CERC assay has been used successfully to identify potential developmental toxins, it also will be used to evaluate the alkaline hydrolysis product of fumonisin B.

Macromolecular Effects on Biochemical Parameters

Examining these effects entails adapting, developing, and utilizing available techniques to study subtle effects of natural toxicants on macromolecular composition and metabolism in animal cells. Specific measurement, include turnover and transformation of RNA, DNA, and protein to predict the action of toxins acting either individually or in combination to produce deleterious changes in the function and morphology of target organs. By employing sensitive endpoints to detect biochemical changes in cells in vitro, suspect toxicants or combinations of toxicants (e.g., those found in crude mold or herbal extracts) can be detected in small amounts. Additionally, the mechanisms of toxicity can be elucidated to facilitate interpretation of animal data, and possibly its extrapolation to humans.

Fumonisins, a group of naturally occurring toxicants produced by the fungus *Fusarium moniliforme* and closely related species, are believed to be the etiologic agent of several animal diseases associated with consumption of corn-based feeds (e.g., porcine pulmonary edema and equine leukoencephalomalacia). In rats, hepatic and renal toxicity as well as hepatic neoplasms are induced with both contaminated feed and pure fumonisin B1. Although the mechanisms underlying these fumonisin-induced diseases are not clear, fumonisins B1 and B2 are potent inhibitors of sphingolipid biosynthesis, via action on sphingosine and sphinganine *N*-acyltransferase, in cultured cells including primary hepatocytes.[1] It has been postulated that depletion of complex sphingolipids could alter the permeability property of cell membranes and thus have profound effects on cell function. Although the inhibition of de novo sphingolipid biosynthesis and cytotoxicity of fumonisin B1 are well correlated in cultures of kidney epithelial and some other cells, the former effect but not the latter has been observed in primary rat hepatocytes (i.e., these cells are resistant to lethal effects of the toxicant). However, expression of certain toxin-induced hepatotoxicities has been shown to require the presence of other liver cells (e.g., Kupffer cells) in association with parenchymal cells, the predominant cell type in typical hepatocyte preparations. Thus, the effect of fumonisins on the liver may be best studied using intact liver slices in which the almost normal architecture and cell–cell interaction of the liver lobule is preserved.

Biochemical and Analytical Toxicology Branch

This branch addresses immunotoxicology issues, and employs a combination of in vitro and in vivo techniques to investigate the molecular mechanisms of toxicity with emphasis on carcinogenesis. The experimental approaches include: (1) measurement of specific carcinogen–DNA–RNA–protein adducts in studies in vitro as well as in the carcinogen target tissues; (2) development of rapid techniques to measure specific biomarkers of exposure and susceptibility; and (3) development of procedures to measure biomarkers of carcinogenesis (e.g., differential gene expression, oncogenes and tumor suppressor genes).

Immunotoxicology

This research focuses on identifying and evaluating test strategies for assessing sensitive methods for detection of DNA adducts, and development of a rodent model to assess allergic potential. Aflatoxin B1 is being used as a model compound to develop, in collaboration with the National Center for Toxicological Research (NCTR), a highly sensitive ELISA (enzyme-linked immunosorbent assay) for the detection of aflatoxin B1–DNA adducts. The adducts and immunotoxic potential of aflatoxin B1 are being analyzed during a short-term subchronic study with intermittent and continuous dosing. The data will be used for the design of a chronic study. Studies to develop an "asthmatic" animal model, in collaboration with the Center for Drug Evaluation and Research (CDER), involve assessment of pulmonary and immunologic endpoints after sensitization in the rat.

Molecular Mechanisms of Carcinogenesis

Epidemiological studies have established that women in Asian countries consuming predominantly soy-based vegetarian diets have a significantly lower incidence of breast cancer than women in Western countries. Phytoestrogens such as soy- and flaxseed-derived isoflavones and lignans, respectively, are components of the vegetarian diet that are hypothesized to inhibit breast tumor cell growth by modulating the expression of estrogen-responsive, growth-regulatory genes. Thus, the primary objective of one research effort is the identification and development of these genes as surrogate genetic markers of dietary phytoestrogen-regulated human breast tumor growth inhibition. To accomplish this effort, established cell lines of human breast carcinoma will be used; proliferation of cells will be measured by direct cell counting and/or colorimetric assay. The potent antiestrogenic compounds tamoxifen and the negative growth regulator TGF beta 1 will be included in the study as positive controls. The leaves of the natural antioxidant chaparral have been used as dietary supplements in the form of herbal tea, capsules, and tablets; however, ingestion of high levels of these products for prolonged periods of time may result in liver damage, jaundice, and hepatitis.[2] Chaparral leaves have a high content of phenolic compounds such as flavonoids and nordihydroguaiaretic acid[3] that are easily oxidized to their respective quinones. The quinones are known to undergo redox cycling, with the production of reactive oxygen species that are potentially capable of inducing oxidative stress in living organisms.[4,5] Because the liver appears to be the target organ of chaparral toxicity in animal studies, isolated rat liver nuclei have been used as an in vitro test system to measure lipid peroxidation of the nuclear membrane and oxidative DNA damage as indicators of hepatotoxicity. Studies are now ongoing to determine whether similar results can be obtained using liver nuclei isolated from treated animals. If similar results are obtained using nuclei from treated and untreated animals, this in vitro test system may provide a short-term in vitro assay with potential applicability for the detection of food-borne toxicants, including mutagens and carcinogens, that induce lipid peroxidation or oxidative DNA damage in vivo.

Molecular Biomarkers

In collaboration with the FDA National Center for Toxicological Research (NCTR), DNA damage (assessed by quantitation of DNA adducts) and phase II liver detoxifying enzymes will be evaluated following intermittent exposure of rats to a model carcinogen, aflatoxin B1. The primary purpose of this study is to test the hypothesis that tumor incidence is a function of the accumulated lifetime exposure, and predictable from the average daily dose for both continuous and intermittent exposures. If the accumulated level of DNA damage is not significant following intermittent exposures, one can predict that the cancer risk from intermittent exposure to genotoxic compounds may be significantly lower than would be estimated from chronic bioassay data generated under conditions of continuous exposure. Results from this study also will help determine whether phase II liver detoxifying enzymes play an active role in achieving any observed reduction of risk.

Pharmacokinetics and Metabolism Branch

The Pharmacokinetics and Metabolism Branch conducts interspecies comparative metabolism and pharmacokinetic studies and studies to define the absorption, distribution, metabolism, and excretion of food-borne xenobiotics. Such studies are conducted to provide information for toxicological evaluation of specific compounds, and to validate or to define parameters for use in pharmacokinetic and pharmacodynamic models.[6]

Pharmacokinetic and Pharmacodynamic Models

A physiologically based pharmacokinetic (PBPK) model is a computer simulation model that represents the physiological aspects of the chemical disposition in a biological system. The versatility of PBPK models can provide quantitative information on the disposition of chemicals for variously administered doses, exposure routes, and target species of all ages. A validated PBPK dosimetry model also can be used to predict the experimental time course of a substance in plasma and the dose delivered to target sites. Ideally, an individual model for each compound of interest needs to be constructed for risk assessment of that particular compound; however, this approach requires a substantial resource commitment, and few models are currently available for individual toxicants or drugs. An alternative, and more practical, approach is the use of generic models applicable to evaluation of many compounds of interest. The models under development in our laboratories are:

1. Because a number of food additives and classical neurotoxins are organic acids, PBPK models are currently being developed for single-dose kinetics of a model compound for organic acids (i.e., 2,4-D) in the young and developing brain, and for low-dose, long-term kinetics in the adult brain. The basic approach to this type of work is to develop a PBPK computer model, then conduct validation experiments in animals (in this case, near-term pregnant rabbits).
2. Glutamic acid is an excitatory neurotransmitter, and is present in the highest concentration of any endogenous amino acid in the brain. The effect of seafood toxins (domoic acid and okadaic acid) on the uptake of glutamic acid by the astrocyte to cause neurotoxicity will be tested. Experiments will be carried out to investigate whether seafood toxins such as domoic or okadaic acid cause inhibition of the uptake of glutamate by astrocytes in vitro, which may result in neurotoxicity. An emphasis of this study is to clarify whether endogenous glutamate release rather than external ingestion of glutamate can cause neurotoxicity.
3. We previously developed a mathematical model to predict the formation and fate of aflatoxin B1–DNA adducts and the expected number of mutations in the total genome under a variety of exposure scenarios. We are currently developing, in collaboration with the NCTR, a coupled model for cell death and tissue necrosis that is driven by the level of DNA adducts and mutations that result from them. Several experiments relating to cell death, apoptosis, measurement of DNA adduct repair rates, and related parameters are planned or ongoing with the NCTR. Simulations performed with our models using existing data are being used to interpret results and plan further experiments.
4. Most food chemicals and drugs are metabolized in part to water-soluble glucuronide, sulfate, or glutathione conjugates that can be excreted in the urine and feces. In many cases, the metabolite rather than the parent chemical is the ultimate toxic agent. Therefore, a project has been designed to provide information needed to predict rates of elimination and body burdens of metabolites that are unknown and unpredictable with currently available information. In this effort metabolic conjugates for a set of benchmark chemicals will be prepared in experimental quantities, and uptake and partitioning studies will be performed with perfused tissues or cells in culture. The results will be used to develop structure–activity correlations for each group of conjugates, and to validate an existing metabolite-tracking model that predicts tissue concentrations of these conjugates as they are formed from metabolism of the parent compound.

Toxicological Effects Branch

The Toxicological Effects Branch conducts primarily animal studies in the areas of neurobehavioral and developmental toxicity, including teratology and male and female reproduction studies. The test articles typically are foods/food additives, contaminants, natural toxicants, or metabolites, with the studies designed to evaluate current or emerging regulatory issues.

Developmental Toxicity

Research in this area is addressing issues concerning fumonisin B1, phytoestrogens, and sodium fluoride. Where possible the results of the longer term animal studies are correlated with those obtained using whole rodent embryo cultures or other in vitro tests. Additionally, the Chernoff test, a shorter term in vivo alternative, is conducted when its use is appropriate.

Neurotoxicology

Studies in this area are divided into two primary research efforts. One effort focuses on the development of test strategies and test criteria for identifying and assessing neurotoxic hazards associated with exposure to food-borne contaminants. Specific research activities include, for example, comparison of interspecies sensitivity to a particular chemical, the influence of the dosing regimen on development of toxicity, and correlation of overt behavioral signs of toxicity with neurochemical and/or neuropathological responses. These efforts are not related to alternative testing.

The other research task that is more directly applicable to alternative test methods is the development of either more sensitive or alternative test strategies such as the use of biomarkers that ultimately will guide the continuing refinement of neurotoxicity test guidelines and will provide more accurate and meaningful data for setting allowable limits for neurotoxic contaminants. Much of the assessment of neurotoxicity currently involves histologic screening methods that are capable of detecting overt damage to the nervous system, but that are incapable of detecting more subtle forms of nervous system damage, such as small focal areas of degenerating neurons or neurons that are undergoing physiological stress. The neuroscience community has come to recognize that these more subtle, selective effects of neurotoxicants tend to be the rule rather than the exception, and that the consequences of these lesions in humans can be quite serious. Thus, using Western blotting techniques, the tissues from treated (and control) animals are being analyzed for changes in the expression of a number of "stress" proteins with potential usefulness as markers of neuronal injury. Examples of these proteins include hsp72, c-fos, ubiquitin, and glial fibrillary acidic protein. Using the results of the Western blotting experiments, proteins that show increased expression as a result of exposure to a neurotoxicant will be visualized in tissue sections using immunocytochemical techniques. This enables a correlation between the cellular locations of increased protein expression and subsequent neuronal damage. Identification of useful biomarkers is intended to result in the development of alternate test strategies that are expected to enhance the predictability of animal studies, and that potentially may be applicable to in vitro test systems.

DIFFICULTIES

There have been many successes in the use of alterative tests (e.g., screening of new drugs, investigation of mechanisms of action); however, there are several difficulties inherent in the adoption of alternative tests for determining whether a chemical is toxic and, if so, for assessing its health hazards/risks. Some of these issues are scientific; others involve practical considerations; and still others are a combination of practical and scientific issues. Despite the fact that several of these issues have been discussed at symposia and in the published literature, a few of the primary issues are addressed here. An underlying issue in the development and implementation of alternative tests is the perception of the general public and some scientists that alternative tests can rapidly provide data, often with minimal or no usage of animals. Pressure resulting from this type of perception, in turn, leads to studies using alternative test systems that are readily available, but sometimes poorly or partially characterized, and endpoint measurements that are quickly and easily performed. All too often these circumstances yield data that either do correlate with, or simply are not explainable in light of, data obtained from animal studies or human case reports. While there is no immediate or easy resolution of this issue, such problems might be minimized by (a) better educating the public and end-users of data concerning the appropriate uses and limitations of alternatives, and (b) efforts within the scientific community to focus and consolidate efforts to develop alternative test strategies. A primary issue in the use of alternative test strategies is the selection of an appropriate test or test battery, and selection of appropriate endpoints with which to conduct the evaluation. Selection of the alternative(s) generally is guided by information on the target-organ toxicity or mechanism of action of the chemical under consideration, but becomes more complex if one must evaluate compounds/ substances either of unknown target-organ toxicity or involving confounding factors (e.g., poor solubility with the substance precipitating out of "acceptable" culture media, need to maintain the food or use matrix that somehow influences toxicity). Once the alternative test is selected, one also must determine whether to evaluate one or more selected endpoints or a pattern of responses (e.g., changes in stress proteins). Such measurements typically vary with respect to technical difficulty and resource requirements, as well as in the type and utility of information that will be generated. A critical step in defining an appropriate endpoint(s) or pattern of responses with which to assess toxicity is the need to validate the selected alternative endpoint that correlates with the toxicity expressed in the whole animal or man.

Following selection and "validation" of an appropriate alternative test system, one then is faced with the problem of extrapolating the data to humans—for example, from an established cell line or primary rodent cell culture system to the animal to humans. Some of the extrapolation issues are not unique to alternative test systems; others potentially could be minimized by the use of primary human cell culture or tissue slice systems. Although tissue banks have been established to provide human tissues, a number of factors must be taken into consideration when they are used. These range from practical considerations such as the safety of workers handling the tissues to technical issues such as the potential effect on the cellular/organ slice system of donor age, medical condition, and any medical treatment prior to death; potential effects of the tissue harvesting conditions (e.g., time after death), storage, and transport of the tissue; and the difficulty of establishing primary cultures of some cell types and the low number of passages through which some primary cultures can be maintained.

Last, but not least, the selection, development, and validation of an alternative test strategy that may ultimately replace animal tests for a given toxic endpoint (e.g., hepatotoxicity) are time and resource intensive. The diversity of issues involved in the process also suggests the need for a multidisciplinary approach that draws together expertise in alternative methodologies, traditional toxicology testing, risk assessors, and regulatory toxicologists. Although such an undertaking may appear overwhelming for a given organization, especially with decreased funding of basic research programs, we suggest that a reasonable degree of progress could be made by consortia composed of individuals from academia, government, and the regulated industry. One approach to this type of effort is to (a) define the toxic endpoints of regulatory interest (i.e., hepatotoxicity, pulmonary toxicity, teratogenesis, etc.) and rank the endpoints in decreasing order of priority, possibly based on the frequency of issues involving each endpoint; (b) establish consortiums to address each endpoint beginning with those of greatest concern; (c) on the basis of the published literature, unpublished information, and expertise of the consortium members, define one or more alternative test strategies for the endpoint under consideration; (d) define the specific research that needs to be done to "validate" and understand the limitations of the alternative test strategy(ies); (e) apportion the research efforts across the consortium; and (f) share information as it is developed, with the final product being a report describing the alternative test strategy and other information, as appropriate. In those cases where an alternative test strategy cannot be identified for an endpoint, the report would focus on the scientific issues and future considerations for research that should be recommended by the consortium.

References

1. Yoo, H., Nored, W. P., Wang, E., Merril, A. H., and Riley, R. T. 1992. Fumonisin inhibition of de novo sphingolipid biosynthesis and cytotoxicity are correlated in LLC-PK1 cells. *Toxicol. Appl. Pharmacol.* 114:9–15.
2. Katz, M., and Saibil, F. 1990. Herbal hepatisis: Subacute hepatic necrosis secondary to chaparral leaf. *J. Clin. Gastroeneterol.* 12:203–206.
3. Brinker, F. 1993. *The chaparral handbook.* Portland, OR: Eclectic Medical Publications.

4. Sahu, S., and Washington, M. 1991. Quercetin-induced lipid peroxidation and DNA damage in isolated rat liver nuclei. *Cancer Lett.* 58:75–79.
5. Sahu, S., and Gray, G. 1996. Pro-oxidant activity of flavonoids: Effects on glutathione and glutathione S-transferase in isolated rat liver nuclei. *Cancer Lett.* 104:193–196.
6. Klassen, C. D., and Eaton, D. L. 1991. Principles of toxicology. In *Casarett and Doull's toxicology: The basic science of poisons,* 4th ed., eds. M. O. Admur, J. Doull, and C. D. Klassen, pp. 12–49. New York: Pergamon Press.

INDEX